CLINICAL PHARMACOLOGY

Dr. Shubham Sewariya
and Dr. Aarushi Singh

ALLIED
HEALTH
PRESS

Clinical Pharmacology

Authors: **Dr. Shubham Sewariya and Dr. Aarushi Singh**

Allied Health Press
4164 Lakeshore Road
Burlington ON L7L 1A4
Canada
www.alliedhealthpress.com
Email: orders@arclereducation.com

ISBN: 978-1-77956-797-0

ABOUT THE AUTHORS

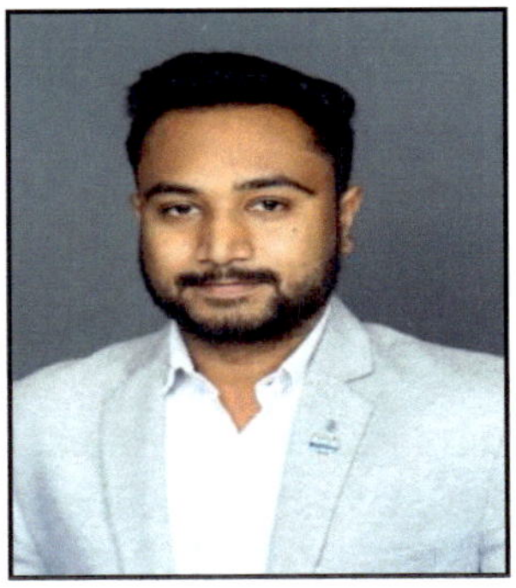

Dr. Shubham Sewariya is a Research Scientist at the University of Delhi, India, with expertise in medicinal chemistry and drug discovery. His research focuses on developing novel anticancer drug leads by combining synthetic chemistry, biological insights, and computational approaches. He holds an Integrated BS–MS degree in Chemistry from the Indian Institute of Science Education and Research (IISER), Thiruvananthapuram, and has completed his Ph.D. jointly at University of Delhi and the University of Lancashire, UK. His doctoral work centers on the discovery and development of secondary metabolites, including noscapinoids and coumarins, as potential anticancer agents. Dr. Sewariya has received several prestigious fellowships and awards, including the Commonwealth Split-site PhD Scholarship (2023–24) funded by the UK Foreign, Commonwealth & Development Office, the CSIR Senior Research Fellowship, and the INSPIRE SHE Fellowship from Department of Science and Technology, Govt of India. He has also presented his work at international platforms such as the American Chemical Society (ACS) conferences in San Francisco and Chicago. With more than a dozen peer-reviewed publications, his contributions span synthetic chemistry, nanomedicine, and biophysical studies, particularly in designing intelligent nanocarriers and molecular probes for cancer therapy. Beyond the laboratory, Dr. Sewariya is deeply committed to advancing translational research that bridges science and medicine for the betterment of human health.

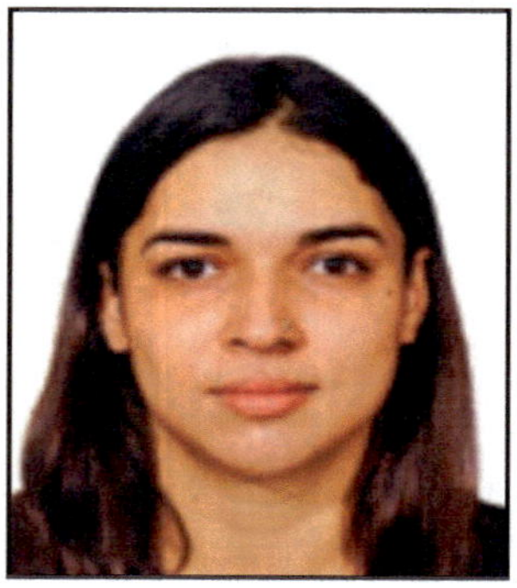

Dr. Aarushi Singh is an accomplished chemist currently serving as an Assistant Professor in the Department of Chemistry at Ramjas College, University of Delhi. She embarked on her academic journey with a B.Sc. in Chemistry from Ramjas College in 2011, followed by a Master's in Chemistry from the University of Delhi in 2013. Driven by a passion for research, Dr. Singh pursued her Ph.D. at the same institution, completing it in 2021. Her doctoral thesis, conducted under the mentorship of Prof. Ramesh Chandra and Dr. Rakeshwar Bandichhor, focused on the synthesis of biologically active Pyrazinoindoles and their mechanistic interaction studies.

Dr. Singh has accumulated significant research experience through various prestigious roles and projects. She worked as a Senior Research Fellow at the Indian Council of Medical Research (ICMR), where she developed inhalable nanomicelles for lung cancer treatment. She has also held positions as a Research Associate at the University of Alberta, Canada, focusing on the synthesis of Piperidinyl allylboronates, and at the Max Planck Institute for Multidisciplinary Sciences in Germany, where she synthesized magnetic resonance contrast agents.

Her international experience includes a stint as a Visiting Scientist at Humboldt Universität zu Berlin, Germany, and as a Ph.D. Exchange Student at the Japan Advanced Institute of Science and Technology (JAIST), where she studied the inhibition of protein aggregation by zwitterionic polymers. These experiences were supported by several prestigious fellowships, including the Shastri Research Student Fellowship and the JASSO Fellowship.

Dr. Singh's research interests are broad and interdisciplinary, encompassing multi-step organic synthesis, heterocyclic synthesis, and the development of biologically active compounds. Dr. Singh has authored one book and published over 15 original scientific research papers in internationally recognized journals. In addition to her research, Dr. Singh is dedicated to teaching and mentoring the next generation of chemists. Her diverse background and international collaborations enrich her teaching, providing students with a global perspective on chemical research and applications.

Dr. Aarushi Singh continues to contribute to the field of chemistry through her innovative research, dedicated teaching, and active participation in the scientific community. Her work aims to bridge the gap between advanced research and practical applications, making complex chemical concepts accessible and impactful.

Brief Table of Contents

Chapter Openers

A list of Chapter Outline is presented providing a brief Introduction to what will be covered in the chapter.

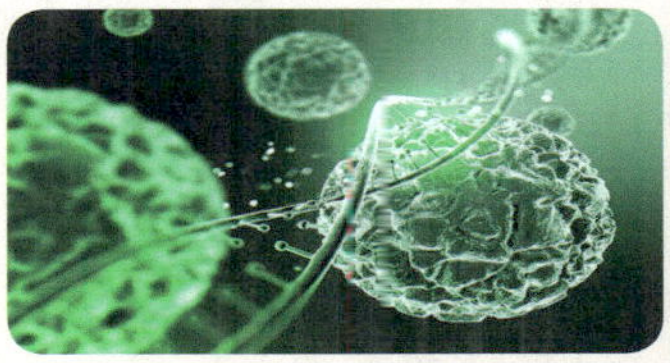

Introduction

Often referred to as the science of life, biology is a broad field of study aimed at comprehending the several kinds of life on Earth, from tiny creatures to sophisticated multicellular entities. Comprising several subfields, including molecular biology, ecology, and evolutionary biology, each of which advances our knowledge of living systems, this field clarifies the mechanisms controlling life events, including development, reproduction, and interaction with the surroundings, which is the central goal of biology. Moreover, biology fills in the void between the natural sciences and medicine by offering a necessary understanding of health, illness, and the interactions between organisms and their environments. Dealing with urgent global issues such as climate change, biodiversity loss, and new diseases depends on an awareness of these complex biological interactions, therefore highlighting the critical part biology plays in modern civilization. Fundamentally, biology explores and tests ideas about the living world using the scientific method. Through methodical observation and experimentation,

LEARNING OBJECTIVES

After studying this chapter, you will be able to:

1. Discuss the scientific method in biology;
2. Explain the cell theory;
3. Discuss the genetics and heredity;
4. Evolution and natural selection;
5. Focus on ecology and ecosystems;
6. Learn about human biology;
7. Evaluate the plant biology;
8. Explain the microbiology;
9. Focus on current trends in biology.

1.1. The Scientific Method in Biology

Learning Outcome

1. Describe the steps of the scientific method;
2. Focus on hypothesis formation;
3. Learn about experimental design.

Learning Outcomes

The beginning of each section of every chapter contains a set of Learning Outcomes that inform students of concepts they should understand. These outcomes help students understand what they should be able to do if they have mastered the material in that section.

Test Your Knowledge

Throughout each chapter, Test Your Knowledge cues you to note which topics have been covered and to self-test your understanding of the material presented.

Test Your Knowledge

1. Explain why correlation does not imply causation in scientific experiments.
2. How does the scientific method help reduce the influence of personal opinions in research?

Chapter Summary

The Summary Section appear at the end of each chapter and summarize main concepts covered throughout the chapter. These points provide key concepts in an engaging and meaningful way.

Summary

The investigation of biological principles highlights the importance of a comprehensive view of life by reflecting the intricate interactions that occur within living systems. The complexity of biology goes beyond individual species or systems, as this essay highlights; it also includes the interactions that mold ecosystems and affect biodiversity. Researchers can conduct in-depth analyses of metabolomic data using sophisticated technologies like MetaboAnalyst, which offer insights into the molecular mechanisms underlying these interactions. As demonstrated by the developments in MetaboAnalyst for example, the integration of diverse omics data promotes a thorough understanding of metabolic pathways and helps identify important biological markers necessary for research on development and disease (Chong et al., 2018). Additionally, the phenomenon of ecological invasions is a key component of biological research and a vital field of study. The introduction of non-native species into unfamiliar habitats has significant ramifications and calls for multidisciplinary management strategies. Examining the origins and effects of these biological incursions, invasion science has become a crucial field that highlights the need to comprehend ecological dynamics and community interactions. As interest in biological invasions increases, new findings are emerging that put conventional ecological theories and practices to the test. The importance of incorporating various scientific viewpoints is shown by this developing discipline, which also highlights how invasive species shape ecosystems and advances our knowledge of ecological resilience (David et al., 2013). When taken as a whole, these discoveries from invasion science and metabolomics highlight the value of multidisciplinary biology research. Fostering cross-disciplinary collaboration and utilizing technological breakthroughs to improve our comprehension of intricate biological interactions are crucial as we look to the future of biological research. In addition to deepening our understanding of the complexities of life, this method lays the groundwork for tackling urgent environmental issues. Future studies can ensure the continued relevance of biology in a world that is constantly changing by acknowledging the interconnection of biological systems and opening the door to creative solutions that support sustainability and biodiversity conservation. We might imagine a thorough comprehension of life that serves both academia and society at large through ongoing investigation and integration of scientific knowledge.

Knowledge Assessment

The chapter includes material designed to review and reinforce each content. It includes Critical Thinking Questions to help test of your understanding of information presented in the chapter and Short answer Questions to review your understanding of the key concepts presented in the chapter.

Critical Thinking Questions

1. **Who is known as the "Father of Modern Biology"?**
   a. Aristotle
   b. Charles Darwin
   c. Gregor Mendel
   d. Louis Pasteur
2. **What is the basic unit of life?**
   a. Atom
   b. Molecule
   c. Cell
   d. Organism
3. **Which branch of biology studies the interaction of organisms with their environment?**
   a. Genetics
   b. Ecology
   c. Physiology
   d. Botany
4. **Which macromolecule is the main source of energy for living organisms?**
   a. Proteins
   b. Lipids
   c. Carbohydrates
   d. Nucleic acids
5. **DNA is primarily responsible for which function in living organisms?**
   a. Energy production
   b. Protein synthesis
   c. Storing genetic information
   d. Regulating body temperature

Short Answer Questions

1. What is biology, and why is it important to study biology?
2. What are the three main domains of life, and how are they different from one another?
3. Define homeostasis and give an example of how it works in living organisms.
4. What is the cell theory, and why is it fundamental to biology?
5. How do autotrophs and heterotrophs differ in the way they obtain energy?
6. What is the scientific method, and how is it applied in biological research?
7. Discuss how biology helps address global challenges such as climate change, disease, and food security.
8. Explain the levels of biological organization from the smallest unit to the largest. Provide examples at each level.
9. Describe the relationship between structure and function in biology, giving specific examples from cells or organs.
10. How has the discovery of genetics shaped our understanding of inheritance and variation among organisms?

Supplementary Materials

Key Terms: A list of key terms is given for quick reference

KEY TERMS FROM THIS CHAPTER

Annotation enrichment analysis	Biological structure	Cell
Cell theory	Cellular structure	Ecology
Ecosystems	Genetics	Human biology
Microbiology	Natural selection	Organism
Plant biology		

Further Resources: Recommendations for additional readings, websites, and multimedia resources.

References

1. Argelaguet, R., Velten, B., Arnol, D., Dietrich, S., Zenz, T., Marioni, J. C., Buettner, F., et al. (2018). Multi-omics factor analysis—A framework for unsupervised integration of multi-omics data sets. *Molecular Systems Biology, 14*. https://doi.org/10.15252/msb.20178124.
2. Bacher, S., Blackburn, T. M., Essl, F., & Genovesi, P. (2017). *Socio-Economic Impact Classification of Alien Taxa (SEICAT)*. https://core.ac.uk/download/286567949.pdf (accessed on 8th March 2025).
3. Barnett, R., Brace, S., Cucchi, T., & Dobney, K. (2013). *Divergent Evolutionary Processes Associated with Colonization of Offshore Islands*. https://core.ac.uk/download/20664364.pdf (accessed on 8th March 2025).

Detailed Table of Contents

CHAPTER 6

Adverse Drug Reactions (ADRs) 151

CHAPTER 7

Drug Interactions 185

CHAPTER 8

Rational Prescribing and Prescription Writing 219

CHAPTER 9

Clinical Pharmacology in Special Populations 251

CHAPTER 10

Pharmacogenetics and Pharmacogenomics 283

CHAPTER 14

LIST OF FIGURES

PREFACE

The study of how medicines affect the human body and how the body, in turn, handles those medicines has never been more vital than in the present era of rapidly evolving healthcare. Advances in technology, the emergence of novel therapeutic agents, and a growing understanding of disease mechanisms have converged to place clinical pharmacology at the forefront of patient management. Clinicians, including physicians and pharmacists, as well as other healthcare providers, require a solid understanding of the fundamental principles that govern drug action, distribution, metabolism, and elimination. Equally essential is an awareness of the complexity of individual patient heterogeneity—encompassing age, genetics, organ function, and comorbidities—that influence both therapeutic responses and risk factors in significant, clinically relevant ways. In this setting, an intimate understanding of pharmacokinetic and pharmacodynamic principles is no longer a theoretical concept but an integral part of safe and efficient patient care.

Concurrently, the discipline has seen an unprecedented shift towards personalized medicine. Pharmacogenetics and pharmacogenomics have revolutionized the one-size-fits-all model, enabling clinicians to tailor prescriptions to an individual's genetic predisposition. Special populations such as children, the elderly, pregnant women, and those with organ dysfunction require special consideration since standard dosing regimens will be contraindicated or unsafe. Stewardship programs, especially those involving antimicrobials, underscore the ethical obligation to balance therapeutic value against the risk of resistance development. Additionally, increased sensitivity to drug side effects and drug–drug interaction complexities requires vigilance at each phase of the drug process, from primary prescription to follow-up and monitoring.

With these challenges and opportunities in mind, *Clinical Pharmacology* is designed to be both a convenient companion and a comprehensive manual. Within a single volume, this book compiles fundamental principles, novel developments, and therapeutic practices. It aims to equip students, practitioners, and researchers with the ability to make informed decisions about drug treatment in a wide range of medical scenarios. The organization of the book reflects the cumulative nature of learning within this field of study, beginning with an introduction to the fundamentals of drug classification and then progressing to advanced subjects such as pharmacogenomics and antimicrobial stewardship.

Chapter 1 provides a systematic introduction to the drug classes and their general characteristics, laying the groundwork for a more comprehensive examination. Chapter 2 is devoted to pharmacokinetic principles—absorption, distribution, metabolism, and elimination—with extensive exposition of compartmental models and clinical applications such as dose adjustment in renal or hepatic failure.

Chapter 3 describes the pharmacodynamics, including drug concentration versus effect, receptor theory, and how target expression variability affects these relationships. Chapter 4 describes drug discovery and the clinical trials process, from preclinical through to Phase I–III trials, post-marketing surveillance, and regulatory issues.

Chapter 5 discusses TDM, describing how drug level measurement directs personal dose adjustment and improves safety. Chapter 6 discusses ADRs, categorizing their mechanism, listing risk factors, and outlining methods of recognition and management.

Chapter 7 describes drug interactions, both pharmacodynamic and pharmacokinetic, and offers practical tips for prevention and minimization. Chapter 8 discusses rational prescribing and writing of prescriptions with a focus on the clinical thinking process, evidence-based decision-making, and proper documentation.

In Chapter 9, the conversation returns to its original topic.to clinical pharmacology, It focuses on special populations, and addresses alterations in pharmacokinetics and pharmacodynamics in pediatrics, geriatrics, pregnancy, and organ impairment. Chapter 10 addresses pharmacogenetics and pharmacogenomics, describing the influence of genetic polymorphisms on drug metabolism and response and noting upcoming applications. Chapter 11 addresses antimicrobial pharmacology and stewardship, explaining the mechanisms of action, emergence of resistance, and guidelines for prudent use.

Chapter 12 provides an overview of cardiovascular drug therapy, including antihypertensives, antiarrhythmics, and heart failure medications, along with case scenarios illustrating therapeutic approaches. Chapter 13 discusses central nervous system (CNS) drug therapy, including antidepressants, antipsychotics, anticonvulsants, and medications for neurodegenerative diseases. Chapter 14 discusses endocrine and metabolic disorders, with descriptions of pharmacotherapy for diabetes, thyroid illness, and lipid diseases.

Lastly, Chapter 15 explores near-future trends in clinical pharmacology, including nanomedicine, biologics, and digital health technologies, which hold the promise to transform drug development and delivery.

This book is intended for medical students, residents, clinical pharmacists, and practicing clinicians who seek an encyclopedic yet concise textbook in pharmacology. It would also serve as a valuable reference for drug development researchers and allied health professionals working in therapeutic drug monitoring, patient safety programs, and related fields. Readers will appreciate how the balance between theoretical principles and practical guidance caters to both academic learning and everyday clinical practice, making them confident in the safe and effective use of medicines. Whether it is the initial approach to the subject or a requirement for a refresher, the book provides a systematic course through the basics and the more advanced topics in clinical pharmacology.

NAMES AND CLASSES OF DRUGS

1

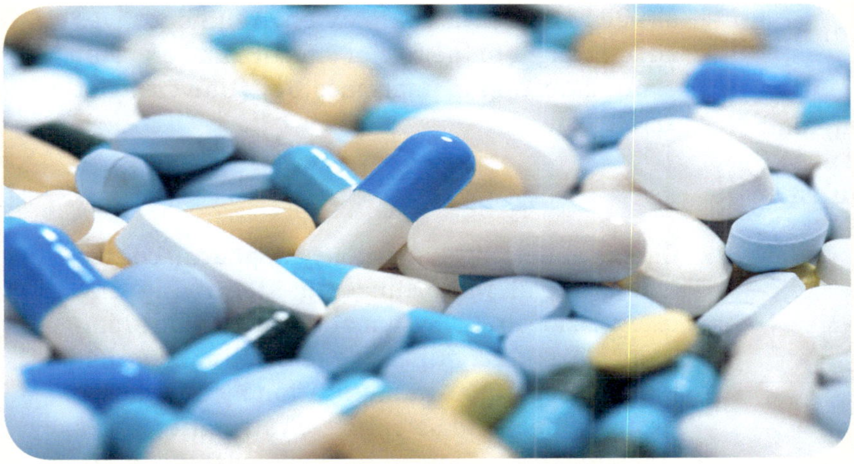

Introduction

The naming of drug classes and names is a crucial field in pharmacology, as it provides the foundation for understanding how drugs are classified and applied in therapeutic practice. Each drug is given a specific name and typically falls within one of numerous different classes based on its chemical nature, mode of action, or therapeutic use. This classification assists the doctors in making well-informed decisions about drug prescriptions and treatment, hence providing proper treatment to the patients. Moreover, the presence of reliable sources of chemical information, such as PubChem, provides improved understanding of such drugs through the provision of comprehensive data about their spectral information and bioactivity profiles (Kim et al., 2018). With drug therapy details being negotiated by health care practitioners, there exists the need to refer to standard guidelines like those given by the ESC and EAS to optimize patient outcome without weakening ethical practice standards (Mach et al., 2019) (Figure 1.1).

LEARNING OBJECTIVES

After studying this chapter, you will be able to:

1. Identify types of drug names
2. Explain major classes of drugs
3. Describe drug classification systems
4. Know the role of drug naming in healthcare

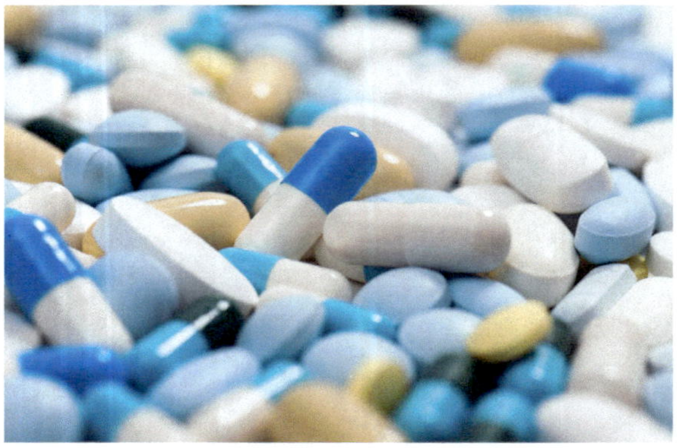

Figure 1.1. Drug classes and medication classification.

Source: https://www.verywellhealth.com/thmb/HXweuW5iQ5_fd0d6Jzoixs_wJAo=/1500x0/filters:no_upscale():max_bytes(150000):strip_icc()/medicine-pills-463594335-ba46b2f34a764be6a9c0e56a308cb938.jpg

1.1. Types of Drug Names

Learning Outcome

1. Know chemical names
2. Focus on generic names
3. Explain brand names and trade names
4. Describe international nonproprietary names (INN)
5. Write the importance of naming consistency
6. Know role of regulatory agencies
7. Identify challenges in drug naming
8. Give examples of well-known drug names

In the category of drug names, there are three types: chemical names, generics, and brand names, with each type serving a distinct purpose in the drug industry. Chemical names convey the molecular structure and makeup of a drug, providing a correct name that is typically complicated and nonsensical to the patient. On the other hand, simpler and more common generic names are given by the United States Adopted Names (USAN) Council for physician-to-physician communication. Brand names, developed by pharmaceutical firms, are created to be appealing and memorable and therefore are designed to influence prescribing practice and consumer education. This connection of these nomenclatures influences drug use, particularly in regions like Africa where traditional medicine and modern medicine exist side by side, as evidenced by the prevalence of African traditional medicine (ATM) and modern therapy occurring together (Diallo et al., 2013). Such a complex environment gives added weight to the role of effective and efficient communication in pharmacology (University et al., 2011).

1.1.1. Chemical Names

Chemical naming, particularly in pharmacology, is of crucial importance in identifying and categorizing drugs. Systematic, generic, and brand names are all significant chemical names that provide accurate communication by healthcare professionals and scientists. Systematic names provide information on the molecular structure and functional groups of a compound and most of the information regarding the chemical properties of the compound. In contrast, generic names offer a simplified, standardized form of identification that facilitates the identification of drugs across various markets.

As has been demonstrated in recent studies, ontologies developed in medicinal chemistry have helped to organize and retrieve vast amounts of information on chemical names and compounds to boost effectively the synthesis of pharmaceutical products (Gómez-Pérez et al., 2013). Further, ethnobotanical research shows the way historical knowledge of plant-based products influences current pharmacological terminology, indicating the application of previous information in drug classification in the present (Hamidova et al., 2019) (Figure 1.2).

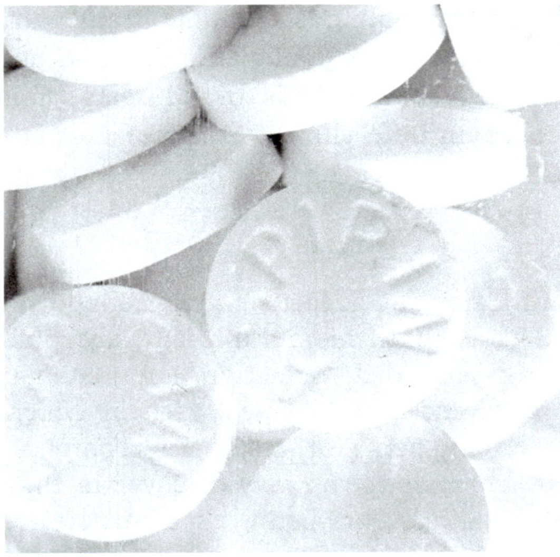

Figure 1.2. The nomenclature of chemicals, particularly in pharmacology, is an essential component in understanding drug identity and classification.

Source: https://upload.wikimedia.org/wikipedia/commons/b/bf/Aspirine_macro_shot.jpg.

1.1.2. Generic Names

In pharmacology, generic names are a critical element, referring to medicines by their active components rather than brand trademarks. Generic names contribute significantly to ensuring clear communication between patients and medical practitioners, as such names typically emerge from chemical names referencing the structure and mechanism of the drug. For instance, the generic name "ibuprofen" points to a drug with anti-inflammatory activity, so its therapeutic function is well-defined in the first place. Besides, generic names are crucial in pharmacogenomics and bioinformatics, communicating drug interactions and their effects on biological pathways. Using databases such as KEGG helps us better understand how drugs interact, including how various drugs affect cellular function and signal pathways. As described, predictive methods utilized in the KEGG resource allow for a complete appreciation of molecular networks whose behavior is regulated by administering drugs, hence the importance of generic names in drug classification as well as in drug therapy (Kanehisa, 2019; Kanehisa et al., 2020).

1.1.3. Brand Names

The function of brand names in the pharmaceutical industry goes beyond the realm of simple advertising; they inform healthcare providers and consumers alike about the function and classification of drugs. Brand names can be helpful in making drugs more memorable, and thereby more easily prescribed and administered particularly for psychotropic drugs when precise identification is the key to successful therapy.

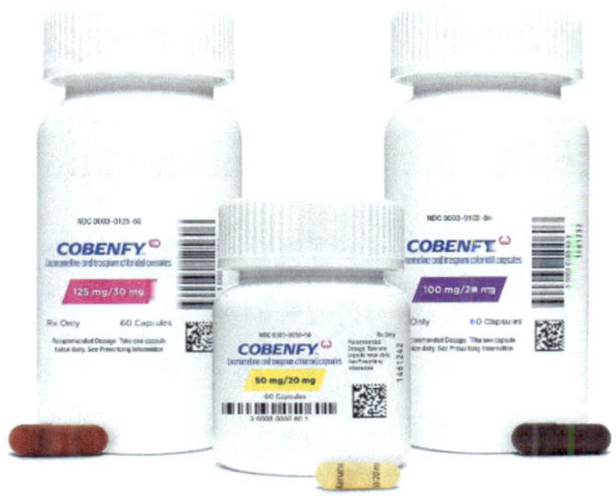

Figure 1.3. Brand names can enhance the memorability of medications, thereby aiding in their prescription and administration, particularly for psychotropic drugs where precise identification is crucial for effective therapy.

Source: https://www.bu.edu/files/2024/10/COBENFY-feat.jpg.

For instance, an in-depth reference such as (Pagliaro et al., 2020) has over 100 prescription psychotropic drugs, their brand names, pharmacological classifications, and dosing information. Furthermore, in the case of synthetic cannabinoids, popular brand names such as Spice and K2 point out how marketing strategies can impact public adoption and usage rates of these substances despite risks outlined in Alves et al. (2020). Thus, brand names hold a prominent place in drug identification and exert influences on both clinical practice and patient choice within the multiple-course complex of drug treatment (Figure 1.3).

1.1.4. Trade Names

Trade names in pharmacy play a crucial role in drug identification and advertisement, distinguishing them from generic drugs. They are typically designed to be both memorable and acceptable, influencing not only patients but also health workers in their drug selection. For instance, a single active drug will be marketed under numerous different brand names, each of which is associated with a specific brand, and this will affect prescribing behavior and patient compliance. It is critical to memorize these names for prescribing psychologists who may discover in clinical practice numerous psychotropic drugs. As noted in the detailed reference listing psychotropic drugs available in North America, each monograph presents a maximum of five common trade names with key differences for prescribing to facilitate well-informed clinical decision (Pagliaro et al., 2020). Additionally, ethical implications regarding trade names mandate healthcare professionals to be vigilant in their prescription practices to ensure patient safety when confronted with brand influence (Visseren et al., 2021).

1.1.5. International Nonproprietary Names (INN)

The provision of International Nonproprietary Names (INN) is a pillar in drug classification, with the function of activating clarity and consistency in pharmaceutical naming.

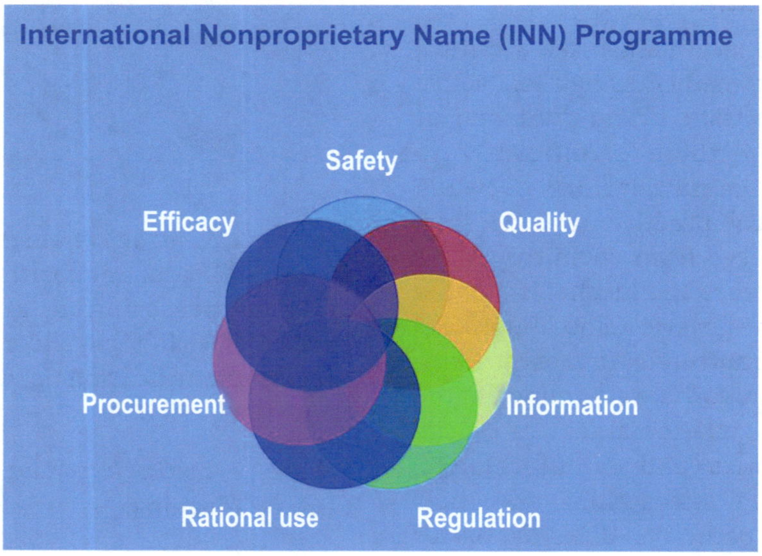

Figure 1.4. The establishment of international nonproprietary names (INN) serves as a crucial framework within the realm of drug classification, promoting clarity and uniformity in pharmaceutical nomenclature.

Source: https://image.slideserve.com/1357241/slide1-l.jpg.

INNs facilitate the identification of active ingredients regardless of languages and regulatory areas, thereby allowing international communication among healthcare professionals, scientists, and regulatory bodies. This systematic process of nomenclature is particularly crucial in drug safety monitoring, where proper mapping of active ingredients to names of drugs can minimize risks of adverse drug reactions (ADRs). As highlighted through the investigation of the adverse event reporting systems, the Diana dictionary significantly improves drug definitions' accuracy and reproducibility, further validating the value of INNs within clinical and regulatory settings (Fusaroli et al., 2024). Furthermore, the international push for the rationalization of drug approval processes, envisioned by the establishment of a Global Medicines Agency, would also complement the role of INNs in facilitating access to critical therapeutics, particularly in developing regions (Niazi, 2023) (Figure 1.4).

1.1.6. Importance of Naming Consistency

The importance of consistency in drug classification naming cannot be overstated, as it is a cornerstone of effective communication among practitioners, researchers, and regulators. Consistency in the names of drugs enhances clarity and reduces the chances of errors in dispensing or prescribing drugs. For instance, where chemical names are named systematically, as in cheminformatics, knowledge retrieval is highly optimized, facilitating easy access to valid chemical data on various platforms and documents (Abacha et al., 2017). On another note, compliances with naming conventions enhance data integration quality, facilitating better mapping of chemical names to respective structures and corresponding biological data. This exercise not only assists in the development of strong chemical knowledge bases but also makes significant contributions to strategic advancements in drug design and delivery systems, particularly in molecular modeling (Buhleier et al., 2014). Finally, adhering strictly to generally accepted nomenclature practices is essential in leading pharmaceutical sciences and patient safety.

1.1.7. Role of Regulatory Agencies

Regulatory agencies are key players in the approval, development, and regulation of medication to ensure that drugs are safe and effective for public use. .

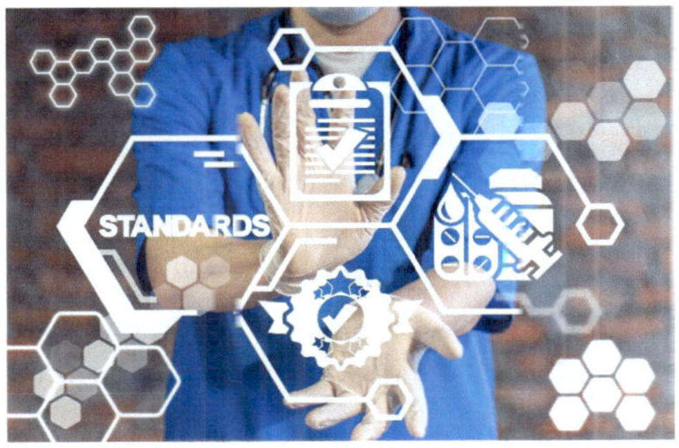

Figure 1.5. Regulatory agencies are crucial in overseeing the development, approval, and monitoring of pharmaceuticals, ensuring that drugs are safe and effective for public use.

Source: https://d2jx2rerrg6sh3.cloudfront.net/images/Article_Images/ImageForArticle_24826_17151698709336463.jpg.

Such agencies, such as the U.S. Food and Drug Administration (FDA) and the European Medicines Agency (EMA), operate under austere rules to review all types of drugs, from prescription medication to over-the-counter drugs. Their role by encompassing not only scientific assessment but also ensuring compliance with legal standards, thereby mitigating the risks associated with drug side effects. As globalization increases, regulatory authorities face the challenge of reconciling standards across borders, as seen in recent moves in global regulation, which at times lean towards industry over public health implications. In emerging markets, such as China, regulatory frameworks need to be adjusted so that they can keep pace with world best practices, particularly since medical innovation demands are emerging very rapidly (Chatwin et al., 2016) (Figure 1.5)

1.1.8. Challenges in Drug Naming

The naming of drugs is a process fraught with difficulty that reflects the complexity of drug development and regulation. The greatest challenge is the selection of names that are not only distinct from one another but also communicate relevant information about the drug's function and class. This means that there is a risk of confusion between close-sounding names that can lead to errors in medication that ultimately affect the safety of patients. Moreover, regulatory bodies have the mandate on their side to ensure that drug names have no misleading implications. This task is made difficult by the extensive range of drug types and classes used today. For instance, antimicrobial resistance (AMR) is demanding the significance of clear communication regarding antibiotic names and usage (Murray et al., 2022). Besides, with nanomaterials joining the pharmaceutical sector, their unique properties demand precise words that will still be in development (Jeevanandam et al., 2018). The quest for good naming practices is thus still a critical aspect in enhancing drug efficacy and safety.

1.1.9. Examples of Well-Known Drug Names

The pharmaceutical scene is enhanced by a rich diversity of familiar drug names, each sorted according to their therapeutic categories and purposes. Analgesics, ibuprofen, and acetaminophen are well known for relieving pain, while penicillin and amoxicillin represent antibiotics that fight bacterial infections. Further, the opioid group, which includes oxycodone and morphine, is distinguished by its efficacy in managing severe pain, albeit with significant risks of respiratory depression and addiction (Phillips et al., 2024). At the other end, psychotropic agents like fluoxetine and sertraline act to manage psychiatric diseases, reflecting the variability of drug names that reflect their pharmacological application. Understanding these categories not only aids in determining their applications but also emphasizes the necessity of safe and informed use of these drugs in clinical practice (Treschow et al., 2024) (Figure 1.6).

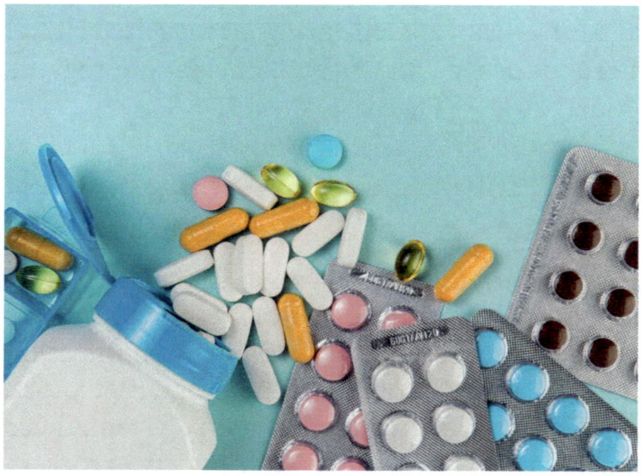

Figure 1.6. Analgesics.

Source: https://www.lahacienda.com/wp-content/uploads/2021/11/examples-of-analgesic-drugs-la-hacienda.jpg.

Test Your Knowledge

1. What are generic drugs?
2. Write a short note on International Nonproprietary Names (INN).

1.2. Major Classes of Drugs

Learning Outcome

1. Explain stimulants, depressants, and hallucinogens
2. Describe opioids
3. Define antidepressants
4. Know antipsychotics
5. Describe antibiotics
6. Understand antihistamines and anesthetics

The knowledge of major drug categories implies the knowledge of both their use for treatment and their consequences in society. The categories, such as stimulants, depressants, hallucinogens, and opioids, each have unique mechanisms of action capable of significantly altering physiological and psychological states. For instance, amphetamines stimulate wakefulness and energy but lead to addiction and cardiovascular disease. Meanwhile, depressants like benzodiazepines and alcohol reduce anxiety but at the risk of dependence and respiratory depression. The sudden growth of new psychoactive substances has also contributed to this scenario, as the Advisory Council on the Misuse of Drugs (ACMD) reports on substances like mephedrone, showing and presenting the urgent need for systemic regulation and public health policy. Hence, the understanding of differences and impacts of these major drug categories is crucial to assist policy development and public health measures (Schenk et al., 1959).

1.2.1. Stimulants

Stimulants, perhaps the most popular drug category, have been a subject of immense interest due to their widespread use and abuse potential. Cocaine, amphetamines, and methamphetamines are some of the drugs that come in this category and primarily impact the central nervous system (CNS) by increasing alertness and energy. Fatal health risks typically follow their use. For instance, stimulant use combined with other drugs, such as opioids, is likely to exacerbate cardiovascular issues and ultimately lead to progressive health complications and increased mortality rates, as reflected in recent research on polynegative use (Arab et al., 2021). The changing patterns of stimulant-related deaths indicate how complex these drugs are; e.g., death related to cocaine in the UK has been rising at an alarming rate and is most commonly linked with polypharmacy overdoses involving opioids (Arendt et al., 2017). Based on this, awareness regarding the dangers of stimulants is vital while making plans for prevention and intervention (Figure 1.7).

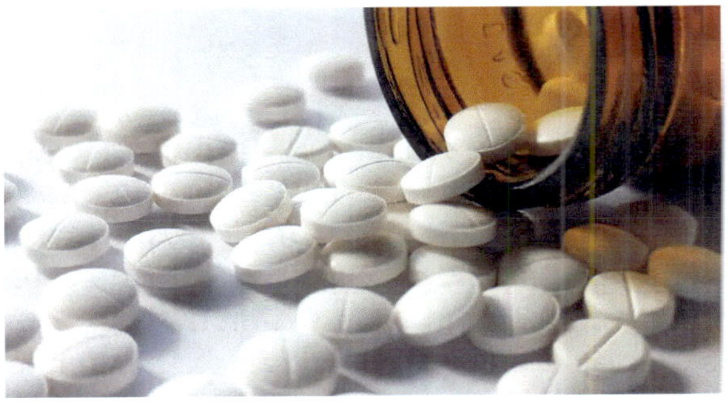

Figure 1.7. Stimulants, a prominent class of drugs, have garnered significant attention due to their widespread use and potential for abuse.

Source: https://neveralonerehab.com/wp-content/uploads/2024/01/are-amphetamines-addictive-th-copy-1.webp.

1.2.2. Depressants

Depressants are a significant category of psychotropic drugs that primarily exert their effect by decreasing the activity of the CNS and slowing it down. This process can result in alleviation of insomnia and anxiety, and thereby, drugs like benzodiazepines prove to be a favorite choice among individuals seeking relief from psychological issues temporarily. Benzodiazepines, such as those mentioned in Edinoff et al. (2021), are characteristically known for their rapid onset and addictive nature, leading to dependency that must be carefully managed upon cessation. Further, even though depressants are commonly known to have a sedative effect, their use may also suppress or mask underlying mental disorders, thereby making treatment protocols more complex.

According to Sakloth et al. (2019), experiments with substances such as LSD, mescaline, and psilocybin show fascinating potential for therapeutic purposes outside from their general classification as hallucinogens, to manage depression and drug dependence.. In conformity, the complexity of depressants points towards their dual nature as both therapeutic and harmful agents.

1.2.3. Hallucinogens

Hallucinogens are a diverse group of drugs that have potent effects on perception, mood, and cognitive function, often resulting in intense psychological experiences. Psilocybin in some mushrooms and synthetic drugs like lysergic acid diethylamide (LSD) are examples of these drugs. Hallucinogens tend to create vivid changes in sensory perceptions and emotional responses, but are accompanied by the risk of side effects, particularly in regard to dermatological disorders.

Multiple skin reactions have been evidenced after hallucinogenic use, with studies discovering correlations between cannabis and MDMA with contact dermatitis and urticaria (Rahman et al., 2024). Importantly, structural diversity within this class, e.g., how MDMA differs from related molecules, illustrates their unique pharmacological profiles; for instance, MDMA produces social bonding effects rather than the expected hallucinogenic experience (Nichols, 2022). Hence, ongoing research is essential to understand their therapeutic significance as well as hazards (Figure 1.8).

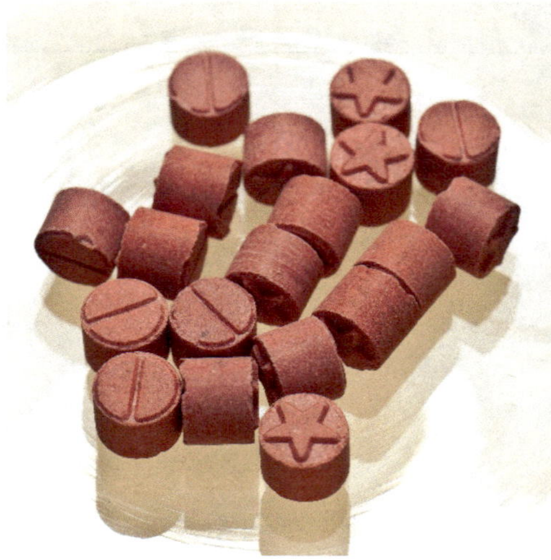

Figure 1.8. Hallucinogens.

Source: https://www.dea.gov/sites/default/files/2023-04/MDMA_Ecstasy_005.jpg.

1.2.4. Opioids

Opioids constitute a critical class of medications, which either occur in the opium poppy or are synthesized in a laboratory to mimic natural opiates. Opioids can be classified into two categories: natural opioids, including morphine and codeine, and semi-synthetic or synthetic opioids, such as oxycodone and fentanyl. The primary application of these medications is their analgesic effect, which proves effective in managing pain in a clinic setting. Yet their potential for addiction and abuse has caused a chronic public health problem, especially in the United States. Two decades of growth in opioid prescriptions have attracted significant attention from healthcare providers, who now see an urgent need for ongoing education about opioids and their impacts. According to recent questionnaires, the majority of healthcare professionals have expressed a desire for more training in new psychoactive drugs, such as opioids, so that they are better able to inform patient management and promote effective harm reduction policy (Bancroft et al., 2020; García Ruiz et al., 2021).

1.2.5. Antidepressants

Antidepressants are a crucial class of drugs ingested to minimize symptoms of depression and other affective disorders, made up of several classes with varying mechanisms of action. Some of the key classes are Selective Serotonin Reuptake Inhibitors (SSRIs) and the older tricyclic antidepressants (TCAs), which function by altering neurotransmitter action in the brain in a manner that boosts mood and emotional sensation. The selection of a specific antidepressant is mainly based on the side effects patients experience because no drug can have therapeutic action without side effects (Agius et al., 2017). Sexual dysfunction is one of the serious side effects that has a great impact on the quality of life and adherence to treatment plans. Identification of these effects is essential for medical practitioners since they not only impact the health of patients but also the overall outcome of depression (Jespersen et al., 2006). Antidepressants should therefore be administered carefully, considering both efficacy and patient-centric results (Figure 1.9).

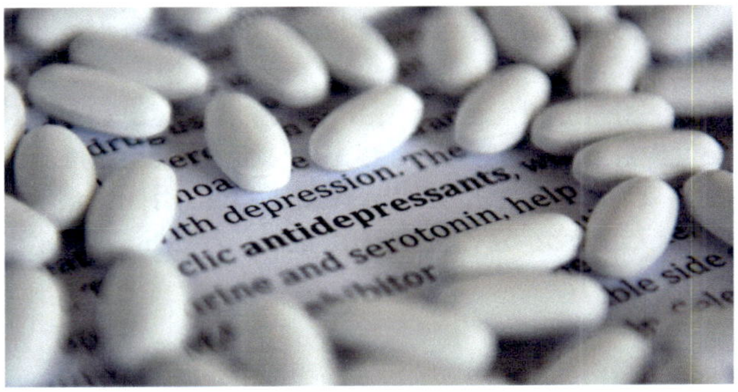

Figure 1.9. Antidepressants.

Source: https://www.ibdrelief.com/uploads/files/mind_antidepressants_depression_cg_image_243.jpg.

1.2.6. Antipsychotics

Antipsychotics are a fundamental class of medication employed primarily in the treatment of psychotic disorders such as schizophrenia and bipolar disorder. Antipsychotics typically come in two categories: typical and atypical antipsychotics. Typical antipsychotics, developed in the mid-20th century, predominantly block the dopamine receptors and, in doing so, lower hallucination and delusion symptoms. On the other hand, newer atypical antipsychotics have a broader mode of action, targeting more neurotransmitter systems, perhaps accounting for their efficiency in treating positive and negative symptoms of psychosis. This class of drugs poses challenges, notably to managing side effects and the emergence of new psychiatric illness related to newer synthesized drugs (Chiappini et al., 2019). Network pharmacology knowledge, such as in the case of the DTome tool, enables the understanding of drug-target networks for antipsychotics and fosters the ability for the effective management of therapeutic strategies (Sun et al., 2012).

1.2.7. Antibiotics

Antibiotics are an essential group of medications that combat bacterial infections through a plethora of mechanisms and have revolutionized the practice of medicine. Agents fall into several categories, including the *penicillins*, tetracyclines, and macrolides, and each exhibits distinct pharmacologic properties and blocks different bacterial functions. The emergence of antibiotic resistance in the form of multi-resistant infections complicates treatment regimens and is a testament to the need for prudent use of antibiotics. Research has shown that exposure to healthcare facilities significantly increases the risk of acquiring multi-resistant infections, underscoring the crucial role healthcare workers play in regulating antibiotic use within these facilities (Ceccarelli et al., 2015).

Further, the complexity of accurately describing medical vocabulary in explaining antibiotic resistance highlights the gap between technological advancement and clinical practice (Singh et al., 1997). Thus, understanding and correct usage of antibiotics are most crucial in stopping resistance spread and effective treatment for patients (Figure 1.10).

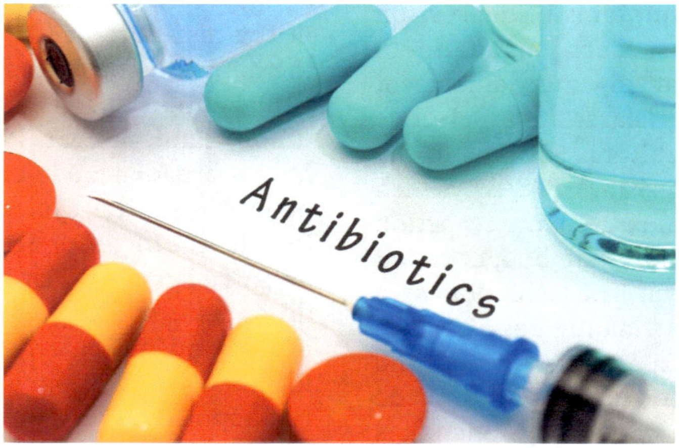

Figure 1.10. Antibiotics.

Source: https://medshadow.org/wp-content/uploads/2020/03/antibiotics-scaled.jpeg.

1.2.8. Antihistamines

In pharmacology, antihistamines are a significant drug class that is primarily employed for neutralizing allergic reactions and symptom relief of diseases such as hay fever and urticaria. Antihistamines work by inhibiting the action of histamine at the H1 receptor sites, thereby reducing symptoms like itching, sneezing, and swelling. The global prevalence of antihistamine-treated conditions underscores the demand for such medicines, with about 20% of individuals having acute urticaria at some point in their lifetime, which has a profound impact on their activity and quality of life (Zuberbier et al., 2021). Moreover, progress in antihistamine drug formulations has developed second-generation drugs with reduced sedation effects and improved safety profiles compared to first-generation drugs. Therefore, an understanding of the mechanisms and classification of antihistamines is paramount for optimizing therapeutic control of allergy in consideration of its broader implications for public health (Pępnicki et al., 2018).

1.2.9. Anesthetics

Anesthetics are a common group of pharmacologic agents for establishing a state of controlled unconsciousness and facilitating the performance of surgical interventions. The drugs fall primarily into the categories of general and local anesthetics, each serving to achieve specific clinical objectives. General anesthetics, such as propofol, induce profound unconsciousness and are generally administered through intravenous or inhalation routes. Local anesthetics, e.g., lidocaine, block sensation in a particular location by blocking nerve conduction. The improvement in anesthetic techniques, particularly the arrival of target-controlled infusions (TCI), has transformed anesthetic procedures to administer the anesthetic with precise control in line with the needs of the patient (Shafer et al., 2015). Moreover, the role of neuromuscular blocking agents (NMBAs) has become an integral aspect of muscle relaxation surgery, as NMBAs act upon the neuromuscular junction to block muscle contraction, thus intensifying the efficacy of anesthesia (Keegan, 2015). Such advances reflect the complexity and evolution of anesthetic agents in the broader pharmacological picture (Figure 1.11).

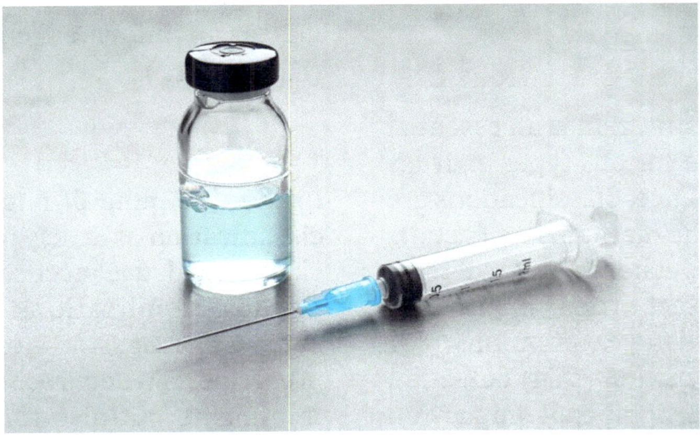

Figure 1.11. Anesthetics.

Source: https://maineanesthesiaservices.com/wp-content/uploads/2024/03/localanestheticsregionalanesthesia-1080x675.jpeg.

Test Your Knowledge

1. What are opioids?
2. Give some examples of antidepressants.

1.3. Drug Classification Systems

Learning Outcome

1. Understand pharmacological classification and therapeutic classification
2. Know the mechanism of action
3. Explain legal classification (controlled substances)
4. Focus on prescription vs. over-the-counter
5. Explain the role of the World Health Organization
6. Describe national classification systems
7. Learn the importance of classification in treatment
8. Identify challenges in drug classification

As one can see when looking at the drug classification systems within the context of the framework, drug classification systems within the framework are double-purpose: controlling the abuse of drugs while maintaining access for lawful medical uses. In other jurisdictions, such as the USA, UK, Canada, New Zealand, and Australia, legal systems separately classify drugs based on their cultural and social conception of drug use. For instance, Atik et al. (2020) illustrate how Australia treats controlled drugs differently, citing its uniqueness in punishing according to the quantity of the drugs rather than solely categorizing strictly. Additionally, the incorporation of indigenous medicinal practice into modern systems, as illustrated in Diallo et al., (2013), highlights the requirement to combine disparate knowledge for greater therapeutic potential. This dynamic tension between regulation and practice underscores the complexity of drug classification, and the necessity for ongoing dialogue and adaptation in light of shifting societal requirements.

1.3.1. Pharmacological Classification

Pharmacologic drug classification is an essential system for organizing the various types of drugs prescribed in clinical practice. Classifications are commonly grounded in the mechanism of action, therapeutic effect, and chemical structure, enabling clinicians to select proper medication and forecast potential drug interactions. For instance, drug-drug interaction (DDI) detection is crucial since it has a significant impact on patient outcomes, typically leading to morbidity and mortality (Kolchinsky et al., 2012).

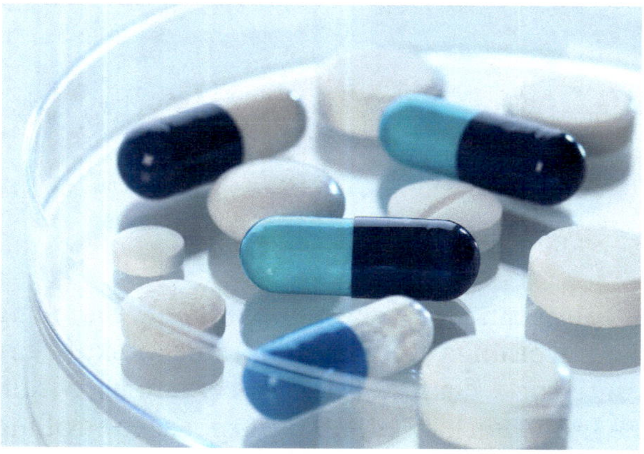

Figure 1.12. The pharmacological classification of drugs serves as a critical framework for understanding the various categories of medications used in clinical practice.

Source: https://images.ctfassets.net/o78em1y1w4i4/2Erx22h1T2BvLwINhv0GTw/ef9618830bef739c06d02796c3baa540/Drug-repurposing-banner-landscape.jpg.

While some may be region- and culture-specific, such a classification system not only facilitates systematic drug efficacy research but also improves pharmacovigilance, especially when it comes to harmonizing traditional and mainstream medicine (Diallo et al., 2013). Accordingly, a robust pharmacological classification thus augments sound therapeutic strategies and maximizes patient safety as a matter of informed clinical decision-making (Figure 1.12).

1.3.2. Therapeutic Classification

In the discipline of pharmacology, therapeutic classification is a key organizing system that classifies drugs according to their intended medical applications and mechanisms of action. The classification is crucial not just for prescribers when recommending appropriate treatments but also for pedagogical purposes since it enables students and practitioners to know the therapeutic action and potential side effects of drugs. For instance, the European Society of Cardiology and European Atherosclerosis Society (ESC/EAS) Guidelines identify the degree to which effective therapeutic categorization influences medical decisions and the implementation of treatment strategies, thereby ensuring healthcare practitioners can make appropriate decisions based on special patient needs (Mach et al., 2019). Moreover, the typical attributes of drugs in these categories can significantly impact their safety and efficacy profiles, illustrating the necessity for effective classification systems within medicine (Khan et al., 2017). Therapeutic classification is thus an essential component of acquiring information about and making effective use of pharmacological agents in the healthcare sector.

1.3.3. Mechanism of Action

The mechanism of action is significant in demonstrating how various drugs have their therapeutic effect, hence defining their categorization and application in clinical practice. It is the specific biochemical interaction whereby a drug operates its pharmacologic effect, either by receptor binding, enzyme inhibition, or physiologic process alteration.

For instance, antipsychotic medications work primarily through acting on neurotransmitter mechanisms in the brain, by blocking dopamine receptors, as a part of their therapeutic action for the treatment of psychotic disorders. Furthermore, research highlights the importance of active student participation in studying such mechanisms, for example, through innovative methods like storytelling, which can lead to enhanced comprehension of intricate pharmacological concepts (Elango et al., 2022). Understanding mechanisms of action is crucial not only for ideal treatment planning, but it is also essential for predicting potential side effects and drug interactions, thereby emphasizing the interdisciplinary nature of pharmacology (Figure 1.13).

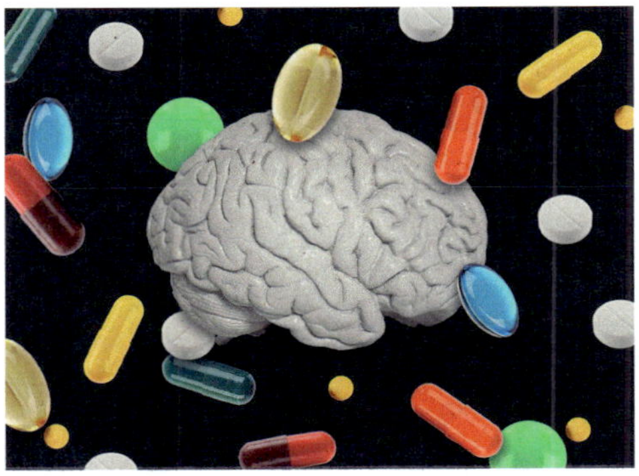

Figure 1.13. Antipsychotic medications.

Source: https://www.wondermind.com/wp-content/uploads/2024/02/Heres-What-Experts-Want-You-to-Know-About-Antipsychotics1.jpg?w=960.

1.3.4. Legal Classification (Controlled Substances)

Controlled substance legal status is the core component of drug policy that varies extensively from one jurisdiction to another. It not only helps to prevent drug abuse, but also allows them to be used medically safely. Each country has its legislative mechanisms for categorizing substances that reflect its cultural orientation and health concerns. For instance, the Australian model focuses more on quantity-based penalties, which leave space for enforcement flexibility. At the same time, the UK and Canada have shown to be more flexible models that deal with therapeutic and recreational use equally effectively.

The emergence of new psychoactive substances, popularly referred to as legal highs, has further obscured this scenario. The ACMD identifies the necessity of governments to adapt their approaches to mitigate the threats posed by these drugs, ultimately demanding collaborative efforts between various departments of government (Atik et al., 2020).

1.3.5. Prescription vs. Over-the-Counter

The distinction between over-the-counter (OTC) and prescription drugs is significant in the understanding of drug names and classifications available to consumers. Prescription drugs are tightly regulated and require a physician's approval, such that their administration is tailored for a patient's specific health circumstances. Such levels of concern are especially relevant in the management of chronic disease, like Alzheimer's, where drugs can significantly impact disease patterns and quality of life. On the other hand, OTC medications are considered safe and effective for use by the general public without the supervision of a healthcare provider, enabling self-medication for everyday conditions such as a headache or an allergy (Johnston et al., 2020).

This ease of access, however, poses a threat of abuse or excessive intake, enhancing the need for consumer education regarding safe drug use. Knowingly recognizing these categorizations helps make informed choices, eventually influencing general health results and drug safety (Figure 1.14).

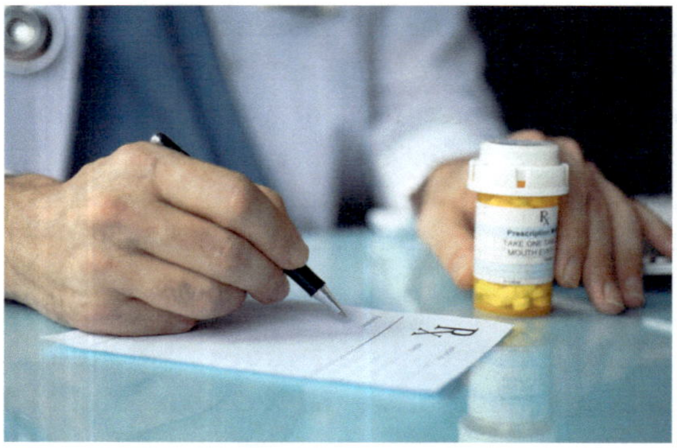

Figure 1.14. Prescription medications are specifically regulated and require a doctor's authorization, ensuring that their use is appropriate for a patient's unique health circumstances.

Source: https://www.inspirahealthnetwork.org/sites/default/files/2022-09/iStock-1190193669.jpg.

1.3.6. Role of the World Health Organization

The World Health Organization (WHO) plays an integral part in setting global health policies and practices, particularly in drug classification and standardization. By establishing comprehensive classifications for drugs, the WHO facilitates international cooperation and helps countries maximize the use of health resources. It is essential at a time when several varied naming systems and terminologies make drug identification and application more difficult, as has been experienced with the intricacy of drug names. Furthermore, the WHO's focus on controlled vocabularies supports greater integration of information from disparate health information systems, so critical to personalized medicine initiatives where genomics and clinical information converge. The efforts highlight the importance of a single drug classification methodology that promotes both interoperability and availability in healthcare, thereby offsetting inequalities resulting from variations in terminology and practices. As such, the WHO's power goes beyond policy formulation to tangible applications that improve world health outcomes (Bodenreider et al., 2004; Ceusters et al., 2007).

1.3.7. National Classification Systems

National drug classification systems play a significant role in classifying and regulating drugs, establishing a system that facilitates the identification and control of drugs. They are crucial in the establishment of public safety and adequate provision of healthcare because they categorize drugs according to their application in therapy, chemical structure, and potential for abuse.

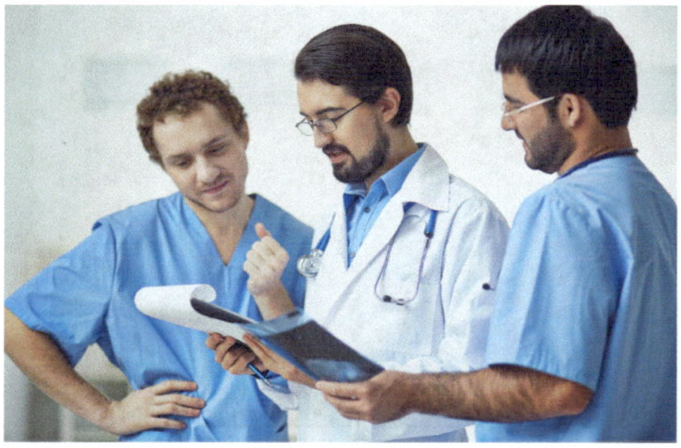

Figure 1.15. National classification systems play a crucial role in the regulation and categorization of drugs, establishing a framework that aids in the identification and management of pharmaceuticals.

Source: https://cdn.sanity.io/images/9dzxez9p/production/53d8aeafed09ad0dfe39ad0ca8fe1a8b10f51ef3-1200x800.png.

For instance, the WHO drug classification system classifies drugs into various classes, making communication between health workers easier and enhancing the prescription practices. Furthermore, understanding the consequences of AMR is essential, as they significantly influence healthcare resources and inform policy decision-making due to the growing threats of drug-resistant infections (Murray et al., 2022). Moreover, adhering to national recommendations, such as those presented by the ESC, emphasizes the need for experts to make informed therapeutic choices according to established protocols, thus aiming to optimize patient outcomes (Visseren et al., 2021) (Figure 1.15).

1.3.8. Importance of Classification in Treatment

Optimal drug categorization is of critical value in optimizing treatment response for a variety of medical conditions. The recent breakthrough in antiepileptic drug classification, for instance, shows how particular treatment approaches can maximize seizure control for epilepsy sufferers. By the description of seizure type etiology, clinicians can apply the most effective medication, thereby increasing the prospects of achieving seizure freedom in approximately two-thirds of the patients (Perucca et al., 2018). Furthermore, pharmacogenetic profiling in the case of TCAs demonstrates how differential gene expression, e.g., CYP2D6 and CYP2C19, primarily influences drug metabolism as well as patient response. These genetic discoveries enable clinicians to customize TCA treatment, decreasing the risk of treatment failure and toxicity (Hicks et al., 2015). Thus, classification is not merely a systemic categorization but a foundation for precision medicine to optimize interactions between therapeutic agents and patient heterogeneity.

1.3.9. Challenges in Drug Classification

The complexities of drug classification bring on serious challenges, particularly about pharmaceutical drug safety and efficacy. One of the principal challenges lies in the variety of side effects documented across various groups; despite the rigorous clinical trials, there are always some adverse effects that hide until after drug launch.

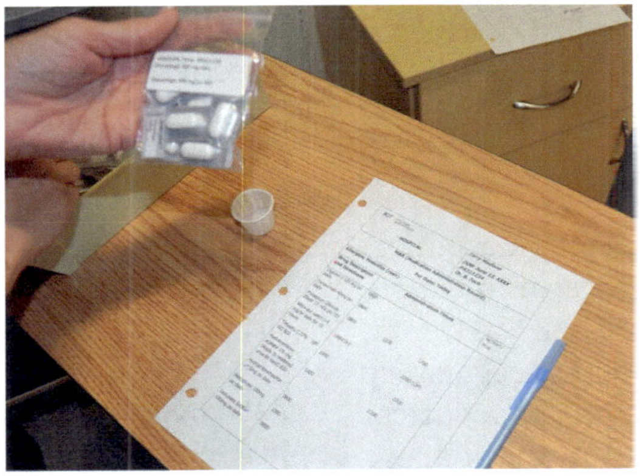

Figure 1.16. The complexities of drug classification present significant challenges, particularly as they pertain to the efficacy and safety of pharmaceutical treatments.

Source: https://wtcs.pressbooks.pub/app/uploads/sites/29/2020/10/DSC_17601-1024x764.jpg.

This information gap necessitates innovative solutions, including the use of social media data to identify real-world side effects of drugs effectively. Newest advances in data processing, such as techniques like Apache Spark, allow researchers to quickly and precisely process huge amounts of data, which strengthens our understanding of the drug effect (Hsu et al., 2017). Also, cultural variability in the practice of traditional medicine, which significantly varies from culture to culture, contributes to the intricacies of drug classification since they tend to rely heavily on oral traditions and local differences in medicinal plants. Merging these contrasting methods could enhance conventional and traditional treatments while reducing risks that occur with faulty drug classification (Diallo et al., 2013) (Figure 1.16).

Test Your Knowledge

1. What are over-the-counter drugs?
2. Write short note on national classification systems.

1.4. The Role of Drug Naming in Healthcare

Learning Outcome

1. Give importance to healthcare professionals
2. Know the impact on patient safety
3. Explain the role in prescribing practices
4. Understand the influence on patient adherence
5. Know misunderstandings due to naming
6. Describe education and training for healthcare providers
7. Learn case studies of naming errors
8. Identify strategies to improve drug name clarity
9. Know future trends in drug naming

In the intricate field of medicine, pharmaceutical nomenclature is the identifying term to enable correct communication between patients, medical practitioners, and medicines regulatory authorities. Not only does pharmaceutical nomenclature allow the identification of drugs but also their pharmacological properties and therapeutic use, which makes them eligible for prescription and dispensation. As has been witnessed in the rising medical translation literature, the challenges of heterogeneous terminologies pose the imperative of standard naming conventions as a solution against clinician-to-clinician miscommunication (Azizova et al., 2023). Secondly, drug development and user interaction pose an increased focus on making drug names more intuitive to patients and thereby facilitating them to comprehend their drugs in a better way (Penati et al., 2024). Hence, sensitive consideration of drug naming is pivotal to enhancing patient safety, adherence, and overall successful delivery of healthcare.

1.4.1. Importance for Healthcare Professionals

Given the changing dynamics of healthcare, it is crucial for healthcare practitioners to thoroughly understand the names and classifications of drugs. The knowledge is not only critical for effective patient treatment but also for safe prescribing practices. As the ESC/EAS Guidelines stress, it is the individual responsibility of healthcare professionals to use clinical judgment to ensure treatment schedules align with established guidelines and take into account the unique health condition of each patient (Mach et al., 2019). In addition, the challenge of AMR necessitates that medical practitioners use prudence when prescribing because improper use will lead to a serious public health issue (Will, 2018). By learning the intricacies of pharmacology, including drug mechanisms and classifications, medical practitioners can better master the complexities of these events and eventually improve the outcome for patients towards the larger goal of responsible drug control (Figure 1.17).

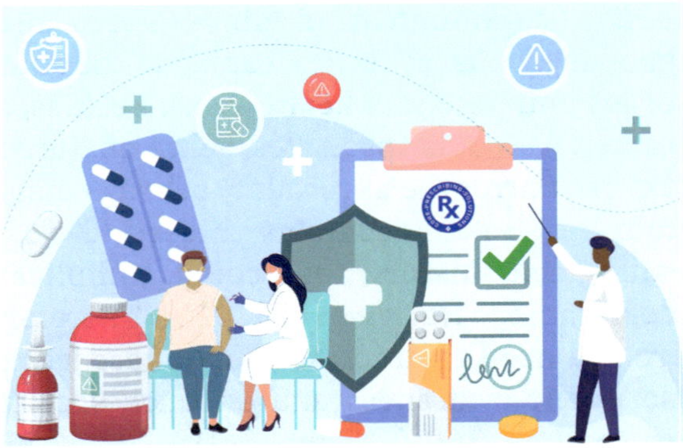

Figure 1.17. In the evolving landscape of healthcare, the importance of understanding the names and classes of drugs cannot be overstated for healthcare professionals.

Source: https://coreprescribingsolutions.co.uk/wp-content/uploads/2023/12/MEDICATION-SAFETY-scaled.jpg.

1.4.2. Impact on Patient Safety

Patient safety is greatly influenced by the dispensing and classification of various drugs, particularly for mental illness and chronic diseases. Misusing drugs like psychotropic and analgesic drugs will lead to severe health complications, including dependence and overdose.

For instance, the ramifications of the Brady Handgun Violence Prevention Act illustrate greater awareness of mental health collaboration and patient safety dynamics with the need for strict data collection and background checks to avoid potential pitfalls in prescriptive measures (Atwell et al., 1998). Second, the provision of standardized guidelines for monitoring drug efficacy and safety emphasizes the necessity for harmonization of information collection across acute and chronic illnesses, as can be observed through improving the treatment of diseases such as atopic eczema (Apfelbacher et al., 2019). This is crucial in preventing treatment from inadvertently compromising patient safety.

1.4.3. Role in Prescribing Practices

The role of prescribing practice is significantly influenced by diverse patient populations and healthcare needs indicators (HCNIs), which in turn impact the therapeutic setting for various classes of medicines. Researches point out significant variations in levels of prescribing among general practitioners, which suggests that age, ethnicity, and socioeconomic status can lead to differences in care provision. For example, prescription rates of such vital medications as statins and ACE inhibitors were remarkably impacted by the age profile of the patient population, with more advanced age groups being likely to receive suboptimal treatment (Gibson et al., 2005). Moreover, ischemic heart disease research reveals that the most commonly prescribed drug classes, such as antiplatelets and hypolipidemic, not only reflect the disease prevalence but also population demographics regarding age (Jadhav et al., 2019).

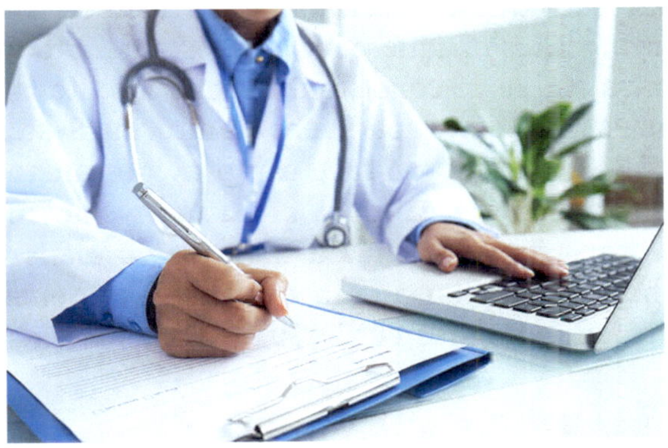

Figure 1.18. Various patient demographics critically influences the role of prescribing practices and healthcare needs indicators (HCNIs), shaping the therapeutic landscape for different drug classes.

Source: https://www.outsourcestrategies.com/wp-content/uploads/2022/06/prior-authorization-for-prescription-drugs.jpg.

This implies that optimal prescribing is not just a matter of selecting the appropriate drug classes but even requires attention to the broader social determinants that influence patient outcomes (Figure 1.18).

1.4.4. Influence on Patient Adherence

The effect on patient compliance is a multifaceted issue that will have a significant influence on the efficacy of pharmacotherapy, particularly when managing chronic diseases such as HIV and mental illness. Cognitive function, especially in terms of verbal episodic memory, was found to have a linear relationship with the level of patient compliance. HIV-positive patients with impaired recall of memory may fail to remember drug regimen, thus leading to greater non-compliance. Specifically, individuals with impaired free recall have significantly greater chances of non-adherence than individuals with better memory profiles (Casaletto et al., 2015). Similarly, when speaking of psychiatric drugs for depression and schizophrenia, pharmacokinetic variability, as reflected in varying rates of adherence, is a testament to the central value of consistent dosage monitoring. The use of Medication Event Monitoring System (MEMS) data in this case can provide valuable insight into the conduct of patients, showing the need for coordinated therapeutic plans to enhance compliance and optimize the benefit of treatment (Bies et al., 2011).

1.4.5. Misunderstandings Due to Naming

The complexity of naming drugs typically leads to colossal misconceptions, particularly in terms of categorizing them and how they affect people. It is compounded by the vagueness between words used in science and colloquial language, which can make consumers just as baffled as experts in the healthcare sector. For instance, an illegal drug can use different names—its chemical name, brand name, and street name—each of which has various meanings and degrees of legitimacy. Such multiple naming can hamper effective communication since users may unknowingly misuse terms, leading to the abuse of drugs and potential health risks. Besides, as Enrique Vila-Matas speculates, genre mixture in books can mirror the uncertainty of drug naming because each name contains crossed levels of meaning and history that could complicate understanding (Hurley et al., 2011). Therefore, there is a need to describe such differences to raise public awareness and enhance security (Caruso et al., 2008) (Figure 1.19).

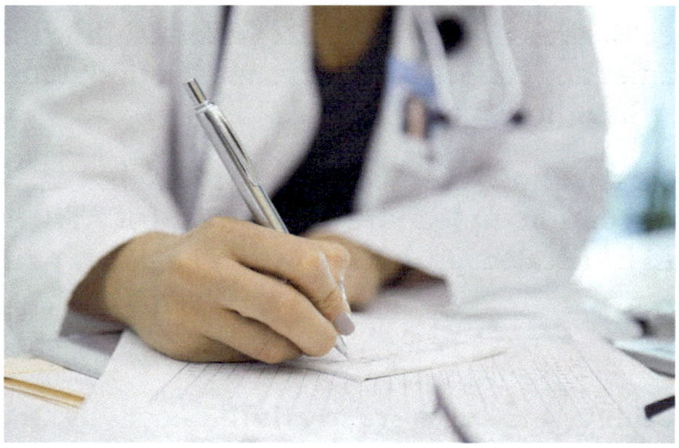

Figure 1.19. The complexities surrounding the naming of drugs often lead to significant misunderstandings, particularly in the context of their classification and effects.

Source: https://www.verywellhealth.com/thumb/LNJRFRlHlpX7cgydJIaEJ_d5Z9I=/1500x0/filters:no_upscale():max_bytes(150000):strip_icc()/prescription-56a68fa63df78cf7728eff7e.jpg.

1.4.6. Education and Training for Healthcare Providers

Accurate education and training of health care practitioners are vital to ensuring safe and competent patient care, particularly about drug therapy. The education must cover not only pharmacological information about various drug classes but also the ethical considerations that govern their administration. For instance, knowledge of the latest clinical guidelines, those articulated by leading health organizations, can potentially equip providers with better, more tailored decisions catering to the unique patient needs (Cosentino et al., 2019). Further, emerging technologies, including massive language models like ChatGPT, hold promising value in improving medical education by providing instant access to vast amounts of information and decision-support systems (Kung et al., 2023). Such innovations would add to traditional learning methods, updating providers with evolving drug therapies and aligning with best practices. Last but not least, a robust education system constructs an efficient healthcare workforce that can handle the complexities involved in drug management more effectively (Figure 1.20).

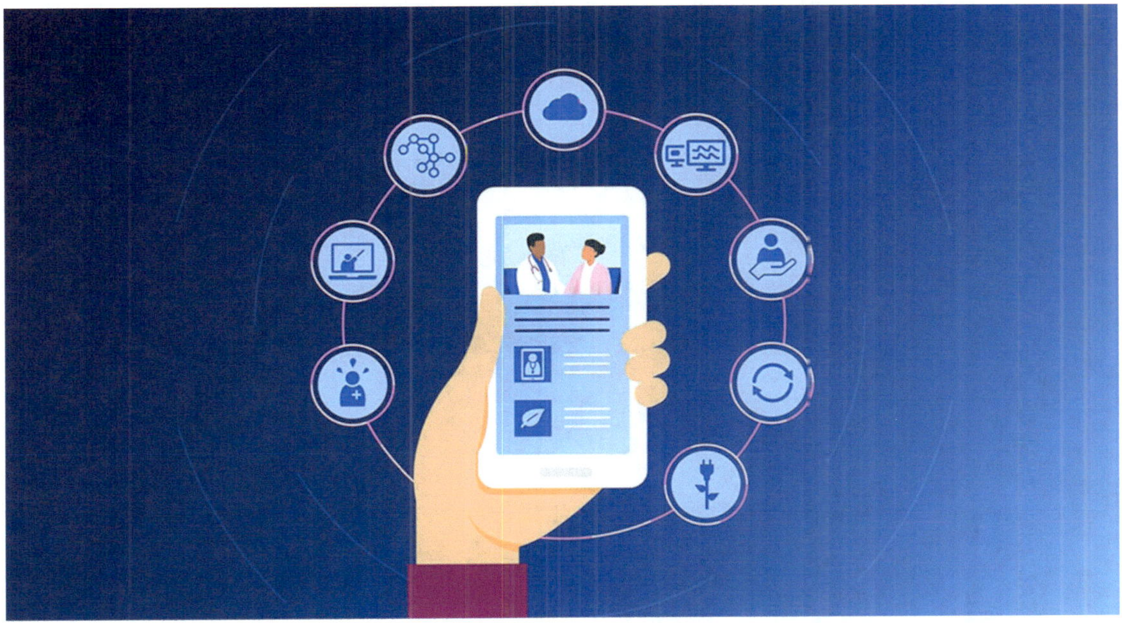

Figure 1.20. Effective education and training for healthcare providers is paramount to ensure safe and competent patient care, particularly in the context of drug therapy.

Source: https://www.philips.com/c-dam/corporate/innovation-and-you/global/dec-2023/hero-2023-healthcare-technology-trends.jpg.

1.4.7. Case Studies of Naming Errors

When analyzing pharmacology name errors case studies, it is essential to understand how the errors impact medication efficacy and patient safety. Name errors may be due to sounding drug names or unclear abbreviations, leading to confusion and risking unsafe medication errors. For instance, the cross-over of methicillin-resistant Staphylococcus aureus with other pathogens of the same name shows the foreboding consequences of clinical error, particularly in the field of AMR (Murray et al., 2022). Secondly, medical artificial intelligence also underscores the importance of proper drug nomenclature, particularly how machine learning (ML) techniques are applied to rationalize drug classification and minimize errors in prescriptions (Jiang et al., 2017). Appreciation is obtained through the examination of such case studies for the systematic issues involving conventions for drug names, as well as persistent problems with the proper administration of medication.

1.4.8. Strategies to Improve Drug Name Clarity

Enhancing drug name clarity is crucial for reducing drug errors and ensuring patient safety. One possible approach is to reduce look-alike and sound-alike names, which are a common source of errors among healthcare providers and patients alike. Tighter drug nomenclature guidelines, suggested by clinical professionals, would greatly influence recognition and recall (Dennison et al., 2020). Moreover, newer technology such as Knowledge Discovery in Databases (KDD) can be used to discover patterns for medication errors that are rooted in naming issues. Trends can be found by healthcare professionals using big data sets and applied to areas of confusion where they can utilize them to educate medication naming processes (Taft et al., 2010). Also, training health professionals in the importance of proper drug names in clinical settings can instill a culture of safety, which will, in turn, enhance the practice of medication administration and patient outcomes (Figure 1.21).

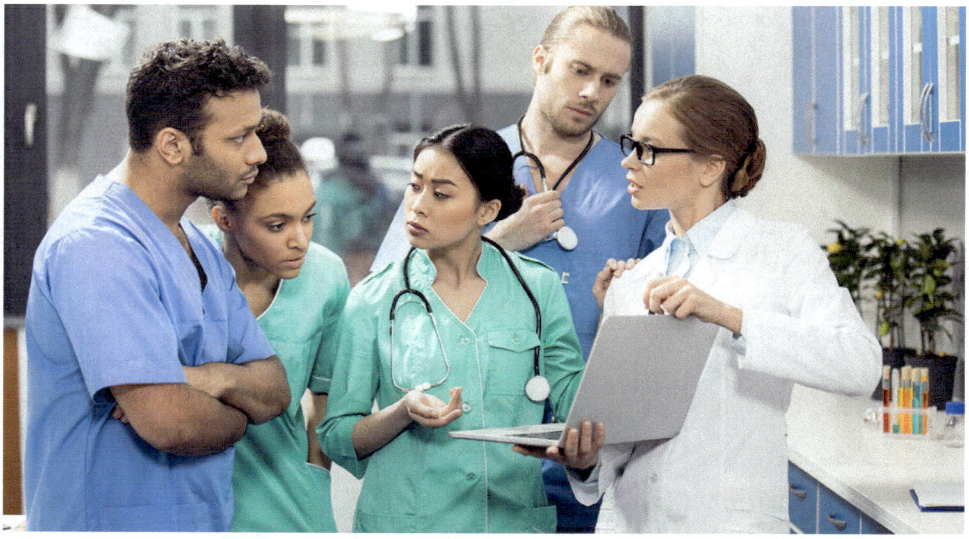

Figure 1.21. Enhancing drug name clarity is paramount for ensuring patient safety and reducing medication errors.

Source: https://images.squarespace-cdn.com/content/v1/56a042fb25981d9326c9bbdb/9c769d51-0081-4ae2-a363-85ab65d1afc5/Top+Benefits+of+GCP+Training+for+Healthcare+Professionals.png.

1.4.9. Future Trends in Drug Naming

With the new pharma industry face, it is a trend in drug naming that awaits an awe-inspiring transformation with science and technology advances. Drug names in the future would most likely have elements expressing their action or therapeutic category as a means of inducing a better impression of their action and uses among healthcare professionals and patients. Development of AMR and the necessity of effective antibiotics make precise and comprehensive nomenclature even more critical to note, with evidence from growing rates of drug-resistant infections being reported worldwide (Murray et al., 2022). Furthermore, novel technologies such as lipid nanoparticles are revolutionizing drug delivery systems, and drug names will begin to place greater emphasis on such new preparations and their biopharmaceutical properties (Montoto et al., 2020). Ultimately, the future drug names will also take relevance and clarity into consideration so that the names will directly indicate both the roles of drugs and their efficacy in disease treatment.

Test Your Knowledge

1. How can confusing drug names affect patient adherence to treatment?
2. In what ways can pharmacists assist patients in understanding the difference between generic and brand names?

Summary

The drug classes and pharmacology capture the intricate relationship between therapeutics and pharmacology, highlighting the need to understand such interaction to deliver quality patient care. Generic vs. brand names is of relevance in prescribing, having implications for availability as well as cost-effectiveness of drugs. Besides, as with the case of the cancer therapies, including the positive impacts of CDK4/6 inhibitors for advanced breast cancers, certain types of drugs can have a considerable effect on the condition of patients and are therefore closely watched for their toxicities (Sollena et al., 2023). Thus, the limitations imposed on the use of radiomics to identify metastasis in cancer validate the continuity of problems to pharmacological research and its applicability (Pullen et al., 2023). Therefore, a deeper understanding of drug classes not only improves medical data but also facilitates rational clinical decision-making, ultimately improving patient management as well as the efficiency of treatments.

In outlining the main findings, it is necessary to highlight once again the intricacy involved in the categorical distinctions and the implications that the distinctions have for medicine and sociocultural environments. The chapter outlines how drugs are categorized in terms of their pharmacological action and therapeutic uses, such as analgesics, anxiolytics, and stimulants. Also, the debate is carried over to the social views of these classes and how public opinion may strongly impact policy and health. This kind of multi-dimensional analysis is needed to further knowledge in the area, as even simple cases provide a demanding model of interpretation, especially in biological instances in which drug safety and efficacy matter strongly (Nazarenko et al., 2005). Furthermore, social dynamics such as communication patterns between communities engaged in illicit drug use emphasize the need for specialized law enforcement tactics (Balasuriya et al., 2016).

KEY TERMS FROM THIS CHAPTER

- Lant-based products
- Psychotropic drugs
- Regulatory authorities
- Researchers
- Scientists
- Sertraline
- Standard guidelines
- Synthetic cannabinoids
- Target-controlled infusions (TCI)
- Therapeutic function
- Practitioners
- Rationalization
- Regulatory frameworks
- Scientific assessment
- Selective Serotonin Reuptake Inhibitors
- Spice
- Stimulants
- Systematic names
- Tetracyclines
- Therapeutic practice

Critical Thinking Questions

1. **Why is the use of generic drug names encouraged in healthcare settings?**
   a. Generic names are easier to pronounce
   b. Generic names are more expensive
   c. Generic names reduce confusion and ensure consistency
   d. Generic names are brand-specific
2. **Which of the following best describes a generic drug name?**
   a. A name given by the manufacturer for marketing
   b. A patented name exclusive to a company
   c. A standard, universally accepted scientific name
   d. A street name used in informal settings
3. **Which organization is primarily responsible for assigning generic drug names internationally?**
   a. FDA
   b. WHO (World Health Organization)
   c. USP
   d. CDC
4. **A risk of similar-sounding drug names (e.g., Celebrex vs. Celexa) is:**
   a. Branding issues
   b. Delayed drug approval
   c. Medication errors
   d. Reduced drug potency
5. **What is the primary purpose of a brand (trade) name for a drug?**
   a. To classify it chemically
   b. To identify the country of origin
   c. For marketing and recognition by healthcare providers and patients
   d. To ensure safety in hospitals

Answers to Critical Thinking Questions

1. (c); 2. (c); 3. (b); 4. (c); 5. (c).

Short Answer Questions

1. What is the difference between a drug's generic name and its brand name?
2. What drug class does ibuprofen belong to?
3. Name two drugs that belong to the ACE inhibitor class.
4. What class of drugs does amoxicillin belong to?
5. Which drug class is primarily used to reduce cholesterol levels?

References

1. Krallinger, M., Rabal, O., Lourenço, A., Oyarzabal, J., & Valencia, A. (2017). Information retrieval and text mining technologies for chemistry. *Chemical Reviews, 117*(12), 7673–7761. https://doi.org/10.1021/acs.chemrev.6b00851Advisory Council on the Misuse of Drugs. (2011). *Consideration of the Novel Psychoactive Substances ('Legal Highs')*. https://core.ac.uk/download/1643031.pdf (accessed on 10th June 2025).
2. Agius, M., & Bonnici, H. (2017). *Antidepressants in Use in Clinical Practice*. https://core.ac.uk/download/512491574.pdf (accessed on 10th June 2025).
3. Alcock, B., Raphenya, A. R., Lau, T. T. Y., Tsang, K. K., Bouchard, M., Edalatmand, A., Huynh, W., et al. (2019). CARD 2020: Antibiotic resistome surveillance with the Comprehensive Antibiotic Resistance Database. *Nucleic Acids Research*. https://doi.org/10.1093/nar/gkz935.
4. Alves, V. L., Gonçalves, J., Aguiar, J., Teixeira, H. M., & Câmara, J. S. (2020). The synthetic cannabinoids phenomenon: From structure to toxicological properties. A review. *Critical Reviews in Toxicology, 50*, 359–382. https://doi.org/10.1080/10408444.2020.1762539.
5. Apfelbacher, C. J., Arents, B. W. M., Barbarot, S., et al. (2019). TREatment of ATopic eczema (TREAT) Registry Taskforce: Consensus on how and when to measure the core dataset for atopic eczema treatment research registries. https://core.ac.uk/download/323310740.pdf (accessed on 10th June 2025).
6. Arab, A. Z., Baldacchino, A., Conti, A. A., et al. (2021). Relationship between cardiovascular disease pathology and fatal opioid and other sedative overdose: A post-mortem investigation and pilot study. https://core.ac.uk/download/481494184.pdf (accessed on 10th June 2025).
7. Archibuigi, D., Augsdorfer, P., Bijker, W. E., Bowker, G., Freeman, C., Headrick, D., et al. (2013). Just how difficult can it be counting up R&D funding for emerging technologies (and is tech mining with proxy measures going to be any better?). https://core.ac.uk/download/16413077.pdf (accessed on 10th June 2025).
8. Arendt, M., Goodair, C., Cregler, L. L., Schifano, F., Claridge, H., Corkery, J. M., et al. (2017). An exploratory study of information sources and key findings on UK cocaine-related deaths. https://core.ac.uk/download/84342133.pdf (accessed on 10th June 2025).
9. Atik, S., Gallagher, C., Isse, L., et al. (2020). Doctor or drug dealer? International legal provisions for the legitimate handling of drugs of abuse. https://core.ac.uk/download/287582629.pdf (accessed on 10th June 2025).
10. Atwell, C., Barnes, A. R., & Trostle, L. C. (1998). *Brady Statute Data: Establishing Noncriminal Classifications for the Alaska Department of Public Safety*. https://core.ac.uk/download/162576293.pdf (accessed on 10th June 2025).
11. Azizova, S. (2023). *Challenges of Medical Translation in the 21st Century from English into Azerbaijani*. https://core.ac.uk/download/614441920.pdf (accessed on 10th June 2025).
12. Balasuriya, L., Doran, D., Sheth, A., et al. (2016). Finding street gang members on Twitter. https://arxiv.org/abs/1610.09516 (accessed on 10th June 2025).
13. Bancroft, A., Corkery, J. M., Felice, A. M., et al. (2020). Exploring the baseline knowledge and experience of healthcare professionals in the United Kingdom on novel psychoactive substances. https://core.ac.uk/download/287582648.pdf (accessed on 10th June 2025).

14. Bender, E. M., Gebru, T., McMillan-Major, A., & Shmitchell, S. (2021). On the dangers of stochastic parrots. https://doi.org/10.1145/3442188.3445922.

15. Bies, R. R., Feng, Y., Frank, E., Gastonguay, et al. (2011). Performance of Cpred/Cobs concentration ratios as a metric reflecting adherence to antidepressant drug therapy. https://core.ac.uk/download/12213831.pdf (accessed on 10th June 2025).

16. Bodenreider, O., Burgun, A., Kumar, A., et al. (2004). Investigating subsumption in DL-based terminologies: A case study in SNOMED CT. https://core.ac.uk/download/131216167.pdf (accessed on 10th June 2025).

17. Buhleier, Carbone, Florida, H., Florindo, H., Klajnert, Hess, Silva, L., et al. (2014). Molecular modeling to study dendrimers for biomedical applications. https://core.ac.uk/download/29849184.pdf (accessed on 10th June 2025).

18. Caruso, D. R., Mayer, J. D., & Salovey, P. (2008). Emotional intelligence: New ability or eclectic traits? https://core.ac.uk/download/215529979.pdf (accessed on 10th June 2025).

19. Casaletto, K. B., Grant, I., HIV Neurobehavioral Research Program Group, Morgan, E. E., et al. (2015). Antiretroviral non-adherence is associated with a retrieval profile of deficits in verbal episodic memory. https://core.ac.uk/download/305124046.pdf (accessed on 10th June 2025).

20. Ceccarelli, G., Di Gregorio, V., Falcone, M., et al. (2015). The spread of multi-drug-resistant infections is leading to an increase in the empirical antibiotic treatment failure in cirrhosis: A prospective survey. https://core.ac.uk/download/54521158.pdf (accessed on 10th June 2025).

21. Ceusters, W., & Smith, B. (2007). Ontology as the core discipline of biomedical informatics: Legacies of the past and recommendations for the future direction of research. https://core.ac.uk/download/131212555.pdf (accessed on 10th June 2025).

22. Chatwin, C., Lui, R., & Zhang, W. (2016). Marketing authorization of medical devices in China. https://core.ac.uk/download/42578571.pdf (accessed on 10th June 2025).

23. Chiappini, S., Corkery, J. M., De Berardis, D., et al. (2019). The bridge between classical and 'synthetic'/chemical psychoses: Towards a clinical, psychopathological and therapeutic perspective. https://core.ac.uk/download/287582435.pdf (accessed on 10th June 2025).

24. Cook-Deegan, R., Perin, N. C., & Wiechers, I. R. (2013). The emergence of commercial genomics: Analysis of the rise of a biotechnology subsector during the Human Genome Project, 1990 to 2004. https://core.ac.uk/download/323073877.pdf (accessed on 10th June 2025).

25. Cosentino, F., Grant, P. J., Aboyans, V., Bailey, C. J., Ceriello, A., Delgado, V., Federici, M., et al. (2019). 2019 ESC Guidelines on diabetes, pre-diabetes, and cardiovascular diseases developed in collaboration with the EASD. *European Heart Journal, 41*, 255–323. https://doi.org/10.1093/eurheartj/ehz486.

26. Dennison, S., Freeman, M. A., Giannotti, N., et al. (2020). An evidence-based framework for reporting student nurse medication incidents: Errors, near misses and discovered errors. https://core.ac.uk/download/352935267.pdf (accessed on 10th June 2025).

27. Diallo, G., Foguem, C., & Kamsu-Foguem, B. (2013). Conceptual graph-based knowledge representation for supporting reasoning in African traditional medicine. https://core.ac.uk/download/12044019.pdf (accessed on 10th June 2025).

28. Edinoff, A. N., Nix, C. A., Hollier, J. W., Sagrera, C. E., Delacroix, B. M., Abubakar, T., Cornett, E. M., et al. (2021). Benzodiazepines: Uses, dangers, and clinical considerations. *Neurology International, 13*, 594–607. https://doi.org/10.3390/neurolint13040059.

29. Elango, D. M. (2022). It is story time!! Storytelling–Narrative session by medical students, an effective way of reflection of learning pharmacology. *National Journal of Physiology, Pharmacy and Pharmacology*. https://www.semanticscholar.org/paper/4d1b23629296fb0ef3434c259cb4f600d7937c92 (accessed on 10th June 2025).

30. Fusaroli, M., Giunchi, V., Battini, V., Puligheddu, S., Khouri, C., Carnovale, C., Raschi, E., et al. (2024). Enhancing transparency in defining studied drugs: The open-source living DiAna dictionary for standardizing drug names in the FAERS. *Drug Safety, 47*, 271–284. https://doi.org/10.1007/s40264-023-01391-4.

31. García Ruiz, C., Matey Cabañas, J. M., Montalvo García, G., et al. (2021). Chemical classification of new psychoactive substances (NPS). https://core.ac.uk/download/578288053.pdf (accessed on 10th June 2025).

32. Gibson, A., Majeed, A., Williams, A., Tod, A. M., St Leger, A. S., et al. (2005). *Exploring The Equity of GP Practice Prescribing Rates for Selected Coronary Heart Disease Drugs: A Multiple Regression Analysis with Proxies of Healthcare Need*. https://core.ac.uk/download/57783.pdf (accessed on 10th June 2025).

33. Gómez-Pérez, A., Martínez-Romero, M., Rodríguez-González, A., et al. (2013). Ontologies in medicinal chemistry: Current status and future challenges. https://core.ac.uk/download/83115523.pdf (accessed on 10th June 2025).

34. Halverson, C. M. E. (2019). Standards and legacies: Pragmatic constraints on a uniform gene nomenclature. https://core.ac.uk/download/299809057.pdf (accessed on 10th June 2025).

35. Hamidova, L. F. (Laman). (2019). The analysis of existing experience for the ethnobotanical information system. https://core.ac.uk/download/322516410.pdf (accessed on 10th June 2025).

36. Hicks, J. K., Sangkuhl, K., Swen, J. J., Ellingrod, V. L., Müller, D. J., Shimoda, K., Bishop, J. R., et al. (2016). Clinical Pharmacogenetics Implementation Consortium guideline (CPIC) for *CYP2D6* and *CYP2C19* genotypes and dosing of tricyclic antidepressants: 2016 update. *Clinical Pharmacology & Therapeutics, 102*, 37–44. https://doi.org/10.1002/cpt.597.

37. Hsu, D. (2017). Mining frequency of drug side effects over a large Twitter dataset using Apache Spark. https://core.ac.uk/download/70406921.pdf (accessed on 10th June 2025).

38. Hurley, U. K. (2011). Walking in the world of ruins: Explorations in the processes and products of autobiographical fiction. https://core.ac.uk/download/1667056.pdf (accessed on 10th June 2025).

39. Jadhav, R. R., Padwal, S. L., Pise, H. N., et al. (2019). Study of drug prescription pattern in ischemic heart disease patients. https://core.ac.uk/download/539896941.pdf (accessed on 10th June 2025).

40. Jeevanandam, J., Barhoum, A., Chan, Y. S., Dufresne, A., & Danquah, M. K. (2018). Review on nanoparticles and nanostructured materials: History, sources, toxicity and regulations. *Beilstein Journal of Nanotechnology, 9*, 1050–1074. https://doi.org/10.3762/bjnano.9.98.

41. Jespersen, S. (2006). Antidepressant induced sexual dysfunction part 2: Assessment and

management. https://core.ac.uk/download/478366896.pdf (accessed on 10th June 2025).

42. Jiang, F., Jiang, Y., Zhi, H., Dong, Y., Li, H., Ma, S., Wang, Y., et al. (2017). Artificial intelligence in healthcare: Past, present and future. *Stroke and Vascular Neurology, 2*, 230–243. https://doi.org/10.1136/svn-2017-000101.

43. Johnston, L. D., Miech, R. A., & O'Malley, P. M. (2020). *Monitoring the Future National Survey Results on Drug Use, 1975–2019: Overview, Key Findings on Adolescent Drug Use.* https://doi.org/10.3998/2027.42/162579.

44. Kanehisa, M. (2019). Toward understanding the origin and evolution of cellular organisms. *Protein Science, 28*, 1947–1951. https://doi.org/10.1002/pro.3715.

45. Kanehisa, M., Furumichi, M., Sato, Y., Ishiguro-Watanabe, M., & Tanabe, M. (2020). KEGG: Integrating viruses and cellular organisms. *Nucleic Acids Research, 49*, D545–D551. https://doi.org/10.1093/nar/gkaa970.

46. Keegan, R. D. (2015). Muscle relaxants and neuromuscular blockade. https://doi.org/10.1002/9781119421375.ch14.

47. Khan, I., Saeed, K., & Khan, I. (2017). Nanoparticles: Properties, applications and toxicities. *Arabian Journal of Chemistry, 12*, 908–931. https://doi.org/10.1016/j.arabjc.2017.05.011.

48. Kim, S., Chen, J., Cheng, T., Gindulytė, A., He, J., He, S., Li, Q., et al. (2018). PubChem 2019 update: Improved access to chemical data. *Nucleic Acids Research, 47*, D1102–D1109. https://doi.org/10.1093/nar/gky1033.

49. Kolchinsky, A., Li, L., Lourenço, A., et al. (2012). Evaluation of linear classifiers on articles containing pharmacokinetic evidence of drug-drug interactions. http://arxiv.org/abs/1210.0734 (accessed on 10th June 2025).

50. Kouper, I. (2025). Mental disorders over time: A dictionary-based approach to the analysis of knowledge domains. https://core.ac.uk/download/158312470.pdf (accessed on 10th June 2025).

51. Kung, T. H., Cheatham, M., Medenilla, A., Sillos, C., De Leon, L., Elepaño, C., Madriaga, M., et al. (2023). Performance of ChatGPT on USMLE: Potential for AI-assisted medical education using large language models. *PLOS Digital Health, 2*, e0000198. https://doi.org/10.1371/journal.pdig.0000198.

52. Lemmens, A., & Stremersch, S. (2025). Sales growth of new pharmaceuticals across the globe: The role of regulatory regimes. https://core.ac.uk/download/pdf/6906001.pdf (accessed on 10th June 2025).

53. Mach, F., Baigent, C., Catapano, A. L., Koskinas, K. C., Casula, M., Badimón, L., Chapman, M. J., et al. (2019). 2019 ESC/EAS Guidelines for the management of dyslipidemias: Lipid modification to reduce cardiovascular risk. *European Heart Journal, 41*, 111–188. https://doi.org/10.1093/eurheartj/ehz455.

54. Mitchell, W., Richman, B. D., Schulman, K., et al. (2017). Pharmaceutical M&A activity: Effects on prices, innovation, and competition. https://core.ac.uk/download/84098980.pdf (accessed on 10th June 2025).

55. Murray, C. J. L., Ikuta, K. S., Sharara, F., Swetschinski, L. R., Robles Aguilar, G., Gray, A. P., Han, C., et al. (2022). Global burden of bacterial antimicrobial resistance in 2019: A systematic analysis. *The Lancet, 399*, 629–655. https://doi.org/10.1016/s0140-6736(21)02724-0.

56. Nazarenko, A., & Nédellec, C. (2005). Ontologies and information extraction. http://arxiv.org/abs/cs/0609137 (accessed on 10th June 2025).

57. Niazi, S. K. (2023). A proposed Global Medicines Agency (GMA) to make biological drugs accessible: Starting with the League of Arab States. *Healthcare, 11*, 2075. https://doi.org/10.3390/healthcare11142075.

58. Nichols, D. (2022). Entactogens: How the name for a novel class of psychoactive agents originated. *Frontiers in Psychiatry, 13.* https://www.semanticscholar.org/paper/28b48be20203c18676bb7299310b6cda7351e5f4 (accessed on 10th June 2025).

59. Pagliaro, L. A., & Pagliaro, A. M. (2020). *Psychologists' Psychotropic Drug Reference.* https://doi.org/10.4324/9781315825731.

60. Penati, A. V. (2024). *In-Home Medication: Integrating Multidisciplinary Perspectives in Design-Driven Pharma Practices.* https://core.ac.uk/download/638781703.pdf (accessed on 10th June 2025).

61. Perucca, P., Scheffer, I. E., & Kiley, M. (2018). The management of epilepsy in children and adults. *The Medical Journal of Australia, 208*, 226–233. https://doi.org/10.5694/mja17.00951.

62. Phillips, R., & Baertsch, N. (2024). Dissecting the interaction of pain and respiration at the level of the rostral ventromedial medulla via cell-type specific manipulations. *Physiology.* https://www.semanticscholar.org/paper/e54c4408b2a29d73c20eadfe00793e6e078b0b0f (accessed on 10th June 2025).

63. Pullen, L. C. E., Noortman, W. A., Triemstra, L., de Jongh, C., Rademaker, F. J., Spijkerman, R., Kalisvaart, G. M., et al. (2023). Prognostic value of [18F]FDG PET radiomics to detect peritoneal and distant metastases in locally advanced gastric cancer—A side study of the prospective multicenter PLASTIC study. *Cancers, 15.* https://www.semanticscholar.org/paper/ea19fa74316d253125e6d396fa07b3262863babc (accessed on 10th June 2025).

64. Rahman, S. M., Salem, Y., & Hussain, A. (2024). Trips through the skin: Reviewing cutaneous drug reactions to psychedelics and hallucinogens. *Dermatitis: Contact, Atopic, Occupational, Drug.* https://www.semanticscholar.org/paper/80939c30ae4c0da8b28c2726b5dd2f7319f98269 (accessed on 10th June 2025).

65. Sakloth, F., Leggett, E., Moerke, M. J., Townsend, E. A., Banks, M. L., & Negus, S. S. (2019). Effects of acute and repeated treatment with serotonin 5-HT2A receptor agonist hallucinogens on intracranial self-stimulation in rats. *Experimental and Clinical Psychopharmacology, 27*, 215–226. https://doi.org/10.1037/pha0000253.

66. San Jose State University, School of Journalism and Mass Communications. (2011). *Spartan Daily May 10, 2012.* https://core.ac.uk/download/70410787.pdf (accessed on 10th June 2025).

67. Schenk, K. (1959). A study to determine if facts about drugs and drug therapy can be learned as effectively by a patient-centered approach as by classroom presentation. https://open.bu.edu/bitstream/2144/21940/1/Schenk_Katharine_1959_web.pdf (accessed on 10th June 2025).

68. Scioli Montoto, S., Muraca, G., & Ruiz, M. E. (2020). Solid lipid nanoparticles for drug delivery: Pharmacological and biopharmaceutical aspects. *Frontiers in Molecular Biosciences, 7.* https://doi.org/10.3389/fmolb.2020.587997.

69. Shafer, S. L., & Egan, T. D. (2015). Target-controlled infusions. *Anesthesia & Analgesia, 122*, 1–3. https://doi.org/10.1213/ane.0000000000001061.

70. Shen, Y. X., Lee, P. S., Wang, C. C., Teng, M. C., Huang, J. H., & Fan, H. F. (2024). Exploring the cellular impact of size-segregated cigarette aerosols: Insights into indoor particulate matter toxicity and potential therapeutic interventions. *Chemical Research in Toxicology, 37*, 1171–1186. https://www.semanticscholar.org/paper/c3422e6ae74a559b28aecf78c8c9ba215c2d100e (accessed on 10th June 2025).

71. Simons-Linares, C. R., Elkhouly, M. A., & Salazar, M. (2019). Drug-induced acute pancreatitis in adults. *Pancreas, 48*, 1263–1273. https://doi.org/10.1097/MPA.0000000000001428.

72. Singh, M. (1997). *Object Oriented Partitioning for A Medical Vocabulary Based on Semantic Network*. https://core.ac.uk/download/232276144.pdf (accessed on 10th June 2025).

73. Sollena, P., Nikolaou, V., Kotteas, E., Stratigos, A., Fattore, D., Orlandi, A., Mannino, M., et al. (2023). Cyclin-dependent kinase 4/6 inhibitors and dermatologic adverse events: Results from the EADV Task Force "Dermatology for Cancer Patients" international study. *Cancers, 15*. https://www.semanticscholar.org/paper/9a39643ae0be8ac1f5cd4c14c6d1aa20fefea468 (accessed on 10th June 2025).

74. Stępnicki, P., Kondej, M., & Kaczor, A. A. (2018). Current concepts and treatments of schizophrenia. *Molecules, 23*, 2087. https://doi.org/10.3390/molecules23082087.

75. Sun, J., Wu, Y., Xu, H., Zhao, X., et al. (2012). DTome: A web-based tool for drug-target interactome construction. https://core.ac.uk/download/pdf/8738599.pdf (accessed on 10th June 2025).

76. Taft, L. M. (2010). *Doctor of Philosophy*. https://core.ac.uk/download/276264399.pdf (accessed on 10th June 2025).

77. Treschow, A. F., Valente, M. J., Lauschke, K., Holst, B., Andersen, A. R., & Vinggaard, A. (2024). Investigating the applicability domain of the hiPSC-based PluriLum assay: An embryotoxicity assessment of chemicals and drugs. *Archives of Toxicology, 98*, 1209–1224. https://www.semanticscholar.org/paper/2ee0cb8d2ec38721026ee035dfef0cd095ee9350 (accessed on 10th June 2025).

78. Visseren, F. L. J., Mach, F., Smulders, Y. M., Carballo, D., Koskinas, K. C., Bäck, M., Bénétos, A., et al. (2021). 2021 ESC Guidelines on cardiovascular disease prevention in clinical practice. *European Heart Journal, 42*, 3227–3337. https://doi.org/10.1093/eurheartj/ehab484.

79. Will, C. (2018). Editorial: Beyond behavior? Institutions, interactions and inequalities in the response to antimicrobial resistance. *Sociology of Health & Illness, 40*. https://doi.org/10.1111/1467-9566.12735.

80. Wu, Z., Pan, S., Chen, F., Long, G., Zhang, C., & Yu, P. S. (2020). A comprehensive survey on graph neural networks. *IEEE Transactions on Neural Networks and Learning Systems, 32*, 4–24. https://doi.org/10.1109/tnnls.2020.2978386.

81. Yazdani, A., Bornet, A., Zhang, B., Khlebnikov, P., Amini, P., & Teodoro, D. (2024). CT-ADE: An evaluation benchmark for adverse drug event prediction from clinical trial results. *arXiv*, abs/2404.12827. https://www.semanticscholar.org/paper/443be6edc1fcd77b934649001a03c2cc8f0ad718 (accessed on 10th June 2025).

82. Zuberbier, T., Abdul Latiff, A. H., Abuzakouk, M., Aquilina, S., Asero, R., Baker, D. R., Ballmer-Weber, B., et al. (2021). The international EAACI/GA²LEN/EuroGuiDerm/APAAACI guideline for the definition, classification, diagnosis, and management of urticaria. *Allergy, 77*, 734–766. https://doi.org/10.1111/all.15090.

PRINCIPLES OF PHARMACOKINETICS

2

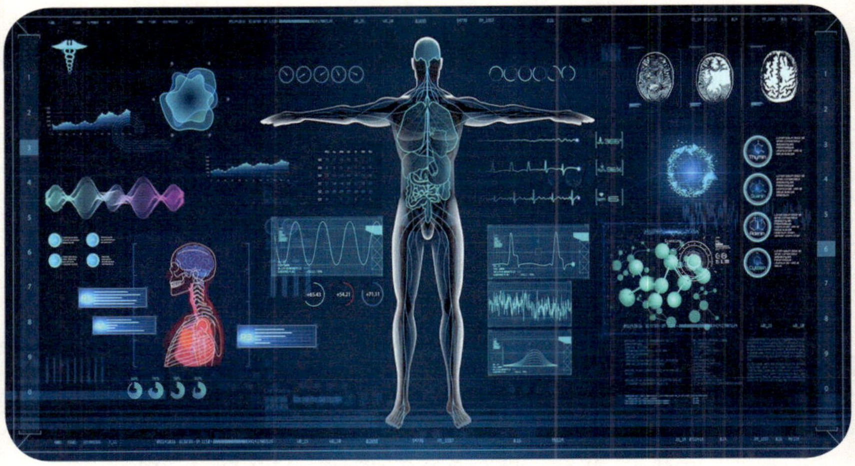

LEARNING OBJECTIVES

After studying this chapter, you will be able to:

1. Understand absorption
2. Explain distribution
3. Discuss metabolism
4. Focus on excretion

Introduction

Pharmacokinetics is an essential platform for studying drug disposition in the human body, including processes such as absorption, distribution, metabolism, and excretion. Pharmacokinetic principles enable the clinician to forecast medication activity and efficiently tailor the treatment to each patient's unique demands as the need for tailored therapy grows. With the use of population pharmacokinetic (popPK) methods, researchers have been able to make tremendous progress in the capacity to comprehend variability in drug response between populations, and thus the clinical utility of such models in therapeutic drug monitoring (TDM) and personalized medicine (Guidi et al., 2020). New analysis techniques and technology also proceed to advance pharmacokinetic practice further, enabling ever-growing accuracy in the measurement of drug dynamics. But all challenges remain, particularly in computational and numerical accuracy, as indicated in recent testing of tools like ChatGPT, where rampant error in computations overwhelms its potential as a productivity tool in pharmacokinetic data analysis (Shin et al., 2023) (Figure 2.1).

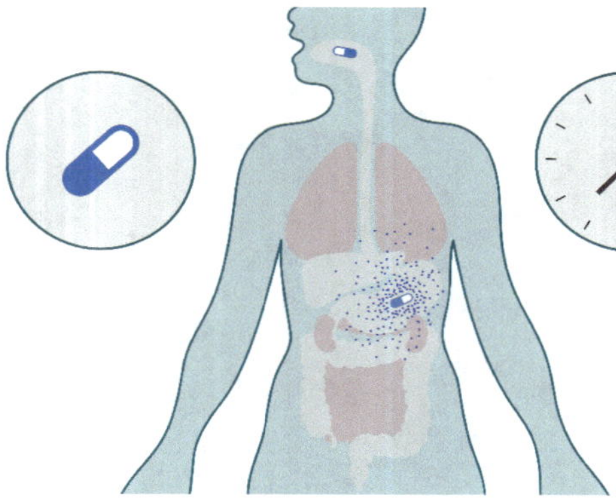

Figure 2.1. Pharmacokinetics.

Source: https://mrctcenter.org/wp-content/uploads/2024/03/pharmacokinetics-Study-PK-study-2023-08-09-1.png.

2.1. Absorption

Learning Outcome

1. Understand mechanisms of drug absorption
2. Identify factors affecting absorption
3. Know routes of drug administration
4. Explain bioavailability and its significance
5. Focus on first-pass metabolism
6. Describe the role of ph in absorption
7. Know the influence of food on absorption
8. Discuss drug formulation and absorption
9. Explain the clinical implications of absorption

Absorption is likewise a major driver of the pharmacokinetics of drugs, as it determines the rate and extent to which active pharmaceutical ingredients can enter systemic circulation. Understanding the Biopharmaceutics Classification System (BCS) is crucial, especially for Class III drugs, with high solubility but low permeation. These drugs are expected to encounter high absorption barriers, whereby their low permeability in many instances is the bioavailability rate-limiting step (Dave et al., 2016). Besides, conditions such as acute kidney injury (AKI) may further challenge absorption dynamics; evidence indicates that AKI patients exhibit decreased hepatic cytochrome P450 enzyme activity, which further can hinder drug metabolism and alter pharmacokinetic profiles (Abosaif et al., 2014). Therefore, specific interventions to enhance absorption, for example, the use of permeation enhancers or new drug forms, are imperative to maximize therapeutic gains, particularly in vulnerable patient populations. These factors emphasize the relevance of personalized medicine in pharmacotherapy.

2.1.1. Mechanisms of Drug Absorption

Understanding the mechanism of drug absorption is necessary in designing and administering drugs correctly because drug absorption influences the therapeutic action of drugs. Drug absorption occurs primarily through passive diffusion, facilitated diffusion, and active transport, depending upon which process employs the properties of the drug as well as the biological compartment into which the drug is administered. For instance, lipophilic drugs easily pass through cellular membranes through passive diffusion, while polar or charged drugs may rely on transporters for access to systemic circulation. Individual variation due to age, genetics, and underlying diseases can transform these absorption mechanisms significantly, thereby modifying drug efficacy and safety profiles (Bailey et al., 2018). Apart from this, in some clinical scenarios, such as patients undergoing ECMO therapy, a physiological parameter change can lead to unpredictable pharmacokinetic change, reflecting the complexity of drug absorption and the necessity for customized therapeutic regimens (Aebi et al., 2017) (Figure 2.2).

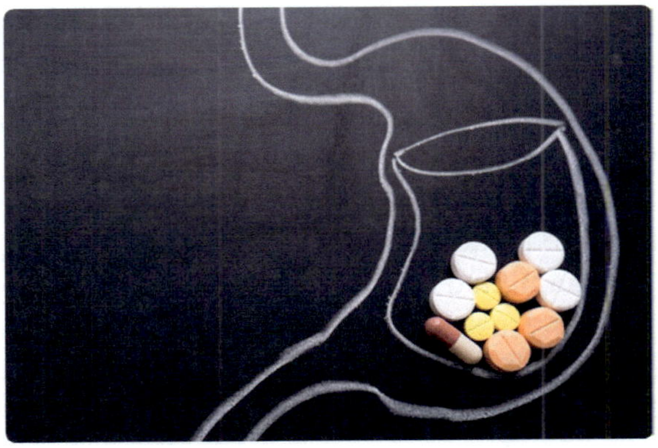

Figure 2.2. Drug absorption is crucial for the effective design and administration of pharmaceuticals, as this process directly influences the therapeutic outcomes of medications.

Source: https://d2jx2rerrg6sh3.cloudfront.net/image-handler/picture/2019/6/shutterstock_1185054181.jpg.

2.1.2. Factors Affecting Absorption

Absorption, being a crucial phase of pharmacokinetics, is controlled by various physiological and pathological determinants, which have the potential to affect the drug's bioavailability significantly. Parameters like route of administration, formulation of the drug, and physiological conditions like pH levels and gastrointestinal motility all determine the efficiency with which a drug gets absorbed into systemic circulation. For instance, acute illnesses such as AKI can potentially impair the drug metabolizing function of the liver and thus alter the pharmacokinetic parameters and drug absorption profiles; studies have indicated that AKI inhibits the functioning of the cytochrome P450 (CYP) enzyme system that is tasked with metabolizing drugs (Abosaif et al., 2014). In addition, the prevalence of comorbidities such as diabetes mellitus can even make such dynamics more complex, as is suggested by studies that identify reduced metabolism of antiplatelet drugs in specific patient populations (Ibanez et al., 2018). In this regard, awareness of these determinants is also essential for optimizing pharmacotherapy.

2.1.3. Routes of Drug Administration

The routes of administration of drugs play an role in pharmacokinetics, as they influence the absorption, distribution, metabolism, and excretion patterns of drugs. The various routes, oral, intravenous, subcutaneous, and rectal, are capable of significantly affecting the bioavailability as well as the therapeutic activity of a drug. For instance, the Asian elephant levofloxacin study demonstrated that rectal and oral routes had adequate plasma concentrations, thereby highlighting the importance of route selection in achieving desired pharmacodynamics (Kilburn et al., 2023).

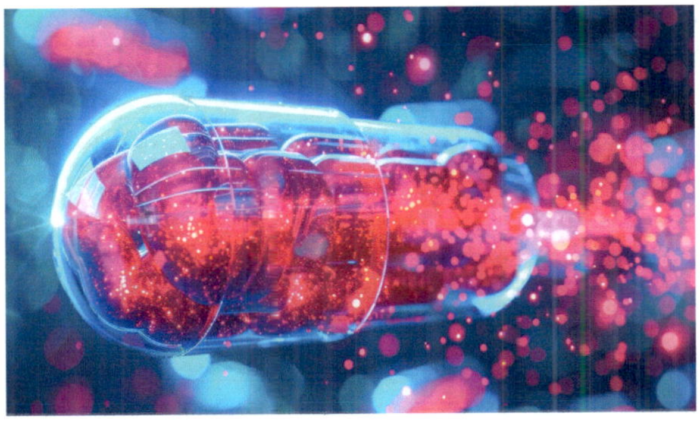

Figure 2.3. The routes of drug administration play a critical role in pharmacokinetics, influencing the drugs absorption, distribution, metabolism, and excretion profiles.

Source: https://www.allucent.com/wp-content/uploads/2022/04/23-1.webp.

Similarly, in respiratory infections caused by Pseudomonas aeruginosa, the choice of an appropriate route is crucial; treatment regimens require that antibiotics be given in formulations that maximize lung levels, particularly in serious infections, to treat resistant states. Lastly, awareness of the nuances of various routes of administration allows clinicians to customize treatment, enhancing effectiveness and minimizing toxicity in the frameworks of pharmacokinetics (Figure 2.3).***2.1.4. Bioavailability and Its Significance***

The word bioavailability is crucial in the field of pharmacokinetics since it determines the extent and rate at which an active drug component or active moiety is absorbed and made accessible to the action site. It is a must that the area of bioavailability is understood not only in order to maximize therapeutic efficacy but also to minimize unwanted side effects. A drug's bioavailability is significantly influenced by drug formulation, route of administration, and patient factors. For example, emerging techniques like nanotechnology enhance drug delivery systems with increased bioavailability by targeted release and high solubility of therapeutic agents. With materials that facilitate effective delivery and control drug release, scientists are fighting against severe challenges in pharmacotherapy (Chenthamara et al., 2019). Besides that, the need for new drug options with increasing AMR underscores the importance of excessive bioavailability in new antibiotic drug discovery approaches (Miethke et al., 2021). Such developments are and essential to public health as well as therapeutic outcomes in the future.

2.1.5. First-Pass Metabolism

First-pass phenomenon is a significant concept of pharmacokinetics that primarily affects the bioavailability of an orally administered drug. It refers to the metabolism through which drugs are absorbed from the gastrointestinal tract and delivered by portal circulation to the liver, where they undergo enzymatic alteration that can significantly reduce the concentration of the active drug before it enters systemic circulation. For example, investigations involving midazolam have shown that about 75% of its dose is still present in portal blood, depicting a significant hepatic first-pass effect that reduces its systemic bioavailability (Li et al., 2023).

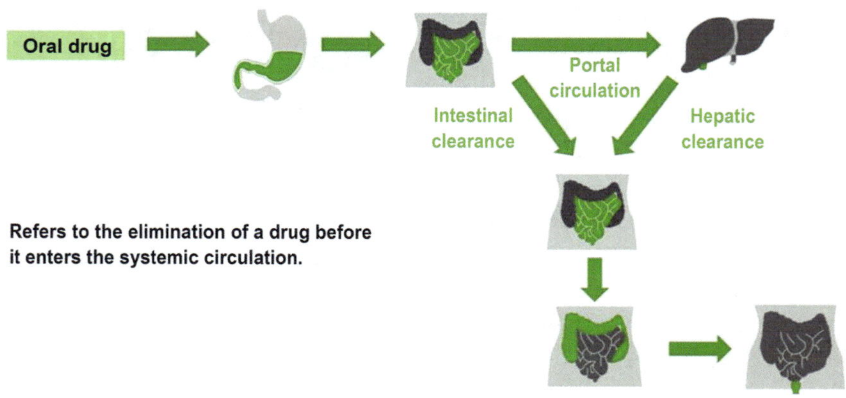

Figure 2.4. The phenomenon of first-pass metabolism plays a pivotal role in pharmacokinetics, primarily affecting the bioavailability of orally administered drugs.

Source: https://cdn.lecturio.com/assets/drug-undergoing-the-first-pass-metabolism.jpg.

Conversely, some drugs, like garcinol, have relatively low first-pass metabolism, with only 6% being hepatically processed, thus enabling a larger proportion to enter systemic circulation (Gajula et al., 2023). Knowledge of such dynamics serves to optimize drug dosing regimens and enhance therapeutic efficiency, which speaks of the importance of first-pass metabolism in pharmacokinetic principles (Figure 2.4).

2.1.6. Role of pH in Absorption

The role of pH in absorption is a crucially significant pharmacokinetic characteristic, defining the solubility and permeability of drugs under physiological conditions. In the gastrointestinal system, for instance, pH can vary significantly, with the stomach acidic and the small intestine slightly alkaline to neutral. The shift affects the ionization of drug molecules, thereby affecting their ability to move across cell membranes. Weak acids are absorbed more in acidic pH, as they are predominantly present in un-ionized form, whereas weak bases are favored under alkaline pH, where they are un-ionized. Therefore, the understanding of pH-dependent absorption properties assists in the prediction of drugs' bioavailability. Moreover, pH also plays a pivotal role in the characterization of drug delivery systems like polymeric micelles, which can enhance poor water solubility and enhance drug permeability across biological barriers (Ghezzi et al., 2021; Lyon et al., 2022). Therefore, pH is not only a physiological parameter but also a factor in the efficacy of pharmacotherapy.

2.1.7. Influence of Food on Absorption

Food-drug interaction is an essential aspect of pharmacokinetics, influencing the therapeutic and toxic effects of drugs. Food can profoundly modify the gastric pH, increase or decrease gastrointestinal motility, and alter drug solubility, thus affecting bioavailability.

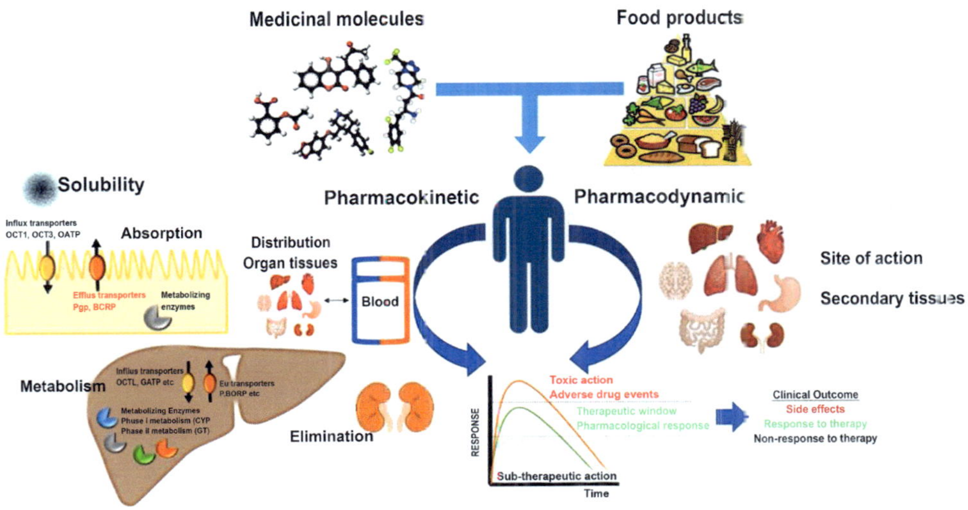

Figure 2.5. The interaction between food and drug absorption plays a crucial role in pharmacokinetics, affecting the efficacy and safety of therapeutic agents.

Source: https://www.mdpi.com/applsci/applsci-12-10207/article_deploy/html/images/applsci-12-10207-g001.png.

For instance, the presence of certain fatty foods can increase the bioavailability of lipophilic drugs. At the same time, a diet rich in specific fibers can decrease the absorption of certain medications due to the binding ability of fibers. Moreover, food constituents can interact with drug transporters and also the extent to which drugs get absorbed into the systemic circulation. These encounters point to the necessity of considering food availability and eating behaviors when dispensing medications because variations in nutrient intake lead to unforeseen therapeutic outcomes (Steffel et al., 2021).

Moreover, the effects are not just isolated to individual choices; public health programs must investigate the complex dynamic relationship between diet, drug use, and overall well-being in order to fight the risk of adverse effects and drug resistance caused by poor absorption (Manyi-Loh et al., 2018) (Figure 2.5).

2.1.8. Drug Formulation and Absorption

A thorough understanding of drug absorption and formulation is of the highest priority in optimizing the pharmacotherapeutic strategy in a broader context of pharmacokinetics. Improved drug delivery systems such as polymeric micelles are state-of-the-art solutions to addressing issues such as low solubility and limited permeability of therapeutic molecules. These self-assembled colloidal architectures are capable of promoting the bioavailability of drugs by increasing the drug's water solubility, a critical need in the battle against the growing issue of AMR, as suggested by the urgent need for novel drugs with novel mechanisms of action (Miethke et al., 2021).

Besides, structural characterization of micelles through various techniques allows for an in-depth understanding of their behavior in biological systems and ultimately their safety and effectiveness in therapeutic applications (Ghezzi et al., 2021). With scientists developing innovative formulations enhancing drug absorption, the incorporation of such methodologies will be key to the effective translation of pharmacological breakthroughs into effective therapies.

2.1.9. Clinical Implications of Absorption

The clinical significance of absorption is most significant in the case of pharmacokinetics, as the extent and rate of absorption significantly affect the therapeutic efficacy. Variations in absorption could occur because of drug formulation, the physiology of the patient, and concomitant ingestion of food, so that all these variables should be evaluated with great caution in clinical scenarios. For instance, with anticoagulants like rivaroxaban, the profile of absorption can decide dosing in special populations like the elderly or patients with renal impairment to ensure effectiveness while minimizing bleeding risks (Steffel et al., 2021).

Besides, improper understanding of absorption can lead to issues such as antibiotic resistance, particularly when considering the effectiveness of absorbed chemicals in the gut and how they affect microbial flora (Manyi-Loh et al., 2018). Therefore, healthcare providers must consider these processes of absorption to ensure pharmacotherapy that is effective and safe across different patient populations (Figure 2.6).

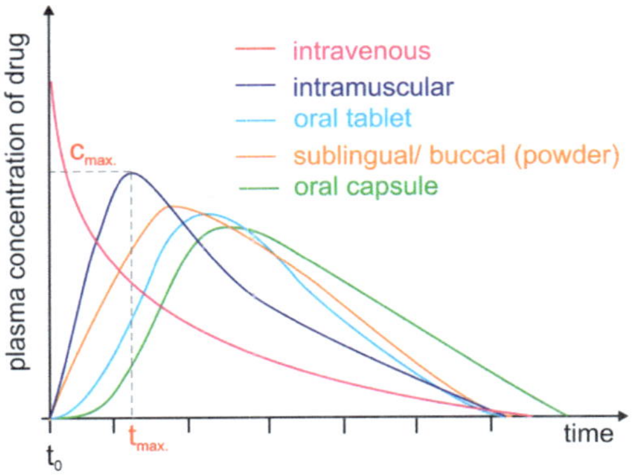

Figure 2.6. The clinical implications of drug absorption are critical in the context of pharmacokinetics, as the rate and extent of absorption significantly influence therapeutic outcomes.

Source: https://www.mdpi.com/molecules/molecules-28-08038/article_deploy/html/images/molecules-28-08038-g001-550.jpg.

Test Your Knowledge

1. How does the route of administration affect drug absorption?
2. Explain the concept of "first-pass metabolism" and how it affects oral drug bioavailability.

2.2. Distribution

Learning Outcome

1. Understand volume of distribution (Vd)
2. Identify factors influencing drug distribution
3. Explain protein binding and its effects
4. Describe the blood-brain barrier and drug penetration
5. Identify tissue distribution patterns
6. Know the impact of age and gender on distribution
7. Discuss pharmacogenomics and distribution variability
8. Explain clinical considerations in distribution
9. Learn case studies on distribution

The distribution principle is at the core of the pharmacokinetic model because it captures the way a drug distributes across the body tissues and fluids following administration. Factors such as blood flow, tissue permeability, and the drug's physicochemical properties play significant roles in influencing this effect. Surprisingly, AKI has the potential to cause substantial pharmacokinetic changes and influence drug distribution and metabolism. Recently, studies have shown that AKI interferes with the hepatic cytochrome P450 activity, thus necessitating proper attention in drug dosage for such individuals, particularly CKD patients (Abosaif et al., 2014). In addition, the relationship between drug exposure and therapeutic effects in chronic diseases such as HIV points to distribution as central to treatment efficacy. There is potential for some instability in drug concentrations to compromise long-term antiretroviral treatment through adherence and drug resistance, underlining the delicate balance in drug distribution necessary for virological success (Huang et al., 2009).

2.2.1. Volume of Distribution (Vd)

It is essential to comprehend the volume of distribution (Vd) concept to appreciate how drugs distribute within the body and become therapeutically effective. Vd may be explained as the theoretical volume in which the whole amount of a drug within the body would be contained at the same concentration as in plasma. A large Vd means extensive distribution of the drug into body tissues, and this makes dosing schedules more complex and interferes with therapeutic action. For example, physiologic changes brought on by extracorporeal membrane oxygenation (ECMO) impact medication pharmacokinetics, changing Vd dynamics and potentially decreasing efficacy or increasing side effects (Aebi et al., 2017). Similarly, drug distribution alterations may be observed in conditions such as peritoneal dialysis, where empiric dosing of vancomycin is facilitated based on its disposition in the patients, reflecting the intricacy of Vd in the clinical setting (Kraft et al., 2020) (Figure 2.7).

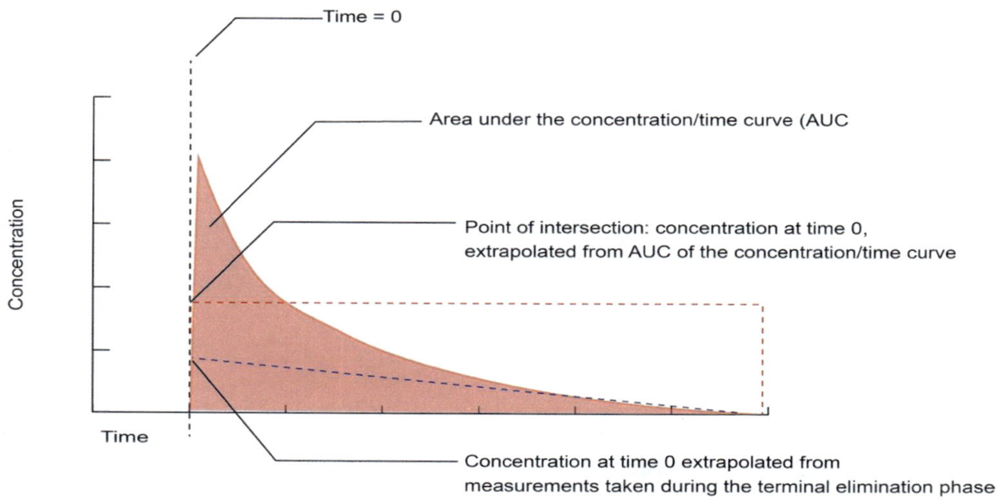

Figure 2.7. Understanding the concept of Volume of Distribution (Vd) is crucial for comprehending how drugs disperse throughout the body and achieve therapeutic effects.

Source: https://www.derangedphysiology.com/main/sites/default/files/sites/default/files/CICM%20 Primary/B%20Pharmacokinetics/v%28area%29%20volume%20of%20distribution%20graph.JPG.

2.2.2. Factors Influencing Drug Distribution

The process of distribution is greatly influenced by a range of related factors, which play an essential role in determining the therapeutic effect of drugs. Foremost among these are the physicochemical properties of drugs like solubility, molecular weight, and ionization that govern their permeation through biological membranes. Furthermore, the route of administration of the drug significantly affects distribution; intravenous drugs are characterized by quicker and more uniform distribution compared to drugs administered per os. Host variables, including tissue blood flow and transport proteins, as well as patient variables such as age, gender, and comorbidities, also alter distribution patterns. The intricate interaction of drug pharmacokinetics in diseases such as central nervous system (CNS) tumors highlights the role of effective drug delivery devices that can overcome bio-obstacles. These areas of knowledge are required to optimize the therapeutic effects and address matters of drug interaction and safety issues (Straehla et al., 2020; Hughes, 2014).

2.2.3. Protein Binding and Its Effects

The understanding of protein binding is essential in the knowledge of pharmacokinetic concepts since it greatly influences the efficacy and safety profile of a drug. After administration, certain portions of the drug become bound to plasma proteins, acting as a reservoir, keeping the drug in supply while avoiding toxicity. It will alter the distribution of the drug within the body, affecting concentration at sites of action and ultimately therapeutic effects. For instance, in the case of NOACs, protein binding variability can lead to different anticoagulation effects among patients, and dosing schedules become more complicated and responses hard to predict (Steffel et al., 2018). Additionally, drug delivery systems, such as nanoparticles, emphasize the role of protein interactions as these platforms can enhance targeted delivery and reduce side effects (Rizvi et al., 2017). A satisfactory knowledge of protein binding processes, therefore, becomes critical towards optimizing pharmacotherapy and desired clinical effects (Figure 2.8).

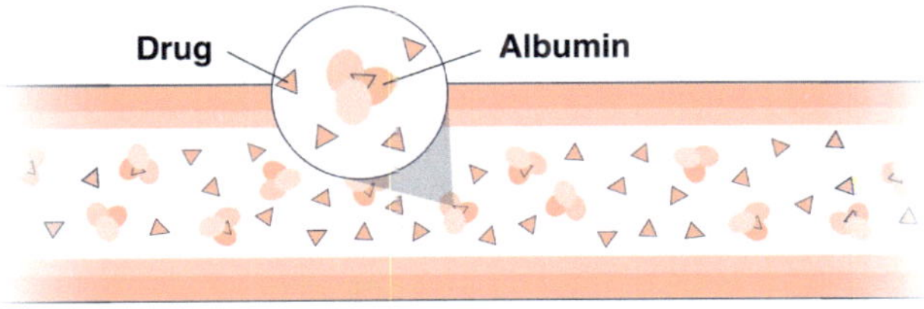

Figure 2.8. Understanding protein binding is essential for grasping the principles of pharmacokinetics, as it significantly influences a drugs efficacy and safety profile.

Source: https://www.mdpi.com/antibiotics/antibiotics-11-00923/article_deploy/html/images/antibiotics-11-00923-g001.png.

2.2.4. Blood-Brain Barrier and Drug Penetration

The blood-brain barrier (BBB) is a critical protective mechanism that regulates the passage of substances into the CNS and its homeostasis. It is a selectively permeable barrier that appropriately blocks approximately 99% of xenobiotics, which presents significant challenges to the pharmacotherapy of CNS disorders such as neurodegenerative diseases and epilepsy. For instance, even though a variety of treatments exist for illnesses like Alzheimer's and Parkinson's, their role is restricted to the relief of symptoms since they cannot penetrate the BBB properly, limiting therapeutic utility aimed at disease modification (Lamptey et al., 2022). The same issue is also exposed in the management of epilepsy, where nearly one-third of epileptic patients have refractory seizures despite the creation of over 20 antiseizure drugs (Löscher et al., 2020). As a result, novel strategies—such as the creation of nanotherapeutics—are being investigated for their potential to improve medication delivery through this daunting obstacle in the hopes of providing patients with these debilitating illnesses with greater clinical benefit.

2.2.5. Tissue Distribution Patterns

The concept of tissue distribution patterns is a fundamental aspect of pharmacokinetics as it governs the way drugs spread in various organs and tissues upon administration. Distribution is influenced by factors such as blood flow, permeability of tissues, and plasma protein binding, all of which interact to influence drug concentration at the site of action. Certain drugs have been found to bind preferentially to tissues with high lipid composition or with very high concentrations of specific receptors, often leading to ambivalent therapeutic and toxicological consequences. An example is the intricate interaction between per- and polyfluoroalkyl compounds (PFAS) and biological systems, which has given valuable information on their tissue distribution and ensuing health implications, as noted in the new toxicological literature (Fenton et al., 2020). Besides, the necessity for new antimicrobial medication is emphasized by the necessity to understand their distribution to address resistance maximally (Miethke et al., 2021). An in-depth knowledge of tissue distribution patterns thus remains crucial in guaranteeing drug efficacy and safety (Figure 2.9).

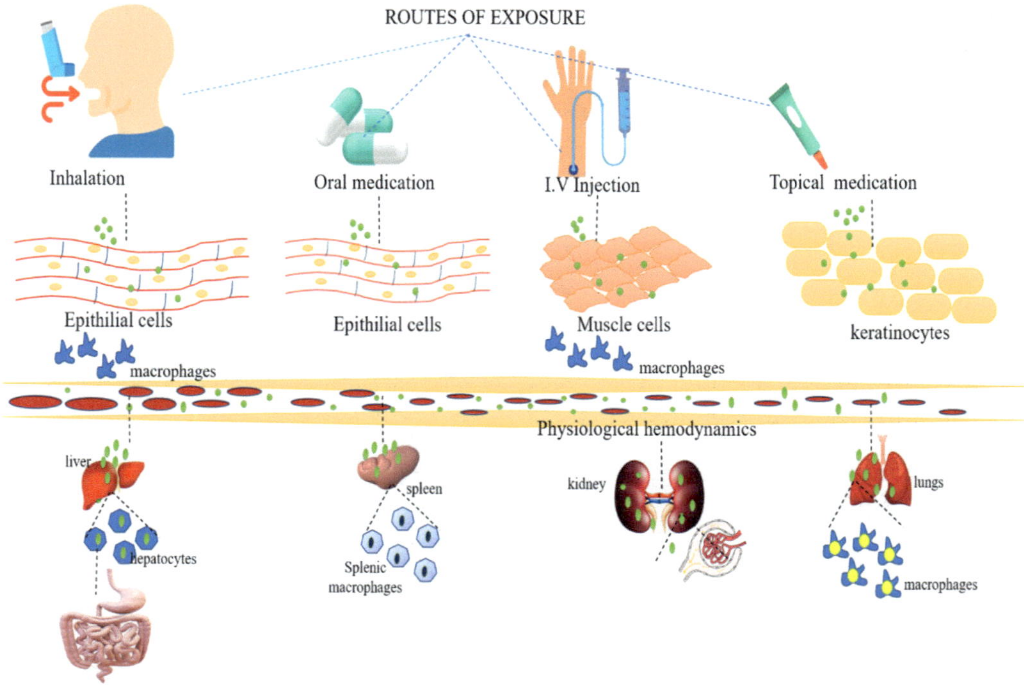

Figure 2.9. The concept of tissue distribution patterns is a pivotal aspect of pharmacokinetics, as it dictates how drugs disperse throughout various organs and tissues after administration.

Source: https://media.springernature.com/lw1200/springer-static/image/art%3A10.1186%2Fs43094-023-00569-y/MediaObjects/43094_2023_569_Fig6_HTML.png.

2.2.6. Impact of Age and Gender on Distribution

Understanding the influence of age and gender on drug distribution is crucial in the principles of pharmacokinetics because both have a significant impact on how the body processes drugs. Age-related physiological changes may alter the structure and function of tissues and hence contribute to drug distribution variability. For instance, the elderly will have a decrease in lean body mass and body water, affecting the volume of distribution of lipophilic drugs and hydrophilic drugs, respectively. Gender cannot be overlooked either; variability in biological parameters such as hormonal variations and fat deposition can result in gender-related pharmacokinetic variations among men and women. This is especially relevant in the context of precision medicine, where the incorporation of sex- and gender-specific factors can lead to more effective and tailored regimens for treatment. As underscored in more recent guidelines, these factors must be integrated into systems of therapeutic decision-making to consistently ensure improved patient outcomes, thus providing optimal access to care (Lyon et al., 2022; Pichhadze et al., 2023).

2.2.7. Pharmacogenomics and Distribution Variability

The interfacing of pharmacogenomics with distribution heterogeneity provides the best example of the application of personalized medicine in pharmacokinetics. The genetic variation among individuals can substantially influence drug metabolism and distribution, altering the trajectory of therapeutic activity. Pharmacogenomic testing, for instance, can identify specific genetic markers that predict how an individual metabolizes specific drugs, thus allowing for tailoring of dosage levels to provide enhanced efficacy while reducing side effects. While promising, the integration of pharmacogenomics into practice is in its infancy. Review of clinical trials indicates that although pharmacogenomic findings are frequently utilized in academic institutions, drug developers have been reluctant to use them (Burt et al., 2013). Moreover, knowledge gaps in pharmacy curriculum are responsible for the underutilization of pharmacogenomics within clinical practice, and the focus on further training and instructional resources in this critical area (Freeman et al., 2022). It is essential to address these issues to achieve the full potential of pharmacogenomics to maximize drug distribution and effectiveness (Figure 2.10).

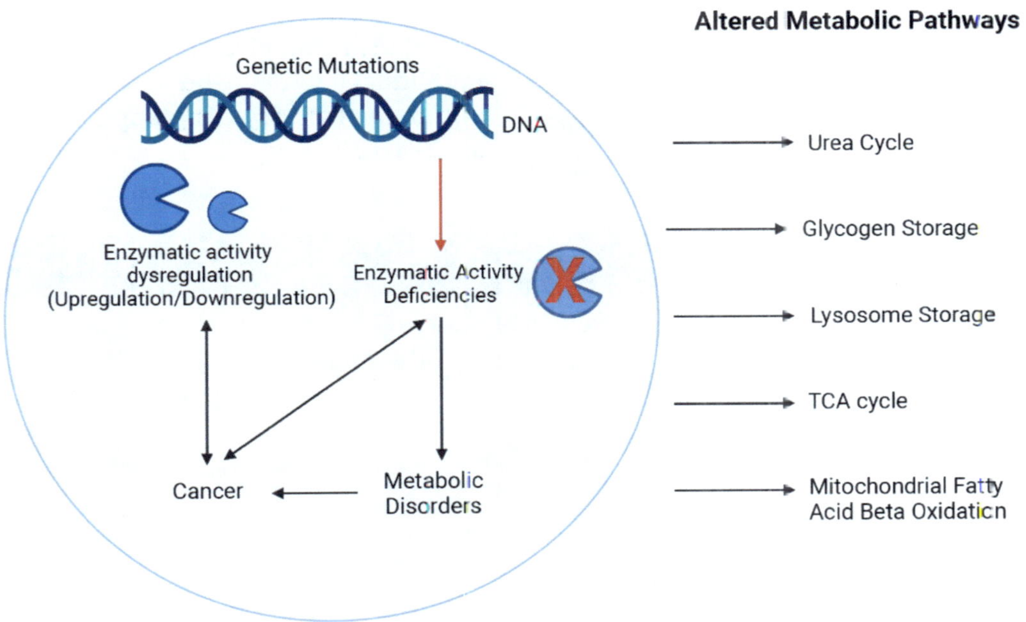

Figure 2.10. Genetic variations among individuals can substantially influence drug metabolism and distribution, leading to diverse therapeutic responses.

Source: https://www.frontiersin.org/files/Articles/1230934/fonc-13-1230934-HTML/image_m/fonc-13-1230934-g001.jpg.

2.2.8. Clinical Considerations in Distribution

Knowledge of clinical considerations in drug distribution is relevant to optimize therapeutic effect and restrict unwanted effects. Distribution is the process by which a drug diffuses throughout body fluids and tissues, dependent on factors such as blood flow, tissue permeability, and the physicochemical properties of the drug itself. A consideration is how disease states such as kidney disease can radically alter pharmacokinetics. For instance, alterations in kidney function can lead to variations in drug clearance and volume of distribution, necessitating modification of the dosing regimen to avoid overdosing or underdosing (Roberts et al., 2018). Additionally, novel drugs, such as small interfering RNA (siRNA) drugs, pose new challenges due to a limited understanding of their absorption and distribution attributes, which may hinder their effective utilization (Humphreys et al., 2020). Therefore, adopting an integrated approach that encompasses patient individuality, as well as pathological conditions, is vital to ensuring efficacy and safety in the process of pharmacotherapy.

2.2.9. Case Studies on Distribution

A closer examination of pharmacokinetics presents the forefront role of drug distribution, particularly highlighted by many case studies. These case studies offer individual observations on how various therapeutic conditions can affect the bioavailability and potency of drugs. As an illustration, the complexity of ECMO therapy presents how changes in physiological conditions affect drug pharmacokinetics. As noted, ECMO requires the administration of multiple drugs, and the therapy's physiologic changes can generate both reduced efficacy and enhanced side effects, thereby showing the necessity for careful drug dosing consideration (Aebi et al., 2017). Additionally, the debates concerning population variability in pharmacokinetic responses underscore the necessity for a personalized drug administration strategy. With the incorporation of available pharmacokinetic information through modeling and simulation resources, scientists can better predict how the pharmacological response is affected by individual factors, and this is important for optimal veterinary drug application (Bailey et al., 2018).

Test Your Knowledge

1. What is the volume of distribution (Vd), and what does it tell us about a drug?
2. Why do lipid-soluble drugs have a wider distribution than water-soluble drugs?

2.3. Metabolism

Learning Outcome

1. Identify phases of drug metabolism
2. Explain the role of the liver in metabolism
3. Describe enzyme systems involved in metabolism
4. Discuss factors affecting drug metabolism
5. Focus on genetic variability in metabolism
6. Explain drug interactions and metabolism
7. Learn clinical implications of metabolism
8. Understand metabolite activity and toxicity
9. Discuss case examples of metabolic pathways

Metabolism is a key feature of pharmacokinetics that has a direct bearing on drug safety and efficacy. Metabolism is defined as the biochemical transformation of drugs into their metabolites, which can yield active therapeutic effects or inactive byproducts. Complexity in metabolic pathways is catered to by the availability of enzymes and transporters, which recognize the absorption, distribution, and elimination of drugs within the body. Recent developments have reaffirmed the significance of elucidating DDIs and their impact on metabolism and designing new drug candidates, including peptides and antibody-drug conjugates, with unique metabolic properties (Lai et al., 2022). Besides, newer techniques like positron emission tomography (PET) enable assessment of a drug's pharmacokinetic properties by elucidation of its distribution and metabolism in real-time, particularly useful in the case of CNS drug development (Piel et al., 2014). Since metabolism is an essential determinant of drug disposition, more emphasis in this regard is needed for maximizing therapeutic action.

2.3.1. Phases of Drug Metabolism

Understanding drug metabolism phases is and vital in pharmacokinetics because these determine the pharmacologic effect and safety of the drugs. Nearly all drug metabolism occurs in two phases: Phase I and Phase II. Phase I reactions typically entail drug molecule modification in structure by oxidation, reduction, or hydrolysis, most commonly through cytochrome P450 enzymes. This is a significant step because it introduces or unveils functional groups, which render the drug polar and therefore more water-soluble, permitting it to be excreted more easily.

Phase II reactions then include conjugation, whereby the drug or its Phase I metabolites are further changed, usually by attachment of a glucuronide, sulfate, or other similar moiety, increasing solubility for renal or biliary excretion.

The complexity of such phases is due to the need for profound comprehension, especially regarding population heterogeneity that could influence drug response and safety profiles (Bailey et al., 2018). Knowledge of these metabolic pathways informs drug design and monitoring practices in clinics (Howland et al., 2009) (Figure 2.11).

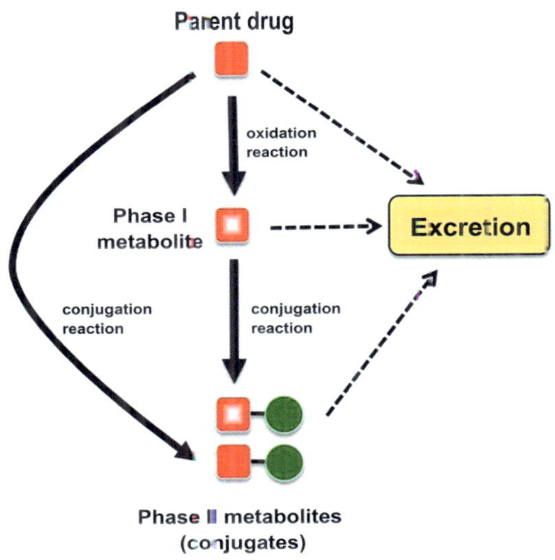

Figure 2.11. Phases of drug metabolism.

Source: https://www.abdn.ac.uk/medical/elf/coursefiles/pharmacokinetics-i/1/img/p12.png.

2.3.2. Role of the Liver in Metabolism

The liver is a central organ in metabolic processes and is the primary organ involved in conducting drug metabolism, synthesis, and the regulation of various biochemical compounds. It performs essential functions such as detoxification of waste material, bioactivation of prodrugs, and xenobiotic metabolism, ultimately influencing the pharmacokinetics of a therapeutic agent. The unique structure of this organ facilitates efficient processing of the gastrointestinal tract's blood to facilitate first-pass metabolism, in which drugs are metabolized before entering systemic circulation. Pertinent studies have determined correlations with liver disease and altered pharmacokinetic profiles, underscoring hepatic clearance as a key factor for therapeutic effect (Fenton et al., 2020). One of the key components of medication design and evaluation is the understanding of hepatic metabolism, and scientists are working to increase the accuracy of human pharmacokinetic predictions from animal data by using sophisticated predictive models (Davies et al., 2020). Understanding the liver's role in these processes is essential for optimizing drug effect and minimizing unwanted effects.

2.3.3. Enzyme Systems Involved in Metabolism

Enzyme systems play a key role in drug metabolism with extensive effects on pharmacokinetic profiles. The cytochrome P450 (CYP) enzyme system is especially of interest in drug structure-altering biotransformation reactions and, consequently, efficacy and elimination.

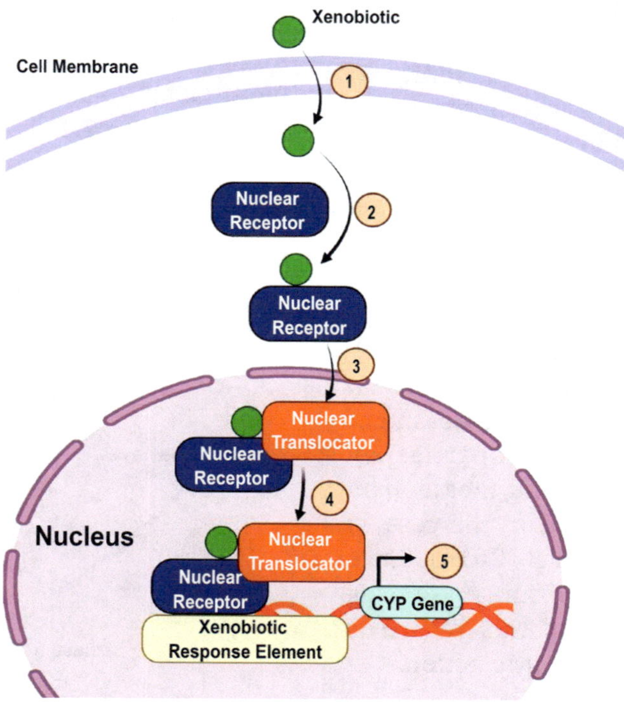

Figure 2.12. Enzyme systems play a crucial role in the metabolism of drugs, significantly influencing their pharmacokinetic profiles.

Source: https://www.mdpi.com/biomedicines/biomedicines-12-01467/article_deploy/html/images/biomedicines-12-01467-g001.png.

Disruption of these enzyme systems, as is the case in conditions such as AKI, can result in impaired drug metabolism and present challenges to effective dosing strategies in vulnerable patient populations. There is evidence that AKI may impair hepatic CYP function, especially of the CYP3A subtypes, and thereby create problems regarding drug dosing recommendations extrapolation from CKD-derived data to AKI patients, as the underlying mechanisms are very distinct (Abosaif et al., 2014). In addition, genetic expression variations in enzymes such as CYP3A5 can influence individuals' reactions to drugs, and therefore, a tailored method to pharmacotherapy must be developed to render it safe and efficacious (Bailey et al., 2018) (Figure 2.12).

2.3.4. Factors Affecting Drug Metabolism

Drug metabolism is regulated by a wide variety of factors, which influence the pharmacokinetic profile and therapeutic action of drugs. Organ function, more so hepatic and renal function, has a direct impact on the clearance and half-life of drugs. For instance, patients who suffer from liver damage can experience reduced activity of the liver cytochrome P450 enzymes, resulting in altered drug metabolism and potentially increased toxicity or no effect (Dudhat, 2022). In addition, genetic variations in drug transporters can result in interindividual variability of drug action, demonstrating the necessity for precision medicine considering these differences (Ahire et al., 2022). These are also complicated by other variables, such as age, genetic polymorphisms, and concomitant medications, and healthcare professionals must appreciate the processes involved in drug disposition and efficacy. Understanding these factors allows practitioners to maximize dosing regimens for drugs to enhance therapeutic effects.

2.3.5. Genetic Variability in Metabolism

The basis of metabolic genetic variation is at the core of understanding the principles of pharmacokinetics, as it directly contributes to modulating an individual's reaction to therapeutic drugs. Genetic factors contribute considerably to drug metabolism to produce heterogeneity in the pharmacokinetic profile of patients. This heterogeneity can be responsible for suboptimal therapeutic effects or toxic effects when conventional doses are being administered, thus mandating the concept of personalized medicine.

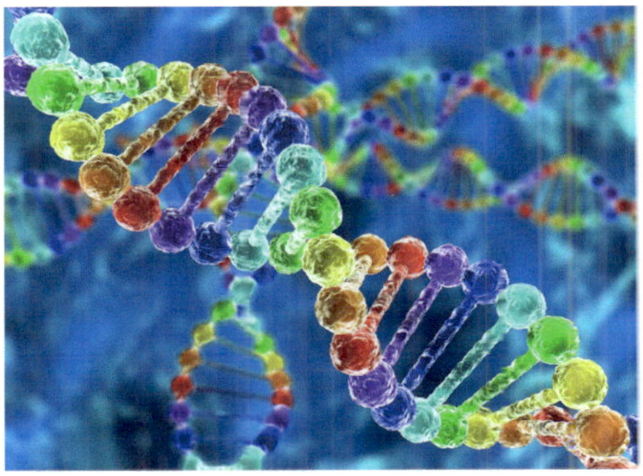

Figure 2.13. Genetic factors significantly affect drug metabolism, leading to variability in the pharmacokinetic profiles observed among patients.

Source: https://domf5oio6qrcr.cloudfront.net/medialibrary/9045/iStock-473718564.jpg.

Recent developments in pharmacometabolomics enable the inclusion of genetic and environmental factors, enabling the prediction of drug response with greater accuracy from pre-drug levels of metabolism. Furthermore, exploration of pharmacokinetics as it concerns endogenous metabolites provides key information regarding personalized therapy, allowing clinicians to modify drug treatments to achieve maximal therapeutic effect (Jian et al., 2023). As evidenced by the incorporation of systematic reviews within clinical guidelines, recognition of this genetic variation is critical to the safe and effective management of testosterone therapy, enhancing treatment plans and patient results (Bhasin et al., 2018) (Figure 2.13).

2.3.6. Drug Interactions and Metabolism

Drug interaction and metabolism knowledge is essential in the field of pharmacokinetics because these conditions play a significant role in therapy effectiveness and patient safety. Drug interaction can be caused by several mechanisms, including altered absorption, distribution, metabolism, and excretion as a result of interaction among many substances within the body. For instance, the metabolic pathways can be controlled by several variables like the physicochemical characteristics of drugs as well as their drug formulations, eventually influencing their bioavailability and pharmaceutical activity (Frijlink et al., 2023). Additionally, variation between populations in pharmacokinetic responses can pose additional challenges in finding optimal dosing regimens. Utilizing modeling and simulation software, considering drug properties as well as physiological variations, the researchers can predict more precisely the relevance of drug interactions (Bailey et al., 2018). This understanding facilitates improved drug development as well as safer therapeutic practices, emphasizing the fine connection between pharmacokinetics and patient care.

2.3.7. Clinical Implications of Metabolism

Metabolism plays a very critical role in pharmacokinetics because it directly determines the therapeutic significance of drug therapy. Metabolic processes determine how drugs are metabolized to be active or inactive and greatly influence drug efficacy and safety. Testosterone therapy in hypogonadal men, for instance, relies on accurate diagnosis of hypogonadism and understanding the drugs' metabolism within the body. The practitioners must measure levels of testosterone with high precision, considering serum concentrations affected by metabolic changes, to avoid adverse effects and establish therapeutic efficacy (Bhasin et al., 2018). Moreover, the pharmacokinetics of NOACs emphasize metabolism, as drug metabolism differences among individuals may cause significant clinical effects among patients with atrial fibrillation who are non-valvular (Steffel et al., 2018). Thus, understanding metabolic pathways is essential to optimize drug selection and dosing, thereby improving patient outcomes and minimizing risk (Figure 2.14).

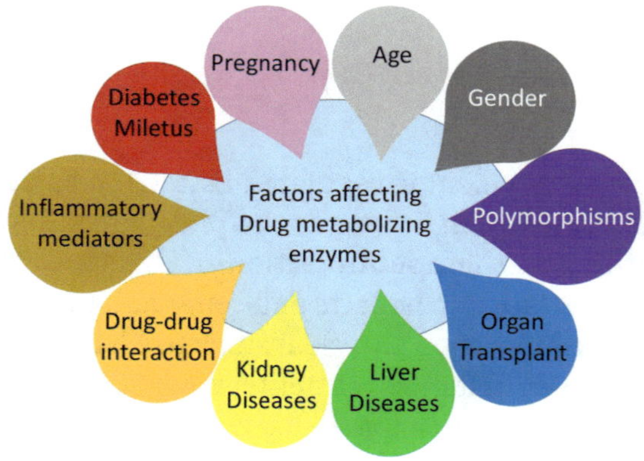

Figure 2.14. Metabolism plays a crucial role in pharmacokinetics, directly influencing the clinical implications of drug therapy.

Source: https://www.liver.theclinics.com/cms/10.1016/j.cld.2016.08.001/asset/fdde489e-f326-4feb-8f9f-1073fdf5611c/main.assets/gr4_lrg.jpg.

2.3.8. Metabolite Activity and Toxicity

Identification of the relationship between metabolite activity and toxicity is crucial in pharmacokinetic research, particularly in defining drug efficacy and safety. The end products of drug metabolism, metabolites, can be either therapeutic or toxic in their activity. For instance, after drug poisoning, the plasma concentration of such metabolites in blood plasma can provide a superior measurement of clinical severity compared to the dose administered. This illustrates the importance of comprehensive data on therapeutic and toxic plasma levels, as evidenced by a recent compilation of over 1,000 xenobiotics, which aids in predicting outcomes in poisoning and drug monitoring (Andresen et al., 2012). Furthermore, studies such as those analyzing *abemaciclib* demonstrate drug interaction intricacies where metabolites can alter pharmacokinetic profiles of co-administered drugs, both with regard to efficiency as well as safety (Beckmann et al., 2018). Ultimately, the intricacies of metabolite functionality must be understood extensively to optimize pharmacotherapy (Figure 2.15).

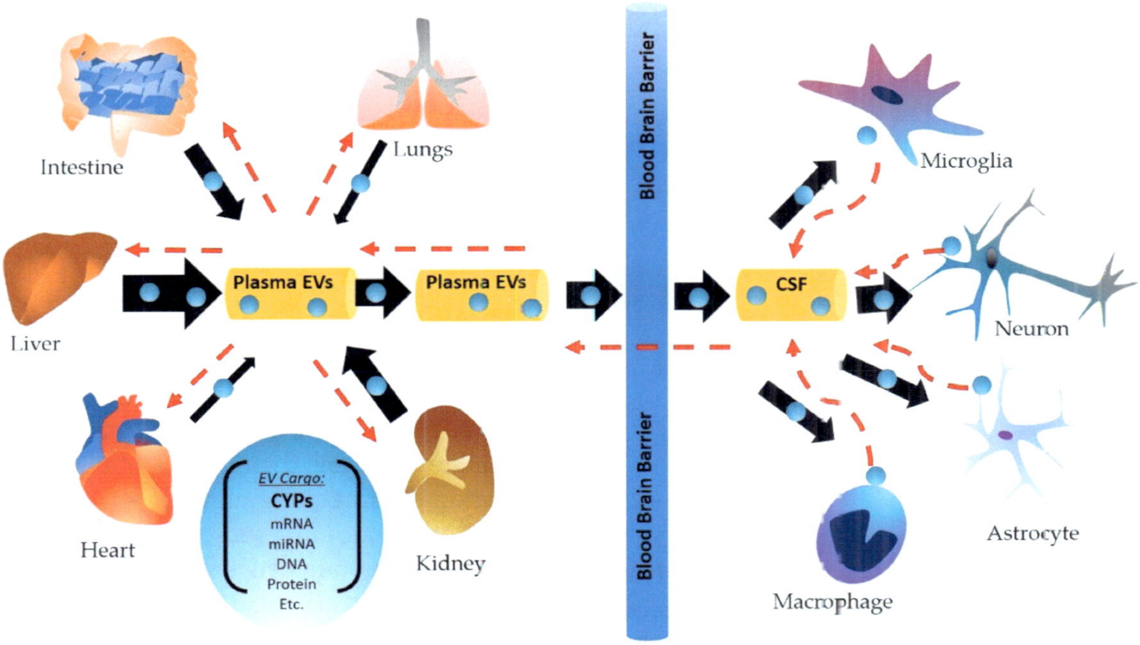

Figure 2.15. Metabolites, the products of drug metabolism, can exhibit varying degrees of activity, which may be either therapeutic or toxic.

Source: https://pub.mdpi-res.com/ijms/ijms-20-06178/article_deploy/html/images/ijms-20-06178-g001.png?1577774168.

2.3.9. Case Examples of Metabolic Pathways

A complete understanding of metabolic pathways is essential in drug pharmacokinetic behavior, as exemplified by several case examples. For instance, the metabolic clearance of a candidate drug can be predicted by scaling from preclinical data, which allows investigators to establish its pharmacokinetic profile before initiating human trials. AstraZeneca's exemplary strategy demonstrates that 83% of their drug development projects can advance to the clinic effectively without issues of pharmacokinetics, which shows the effectiveness of their predictive approach (Davies et al., 2020) TDM is also still a valuable instrument in the optimization of pharmacotherapy, particularly in polymorphic patient groups at risk of pharmacokinetic variability, such as the elderly or mentally handicapped persons. Through integrating TDM into treatment procedures, clinicians optimize therapeutic outcomes and improve patient recovery rates, thus demonstrating the importance of understanding metabolic pathways in pharmacokinetics (Hiemke et al., 2017).

Test Your Knowledge

1. Differentiate between Phase I and Phase II reactions in drug metabolism.
2. What is the significance of cytochrome P450 enzymes in pharmacokinetics?

2.4. Excretion

Learning Outcome

1. Understand the mechanisms of drug excretion
2. Explain renal excretion processes
3. Focus on biliary excretion and its role
4. Identify factors influencing excretion
5. Explain half-life and its clinical relevance
6. Know the impact of disease on excretion
7. Learn methods for assessing excretion
8. Discuss environmental considerations in excretion
9. Describe case studies on excretion

Excretion is a critical process of pharmacokinetics, being the final phase of drug elimination from the body. The effectiveness of excretion directly affects the concentrations of drugs and thus therapeutic efficacy and safety. Predominantly mediated by the liver and kidneys, excretion has various mechanisms attached to it, e.g., passive diffusion and active transport, which can affect the overall pharmacokinetic profile of the drug. Renal clearance is particularly significant since it is influenced by the glomerular filtration rate (GFR) and drug binding to plasma proteins, thereby leading to a large degree of interindividual variation (IV) in drug action. Furthermore, the dynamic interplay between transporters and drug-metabolizing enzymes strengthens the science of drug disposition and highlights the need for accuracy in drug development and management strategies. As ongoing research continues to elucidate these processes, our capacity to predict and optimize drug excretion will enhance therapeutics and minimize side effects, and therefore demonstrate its very critical role in pharmacokinetics (Tirona et al., 2016; Davies et al., 2020).

2.4.1. Mechanisms of Drug Excretion

Drug excretion processes are pivotal to the pharmacokinetic profile of drugs in the body. Primarily through the kidneys, drug excretion is facilitated by filtration, secretion, and reabsorption mechanisms that effectively eliminate drugs and their metabolites. Glomerular filtration eliminates small water-soluble agents, with active tubular secretion increasing the clearance of certain drugs such that their plasma concentrations are maintained at therapeutic levels. Of particular note is the interaction between drug transporters and metabolism as a potent determinant of the efficiency of excretion, and which can produce broad IV in sensitivity to drugs. Clinical observations of pharmacology underscore the significance of understanding these mechanisms because they can affect dosing and therapeutic action of numerous medications, which underlines the significance of healthcare providers considering these factors while making treatment plans (Cosentino et al., 2019). In the wake of pharmacogenomics development, the intricate management of excretory pathways is still irreplaceable in inpatient care optimization (Tirona et al., 2016) (Figure 2.16).

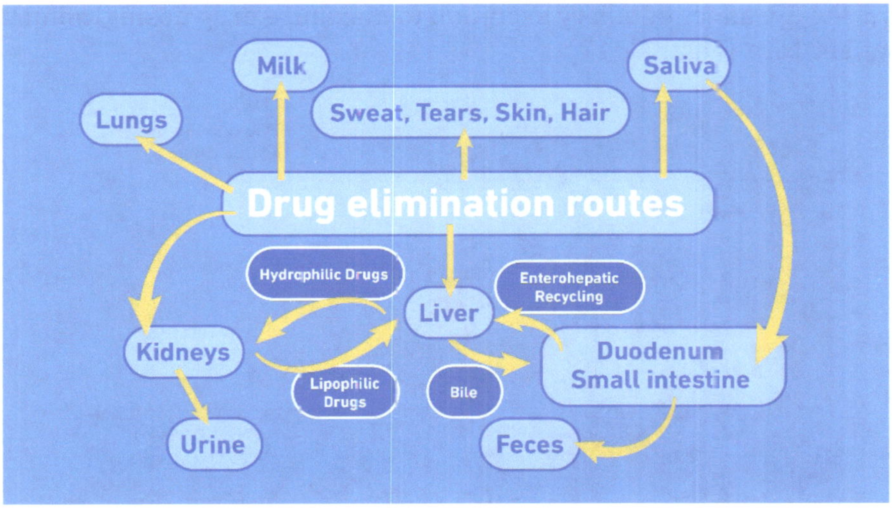

Figure 2.16. The mechanisms of drug excretion play a pivotal role in determining the pharmacokinetic profile of pharmaceuticals within the body.

Source: https://cdn.technologynetworks.com/tn/images/body/dmpk31612794320855.jpg.

2.4.2. Renal Excretion Processes

An understanding of renal excretion mechanisms is required to use pharmacokinetics appropriately since renal excretion mechanisms dictate the fate of a drug in the body after its administration. Renal excretion primarily occurs via glomerular filtration, tubular secretion, and tubular reabsorption, which are all involved in the clearance of drugs from systemic circulation. Glomerular filtration relies on drugs fraction unbound in plasma and GFR, while secretion is with active transport mechanisms whereby substances may be eliminated even against a concentration gradient. Notably, the reabsorption phase is essentially passive with considerable impact on the elimination of lipid-soluble drugs since such drugs are reabsorbed back into the bloodstream. Understanding such processes is not only essential to the prediction of drug excretion but also to the understanding of the impact of renal impairment on drug therapy, as highlighted by recent findings on per- and polyfluoroalkyl substances (PFAS) indicating significant kidney-related health effects, particularly of specific compounds (Fenton et al., 2020; Davies et al., 2020).

2.4.3. Biliary Excretion and Its Role

Biliary excretion is a significant process in the pharmacokinetics of numerous drugs and plays a critical role in the absorption, distribution, metabolism, and elimination of drugs. Biliary excretion is significant in the case of drugs that undergo extensive metabolism within the liver, whereby drug metabolites are transported into the bile by hepatic transporters, thereby contributing to their body elimination. For instance, bosentan, a receptor antagonist of endothelin-1 in pulmonary arterial hypertension, shows the significance of biliary excretion in the disposition of drugs since cytochrome P450 enzymes, which extensively metabolize it and rely on hepatic transporters for elimination (Srinivas, 2016). Changes in biliary excretion can play an essential role in a drug's pharmacokinetics and thereby affect bioavailability and therapeutic efficacy (Li et al., 2018). It is essential to know the dynamics of biliary excretion to maximize drug dosing, minimize side effects, and optimize patient care (Figure 2.17).

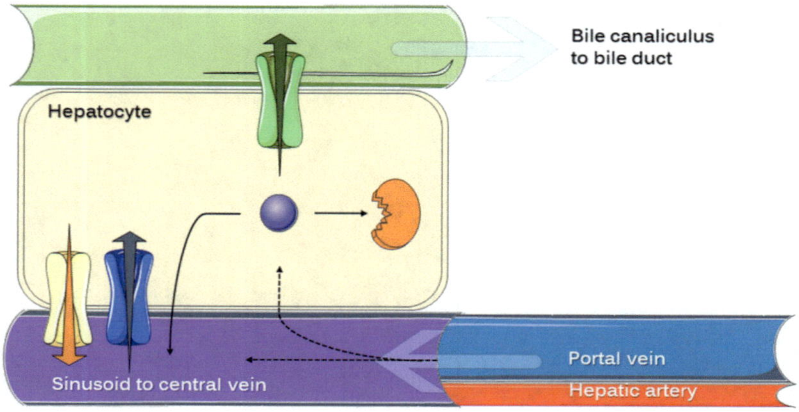

Figure 2.17. Biliary excretion is a critical process in the pharmacokinetics of various drugs, significantly influencing their absorption, distribution, metabolism, and elimination.

Source: https://media.springernature.com/full/springer-static/image/art%3A10.1038%2Fs41598-021-85174-w/MediaObjects/41598_2021_85174_Fig1_HTML.png.

2.4.4. Factors Influencing Excretion

Excretion, which is a crucial component of pharmacokinetics, is subject to various interlinked factors such as drug physicochemical properties, metabolism, and individual differences between patients. Molecular size, polarity, and ionization of the drugs determine to a large extent their clearance from the body and affect renal as well as biliary mechanisms of excretion. Furthermore, the availability and activity of specific transporters, such as organic anion transporters, can increase or reduce renal clearance of the drugs and their metabolites. Furthermore, certain individual factors such as age, gender, and genetic variation may alter pharmacokinetic profiles, resulting in different rates of excretion among individuals. Understanding these factors is critical in predicting drug behavior and realizing maximum therapeutic efficacy at a minimal level of toxicity. The complexity of mechanisms of excretion emphasizes the necessity for robust prediction models which consider these biological variations, as argued in the study of toxicokinetic characteristics of chemicals, e.g., PFAS, which demonstrates the relationship between drug characteristics and excretion kinetics (Fenton et al., 2020; Davies et al., 2020).

2.4.5. Half-Life and Its Clinical Relevance

The half-life is a key concept in the pharmacokinetics of drugs, particularly in determining their dosing regimen and their therapeutic effect. The half-life is the duration required by the drug concentration in the body to drop to half its initial level, and it directly affects the action time and the frequency of administration. For instance, in anticoagulation treatment, such as in the case of vitamin K antagonists, knowing the half-life enables clinicians to optimally manage their patients' thromboembolic risk, especially in instances where they require surgery (Steffel et al., 2021). Furthermore, such drugs with shorter half-lives may need to be administered more regularly to maintain therapeutic levels, hence influencing patients' compliance and treatment outcomes in general (Muratov et al., 2020). Therefore, improved understanding of half-life not only enhances clinical decision-making but also optimizes the safety and efficacy of pharmacotherapeutic interventions (Figure 2.18).

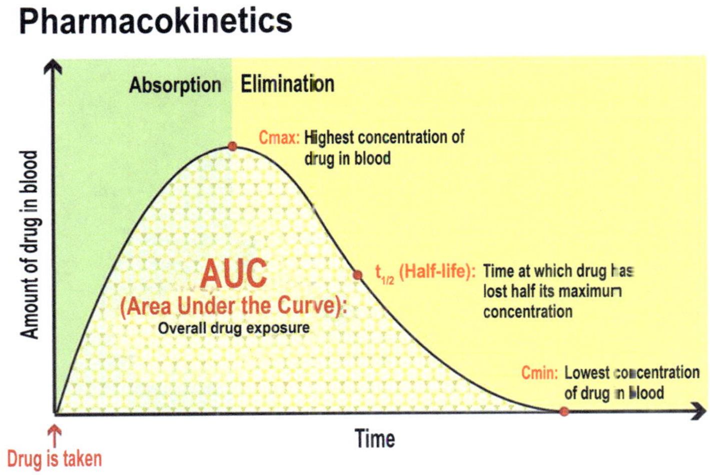

Figure 2.18. Half-life is integral to understanding the pharmacokinetics.

Source: https://clinicalinfo.hiv.gov/sites/default/files/glossaries/images/Pharmacokinetics-800.jpg.

2.4.6. Impact of Disease on Excretion

The influence of disease on excretion is a highly significant aspect of pharmacokinetics, as the body's drug-eliminating capacity can be drastically altered through various pathologies. Most notable in the context of renal disease, the process of excretion can be severely compromised so that drug and drug metabolite accumulation takes place in the blood. This deposition not only increases the risk of harmful side effects but also degrades the efficacy of treatments, necessitating dosing regimen modifications. Furthermore, cardiovascular diseases can affect the metabolism of drugs by altering blood circulation, thereby disrupting the distribution and excretion processes essential in maintaining therapeutic levels of medication, as in the patient's response to anticoagulants like rivaroxaban (Steffel et al., 2021). Moreover, the urgency for novel antibiotics in the context of escalating resistance underscores the necessity for understanding how the pharmacokinetic profiles of various agents are modulated by illness (Miethke et al., 2021).

2.4.7. Methods for Assessing Excretion

Excretion measurement is crucial in pharmacokinetic studies since it has a direct influence on the information obtained on drug clearance and half-life. Various processes are employed to determine excretion, including urine collection, fecal monitoring, and blood sample protocols. In order to determine how medications are removed from the body, urine analysis is crucial since it can reveal metabolites and provide information on renal clearance. This is paramount in a therapeutic setting, especially in chronic disease, where treatment regimens may involve tumor necrosis factor inhibitors (TNFi) for the treatment of conditions such as psoriatic arthritis. The pharmacokinetics of TNFi are such that variability in the rate of excretion is anticipated, making personalized medicine essential (Kraft et al., 2017). Also, the inclusion of physiologically based pharmacokinetic (PBPK) modeling allows scientists to predict individual variations in drug excretion and then address population heterogeneity and susceptibility for successful therapy (Bois et al., 2010). Understanding these methods enhances the overall picture of drug behavior within the organism (Figure 2.19).

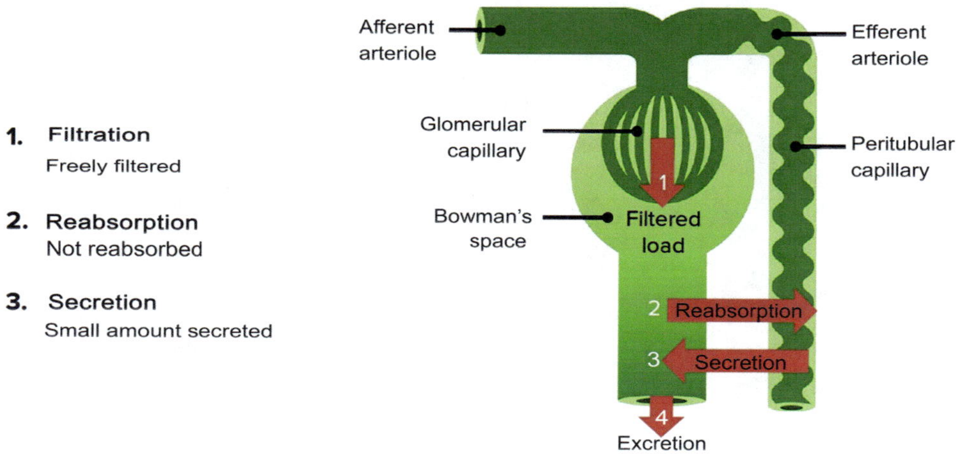

Figure 2.19. Assessing excretion is crucial in the study of pharmacokinetics, as it directly influences the understanding of drug clearance and half-life.

Source: https://cdn.lecturio.com/assets/Creatinine-filtration.jpg.

2.4.8. Environmental Considerations in Excretion

The process of excretion is a vital part of pharmacokinetics, but is also increasingly viewed as a significant environmental problem. The metabolites that are excreted during drug metabolism can reach the environment through wastewater and runoff and constitute a potential environmental hazard to terrestrial and aquatic systems. The environmental persistence of certain chemicals, like per- and PFAS, raises significant health questions. Research indicates that PFAS exposure has been connected with various health effects, including liver and thyroid injury, immune alterations, and even cancer, which suggests the importance of understanding the toxicological effect of such chemicals on the ecosystem (Fenton et al., 2020). Additionally, as therapy development advances, pharmaceutical resistance in illnesses such as epilepsy makes the drug scenario more complicated, and further examination of the potential for excretion pathways to affect both patient-specific outcomes and broader ecological well-being ensues (Löscher et al., 2020). It is therefore essential to address such environmental concerns to move forward with the continued use of pharmacological agents.

2.4.9. Case Studies on Excretion

Excretion case studies form the core of pharmacokinetic research, particularly about renal and hepatic function roles in drug metabolism. The AKI is a critical area of study because it significantly impacts the pharmacokinetic properties of most drugs. Evidence indicates that AKI reduces hepatic metabolism through the cytochrome P450 (CYP) enzyme system, which questions the accuracy of drug dosing recommendations extrapolated from CKD research. While it is recognized that patients with CKD are likely to have changed drug clearance, the multi-factorial character of AKI introduces complicating factors that need adjusted drug management strategies (Abosaif et al., 2014). Furthermore, studies have identified drug transport mechanisms, such as drug induction of the P-glycoprotein (Pgp) efflux transporter by drugs such as pregnenolone 16α-carbonitrile, as capable of modifying drug bioavailability and clearance, and therefore the requirement for personalized pharmacotherapy approaches (Ungell A-et al., 2010).

Test Your Knowledge

1. How does renal function affect drug clearance?
2. How can changes in urinary pH affect drug excretion?

Summary

In combining the pharmacokinetic concepts, one has to respect the unique place that advanced techniques have in deciphering the drug behavior within biological systems. The study of reactive oxygen and nitrogen species (RONS) through state-of-the-art methods, such as ion chromatography, is a good case in point. By equating pharmacokinetic principles to the examination of RONS that are created in plasma-treated solutions, researchers can account for the kinetic profiles and the biological impact of such species, thereby enhancing therapeutic interventions' effectiveness (Locatelli et al., 2025). In addition, the incorporation of nanotechnology into drug delivery is a revolution in oncology that has addressed key problems with target therapy by providing better drug biodistribution and safety profiles (Seliverstov et al., 2024). Overall, all these advances reflect the continued evolution of pharmacokinetic studies, which remain a key constituent in the refinement of drug formulations and therapeutic approaches for improved clinical effects.

It is essential to have a general perception of the principles of pharmacokinetics to optimize drug development and therapeutic action. The essence of these principles is the ADME theory, abbreviated as absorption, distribution, metabolism, and excretion. These factors are essential in defining the bioavailability and drug concentration at the site of action to set their therapeutic actions. Besides, with the increasing prevalence of drug-resistant pathogens, there is an urgent need for novel pharmacologically guided therapeutic agents. The strategic framework presented by researchers provides opportunities for enhancing new antibiotic discovery and development and bridging the gaps between academic centers, industry, and policy-makers (Miethke et al., 2021). Furthermore, understanding the individual pharmacokinetic characteristics, i.e., in the case of non-vitamin K antagonist oral anticoagulants, can maximize treatment behaviors and ensure enhanced patient outcomes (Steffel et al., 2021). Through these principles, the pharmaceutical sector can effectively combat emerging health conditions.

KEY TERMS FROM THIS CHAPTER

- Absorption
- Bioavailability
- Blood flow
- Drug solubility
- Food-drug interaction
- Infections
- Active transport
- Biological compartment
- Cellular membranes
- Excretion
- Gastrointestinal motility
- Lipophilic drugs
- Acute kidney injury (AKI)
- Biological systems
- Drug formulation
- First-pass phenomenon
- Genetics

Critical Thinking Questions

1. **Which of the following processes is NOT part of pharmacokinetics?**
   a. Absorption
   b. Distribution
   c. Metabolism
   d. Receptor binding
2. **The 'first-pass effect' primarily affects which route of drug administration?**
   a. Intravenous
   b. Subcutaneous
   c. Oral
   d. Inhalation
3. **Which organ is primarily responsible for drug metabolism?**
   a. Kidney
   b. Liver
   c. Lung
   d. Stomach
4. **The term "bioavailability" refers to:**
   a. The rate of drug elimination
   b. The percentage of drug bound to plasma proteins
   c. The fraction of an administered dose that reaches systemic circulation
   d. The volume in which the drug is distributed
5. **What does a large volume of distribution (Vd) indicate about a drug?**
   a. It remains mainly in the plasma
   b. It is widely distributed into tissues
   c. It is rapidly excreted
   d. It has a short half-life

Answers to Critical Thinking Questions

1. (d); 2. (c); 3. (b); 4. (c); 5. (b).

Short Answer Questions

1. What is pharmacokinetics and how does it differ from pharmacodynamics?
2. Define the term ADME in the context of pharmacokinetics.
3. Why is understanding pharmacokinetics important in clinical practice?
4. What factors influence the rate and extent of drug absorption?
5. How do plasma protein binding and tissue affinity affect drug distribution?
6. What role does the liver play in drug metabolism?
7. What are the main routes of drug excretion?

References

1. Dixon, J., Lane, K., MacPhee, I., & Philips, B. (2014). Xenobiotic metabolism: The effect of acute kidney injury on Non-Renal drug clearance and hepatic drug metabolism. *International Journal of Molecular Sciences, 15*(2), 2538–2553. https://doi.org/10.3390/ijms15022538Aebi, S., Shah, A. G., Anderson, C., Arlt, W., Barr, J., Barthelemy, H., Beiderlinden, M., et al. (2017). *Medication Complications in Extracorporeal Membrane Oxygenation*. https://core.ac.uk/download/129191716.pdf (accessed on 10th June 2025).
2. Ahire, D. S., Kruger, L., Sharma, S., Mettu, V., Basit, A., & Prasad, B. (2022). Quantitative proteomics in translational absorption, distribution, metabolism, and excretion and precision medicine. *Pharmacological Reviews, 74*, 771–798. https://www.semanticscholar.org/paper/20f1605340019512b5f532e2427200dc05295a3d (accessed on 10th June 2025).
3. Aijaz, A., Vaninov, N., Allen, C., Bárcia, R. N., & Parekkadan, B. (2019). Convergence of cell pharmacology and drug delivery. *Stem Cells Translational Medicine, 8*, 874–879. https://doi.org/10.1002/sctm.19-0019.
4. Andresen, H., Iwersen-Bergmann, S., Schmoldt, A., & Schulz, K. (2012). *Therapeutic and Toxic Blood Concentrations of Nearly 1,000 Drugs and Other Xenobiotics*. https://core.ac.uk/download/14525457.pdf (accessed on 10th June 2025).
5. Arav, Y. (2024). Advances in modeling approaches for oral drug delivery: Artificial intelligence, physiologically based pharmacokinetics, and first-principles models. *Pharmaceutics, 16*. https://www.semanticscholar.org/paper/a6aa41f351f74ce95bb3ea40062f698b4c998895 (accessed on 10th June 2025).
6. Bailey, A., Bon, C., Cox, B., Darwich, A., Dorey, R., Duwal, S., Ette, E., et al. (2018). *Population Variability in Animal Health: Influence on Dose-Exposure-Response Relationships. Part II: Modeling and Simulation*. https://core.ac.uk/download/159992803.pdf (accessed on 10th June 2025).
7. Beckmann, R., Garrido, P., Goldman, J. W., & Gutierrez, M., et al. (2018). *Abaculi in Combination with Single-Agent Options in Patients with Stage IV Non–Small Cell Lung Cancer: A Phase IB Study*. https://core.ac.uk/download/227054197.pdf (accessed on 10th June 2025).
8. Bhasin, S., Brito, J. P., Cunningham, G. R., Hayes, F. J., Hodis, H. N., Matsumoto, A. M., Snyder, P. J., et al. (2018). Testosterone therapy in men with hypogonadism: An Endocrine Society clinical practice guideline. *The Journal of Clinical Endocrinology & Metabolism, 103*, 1715–1744. https://doi.org/10.1210/jc.2018-00229.
9. Bois, F. Y., Clewell, H. J., & Jamei, M. (2010). *PBPK Modeling of Inter-Individual Variability in The Pharmacokinetics of Environmental Chemicals*. https://core.ac.uk/download/52669006.pdf (accessed on 10th June 2025).
10. Burt, T., & Dhillon, S. (2013). *Pharmacogenomics in Early-Phase Clinical Development*. https://core.ac.uk/download/pdf/37750487.pdf (accessed on 10th June 2025).
11. Chehelgerdi, M., Chehelgerdi, M., Allela, O. Q. B., Pecho, R. D. C., Narayanan, J., Rao, D. P., Thamaraikani, T., et al. (2023). Progressing nanotechnology to improve targeted cancer treatment: Overcoming hurdles in its clinical implementation. *Molecular Cancer, 22*. https://doi.org/10.1186/s12943-023-01865-0.
12. Chenthamara, D., Sadhasivam, S., Ramakrishnan, S. G., Krishnaswamy, S., Essa, M. M., Lin, F. H.,

& Qoronfleh, M. W. (2019). Therapeutic efficacy of nanoparticles and routes of administration. *Biomaterials Research, 23*. https://doi.org/10.1186/s40824-019-0166-x.

13. Cosentino, F., Grant, P. J., Aboyans, V., Bailey, C. J., Ceriello, A., Delgado, V., Federici, M., et al. (2019). 2019 ESC Guidelines on diabetes, pre-diabetes, and cardiovascular diseases developed in collaboration with the EASD. *European Heart Journal, 41*, 255–323. https://doi.org/10.1093/eurheartj/ehz486.
14. Dave, V. S., Gupta, D., Varghese, S., Nguyen, M., et al. (2016). *Current and Evolving Approaches for Improving the Oral Permeability of BCS Class III or Analogous Molecules*. https://core.ac.uk/download/81665712.pdf (accessed on 10th June 2025).
15. Davies, M., Jones, R. D. O., Grime, K., Jansson-Löfmark, R., Fretland, A. J., Winiwarter, S., Morgan, P., et al. (2020). Improving the accuracy of predicted human pharmacokinetics: Lessons learned from the AstraZeneca drug pipeline over two decades. *Trends in Pharmacological Sciences, 41*, 390–408. https://doi.org/10.1016/j.tips.2020.03.004.
16. Dowell, D., Ragan, K., Jones, C. M., Baldwin, G., & Chou, R. (2022). CDC clinical practice guideline for prescribing opioids for pain—United States, 2022. *MMWR Recommendations and Reports, 71*, 1–95. https://doi.org/10.15585/mmwr.rr7103a1.
17. Dudhat, K. R. (2022). Basic aspects and the overview on pharmacokinetics and studies on drug distribution: A panoramic review. *Bioequivalence & Bioavailability International Journal*. https://www.semanticscholar.org/paper/2481e68656b189a6705e7bed962b67e461ac2aaf (accessed on 10th June 2025).
18. Fenton, S. E., Ducatman, A., Boobis, A. R., DeWitt, J. C., Lau, C., Ng, C. A., Smith, J. S., et al. (2020). Per- and polyfluoroalkyl substance toxicity and human health review: Current state of knowledge and strategies for informing future research. *Environmental Toxicology and Chemistry, 40*, 606–630. https://doi.org/10.1002/etc.4890.
19. Freeman, C., Krzyzaniak, N., La Caze, A., et al. (2022). Mapping Australian pharmacy school curricula for content related to pharmacogenomics. https://core.ac.uk/download/557050419.pdf (accessed on 10th June 2025).
20. Frijlink, H., Lagarce, F., Touw, D., et al. (2023). Biopharmaceutics. https://core.ac.uk/download/597499024.pdf (accessed on 10th June 2025).
21. Gajula, S. N., Talari, S., Chilvery, S., Chandraiah, G., & Sonti, R. (2023). A unique *in vivo* pharmacokinetic profile, *in vitro* metabolic stability, and hepatic first-pass metabolism of garcinol, a promising novel anticancer phytoconstituent, by liquid chromatography-mass spectrometry. *RPS Pharmacy and Pharmacology Reports*. https://www.semanticscholar.org/paper/c0deac109037d1a348fdb154653f16bd44cdae7f (accessed on 10th June 2025).
22. Ghezzi, M., Pescina, S., Padula, C., Santi, P., Del Favero, E., Cantù, L., & Nicoli, S. (2021). Polymeric micelles in drug delivery: An insight of the techniques for their characterization and assessment in biorelevant conditions. *Journal of Controlled Release, 332*, 312–336. https://doi.org/10.1016/j.jconrel.2021.02.031.
23. Giovannetti, E., & Peters, G. (2021). Beyond animal models: Implementing the 3Rs principles and improving pharmacological studies with new model systems. *Expert Opinion on Drug Metabolism & Toxicology, 17*, 867–868. https://www.semanticscholar.org/paper/cf9244b8ff65ce1376e1700e7209bd9be9c8a07f (accessed on 10th June 2025).

24. Guidi, M., Csajka, C., & Buclin, T. (2020). Parametric approaches in population pharmacokinetics. *Journal of Clinical Pharmacology*. https://www.semanticscholar.org/paper/1c6adcb0a4006024cb0cd9743d18b53804446725 (accessed on 10th June 2025).

25. Hiemke, C., Bergemann, N., Clement, H.-W., Conca, A., Deckert, J., Domschke, K., Eckermann, G., et al. (2017). Consensus guidelines for therapeutic drug monitoring in neuropsychopharmacology: Update 2017. *Pharmacopsychiatry, 51*, 9–62. https://doi.org/10.1055/s-0043-116492.

26. Howland, R. H. (2009). Critical appraisal and update on the clinical utility of agomelatine, a melatonergic agonist, for the treatment of major depressive disease in adults. https://core.ac.uk/download/12213913.pdf (accessed on 10th June 2025).

27. Huang, Y., & Lu, T. (2009). Modeling long-term longitudinal HIV dynamics with application to an AIDS clinical study. http://arxiv.org/abs/0901.3806 (accessed on 10th June 2025).

28. Hughes, G. (2014). A simple introduction to pharmacokinetics: Part 1. *Nurse Prescribing, 12*, 497–503. https://www.semanticscholar.org/paper/6d3833bf800d09b40b5571a39a7f03a677087238 (accessed on 10th June 2025).

29. Humphreys, S. C., Thayer, M. B., Campbell, J., Chen, W., Adams, D., Lade, J. M., & Rock, B. M. (2020). Emerging siRNA design principles and consequences for biotransformation and disposition in drug development. *Journal of Medicinal Chemistry*. https://www.semanticscholar.org/paper/6ee6e163ec59b4d1208fbf06b0a74e469fd18d27 (accessed on 10th June 2025).

30. Ibanez, B., Varenhorst, C., Alexopoulos, D., Aradi, D., Lindholm, D., Zhou, D., Amsterdam, E. A., et al. (2018). *Metabolism of Ticagrelor in Patients with Acute Coronary Syndromes*. https://core.ac.uk/download/287581672.pdf (accessed on 10th June 2025).

31. Jian, J., He, D., Gao, S., Tao, X., & Dong, X. (2023). Pharmacokinetics in pharmacometabolomic: Towards personalized medication. *Pharmaceuticals, 16*, 1568. https://doi.org/10.3390/ph16111568.

32. Joseph, T. M., Mahapatra, D. K., Esmaeili, A., Piszczyk, Ł., Hasanin, M. S., Kattali, M., Haponiuk, J. T., et al. (2023). Nanoparticles: Taking a unique position in medicine. *Nanomaterials, 13*, 574. https://doi.org/10.3390/nano13030574.

33. Kilburn, J. J., Schmitt, D., Kiso, W., Papich, M., & Backues, K. (2023). Pharmacokinetics of rectally and orally administered levofloxacin in Asian elephants (*Elephas maximus*). *Journal of Zoo and Wildlife Medicine, 53*, 670–678. https://www.semanticscholar.org/paper/546a6648f8677de493d457025bcbc430163b10c0 (accessed on 10th June 2025).

34. Kraft, W. K., Lam, E., Lien, Y. T. K., et al. (2020). Vancomycin in peritoneal dialysis: Clinical pharmacology considerations in therapy. https://core.ac.uk/download/322850154.pdf (accessed on 10th June 2025).

35. Kraft, W. K., Mantravadi, S., & Ogdie, A. (2017). Tumor necrosis factor inhibitors in psoriatic arthritis. https://core.ac.uk/download/83049994.pdf (accessed on 10th June 2025).

36. Lai, Y., Chu, X., Di, L., Gao, W., Guo, Y., Liu, X., Lu, C., et al. (2022). Recent advances in the translation of drug metabolism and pharmacokinetics science for drug discovery and development. *Acta Pharmaceutica Sinica B, 12*, 2751–2777. https://doi.org/10.1016/j.apsb.2022.03.009.

37. Lamptey, R. N. L., Chaulagain, B., Trivedi, R., Gothwal, A., Layek, B., & Singh, J. (2022). A review of the common neurodegenerative disorders: Current therapeutic approaches and

the potential role of nanotherapeutics. *International Journal of Molecular Sciences, 23*, 1851. https://doi.org/10.3390/ijms23031851.

38. Li, R., Wang, Q., Liu, Z., Xie, L., Diao, Z., Peng, Y., Wang, G., et al. (2023). Dose-dependent pharmacokinetics of midazolam in rats: Influence of hepatic first-pass metabolism. *Xenobiotic, 53*, 184–192. https://www.semanticscholar.org/paper/79008c33750d795711c3d1e58e2ecc9427158573 (accessed on 10th June 2025).

39. Li, W., Yan, B., Wang, R., & Jia, Z. (2018). [Role of drug transporters in rational use of drugs at high altitude area]. *Zhong Nan Da Xue Xue Bao. Yi Xue Ban = Journal of Central South University. Medical Sciences, 43*(3), 327–332. https://www.semanticscholar.org/paper/bcc1db7a9673a4b3153a89e4ba311f40a993af93 (accessed on 10th June 2025).

40. Locatelli, M., Perrucci, M., Balaha, M., Acharya, T., Kaushik, N., Choi, E., Rapino, M., et al. (2025). Chemical analysis of plasma-activated culture media by ion chromatography. *Pharmaceuticals, 18*. https://www.semanticscholar.org/paper/d85086b8c87b5f99bd9b8fc0298fe4100e065f4c (accessed on 10th June 2025).

41. Löscher, W., Potschka, H., Sisodiya, S. M., & Vezzani, A. (2020). Drug resistance in epilepsy: Clinical impact, potential mechanisms, and new innovative treatment options. *Pharmacological Reviews, 72*, 606–638. https://doi.org/10.1124/pr.120.019539.

42. Lyon, A. R., López-Fernández, T., Couch, L. S., Asteggiano, R., Aznar, M. C., Bergler-Klein, J., Boriani, G., et al. (2022). 2022 ESC Guidelines on cardio-oncology developed in collaboration with the European Hematology Association (EHA), the European Society for Therapeutic Radiology and Oncology (ESTRO), and the International Cardio-Oncology Society (IC-OS). *European Heart Journal, 43*, 4229–4361. https://doi.org/10.1093/eurheartj/ehac244.

43. Manyi-Loh, C. E., Mamphweli, S., Meyer, E. L., & Okoh, A. I. (2018). Antibiotic use in agriculture and its consequential resistance in environmental sources: Potential public health implications. *Molecules, 23*, 795. https://doi.org/10.3390/molecules23040795.

44. Miethke, M., Pieroni, M., Weber, T., Brönstrup, M., Hammann, P., Halby, L., Arimondo, P. B., et al. (2021). Towards the sustainable discovery and development of new antibiotics. *Nature Reviews Chemistry, 5*, 726–749. https://doi.org/10.1038/s41570-021-00313-1.

45. Muratov, E., Bajorath, J., Sheridan, R. P., Tetko, I. V., Filimonov, D., Poroikov, V., Oprea, T. I., et al. (2020). QSAR without borders. *Chemical Society Reviews, 49*, 3525–3564. https://doi.org/10.1039/d0cs00098a.

46. Piel, M., Vernaleken, I., & Rösch, F. (2014). Positron emission tomography in CNS drug discovery and drug monitoring. *Journal of Medicinal Chemistry, 57*, 9232–9258. https://doi.org/10.1021/jm5001858.

47. Rizvi, S. A. A., & Saleh, A. (2017). Applications of nanoparticle systems in drug delivery technology. *Saudi Pharmaceutical Journal, 26*, 64–70. https://doi.org/10.1016/j.jsps.2017.10.012.

48. Roberts, D., Sevastos, J., Carland, J., Stocker, S., & Lea-Henry, T. (2018). Clinical pharmacokinetics in kidney disease: Application to rational design of dosing regimens. *Clinical Journal of the American Society of Nephrology, 13*(8), 1254–1263. https://www.semanticscholar.org/paper/cb4ea9509842ffe01aac4fecc1b3a017698b4f9c (accessed on 10th June 2025).

49. Sapir-Pichhadze, R., & Oertelt-Prigione, S. (2023). P32: A sex- and gender-sensitive model

for evidence-based precision medicine: From knowledge generation to implementation in the field of kidney transplantation. *Kidney International, 103*, 674–685. https://doi.org/10.1016/j.kint.2022.12.026.

50. Seliverstov, P. V., Baksheeva, A. D., Koretskaya, P. S., & Abdusattarov, I. Z. (2024). Use of nanotechnology in the creation of targeted drugs for the treatment of oncological diseases. *Molekulyarnaya Meditsina (Molecular Medicine)*. https://www.semanticscholar.org/paper/c42431c56b70265598b63e22a32d13c30cd0d3ae (accessed on 10th June 2025).

51. Shin, E., & Ramanathan, M. (2023). Evaluation of prompt engineering strategies for pharmacokinetic data analysis with the ChatGPT large language model. *Journal of Pharmacokinetics and Pharmacodynamics*. https://www.semanticscholar.org/paper/5bfd50eb6d5cd6365d98c640c2fc79fdee8281c0 (accessed on 10th June 2025).

52. Singhal, T. S., Jain, J., Tejendra, A. R., Singh, A. J., Saad, J. D., Jain, M. K., Abdul-Zahra, et al. (2024). Eco-design of products and processes: A review on principles and tools for sustainable manufacturing. *E3S Web of Conferences*. https://www.semanticscholar.org/paper/09edee2b72e41355e9b66c899cef86b9e2291420 (accessed on 10th June 2025).

53. Srinivas, N. (2016). Clinical drug-drug interactions of bosentan, a potent endothelial receptor antagonist, with various drugs: Physiological role of enzymes and transporters. *General Physiology and Biophysics, 35*(3), 243–258. https://www.semanticscholar.org/paper/d1af8004d5b6c496ff471d2761be9c1522fc1556 (accessed on 10th June 2025).

54. Steffel, J., Collins, R., Antz, M., Cornu, P., Desteghe, L., Hæusler, K. G., Oldgren, J., et al. (2021). 2021 European Heart Rhythm Association Practical Guide on the use of non-vitamin K antagonist oral anticoagulants in patients with atrial fibrillation. *EP Europace, 23*, 1612–1676. https://doi.org/10.1093/europace/euab065.

55. Steffel, J., Verhamme, P., Potpara, T., Albaladejo, P., Antz, M., Desteghe, L., Hæusler, K. G., et al. (2018). The 2018 European Heart Rhythm Association Practical Guide on the use of non-vitamin K antagonist oral anticoagulants in patients with atrial fibrillation. *European Heart Journal, 39*, 1330–1393. https://doi.org/10.1093/eurheartj/ehy136.

56. Straehla, J. P., & Warren, K. (2020). Pharmacokinetic principles and their application to central nervous system tumors. *Pharmaceutics, 12*. https://www.semanticscholar.org/paper/c8536e99639096fec12d6d3dad266db709c9a0ec (accessed on 10th June 2025).

57. Tirona, R. G., & Kim, R. B. (2016). Introduction to clinical pharmacology. In *Clinical and Translational Science*. https://doi.org/10.1016/b978-0-12-802101-9.00020-x.

58. Ungell, A. L., Bauer, B. M., Fihn, C., Hilgendorf, C., Englund, G., Harrison, F., Haslam, I. S., et al. (2010). *The Effects of Pregnenolone 16α-Carbonitrile Dosing on Digoxin Pharmacokinetics and Intestinal Absorption in The Rat*. https://core.ac.uk/download/30734033.pdf (accessed on 10th June 2025).

59. Zeitlinger, M., Tillotson, G., & Echols, R. (2023). Editorial: Pharmacokinetics, pharmacodynamics (PK/PD) of antibiotics: A reality check. *Frontiers in Pharmacology, 14*. https://www.semanticscholar.org/paper/46d9cd084e687d69dfc3c976d3f60c50aa53c347 (accessed on 10th June 2025).

PHARMACODYNAMICS

3

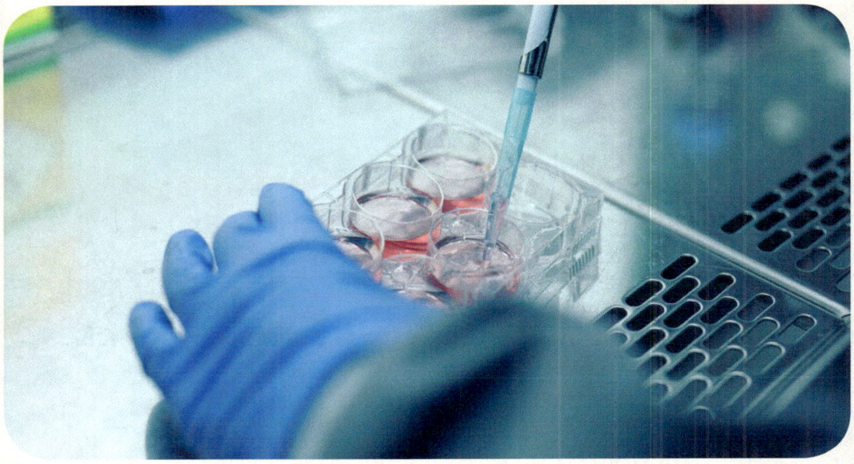

LEARNING OBJECTIVES

After studying this chapter, you will be able to:

1. Understand mechanisms of drug action
2. Identify factors influencing drug response
3. Explain therapeutic applications of pharmacodynamics

Introduction

Pharmacodynamics refers to the field that is crucial for understanding how drugs work within the body, filling the gap between drug administration and therapeutic response. Pharmacodynamics involves the study of drug mechanisms, including how various substances interact at molecular, cellular, and systemic levels to influence physiological processes. A thorough introduction to pharmacodynamics highlights the significance of understanding pharmacological action variables, which could result in more beneficial treatment plans and improved patient outcomes. As we discuss mechanisms of pharmacodynamic concepts, we will see how recent research has utilized new methods, including digital technologies and modeling data, to achieve maximum drug efficacy and safety (Abduvalova et al., 2024). Moreover, increasing demand for postbiotics signals new avenues in the development of drugs, proving the potential of these metabolites in medical use, and it symbolizes the evolving face of pharmacotherapeutics (Kumar et al., 2024) (Figure 3.1).

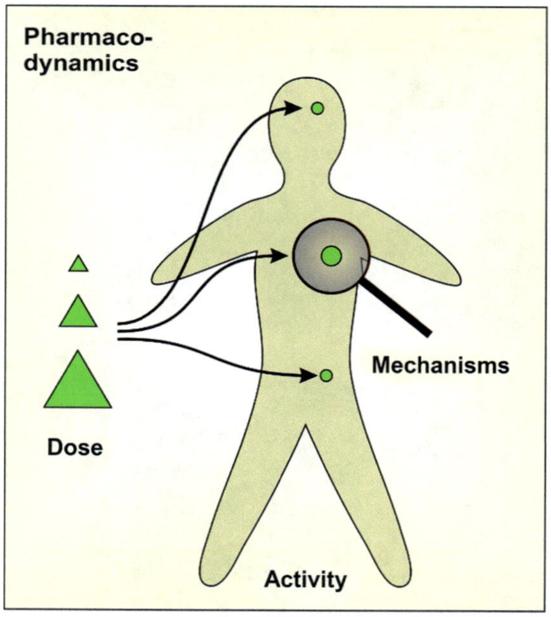

Figure 3.1. Pharmacodynamics.

Source: https://upload.wikimedia.org/wikipedia/commons/thumb/c/c5/Pharmacodynamics.svg/1200px-Pharmacodynamics.svg.png.

3.1. Mechanisms of Drug Action

Learning Outcome

1. Understand receptor theory and drug binding
2. Identify types of receptors
3. Explain agonists vs. antagonists
4. Describe dose-response relationships
5. Focus on signal transduction pathways
6. Describe allosteric modulation
7. Learn enzyme inhibition and activation
8. Discuss pharmacogenomics and individual response
9. Know the role of second messengers.

It is necessary to know the drug action mechanisms in pharmacodynamics because this allows for the development of effective therapeutic interventions and improving patients' outcomes. In most cases, drugs' effects rely on their capacity to interact with some biological targets, e.g., proteins, enzymes, or receptors, which are biologically engaged in the control of physiological processes. For example, antifungals have exhibited diverse mechanisms; azoles inhibit ergosterol synthesis, essential for the integrity of the fungal cell membrane, and echinocandins disrupt the synthesis of β-(1,3)-D-glucan, crucial in the structure of the fungal cell wall. Despite problems, development has persisted, with side effects and resistance being significant issues for treatment protocols (Anália do Carmo et al., 2023). Furthermore, healthcare professionals must balance drug pharmacokinetic and pharmacodynamic profiles against one another to obtain optimal effects with the least harm, thus the importance of guidelines that allow clinical judgment (Visseren et al., 2021).

3.1.1. Receptor Theory and Drug Binding

The intricate dynamics of drug binding and receptor theory are at the core of pharmacodynamics science because they explain how drugs act on the molecular level. Receptor theory is based on the assumption that drugs attach to specific receptor sites so that they can initiate a biological effect, as illustrated using ligand binding models, which focus on occupancy levels of the receptors (Nishtala et al., 2017). The effectiveness of a drug directly correlates with the fraction of receptor occupancy, which emphasizes that higher binding affinity tends to be mirrored in better therapy. This is also demonstrated in conditions such as rheumatoid arthritis, where understanding receptor interaction can inform the development of targeted therapy to enhance therapeutic efficacy and disease progression control (Chaplain et al., 2019). Thus, the appreciation of the nuances of receptor theory not only enhances our theory but also informs actual practice in drug design and therapeutic strategy in pharmacodynamics (Figure 3.2).

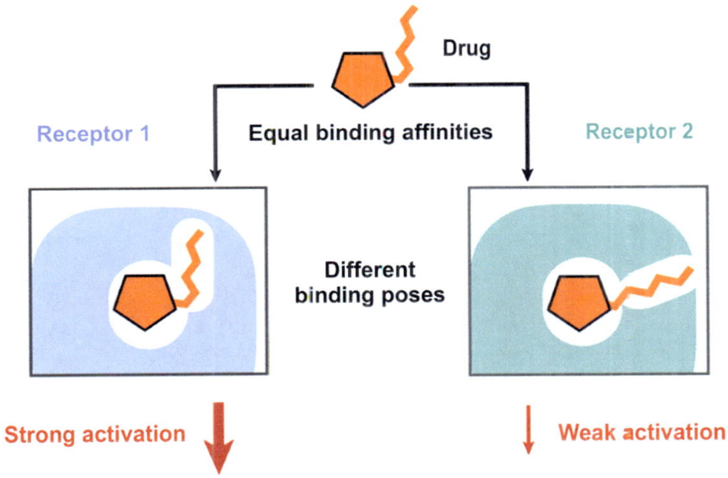

Figure 3.2. Receptor theory and drug binding.

Source: https://media.springernature.com/m685/springer-static/image/art%3A10.1038%2Fs41589-022-01247-5/MediaObjects/41589_2022_1247_Figa_HTML.png.

3.1.2. Types of Receptors (e.g., Ion Channels, GPCRs)

In pharmacodynamics, understanding the types of receptors plays a critical role in describing drug activity and therapeutic actions. Both ion channels and G protein-coupled receptors (GPCRs) are two major receptor categories that play a pivotal role in cellular signaling. Ion channels enable rapid ion movement across membranes, directly influencing cellular excitability and signal cascades. On the other hand, GPCRs, or seven transmembrane receptors, mediate more types of physiological responses, organizing responses to various stimuli such as hormones and neurotransmitters. GPCRs are also particularly significant in the sense that they are the most prominent drug target family, their complex signaling capability allowing them to elicit various kinds of intracellular responses besides mere cell surface interaction (Klauer et al., 2024). This varied repertoire of receptor forms emphasizes the intricate interaction of signaling processes upon which drugs have been seen to tap to have desired therapeutic outcomes (Wang et al., 2022).

3.1.3. Agonists vs. Antagonists

Understanding the distinction between agonists and antagonists is significant in the science of pharmacodynamics because these two classes of drugs act on receptors in quite different ways. Agonists interact with receptors and activate them, resulting in a biological response that will replicate the action of naturally occurring chemicals in the body. Conversely, antagonists engage the same receptors but do not activate them; instead, they block or antagonize the action of the agonist, hence preventing the physiological effect. This functional relationship is significant in the formulation of therapeutic interventions, particularly against the GPCR, which are underutilized in drug discovery despite their capability (Milligan et al., 2017). Ligand binding models also account for the mechanism of such interactions by demonstrating how pharmacological action is dependent on receptor occupation (Nishtala et al., 2017). Such a nuanced comprehension of agonists and antagonists, thus, not only directs the design of drugs but also increases our knowledge of complex physiological mechanisms and disease mechanisms (Figure 3.3).

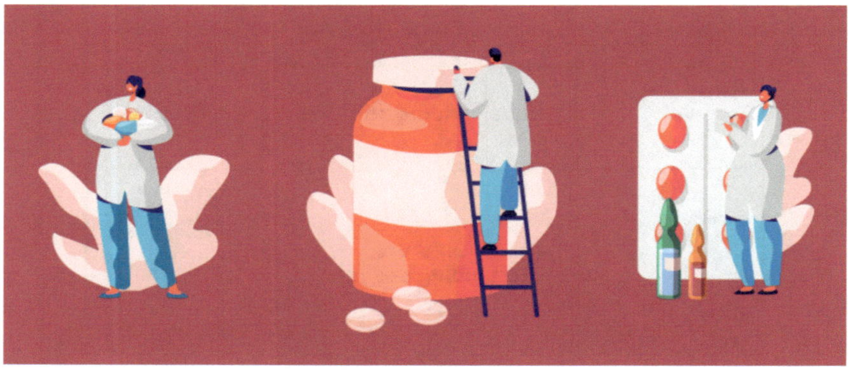

Figure 3.3. Understanding the distinction between agonists and antagonists is crucial in the field of pharmacodynamics, as these two classes of drugs interact with receptors in fundamentally different ways.

Source: https://buzzrx.s3.amazonaws.com/fb40e722-d4c0-4a45-b210-9d5892c46f35/Antagonist.png.

3.1.4. Dose-Response Relationships

Dose-response relationships are the foundation of pharmacodynamics as they establish the relationship between the concentration of the drug and the produced pharmacological effect in the patient. Such relationships are highly critical in optimizing therapeutic regimens, particularly in complex treatments like those involving bispecific antibodies like ABBV-383. A thorough analysis of response rates and dose escalation clinical studies has revealed that specific dosing techniques, such as step-up dosing (SUD), have a significant impact on the safety and efficacy profiles of pharmaceuticals. For instance, in relapsed or refractory multiple myeloma patients, modified dosing schedules were reported to reduce the incidence and severity of side effects like cytokine release syndrome (CRS), thereby enhancing the overall safety profile of ABBV-383, without compromising its ability to achieve desired therapeutic effects (Wang et al., 2024). These findings emphasize the importance of well-defining dose-response relationships to effectively individualize treatments (Mian et al., 2024).

3.1.5. Signal Transduction Pathways

Signal transduction pathways are crucial for cell reactions to external stimuli. They are central to pharmacodynamics, where they have a significant role to play in determining the way drugs exert their therapeutic effect. The pathways involve a sequence of biochemical reactions catalyzed by enzymes and proteins that transmit information from the cell membrane to the interior, which ultimately results in physiological responses. For instance, experiments have validated that Ginkgetin, a bioactive compound derived from Ginkgo biloba extract, binds directly to the STING protein, inhibiting its activation and subsequent signal transduction, which in turn alleviates inflammation and cellular senescence (Liu et al., 2024). Moreover, recognition of various signal pathways, such as PI3K-Akt and MAPK, within the context of different therapeutic applications underscores the complexity and interdependence of these pathways. These findings are indicative of the potential for understanding signal transduction pathways in the development of pharmacological interventions (Liu et al., 2024) (Figure 3.4).

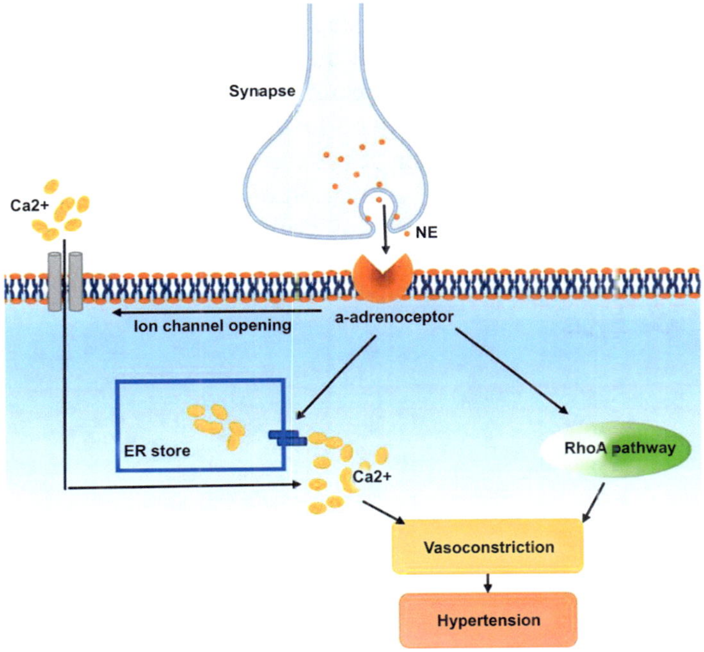

Figure 3.4. Signal transduction pathways are crucial for mediating cellular responses to external stimuli, playing a significant role in pharmacodynamics by determining how drugs exert their therapeutic effects.

Source: https://media.springernature.com/lw1200/springer-static/image/art%3A10.1038%2Fs41392-023-01430-7/MediaObjects/41392_2023_1430_Fig8_HTML.png.

3.1.6. Allosteric Modulation

In the field of pharmacodynamics, allosteric modulation is an essential mechanism by which drug action can be optimized beyond traditional active-site interactions. It involves the binding molecule of an effector at a particular site and thereby inducing conformational alterations that alter the activity of receptors. Allosteric modulators can either enhance or reduce the affinity of the primary ligand towards binding, maintaining an intricate balance between signaling pathways. For example, in cancers that are fueled by the dysregulation of the PI3K/AKT/mTOR (PAM) pathway, allosteric inhibitors targeting entities like AKT have been promising avenues to bypass resistance to treatment, highlighting the ability of non-active site modulation (Glaviano et al., 2023). Besides, allosteric modulation has been gaining more and more popularity in the treatment of neurodegenerative diseases like Alzheimer's disease, where the use of acetylcholinesterase inhibitors (ChE-Is) is also a similar approach to increasing therapeutic efficacy through indirect action (Marucci et al., 2020).

3.1.7. Enzyme Inhibition and Activation

Pharmacodynamic mechanisms of enzyme inhibition and activation play a significant role in ensuring the efficacy and safety of drugs. Synergism between these processes can revolutionize the metabolism of drugs, leading to differential therapeutic effects among patients. For example, inhibitors can block enzyme action, thus lowering the rate of drug metabolism, which can increase the impact of a drug but also make it more toxic, especially in analgesics where genetic differences in enzyme expression influence pain management outcomes. Enzyme activators, on the other hand, can speed up drug metabolism, which can compromise the therapeutic effect of drugs (Abduljalil et al., 2019). In addition, through pharmacogenetic investigations of analgesics, genetic factors inherited by the patient seem to impact their response to drugs and highlight the importance of identifying mechanisms in both inhibition and activation of enzymes in tailor-made pharmacotherapy (Branford et al., 2013). Enzyme modulation is thus still a cornerstone in adjusting drug therapies (Figure 3.5).

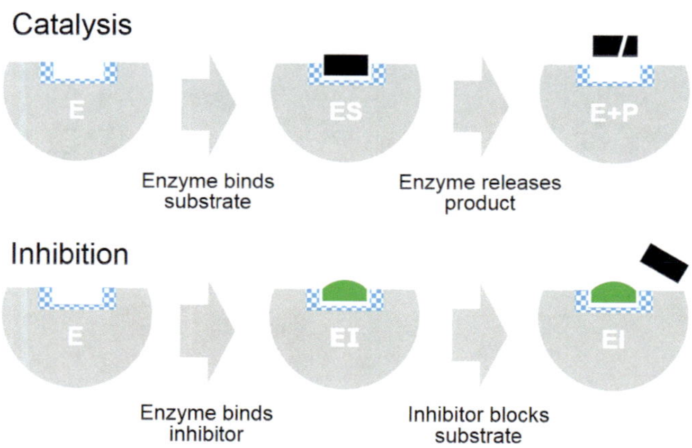

Figure 3.5. Enzyme inhibition and activation are critical processes in pharmacodynamics, influencing drug efficacy and safety.

Source: https://upload.wikimedia.org/wikipedia/commons/d/dd/Enzyme_inhibitors_2.svg.

3.1.8. Pharmacogenomics and Individual Response

Pharmacogenomics application in the practice of medicine has profound implications for describing and maximizing personal drug response, thus enhancing pharmacodynamics. The IV of drug response, where approximately 25–60% of patients exhibit divergent pharmacological effects to a given drug, underscores the impact of genetic determinants, such as single nucleotide polymorphisms (SNPs) and copy number variations (CNVs), on drug safety and efficacy (Sánchez-Pozos et al., 2021). These genetic variations affect not only drug absorption and metabolism mechanisms but also pharmacokinetic and pharmacodynamic effects, resulting in therapeutic efficacy or side effects. As the field of pharmacogenomics improves, it becomes possible to detect key genetic biomarkers, such as opioid response biomarkers, to tailor treatments to individualized profiles, thereby minimizing risks and maximizing therapeutic benefits (Benjeddou et al., 2021). Ultimately, this individualized approach is a step toward precision medicine, wherein treatments are particularly designed to match each patient's unique genetic makeup best.

3.1.9. Role of Second Messengers

Second messengers are in the spotlight of pharmacodynamics to transform extracellular signals into intracellular responses, thereby governing physiological functions. These intracellular messengers, such as cyclic AMP (cAMP) and calcium ions, facilitate the magnification of signals through more than one receptor and run complex cellular processes. For instance, calcium signaling alterations are of great importance in the organophosphate-induced neurotoxicity pathology, whereby elevated intracellular levels of calcium in hippocampal tissue have been observed following exposure, suggesting an extended interfering effect on neuronal function (Battaglia et al., 2016). Likewise, the novel activity of bitter taste receptors as second messengers demonstrates their capacity for causing bronchodilation and modulating inflammatory processes in asthma and COPD, suggesting they are functional therapeutic molecules for the treatment of airway conditions (Deshpande et al., 2019). Second messengers are thus not merely passive carriers but positive forces in pharmacological control of cellular behavior at the heart of both established and yet-to-be therapies (Figure 3.6).

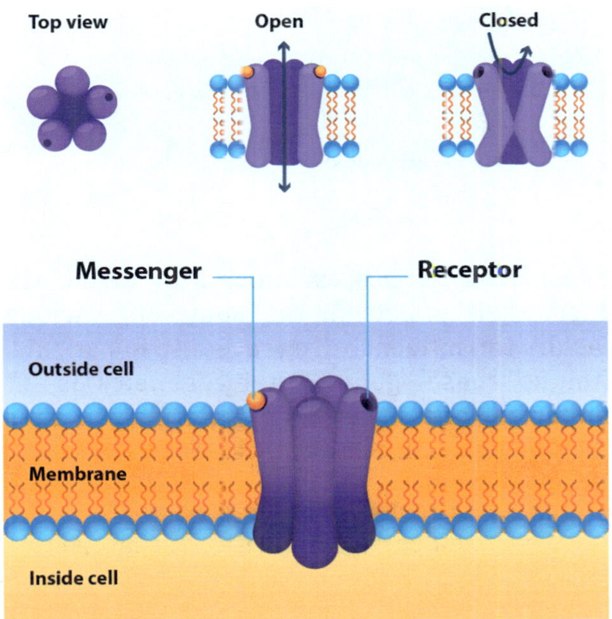

Figure 3.6. Within the realm of pharmacodynamics, second messengers play a pivotal role in translating extracellular signals into intracellular responses, thereby modulating physiological functions.

Source: https://www.oatext.com/img/CRT-9-378-g001.gif.

Test Your Knowledge

1. What is a dose-response curve, and what information does it provide?
2. Differentiate between potency and efficacy.

3.2. Factors Influencing Drug Response

Learning Outcome

1. Identify genetic factors and polymorphisms
2. Explain age and developmental considerations
3. Discuss sex differences in drug metabolism
4. Focus on body weight and composition
5. Describe disease states and comorbidities
6. Identify environmental factors
7. Focus on drug interactions and polypharmacy
8. Explain psychological factors and placebo effects
9. Discuss ethnic and cultural variations in response

Pharmacodynamics examines how medicines exert their effects in the body, but various factors can influence drug response in patients. Among these, genetic heterogeneity is an important one since polymorphisms can alter the pharmacokinetics and pharmacodynamics of medicines.

For instance, it has been seen that genetic variations in drug-metabolizing genes such as the Cytochrome P450 gene family could lead to differential responses of drugs to medications like Donepezil, the most prescribed drug for Alzheimer's disease, with response rates being between 20% and 60% among patients (Lu et al., 2020).

Also, drug effectiveness could be complicated by lifestyle influences like smoking, which has potentially complicated antihypertensive agent effects like beta-adrenergic antagonist effects by the dual mechanism of smoking's impact on blood pressure and drug interaction (Kasim, 2022). Determination of such factors is essential in order to maximize therapeutic response and customize medication regimens in clinical practice.

3.2.1. Genetic Factors and Polymorphisms

The role of genetic influence and polymorphisms in pharmacodynamics is increasingly accepted as a central pillar of targeted or personalized medicine. Variations in the individual's genome can significantly influence the response of drugs to biological processes, both concerning efficacy and the risk of adverse effects. For example, analgesic pharmacology has some genetic variants that affect pain response and response to pain medication. Still, their clinical implication remains to be maximally realized, particularly beyond the highly studied μ-opioid receptor (Branford et al., 2013).

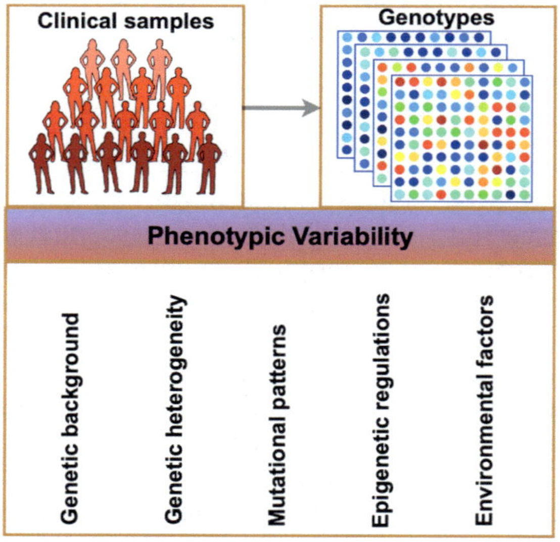

Figure 3.7. The role of genetic factors and polymorphisms in pharmacodynamics is increasingly recognized as a critical aspect of personalized medicine.

Source: https://www.mdpi.com/pharmaceuticals/pharmaceuticals-17-00940/article_deploy/html/images/pharmaceuticals-17-00940-g002.png.

Similarly, diabetic care research has established significant polymorphisms concerning patients' response to basal antihyperglycemic drugs, further supporting the importance of individually targeted therapy based on genetic screening (Andreozzi et al., 2019). This interaction between pharmacodynamics and genetics not only reveals the way to more effective treatment methods but also can lower the risk of complications typically associated with traditional pharmacotherapy (Figure 3.7).

3.2.2. Age and Developmental Considerations

The pharmacodynamics-age interaction is of particular significance in the pediatric category, where drug sensitivity is deeply dependent on developmental stages. Younger children exhibit distinctive pharmacokinetic characteristics in contrast to adults due to the ongoing development of drug-metabolizing and eliminating organs. Most notably, the most significant pharmacokinetic variation is among children less than 2 years old, demonstrating the need for age-specific dosing regimens to optimize efficacy and minimize toxicity (Jovanovi et al., 2022). This is highlighted with newer agents, such as nirmatrelvir/ritonavir for COVID-19, licensed for use in pediatrics. The complexity of compliance and potential drug-drug interactions (DDI) in this age category necessitates careful monitoring and treatment regimens specific to the patient (Yalçın et al., 2022). It is essential to comprehend, therefore, the pharmacodynamic developmental complexities to be able to deliver safe and efficacious therapy among children, necessitating ongoing studies focusing on the changes required in clinical practice.

3.2.3. Sex Differences in Drug Metabolism

Pharmacodynamic science is increasingly recognizing the need for understanding sex differences in drug metabolism, an important area that has implications for therapeutic efficacy and safety profiles.

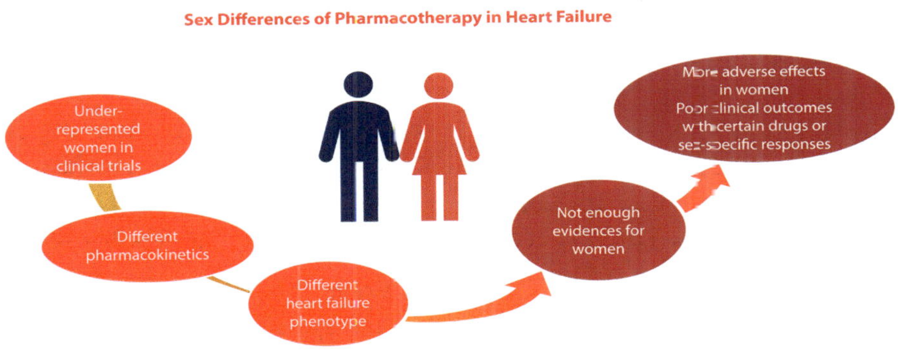

Figure 3.8. The study of pharmacodynamics increasingly recognizes the significance of sex differences in drug metabolism, a crucial area that influences therapeutic outcomes and safety profiles.

Source: https://www.e-emj.org/upload/thumbnails/emj-47-1-3-g2.jpg.

Drug efficacy and toxicity between females and males have been postulated to be due to differential pharmacokinetic parameters, including bioavailability, distribution, metabolism, and elimination processes that are potentially linked to body composition and fluctuations in hormonal status. For instance, it was noted that there are dramatic drug concentration fluctuations within the menstrual cycle, and these primarily concern drugs used in affective disorder treatment, necessitating sex-specific pharmacotherapy (Spadi et al., 2024). Moreover, new data focused on the contribution of sex-related differences in cytochrome P450 activity towards drug metabolism, which emphasized the underlying biology behind such differences (Gandhi et al., 2004). With evidence piling up, it is increasingly critical for clinical practice to adopt these findings to ensure optimal effectiveness of treatment as well as minimize adverse effects for both males and females (Figure 3.8).

3.2.4. Body Weight and Composition

Awareness of body weight and composition is crucial in pharmacodynamics research, particularly about drug efficacy and safety. Variability in body composition can potentially influence the pharmacokinetic profile and therapeutic activity of certain medications, as with the new drug TE-8105. This molecule, through the assistance of multi-arm linker technology, has superior pharmacokinetics and weight-loss activity in animal models of obesity over existing medicines such as semaglutide (Wong et al., 2025). Furthermore, current study shows how dietary ingredients interact with body weight, specifically how the dicarbonyl compounds 3-deoxyglucosone (3-DG) and methylglyoxal (MGO) can influence weight change in European adults (Debras et al., 2024). These findings highlight the complexity of metabolic processes and the possibility of individualized pharmacotherapy based on an individual's body composition and dietary intakes, and therefore the necessity for the integration of metabolic parameters into drug development and clinical practice.

3.2.5. Disease States and Comorbidities

Understanding disease states and comorbidities plays an important role in the study of pharmacodynamics, as these conditions significantly influence drug response and treatment outcomes. Comorbidities such as diabetes or CKD, for instance, tend to complicate drug pharmacokinetics and pharmacodynamics and consequently need to be paid close attention to in therapeutic approaches. For instance, elderly patients with comorbid disease often require tailored immunosuppressive therapy, as their physiological response is unlike that of young patients.

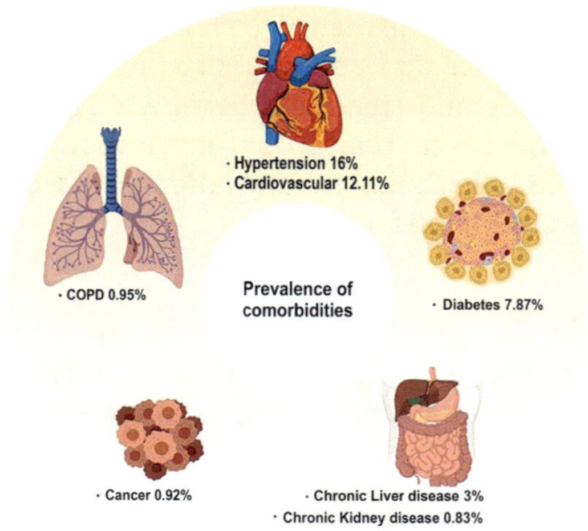

Figure 3.9. An understanding of disease states and comorbidities is essential in the discipline of pharmacodynamics, as these factors significantly influence drug response and treatment outcomes.

Source: https://www.frontiersin.org/files/Articles/567283/fimmu-11-01991-HTML-r1/image_m/fimmu-11-01991-g003.jpg.

This population, particularly those with end-stage renal disease, also presents challenges of its own;. However, they too have a lower rate of acute transplant rejection, their higher risk for infection-related complications requires an accurate balance in immunosuppression (Andrews et al., 2018). In addition, studies have shown that certain drugs, including statins, can increase survival rates in comorbid conditions like pancreatic cancer and potentially create a need for further research on the interaction between specific drug categories and the comorbidities (Demissie et al., 2017) (Figure 3.9).

3.2.6. Environmental Factors (e.g., Diet, Lifestyle)

The impact of environmental factors, e.g., lifestyle and diet, has a big effect on pharmacodynamics, particularly in diseases like psoriasis and rheumatoid arthritis. Nutrition, more importantly, has been identified as a crucial modifiable risk factor in the management of psoriasis because it can exacerbate or mitigate disease severity. For instance, not only does obesity exacerbate clinical manifestations of psoriasis, but it also alters pharmacokinetics and pharmacodynamics of medications used in treatment, making it crucial to have specific dietary guidance to improve patient outcomes (Balato et al., 2016). Similarly, lifestyle components, including diet and exercise, play a pivotal role in the trajectory of rheumatoid arthritis. Identification of such environmental factors allows for the implementation of personalized therapeutic protocols that optimize the effectiveness of pharmacological interventions and address fundamental risk factors (Chaplain et al., 2019). Hence, the inclusion of nutritional and lifestyle changes in the treatment plan is essential to optimize the overall treatment of chronic inflammatory conditions.

3.2.7. Drug Interactions and Polypharmacy

As pharmacodynamics is all about exploring the activity of drugs in biological systems, drug interaction and polypharmacy are critical, particularly in such vulnerable populations as the elderly. The elderly take several drugs simultaneously, and hence are at risk of adverse drug reactions (ADRs), thereby leading to serious morbidity and even hospitalization (Onder et al., 2012).

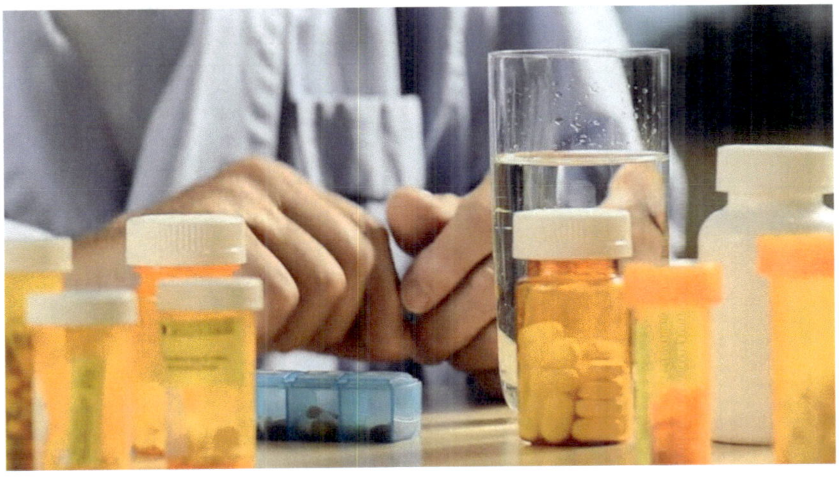

Figure 3.10. As pharmacodynamics explores the effects of drugs on biological systems, understanding drug interactions and polypharmacy is crucial.

Source: https://www.eatg.org/wp-content/uploads/2021/12/polypharmacy.webp.

This enhanced susceptibility is not just a consequence of the polypharmacy but also of age-related alteration of pharmacokinetics and pharmacodynamics. Moreover, challenges of detecting ADRs in patients with such conditions are exacerbated by non-classical presentations, which undermine the capacity of clinicians to intervene. The involvement of clinical pharmacists in healthcare teams has proven to be of value as they can regularly identify and manage drug interactions, particularly in the context of complicated patient conditions such as cancer patients with advanced ages (Khanal et al., 2019). Hence, resolving polypharmacy through improved collaboration and education is required to improve patient outcomes for pharmacological management (Figure 3.10).

3.2.8. Psychological Factors and Placebo Effects

A comprehension of the interaction among psychological factors and placebo effects is especially relevant to the field of pharmacodynamics, as such factors can have an overwhelming influence on the treatment process. The placebo effect, or the phenomenon of a patient's recovery following a therapy with no therapeutic action, demonstrates the place that expectations and beliefs hold in the healing process. For instance, patients with conditions such as Attention Deficit/Hyperactivity Disorder (ADHD) can exhibit diverse reactions to drugs like methylphenidate, which are influenced by psychological traits associated with age and sex (Barke et al., 2010). Similarly, migraine patients are commonly challenged by psychological stressors influencing their condition; thus, awareness of psychological background is essential in determining the effectiveness of drugs like triptans (Calderoni et al., 2001). Through the understanding of such psychological considerations, clinicians can enhance pharmacological interventions, leading to more individualized and effective treatment strategies.

3.2.9. Ethnic and Cultural Variations in Response

Understanding ethnic and cultural differences in response to drugs is crucial in pharmacodynamics, as differences have an impressive impact on therapeutic responses. Research indicates that genes associated with ethnic origins play a role in the pharmacokinetics and pharmacodynamics of drugs, particularly psychotropic drugs.

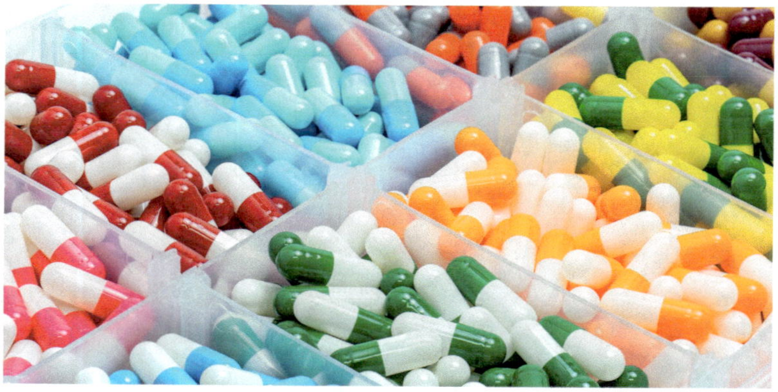

Figure 3.11. Understanding ethnic and cultural variations in response to pharmacological treatments is critical in the field of pharmacodynamics, as these differences can significantly impact therapeutic outcomes.

Source: https://www.allucent.com/wp-content/uploads/2019/03/Intrinsic-and-Extrinsic-Factors-in-Drug-Dev.webp.

For instance, variations in the activity of Cytochrome P 450 (CYP 450) enzymes have been linked with racial differences in drug metabolism and influence on dosage and efficacy across populations (Bakare et al., 2008). Prescribing patterns also point towards how cultural beliefs and practices can shape the treatment approach. One study found that nurses possess varying degrees of cultural competence, which influence their competency in addressing medication reactions unique to every patient's requirement (Virani et al., 2009). Thus, their identification and implementation in practice can enhance the effectiveness of medication as well as care across ethnic populations (Figure 3.11).

Test Your Knowledge

1. How do genetic variations influence an individual's response to drugs?
2. How can genetic polymorphisms in drug-metabolizing enzymes affect drug efficacy and toxicity?

3.3. Therapeutic Applications of Pharmacodynamics

Learning Outcome

1. Understand drug development and clinical trials
2. Explain personalized medicine and tailored therapies
3. Focus on pharmacodynamics in oncology
4. Know the role in pain management
5. Explain applications in infectious diseases
6. Discuss cardiovascular pharmacotherapy
7. Describe neurological disorders and pharmacodynamics
8. Understand antidepressants and mood stabilizers
9. Know implications for chronic disease management

The investigation of therapeutic applications of pharmacodynamics is critical in harmonizing traditional medicinal treatment with scientific research. The plant Holarrhena antidysenterica, for instance, widely utilized in Unani medicine in the treatment of gastrointestinal disorders, has formidable pharmacodynamic characteristics that qualify it for scientific research. Their phytochemical constituents, including alkaloids and flavonoids, are responsible for numerous varying therapeutic effects, including anti-inflammatory and antimicrobial activities, which contribute to their traditional efficacy against diseases such as amoebic dysentery and skin diseases (Sultana et al., 2025). Similarly, the advent of prescription digital therapeutics (PDTs) underscores the need for a pharmacodynamic framework to determine how digital interventions affect clinical outcomes. By applying the principles of pharmacokinetics and pharmacodynamics to such treatments, researchers can prepare parameters like dose and patient interaction, finally ending up with enhanced therapeutic efficacy (Lakhan, 2025). The mentioned examples illustrate the importance of adding pharmacodynamics to both old and emerging treatment types for improved health outcomes.

3.3.1. Drug Development and Clinical Trials

The intricate drug development process and conduct of clinical trials are germane to the quest for effective pharmacological therapy. The process is critical in cancer, where the integration of pharmacological principles such as pharmacodynamics and pharmacokinetics forms the basis of maximizing doses and resulting therapeutic effects. Notably, the FDA launched Project Optimus in 2021 to overcome the limitations of traditional Maximum Tolerated Dose (MTD) approaches, particularly for novel therapies that interact with biological targets differently (Papachristos et al., 2023). The antibacterial drug development case also carries inherent drawbacks, most notably due to rising AMR, making it challenging to establish large-scale randomized trials (Moore et al., 2023). Such advances emphasize the need for adaptive methods involving both preclinical and clinical models to aid not only in the expedience of drug approval but in enhancing the safety and effectiveness of treatments for patients (Figure 3.12).

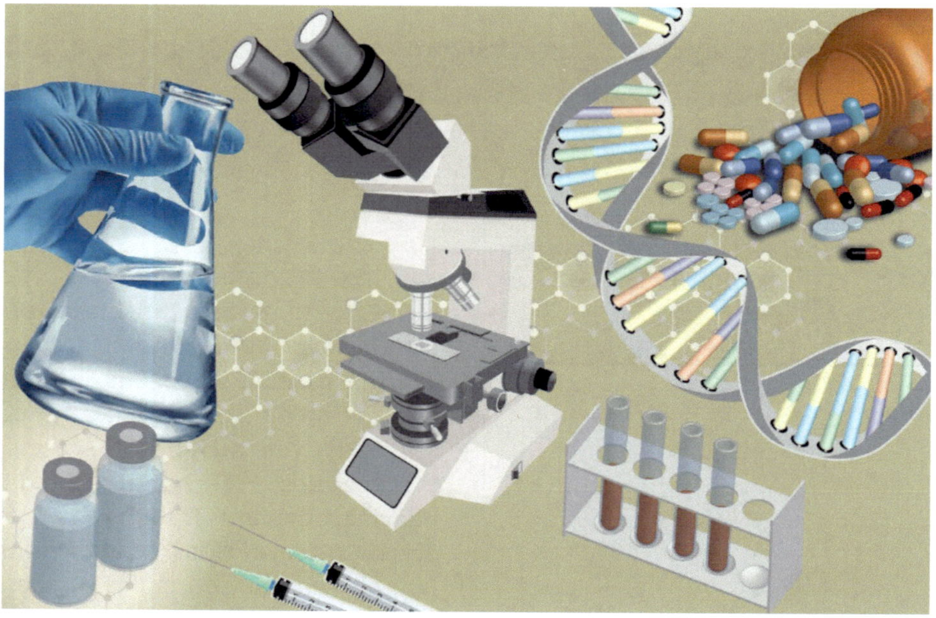

Figure 3.12. The intricate process of drug development and the execution of clinical trials are pivotal in the pursuit of effective pharmacological treatments.

Source: https://www.cbo.gov/sites/default/files/2021-04/57025-home-cover.png.

3.3.2. Personalized Medicine and Tailored Therapies

Personalized therapy and personalized medicine are significant advances in the discipline of pharmacodynamics, since treatment is increasingly adapted to the individual profile of patients. It enhances the therapeutic effect and decreases side effects by considering a patient's genetic, environmental, and life components. New developments highlight the necessity for personalization in complex disorders, such as migraine, whose pathophysiological nuances continue to be complicated and ill-described. For instance, Medication Overuse Headache (MOH) is seen as a significant factor, which was particularly observed by (Martelletti et al., 2018), pointing towards the need for targeted therapies based on the individual histories of the patients rather than generalized regimes. Moreover, gender medicine is at work here; the confluence of the biological and psychosocial determinants necessitates an interest in the sex and gender dimensions of disease presentation and treatment response, as emphasized in Bellini et al. (2019). Personalized medicine thus promises not only improved clinical results but also a fuller appreciation of individual differences in health.

3.3.3. Pharmacodynamics in Oncology

In chemotherapy, the pharmacodynamics is paramount to optimize drug therapy in situations where polypharmacy is common among elderly patients. It has been evidenced that with increasing complexity in cancer treatment, the risk of side effects of drugs greatly increases with polypharmacy, which typically arises from combinations of chemotherapeutic agents and comorbid disease drugs (Khanal et al., 2019). Clinical pharmacist positions have emerged as a key strategy for minimizing such risks, particularly in under-equipped centers, by assisting in monitoring DDI and therapeutic responses. Moreover, some therapies, such as metronomic vinorelbine, also show the necessity to tailor pharmacodynamic rules to patient types by age and overall health status, thereby enhancing efficacy and treatment safety (Bruno et al., 2018). This quiet expansion of pharmacodynamics not only informs wiser therapeutic decisions but also contributes to improved outcomes in the challenging arena of cancer treatment (Figure 3.13).

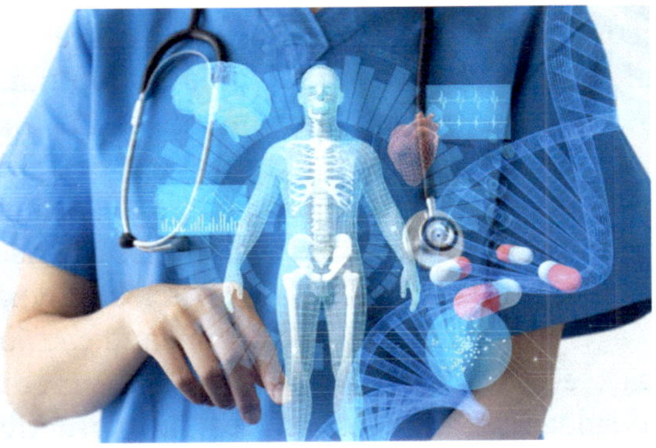

Figure 3.13. Research has demonstrated that as cancer treatment regimens become increasingly complex, the risk of adverse drug reactions rises significantly due to polypharmacy.

Source: https://www.altasciences.com/sites/default/files/inline-images/blogimage_TKPD.png.

3.3.4. Role in Pain Management

Within the realm of pharmacodynamics, the role of opioids in pain control, particularly in cancer patients, is paramount but diverse. Since up to 80% of patients with advanced cancer experience severe pain, its adequate control is significant to ensure maximal quality of life and treatment benefit (Tabin-Barczak et al., 2025). Opioids are recognized as the basis to manage moderate to severe pain, yet substantial risks, including constipation and respiratory depression accompany their pharmacologic action. This emphasizes the importance of a multidisciplinary approach that combines both pharmacologic and non-pharmacologic interventions, ensuring a more cohesive pain management practice (Tabin-Barczak et al., 2025). Furthermore, the pharmacodynamics of adjunct therapeutic approaches, i.e., adjuvants and topical preparations, may provide additional possibilities for pain relief, particularly for neuropathic pain, thereby enabling diversification of treatment to address individual patient requirements. Therefore, optimization of pain control by an optimally balanced and well-informed approach remains a significant objective in pharmacological research.

3.3.5. Applications in Infectious Diseases

Pharmacodynamics is equally relevant in the treatment of infectious diseases since understanding drug-pathogen interaction will shape effective treatment. Disease treatment, such as diffuse telogen alopecia, whose condition may be compounded by infection, underscores this connection. Identification of the underlying cause is critical, as infectious diseases can cause hair loss through various mechanisms, and a careful diagnostic workup is required (Tamrazova et al., 2025). Furthermore, novel imaging modalities, such as hybrid [18F] FDG PET, have been reported to be of value in evaluating infectious and inflammatory processes, allowing clinicians to more accurately measure outcomes of treatment and the effectiveness of therapy (Abikhzer et al., 2024). The integration of pharmacodynamic principles and advanced imaging technologies not only enables personalized therapy but also improves the understanding of disease processes, ultimately leading to improved patient outcomes of infectious disease (Figure 3.14).

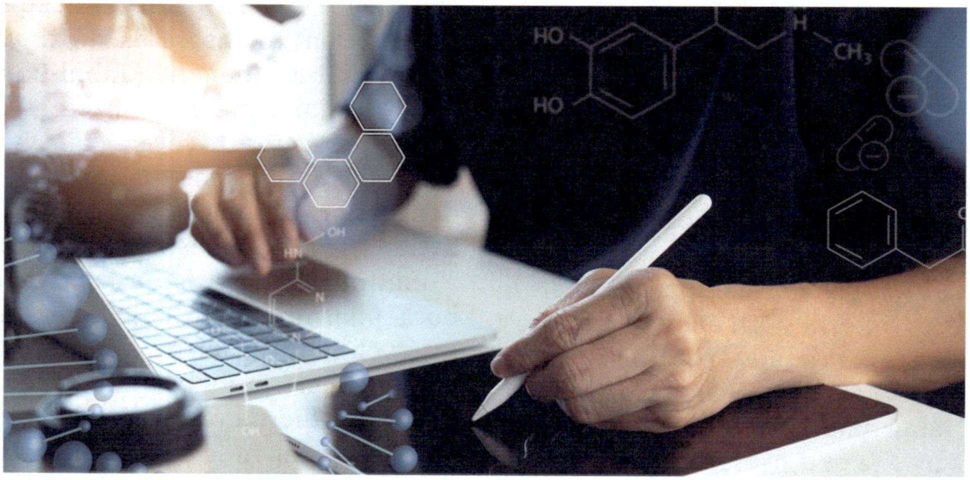

Figure 3.14. Pharmacodynamics plays a significant role in the management of infectious diseases, where understanding drug interactions with pathogens can inform effective treatment strategies.

Source: https://www.allucent.com/wp-content/uploads/2022/12/What-is-pharmadynamics.webp.

3.3.6. Cardiovascular Pharmacotherapy

As cardiovascular pharmacotherapy continues to improve progressively, it becomes more crucial to know the pharmacodynamics of antithrombotic medications in diverse patient populations. Management of antithrombotic therapy in underweight or obese patients, for instance, has unique issues with altered drug pharmacokinetics and pharmacodynamics, highlighted by recent clinical consensus statements (Gigante et al., 2024). These patients display significant physiological changes, which render standard treatment protocols cumbersome; therefore, specialized techniques are needed to enhance therapeutic efficiency. In addition, older individuals exhibit some pharmacodynamic changes as a result of metabolic changes with advancing age, which need to be approached cautiously during drug selection and administration (Popovskaya et al., 2023). These targeted medicine strategies emphasize the necessity of integrating pharmacodynamic principles into practice to improve efficacy and minimize side effects for the treatment of cardiovascular disease, ultimately leading to improved patient care across various populations.

3.3.7. Neurological Disorders and Pharmacodynamics

The intricate relationship between pharmacodynamics and neurological diseases is in sharp relief when consideration is given to the central role that drug activity and drug interactions play in treating these conditions. Neurological diseases, from a wide range of pathologies including epilepsy, Parkinson's disease, and multiple sclerosis, are often in need of pharmacological intervention to alter symptoms and to improve the quality of life. Awareness of the pharmacodynamics of hallucinogens and psychostimulants is critical, since these substances are capable of causing significant neurotoxicity, such as seizures and movement disorders, as depicted in recent publications (Hass et al., 2024). Additionally, the development of new candidate drugs, particularly those involving pyrimidine platforms, has promise in the treatment of neurological disorders through the delivery of increased potency and acceptable pharmacokinetic profiles, which are necessary for optimum improvement in therapy (Nammalwar et al., 2024). As such, the intricate knowledge of pharmacodynamics plays a crucial role in designing effective treatment regimens for patients suffering from neurological ailments (Figure 3.15).

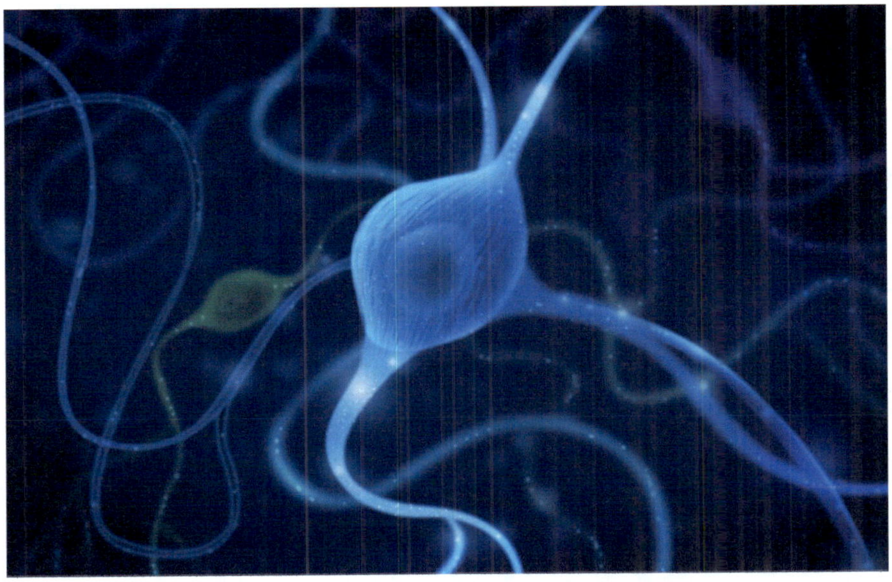

Figure 3.15. Neurological disorders and pharmacodynamics.

Source: https://criver.widen.net/content/t7ajs90alv/jpeg/DS-neurons-no-mea-chips-updated.jpg.

3.3.8. Antidepressants and Mood Stabilizers

Pharmacodynamics of mood stabilizers and antidepressants reveal their pivotal roles in the treatment of mood disorders with emphasis on the differential responses of patients. Antidepressants, such as the selective serotonin reuptake inhibitors (SSRIs), act predominantly through the enhancement of serotonin levels in the synaptic cleft with subsequent mood and emotional modulation. Mood stabilizers like lithium and certain anticonvulsants, on the other hand, modulate mood swings particularly in bipolar disorder (BD). Recent developments in pharmacogenomic testing provide the promise of enhancing drug efficacy; there is evidence that testing of some cytochrome P450 genes can inform selection and dosage of various antidepressants and mood stabilizers, recognized by the International Society of Psychiatric Genetics (Bousman et al., 2020). Furthermore, drugs like cannabidiol (CBD) are also being researched for their anxiolytic as well as neuroprotective potential, which is indicative of the evolving nature of pharmacotherapy in psychiatry (Crippa et al., 2018). Understanding these forces is crucial for maximizing treatment regimens.

3.3.9. Implications for Chronic Disease Management

Long-term disease management is continually demonstrating the complexities involved in taking care of patients, particularly with the emphasis on pharmacodynamics, drawing attention to how drug effects interact with patient responses. Successful management is knowing psychosocial issues, which say a lot about drug treatment adherence and health outcomes, as is highlighted in Tinuoye et al. (2024). Moreover, the integration of telepharmacy in the management of chronic conditions has appeared to close gaps in care and enhance dialogue between patients and healthcare providers. In Hussain et al., (2024), pharmacists play a central role in this transition, assisting in improving medication adherence through individualized interventions as well as alleviating social determinants of health. Thus, a multidisciplinary approach with an integration of both pharmacological and psychosocial interventions is essential in maximizing patient outcomes. This embraces the implications and opens the door to more integrated models of healthcare that facilitate empowering patients to effectively self-manage chronic illness (Figure 3.16).

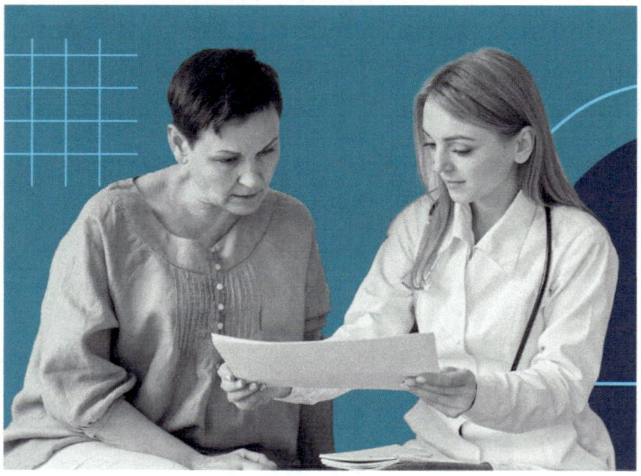

Figure 3.16. Effective management requires a comprehensive understanding of psychosocial factors, which can significantly influence treatment adherence and health outcomes.

Source: https://creyos.com/hubfs/Patient%20 Compliance-1.png.

Test Your Knowledge

1. Why is it important to know the pharmacodynamics of a drug in clinical practice?
2. How can two drugs have the same efficacy but different potencies?

Summary

The science of pharmacodynamics is of critical significance in understanding how drugs work in biological systems, particularly across a heterogeneous population like the elderly population. In the growing population of elderly patients, healthcare providers should remain aware of the enhanced risk factor of perioperative problems, particularly those of neuromuscular blockade (Bertoncello et al., 2017). The complexities of aging further underscore the necessity for vigilant monitoring and reversal treatments, as standard protocols may be insufficient in this risk group. Further, advances in pharmacogenetics with technology offer hope for personalized medicine, with drug responses formulated according to genetic variations, enhancing therapeutic gains and minimizing adverse effects (Fenech et al., 2014). This intersection of pharmacodynamics and the latest scientific knowledge highlights the necessity for continuous research and updating of clinical practice to ensure patient safety and efficacy remain top of the agenda in pharmacology.

In a summary of the key points of pharmacodynamics, the most significant is the realization of the intricate interplay of drug effects and biologic responses. This involves the mechanisms whereby drugs interact with various receptors and enzymes and influence physiology in positive and negative directions. Understanding these interactions is essential to modifying therapeutic strategies to address the specific needs of the individual patient, particularly in response to evolving guidelines. Health practitioners are advised to apply proven guidelines while relying on their clinical judgment in the practice of their profession, according to existing policies that emphasize the practitioners' role in staying informed with the new evidence developed (Mach et al., 2019). Furthermore, the necessity to adhere to the most recent recommendations from public health authorities cannot be overstressed, advocating for the necessity of evidence-based decision-making in prescribing and drug administration (Cosentino et al., 2019). Overall, knowledge of pharmacodynamics is critical to ensuring maximum therapeutic value and minimizing risk for adverse effects in patient treatment.

KEY TERMS FROM THIS CHAPTER

- Genetic heterogeneity
- Ginkgetin
- Ginkgo biloba extract
- Immunosuppression
- Inhibitors
- Ion channels
- Ligand binding models
- Occupancy levels
- Pharmacodynamics
- Pharmacotherapeutics
- Polymorphisms
- Postbiotics signals
- Proteins
- Receptor theory
- Rheumatoid arthritis
- Second messengers
- Sex-specific pharmacotherapy
- Signal transduction pathways

Critical Thinking Questions

1. **The term "efficacy" in pharmacodynamics refers to:**
   a. The ability of a drug to produce a desired therapeutic effect
   b. The concentration of the drug in plasma
   c. The ability of a drug to bind to a receptor
   d. The dose at which a drug produces half its maximum effect
2. **A drug that binds to a receptor and produces a response similar to the naturally occurring substance is called:**
   a. Antagonist
   b. Partial agonist
   c. Agonist
   d. Inverse agonist
3. **Which of the following best describes a competitive antagonist?**
   a. It binds to the receptor and induces a physiological response
   b. It binds to the receptor and blocks the effect of the agonist
   c. It does not affect receptor activity
   d. It causes an opposite physiological effect to the agonist
4. **What is the difference between potency and efficacy?**
   a. Potency refers to the maximum effect a drug can produce, while efficacy refers to the dose required to create that effect
   b. Potency refers to the amount of drug needed for a desired effect, while efficacy refers to the maximum effect a drug can produce
   c. Potency and efficacy are the same concept
   d. Efficacy refers to the dose of the drug, while potency refers to the duration of action
5. **Which of the following best describes a partial agonist?**
   a. It produces a maximal response regardless of the dose
   b. It binds to the receptor but produces a weaker response than a full agonist
   c. It blocks the action of a full agonist
   d. It does not bind to the receptor

Answers to Critical Thinking Questions

1. (a); 2. (c); 3. (b); 4. (b); 5. (b).

Short Answer Questions

1. What is pharmacodynamics, and how does it differ from pharmacokinetics?
2. Define the term "mechanism of action" about pharmacodynamics.
3. What are drug receptors, and why are they essential in pharmacodynamics?
4. Explain the difference between an agonist and an antagonist.
5. What is the significance of receptor selectivity in drug action?

References

1. Aartsma-Rus, A., Ferlini, A., Goemans, N., Pasmooij, A. M., Wells, D. J., Bushby, K., Vroom, E., & Balabanov, P. (2014). Translational and regulatory challenges for EXON skipping therapies. *Human Gene Therapy, 25*(10), 885–892. https://doi.org/10.1089/hum.2014.086Abduljalil, M., Aghazadeh-Habashi, A., Aigrain, S., Aitman, T., Al Za'abi, M., Alegre, M., Alnaqeeb, M., et al. (2019). Current trends in drug metabolism and pharmacokinetics. https://core.ac.uk/download/286361678.pdf (accessed on 10th June 2025).
2. Abduvalova, A., Akhmetzhanova, S., & Eshmakhanova, T. K. (2024). Overview of principles and methods of medical waste management and their application for database design. *Mechanics and Technologies*. https://www.semanticscholar.org/paper/c16d4fd3036a3f50693541fed3aa63415c5db884 (accessed on 10th June 2025).
3. Abikhzer, G., Treglia, G., Pelletier-Galarneau, M., Buscombe, J., Chiti, A., Dibble, E. H., Glaudemans, A., et al. (2024). EANM/SNMMI guideline/procedure standard for [18F]FDG hybrid PET use in infection and inflammation in adults v2.0. *European Journal of Nuclear Medicine and Molecular Imaging, 52*, 510–538. https://www.semanticscholar.org/paper/b8f71b56cbc6ac21c19414fa47416fd484335063 (accessed on 10th June 2025)
4. Allegaert, K., De Cock, P., De Paepe, P., Decaluwe, D., et al. (2019). Dose rationale and pharmacokinetics of dexmedetomidine in mechanically ventilated newborns: Impact of design optimization. https://core.ac.uk/download/227040958.pdf (accessed on 10th June 2025).
5. Al-Saigh, R., Aristea, V., Velegraki, M., Meletiadis, J., Siafakas, N., et al. (2013). Single-dose pharmacodynamics of amphotericin B against *Aspergillus* species in an *in vitro* pharmacokinetic/pharmacodynamic model. https://core.ac.uk/download/30436768.pdf (accessed on 10th June 2025).
6. Andersen, A. H. D., Zhang, Z., Hørsholt, S., Ritschel, T., & Jørgensen, J. B. (2023). Software principles and concepts applied in the implementation of cyber-physical systems for real-time advanced process control. *2023 European Control Conference (ECC)*. https://www.semanticscholar.org/paper/e7546fea5c9bdcdfbaa59d9ee320a262214994ef (accessed on 10th June 2025).
7. Andreozzi, F., Mannino, G. C., & Sesti, G. (2019). Pharmacogenetics of type 2 diabetes mellitus: The route toward tailored medicine. https://core.ac.uk/download/231747878.pdf (accessed on 10th June 2025).
8. Andrews, L. M., van Gelder, T., Hesselink, D. A., Peeters, P. A., et al. (2018). Personalized immunosuppression in elderly renal transplant recipients. https://core.ac.uk/download/154412022.pdf (accessed on 10th June 2025).
9. Androulakis, I. P., Bonate, P., Cheng, L., Cho, H., et al. (2022) Two heads are better than one: Current landscape of integrating QSP and machine learning. https://core.ac.uk/download/541068409.pdf (accessed on 10th June 2025).
10. Bakare, M. O. (2008). Effective therapeutic dosage of antipsychotic medications in patients with psychotic symptoms: Is there a racial difference? https://core.ac.uk/download/pdf/8163851.pdf (accessed on 10th June 2025).
11. Balato, A., Balato, N., Barrea, L., Di Somma, C., et al. (2016). Environmental risk factors in psoriasis: The point of view of the nutritionist. https://core.ac.uk/download/pdf/84246095.pdf (accessed on 10th June 2025).

12. Barke, E., Coghill, D., & Cornforth, C. (2010). Stimulant drug effects on attention deficit/hyperactivity disorder: A review of the effects of age and sex of patients. https://core.ac.uk/download/55797029.pdf (accessed on 10th June 2025).
13. Battaglia, F. P., Campbell, S., Dingeman, A., Filbert, M., Karki, P., Konradsen, F., Moorcraft, P., et al. (2016). Role of the calcium plateau in the neuronal injury and behavioral morbidities following organophosphate intoxication. https://core.ac.uk/download/84402779.pdf (accessed on 10th June 2025).
14. Bellini, T., Bonaccorsi, G., Bramanti, B., Carè, A., et al. (2019). "Bridging the gap": Everything that could have been avoided if we had applied gender medicine, pharmacogenetics and personalized medicine in the gender-omics and sex-omics era. https://core.ac.uk/download/286075866.pdf (accessed on 10th June 2025).
15. Benjeddou, M., & Peiró, A. (2021). Pharmacogenomics and prescription opioid use. *Pharmacogenomics*. https://www.semanticscholar.org/paper/2b022a51a34433ed16be1908d56c0b3d6b28acab (accessed on 10th June 2025).
16. Bertoncello, F., Carron, M., & Ieppariello, G. (2017). Profile of sugammadex for reversal of neuromuscular blockade in the elderly: Current perspectives. https://core.ac.uk/download/158825140.pdf (accessed on 10th June 2025).
17. Bousman, C. A., Bengesser, S., Aitchison, K. J., Amare, A. T., Aschauer, H. N., Baune, B. T., Behroozi Asl, B., et al. (2020). Review and consensus on pharmacogenomic testing in psychiatry. *Pharmacopsychiatry, 54*, 5–17. https://doi.org/10.1055/a-1288-1061.
18. Branford, R., Cregg, R., Gubbay, A., Russo, M., et al. (2013). Pharmacogenetics of analgesic drugs. https://core.ac.uk/download/29416244.pdf (accessed on 10th June 2025).
19. Bruno, P., D'Ascanio, M., Fiorentino, C., Grieco, A., et al. (2018). Metronomic chemotherapy with vinorelbine produces clinical benefit and low toxicity in frail elderly patients affected by advanced non-small cell lung cancer. https://core.ac.uk/download/188825346.pdf (accessed on 10th June 2025).
20. Burt, T., & Dhillon, S. (2013). Pharmacogenomics in early-phase clinical development. https://core.ac.uk/download/pdf/37750487.pdf (accessed on 10th June 2025).
21. Calderoni, D., Galli, F., & Guidetti, V. (2001). Up to date on the use of triptans for child and adolescent migraine: "The state of the art." https://core.ac.uk/download/54380698.pdf (accessed on 10th June 2025).
22. Cashen, A., Al Malki, M. M. A., Stevens, D. A., Muffly, L., Edwin, N., Abadir, E., Tan, P., et al. (2024). WUN101-01: First-in-human (FIH) Phase 1 study of WU-NK-101 (W-NK1) in patients with relapsed or refractory (R/R) acute myeloid leukemia (AML). *Blood*. https://www.semanticscholar.org/paper/a821d05ccb22613fc555616704df020308352dd1 (accessed on 10th June 2025).
23. Chaplain, M. A. J., Eftimie, R., & Macfarlane, F. R. (2019). Quantitative predictive modelling approaches to understanding rheumatoid arthritis: A brief review. https://core.ac.uk/download/286356117.pdf (accessed on 10th June 2025).
24. Chelliah, V., & van der Graaf, P. H. (2022). Model-informed target identification and validation through combining quantitative systems pharmacology with network-based analysis. *CPT: Pharmacometrics & Systems Pharmacology, 11*, 399–402. https://doi.org/10.1002/psp4.12766.

25. Cintron, N. M., & Putcha, L. (2025). Pharmacokinetics and pharmacodynamics in space. https://core.ac.uk/download/pdf/42806060.pdf (accessed on 10th June 2025).

26. Cosentino, F., Grant, P. J., Aboyans, V., Bailey, C. J., Ceriello, A., Delgado, V., Federici, M., et al. (2019). 2019 ESC guidelines on diabetes, pre-diabetes, and cardiovascular diseases developed in collaboration with the EASD. *European Heart Journal, 41*, 255–323. https://doi.org/10.1093/eurheartj/ehz486.

27. Crippa, J. A., Guimarães, F. S., Campos, A. C., & Zuardi, A. W. (2018). Translational investigation of the therapeutic potential of cannabidiol (CBD): Toward a new age. *Frontiers in Immunology, 9*, 2009. https://doi.org/10.3389/fimmu.2018.02009.

28. Debras, C., Córdova, R., Mayén, A. L., Maasen, K., Knaze, V., Eussen, S. J. P. M., Schalkwijk, C. G., et al. (2024). Dietary intake of Di carbonyl compounds and changes in body weight over time in a large cohort of European adults. *British Journal of Nutrition, 131*, 1902–1914. https://www.semanticscholar.org/paper/db25576005942e90d4dab4fa761d832742bbcfa3 (accessed on 10th June 2025).

29. Demissie, K., Jian-Yu, E., Graber, J. M., Lin, Y., et al. (2017). Differential and joint effects of metformin and statins on overall survival of elderly patients with pancreatic adenocarcinoma: A large population-based study. https://core.ac.uk/download/129191624.pdf (accessed on 10th June 2025).

30. Deshpande, D. A., Michael, J. V., Nayak, A. P., Shah, S. A., et al. (2019). Bitter taste receptors for asthma therapeutics. https://core.ac.uk/download/225130683.pdf (accessed on 10th June 2025).

31. do Carmo, A., Rocha, M. J., Pereirinha, P., Tomé, R., & Costa, E. (2023). Antifungals: From pharmacokinetics to clinical practice. *Antibiotics, 12*, 884. https://doi.org/10.3390/antibiotics12050884.

32. Dünser, B., Möller, A., Anđić, B., Lampert, P., Bergmann-Gering, A., & Pany, P. (2024). (Re) growing plant awareness: A Delphi study. *Plants, People, Planet*. https://www.semanticscholar.org/paper/f940f74af8803016e15a2a251796f80505805a67 (accessed on 10th June 2025).

33. Fajria, A. K. (Arsitania), Maziyyah, N. (Nurul), & Nurdianto, A. (Apri). (2018). Identification of potential drug interaction with complementary and alternative medicines among chronic disease outpatients. https://core.ac.uk/download/480549507.pdf (accessed on 10th June 2025).

34. Fenech, A. G., & Grech, G. (2009). *Biotech Drugs: Biological Therapeutic Agents*. https://core.ac.uk/download/46603869.pdf (accessed on 10th June 2025).

35. Gandhi, M., Aweeka, F., Greenblatt, R., & Blaschke, T. (2004). Sex differences in pharmacokinetics and pharmacodynamics. *Annual Review of Pharmacology and Toxicology, 44*, 499–523. https://www.semanticscholar.org/paper/8a2ffe22658c970c92571c2e29f656ca20580734 (accessed on 10th June 2025).

36. García-Cremades, M., Solans, B. P., Strydom, N., Vrijens, B., Pillai, G., Shaffer, C., Thomas, B. V., et al. (2021). Emerging therapeutics, technologies, and drug development strategies to address patient nonadherence and improve tuberculosis treatment. *Annual Review of Pharmacology and Toxicology*. https://www.semanticscholar.org/paper/832b8ac4ddb358eaf5ca110a92d567dffa31eeb5 (accessed on 10th June 2025).

37. Gigante, B., Tamargo, J., Agewall, S., Atar, D., ten Berg, J., Campo, G., Cerbai, E., et al. (2024). Update on antithrombotic therapy and body mass: A clinical consensus statement of the ESC Working Group on Cardiovascular Pharmacotherapy and the ESC Working Group on Thrombosis. *European Heart Journal: Cardiovascular Pharmacotherapy*. https://www.semanticscholar.org/paper/25180e717b5f8fea21de65d1df2b869630ec2ecf (accessed on 10th June 2025).

38. Giovagnoli, A., & Zagoraiou, M. (2025). Simulated clinical trials: Some design issues. https://core.ac.uk/download/pdf/6820410.pdf (accessed on 10th June 2025).

39. Glaviano, A., Foo, A. S. C., Lam, H. Y., Yap, K. C. Y., Jacot, W., Jones, R. H., Eng, H., et al. (2023). PI3K/AKT/mTOR signaling transduction pathway and targeted therapies in cancer. *Molecular Cancer, 22*. https://doi.org/10.1186/s12943-023-01827-6.

40. Gourlay, D., & Heit, H. (2010). The art and science of urine drug testing. *The Clinical Journal of Pain, 26*(4), 358. https://www.semanticscholar.org/paper/66e393caabfc00e4ac65586c59a1ab3777679231 (accessed on 10th June 2025).

41. Halvorsen, S., Mehilli, J., Cassese, S., Hall, T. S., Abdelhamid, M., Barbato, E., De Hert, S., et al. (2022). 2022 ESC Guidelines on cardiovascular assessment and management of patients undergoing non-cardiac surgery. *European Heart Journal, 43*, 3826–3924. https://doi.org/10.1093/eurheartj/ehac270.

42. Hass, R. M., & Stitt, D. W. (2024). Neurological effects of stimulants and hallucinogens. *Seminars in Neurology, 44*, 459–470. https://www.semanticscholar.org/paper/11e119ca927f12666fb9e8e8bd7b224de0b0be56 (accessed on 10th June 2025).

43. Hu, B., Zhong, L., Weng, Y., Peng, L., Huang, Y., Zhao, Y., & Liang, X. J. (2020). Therapeutic siRNA: State of the art. *Signal Transduction and Targeted Therapy, 5*. https://doi.org/10.1038/s41392-020-0207-x.

44. Hussain, A., & Bowen, A. M. (2024). Exploring pharmacist roles in tele pharmacy for chronic disease management in New York State: A qualitative inquiry into improving implementation, patient communication, and healthcare technology support. *Cureus, 16*. https://www.semanticscholar.org/paper/f8905e3c37958f199dd2250e082b73e4d948ae87 (accessed on 10th June 2025).

45. Jiang, X., Kim, J., Menon, A., Ohno-Machado, L., et al. (2012). Doubly optimized calibrated support vector machine (DOC-SVM): An algorithm for joint optimization of discrimination and calibration. https://core.ac.uk/download/323066649.pdf (accessed on 10th June 2025).

46. Jovanović, M., & Vučićević, K. (2022). Pediatric pharmacokinetic considerations and implications for drug dosing. *Arhiv za farmaciju*. https://www.semanticscholar.org/paper/4ce69b7b72da3306780562557512238aeba33347 (accessed on 10th June 2025).

47. Kasim, H. F. (2022). Effects of cigarette smoking on the response of hypertensive patients to beta-adrenergic antagonists: A narrative review. *Journal of Ideas in Health*. https://www.semanticscholar.org/paper/f46918679b953b8bc3be8f92d4747bbbb50d38b1 (accessed on 10th June 2025).

48. Khanal, S., Shrestha, S., & Shrestha, S. (2019). Polypharmacy in elderly cancer patients: Challenges and the way clinical pharmacists can contribute in resource-limited settings. https://core.ac.uk/download/287605655.pdf (accessed on 10th June 2025).

49. Klauer, M. J., Willette, B. K. A., & Tsvetanova, N. G. (2024). Functional diversification of cell

signaling by GPCR localization. *Journal of Biological Chemistry, 300*, 105668. https://doi.org/10.1016/j.jbc.2024.105668.

50. Kumar, A., Green, K. M., & Rawat, M. (2024). A comprehensive overview of postbiotics with a special focus on discovery techniques and clinical applications. *Foods, 13*. https://www.semanticscholar.org/paper/365c66918755cba7f8ef38522982bae7a90fe5dd (accessed on 10th June 2025).

51. Lakhan, S. (2025). Introducing digital pharmacometrics: A pharmacokinetics (PK)/pharmacodynamics (PD) framework for prescription digital therapeutics. *Cureus, 17*. https://www.semanticscholar.org/paper/80f5b30ccdc0a317ab46ffd3653f9070584e0705 (accessed on 10th June 2025).

52. Lee, E. Y., de Lannoy, L., Li, L., de Barros, M. I. A., Bentsen, P., Brussoni, M., Fiskum, T., et al. (2022). Play, learn, and teach outdoors—Network (PLaTO-Net): Terminology, taxonomy, and ontology. *The International Journal of Behavioral Nutrition and Physical Activity, 19*. https://www.semanticscholar.org/paper/71f390908c2502070f05d468f3e72d5ab0431e5a (accessed on 10th June 2025).

53. Li, S., Pan, W., Tao, C., Hu, Z., Cheng, B., Chen, J., & Peng, X. (2024). Small-molecule modulators targeting coactivator-associated arginine methyltransferase 1 (CARM1) as therapeutic agents for cancer treatment: Current medicinal chemistry insights and emerging opportunities. *Journal of Medicinal Chemistry*. https://www.semanticscholar.org/paper/0129f589adc28f134b5a6e8c1d1e5d2cbe385a30 (accessed on 10th June 2025).

54. Liu, C., Fu, C., Sun, J., Lu, Y., Pan, J., Li, Y. J., Wang, Y. L., et al. (2024). Material basis and mechanism of Bletilla Rhizome for melasma, gastrointestinal hemorrhage, lung cancer, and bronchopulmonary inflammation as "homotherapy for heteropathy" based on UHPLC-Q-Exactive Orbitrap HRMS coupled with network pharmacology and molecular docking. *Zhongguo Zhong Yao Za Zhi = China Journal of Chinese Materia Medica, 49*(13), 3552–3565. https://www.semanticscholar.org/paper/40ab017be1bafb717fb82e2ef592b938d0869c12 (accessed on 10th June 2025).

55. Liu, Y., Ye, J., Fan, Z., Wu, X., Zhang, Y., Yang, R., Jiang, B., et al. (2024). Ginkgetin alleviates inflammation and senescence by targeting STING. *Advanced Science, 12*. https://www.semanticscholar.org/paper/00425a95851a6fbc8fbccaa027b3cf938540d006 (accessed on 10th June 2025).

56. Lu, J., Wang, X., Wan, L. L., Fu, J., Huo, Y., Zhao, Y., & Guo, C. (2020). Gene polymorphisms affecting the pharmacokinetics and pharmacodynamics of donepezil efficacy. *Frontiers in Pharmacology, 11*. https://www.semanticscholar.org/paper/75272f1d5bd3c01bbd9c67f2002de36c509d40d9 (accessed on 10th June 2025).

57. Mach, F., Baigent, C., Catapano, A. L., Koskinas, K. C., Casula, M., Badimón, L., Chapman, M. J., et al. (2019). 2019 ESC/EAS guidelines for the management of dyslipidemias: Lipid modification to reduce cardiovascular risk. *European Heart Journal, 41*, 111–188. https://doi.org/10.1093/eurheartj/ehz455.

58. Martelletti, P. (2018). The journey from genetic predisposition to medication overuse headache to its acquisition as sequela of chronic migraine. https://core.ac.uk/download/188821918.pdf (accessed on 10th June 2025).

59. Marucci, G., Buccioni, M., Dal Ben, D., Lambertucci, C., Volpini, R., & Amenta, F. (2020). Efficacy of acetylcholinesterase inhibitors in Alzheimer's disease. *Neuropharmacology, 190*, 108352. https://doi.org/10.1016/j.neuropharm.2020.108352.

60. Mian, H., Baljevic, M., Magen, H., Gatt, M. E., Mazza, I. A., Searle, E., Lichtman, E., et al. (2024). A phase 1b study of step-up dosing with ABBV-383, a B-cell maturation antigen (BCMA) × CD3 bispecific antibody, in patients with relapsed or refractory multiple myeloma. *Blood*. https://www.semanticscholar.org/paper/0434a7b2e0f602274cf86ccbe98ba9b117bb0d7e (accessed on 10th June 2025).

61. Miethke, M., Pieroni, M., Weber, T., Brönstrup, M., Hammann, P., Halby, L., Arimondo, P. B., et al. (2021). Towards the sustainable discovery and development of new antibiotics. *Nature Reviews Chemistry, 5*, 726–749. https://doi.org/10.1038/s41570-021-00313-1.

62. Milligan, G. (2017). G protein-coupled receptors not currently in the spotlight: free fatty acid receptor 2 and GPR35. https://core.ac.uk/download/96883167.pdf (accessed on 10th June 2025).

63. Moore, J. N., Poon, L., Pahwa, S., Bensman, T., Wei, X., Danielsen, Z. Y., & Jang, S. (2023). Animal pharmacokinetics/pharmacodynamics (PK/PD) infection models for clinical development of antibacterial drugs: Lessons from selected cases. *The Journal of Antimicrobial Chemotherapy*. https://www.semanticscholar.org/paper/98b31527112ddb143de8de71545f37eed2b4f430 (accessed on 10th June 2025).

64. Naik, S. R., & Gamare, D. (2025). Evidenced-based phytotherapy overview: Protective role of diverse bioactive phytochemicals in myocardial ischemia through pharmacodynamics and molecular mechanisms. *Journal of Cardiovascular Medicine and Cardiology*. https://www.semanticscholar.org/paper/d8ad6f33026b48ab64a7c0aa4d4d0fd80e4452c3 (accessed on 10th June 2025).

65. Najjar, R. (2023). Redefining radiology: A review of artificial intelligence integration in medical imaging. *Diagnostics, 13*, 2760. https://doi.org/10.3390/diagnostics13172760.

66. Nammalwar, B., & Bunce, R. (2024). Recent advances in pyrimidine-based drugs. *Pharmaceuticals, 17*. https://www.semanticscholar.org/paper/951d743ab701596353f6beafbfb3191621e47a1a (accessed on 10th June 2025).

67. Nishtala, P. S., & Salahudeen, M. S. (2017). An overview of pharmacodynamic modelling, ligand-binding approach and its application in clinical practice. https://core.ac.uk/download/pdf/82752689.pdf (accessed on 10th June 2025).

68. Onder, G., Petrovic, M., & van der Cammen, T. (2012). Adverse drug reactions in older people: Detection and prevention. https://core.ac.uk/download/55848564.pdf (accessed on 10th June 2025).

69. Papachristos, A., Patel, J., Vasileiou, M., & Patrinos, G. (2023). Dose optimization in oncology drug development: The emerging role of pharmacogenomics, pharmacokinetics, and pharmacodynamics. *Cancers, 15*. https://www.semanticscholar.org/paper/d1127377a15830107ed4800ea6cd68939732b788 (accessed on 10th June 2025).

70. Popovskaya, D. P., Shevtsova, V. I., Shevtsov, A. N., & Zuikova, A. A. (2023). Assessment of the rationality of pharmacotherapy in elderly patients with cardiovascular diseases using STOPP/START non-compliance models. *Medical Scientific Bulletin of Central Chernozemic.*

https://www.semanticscholar.org/paper/b688c80ae5db3a10191a520241caab9b7d35e88a (accessed on 10th June 2025).

71. Sánchez-Pozos, K., Granados-Silvestre, M., & Ortiz-López, M. G. (2021). From pharmacogenetics to gene expression: Implications for precision medicine in diabetes. *Drug Metabolism*. https://www.semanticscholar.org/paper/d18a7fd92e3c78ca6cb2cf008a194df45fe6fa04 (accessed on 10th June 2025).

72. Schuessler-Lenz, M., Enzmann, H., & Vamvakas, S. (2019). Regulators' advice can make a difference: European Medicines Agency approval of Zynteglo for beta thalassemia. *Clinical Pharmacology & Therapeutics, 107*, 492–494. https://doi.org/10.1002/cpt.1639.

73. Spadi, J., Scherf-Clavel, M., Leutritz, A. L., Hütz, B., Matentzoglu, M., Nieberler, M., Kurlbaum, M., et al. (2024). Changes in psychotropic drug concentrations across the menstrual cycle: A pilot study. *Therapeutic Drug Monitoring, 46*, 195–202. https://www.semanticscholar.org/paper/f24536e15d25d130918b2fe686560c969ab53daf (accessed on 10th June 2025).

74. Sultana, R., Rahman, M. N., Yusuf, M. S., & Karim, M. S. (2025). Therapeutic potential of Inderjo Talkh (*Holarrhena antidysenterica*) in Unani medicine: An in-depth study. *Journal of Drug Delivery and Therapeutics*. https://www.semanticscholar.org/paper/3017dbc85443ed5b6e31b658a2e2c550c5e31536 (accessed on 10th June 2025).

75. Tabin-Barczak, W., Mazur, M., Waz, D., Szarłowicz, J., Goliszek, Z., Sobek, K. Ł., Sokołowska, A., et al. (2025). Multidisciplinary pain management in oncology: Balancing opioid use and alternative therapies. *Quality in Sport*. https://www.semanticscholar.org/paper/8c220640b7a973ae4d17139b96b7dfc998c2878a (accessed on 10th June 2025).

76. Tamrazova, O. V., & Glukhova, E. A. (2025). Diffuse telogen effluvium: Etiology, pathogenesis, and a comprehensive approach to treatment. *Meditsinskiy Sovet = Medical Council*. https://www.semanticscholar.org/paper/013dbc0fd93c83a2d4c1c36d71d0f915158b70b5 (accessed on 10th June 2025).

77. Terzic, A., & Waldman, S. A. (2017). Process improvement for maximized therapeutic innovation outcome. https://core.ac.uk/download/155271556.pdf (accessed on 10th June 2025).

78. Tinuoye, M. O., Calistus, E., Agbomola, J. O., Ipede, O., Karakitie, L. O., Ogunsina, A. J., Temitope, K., et al. (2024). Psychosocial factors in chronic disease management: Implications for health psychology. *International Journal of Science and Research Archive*. https://www.semanticscholar.org/paper/9467e371bb1a141667e91616f2246e960838a714 (accessed on 10th June 2025).

79. Virani, M. (2009). Assessing culture competence among nurses in an acute care setting. https://core.ac.uk/download/223074332.pdf (accessed on 10th June 2025).

80. Visseren, F. L. J., Mach, F., Smulders, Y. M., Carballo, D., Koskinas, K. C., Bäck, M., Bénétos, A., et al. (2021). 2021 ESC guidelines on cardiovascular disease prevention in clinical practice. *European Heart Journal, 42*, 3227–3337. https://doi.org/10.1093/eurheartj/ehab484.

81. Waddar, S. B., Chalageri, C. C., & Waddar, S. B. (2025). Role of Sarjarasa Malahara in the management of Padadari (Cracked Feet): Case study. *Journal of Ayurveda and Integrated Medical Sciences*. https://www.semanticscholar.org/paper/6872820401d9bd6d87bdb751ee96c8e2f9f6384b (accessed on 10th June 2025).

82. Wang, F., Babel, H., Schmitt, V., Uddin, M. E., Baljevic, M., Voorhees, P., Rodriguez, C., et al.

(2024). Exposure-response (ER) and pharmacokinetic/pharmacodynamic (PK/PD) analyses for optimal step-up dose (SUD) selection to improve cytokine release syndrome (CRS) safety profile of ABBV-383 in patients with relapsed or refractory multiple myeloma (RRMM). *Blood*. https://www.semanticscholar.org/paper/23c73f969fe8ecee6590b9759101ba74bf8ffae8 (accessed on 10th June 2025).

83. Wang, L., Wang, N., Zhang, W., Cheng, X., Yan, Z., Shao, G., Wang, X., et al. (2022). Therapeutic peptides: Current applications and future directions. *Signal Transduction and Targeted Therapy, 7*. https://doi.org/10.1038/s41392-022-00904-4.

84. Wong, M. T., Lin, P. H., Lin, W. C., Peng, C. J., Wright, J. D., Lee, H. J., Chu, H. M., et al. (2025). 2FA-Platform generates dual fatty acid-conjugated GLP-1 receptor agonist TE-8105 with enhanced diabetes, obesity, and NASH efficacy compared to semaglutide. *Journal of Medicinal Chemistry, 68*, 6178–6192. https://www.semanticscholar.org/paper/bc97b09c521160d47419eb7df8a1acaa42205151 (accessed on 10th June 2025).

85. Xing, Y., Czachorowski, A., Lim, J., & Wise, S. (2024). Abstract 6005: Generation of new oncology cell models through long-term acclimation under hypoxic and hyperbaric culture conditions. *Cancer Research*. https://www.semanticscholar.org/paper/0944f477994e91cbee340faacac2ba62749bef79 (accessed on 10th June 2025).

86. Yalçın, N., & Demirkan, K. (2022). Management of drug-related problems including drug–drug interactions caused by nirmatrelvir/ritonavir in pediatric patients with SARS-CoV-2. *Archives of Disease in Childhood, 108*, e16. https://www.semanticscholar.org/paper/cd744bb751c1472c921fbc2510d857ed0c190203 (accessed on 10th June 2025).

87. Zhou, J., Rao, R., Shapiro, M. E., Tania, N., Herron, C., Musante, C., & Hughes, J. H. (2025). Model-informed drug development applications and opportunities in mRNA-LNP therapeutics. *Clinical Pharmacology and Therapeutics*. https://www.semanticscholar.org/paper/917e28039cb93376cf3907e75edca00d0443f795 (accessed on 10th June 2025).

88. Zhou, Y., Wang, F., Tang, J., Nussinov, R., & Cheng, F. (2020). Artificial intelligence in COVID-19 drug repurposing. *The Lancet Digital Health, 2*, e667–e676. https://doi.org/10.1016/s2589-7500(20)30192-8.

DRUG DEVELOPMENT AND CLINICAL TRIALS

4

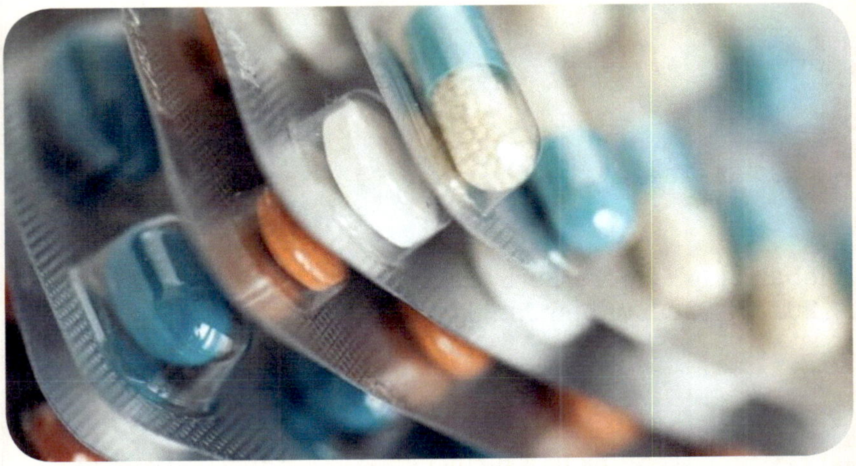

LEARNING OBJECTIVES

After studying this chapter, you will be able to:

1. Understand the drug development process
2. Explain clinical trial design
3. Focus on the regulatory framework
4. Discuss ethical considerations in drug trials

Introduction

Introduction to clinical trials and drug development is characterized by the utmost importance of determining effective therapies in an increasingly complex medical landscape. Traditional preclinical models are often not sufficient to forecast drug efficacy in clinical settings, particularly in oncology, where drugs against cancer are highly heterogeneous in their translation between laboratory results and patient response. As stated, there is an urgent need for preclinical models incorporating the tumor microenvironment (TME) to enhance drug selection efficacy before running clinical trials (Cox et al., 2023). Further, with advances in therapeutic modalities, particularly for inflammatory diseases, a cautious approach is recommended in determining the relative efficacy of newer agents compared to current standards. Despite progress in drug discovery and growth in agents being tried in clinical trials, many new treatments have identical ceilings of efficacy to the treatments of years ago, a reflection of the complexity of mechanisms of disease that demand new strategies such as cutting-edge combination therapies (Danese et al., 2022) (Figure 4.1).

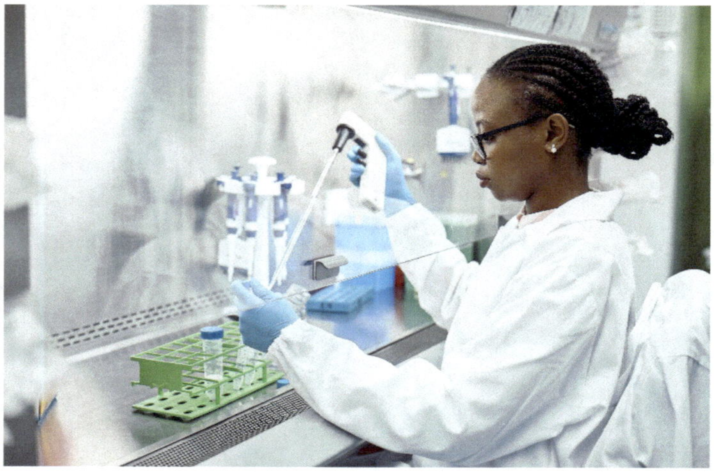

Figure 4.1. Decentralized clinical trials.

Source: https://cdn.aglty.io/phrma/global/blog/import/hero/Decentralized%20clinical%20trials%20and%20the%20future%20of%20drug%20development.jpg.

4.1. The Drug Development Process

Learning Outcome

1. Know the stages of drug development
2. Explain preclinical research and testing
3. Describe investigational new drug (IND) application
4. Learn the phases of clinical trials
5. Understand collaboration with academic institutions
6. Discuss funding and investment in drug development
7. Identify challenges faced during development
8. Know success rates and timelines

The process of developing a drug is a multifaceted and intricate process involving numerous phases, all aimed at ultimately creating new medicines that are effective as well as safe for human use. Following the discovery stage, scientists carry out preclinical testing to screen candidate compounds *in vitro* and *in vivo* before advancing to clinical trials. A significant component of this phase is the gathering and management of clinical trial data that is required to achieve regulatory approval from bodies such as the Food and Drug Administration (FDA). Effective management of data, for example, through electronic data capture, enhances the efficacy and reliability of trials, reducing the time taken as well as the cost of drug development (Banerjee et al., 2016). Furthermore, the advent of quantum computing has paradigm-shifting possibilities to streamline the drug discovery process through rapid molecular simulations and improved predictive modeling, potentially also reducing development times and maximizing therapeutic effect (Hassan et al., 2023).

4.1.1. Stages of Drug Development

Phases of drug development are of prime importance in ensuring the efficacy and safety of drug interventions before reaching the market. Firstly, drug discovery involves the identification of potential therapeutic agents through several approaches, including the identification of natural products that yield a high ratio of successful drug candidates, as cited in Domingo-Fernández et al., (2024). After lead compounds are discovered, they are then subjected to preclinical testing, during which laboratory and animal tests measure their toxicity and biological activity. After proving preclinical efficacy, drugs move into clinical trials, a sequence of three phases to increasingly evaluate safety and efficacy in human populations. The increasing rate of natural products moving towards subsequent stages of clinical trials indicates their pharmacological utility as drug-like molecules, reflecting a shift in paradigm towards more effective pharmacological intervention (Domingo-Fernández et al., 2024). Also, epigenetic advances in the recent past reflect the imperative to determine molecular mechanisms behind disease, ultimately opening the floodgates for improved drug discovery and personalized medicine approaches (Figure 4. 2).

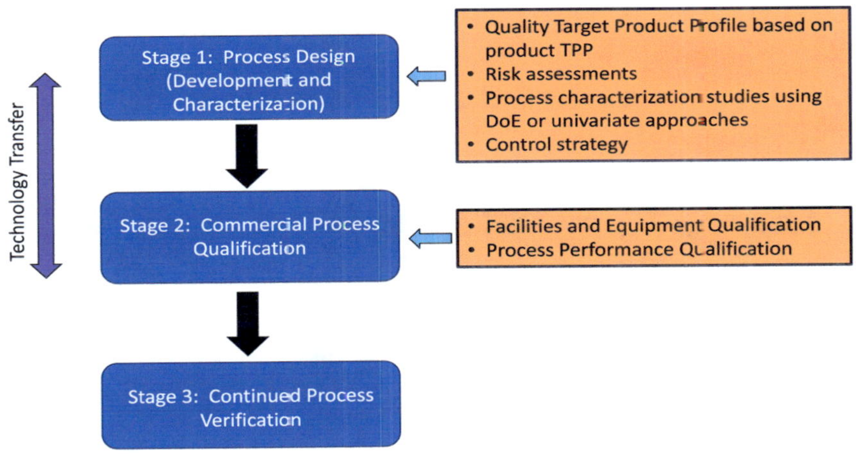

Figure 4.2. The stages of drug development are critical in ensuring the safety and efficacy of pharmaceutical interventions before they reach the market.

Source: https://jpharmsci.org/cms/10.1016/j.xphs.2023.11.004/asset/1e6275ff-b79d-4fc9-a5d8-8d14364c4606/main.assets/gr2_lrg.jpg.

4.1.2. Preclinical Research and Testing

Preclinical studies and experiments are crucial supports of drug development, marking the transition from fundamental research to clinical application. Preclinical experiments generally involve both *in vitro* and *in vivo* experiments that are aimed at assessing the safety and efficacy of a potential drug candidate before transitioning to human trials. According to (Gooneratne et al., 2019), the development cost of drugs ranges from $2 to $3 billion. It lasts for 7 to 12 years, highlighting the need for extensive preclinical trials for risk reduction and regulatory sanction. Moreover, the intricacies involved in the development of drugs against diseases with a high level of complexity, such as diseases of the brain, mandate novel testing strategies. As stated by (Gazerani et al.,

2024), traditional animal models are generally non-translational due to interspecies variability, and therefore, human brain organoids emerged as a helpful alternative. All such progresses can enhance the reproducibility of preclinical assessment and hence facilitate the transition to the clinic.

4.1.3. Investigational New Drug (IND) Application

The Investigational New Drug (IND) filing is a milestone in the pipeline of developing drugs, and it is the gateway through which new drugs come into clinical trials. When submitted, the IND should have sufficient evidence for the safety and efficacy of the drug, which is not only crucial for approval by the regulatory authority, but also for the safety of patients when on trial. In particular, the intracompound complexity of preparing medications for rare diseases adds to these issues, as attested by the FDAs modest approval rate for treatment of such conditions, highlighting remarkable gaps in therapies available (Bannister et al., 2018). There is an imperative for new answers, particularly among patients with terminal illnesses, wherein the necessity for such access to experimental treatments could endanger patients, as in Jolee Mohr's experience, who experienced dangerous side effects in a clinical trial (Sikora et al., 2008). Those kinds of cases highlight the thin line between advancing medical science and safeguarding patient health (Figure 4.3).

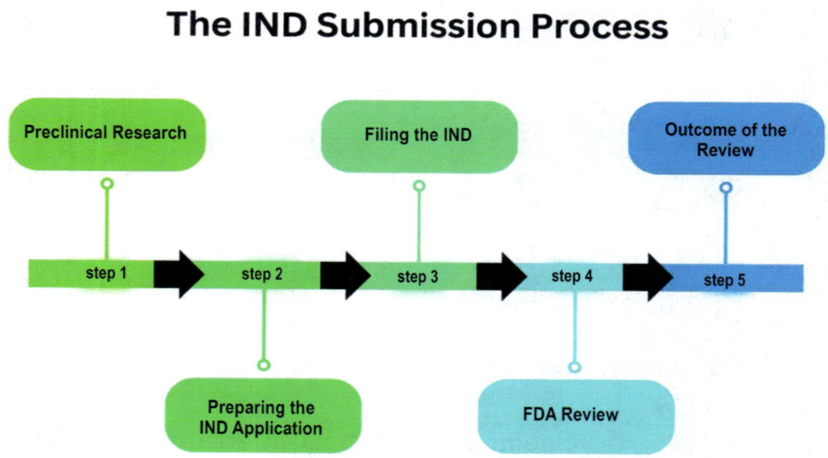

Figure 4.3. The investigational new drug (IND) application represents a critical juncture in the drug development process, serving as the gateway for new therapeutics to enter clinical trials.

Source: https://www.docshifter.com/wp-content/uploads/2025/01/the-ind-submission-process-668bc9a0774a9.webp.

4.1.4. Phases of Clinical Trials

Clinical trials are divided into distinct phases, each with unique goals and regulatory limitations essential to the assessment of new drugs' safety and effectiveness. Phase I clinical trials are primarily designed to assess the safety, pharmacokinetics, and pharmacodynamics of the drug in a small number of healthy volunteers, establishing appropriate dosing and watching for adverse effects. Phase II tests engage a larger number of participants, the focus being on the drug's efficacy and other safety protocols in a large group of patients of the same ailment. Following the success of these phases, Phase III tests involve massive-scale testing across multiple groups to confirm the efficacy and compare it with existing treatments. Of note critically has been the problem of representation by sex in medicine in the setting of these trials, and there is evidence to suggest that women were systematically underrepresented about disease prevalence rates (Dekker et al., 2021). Preclinical pharmacokinetic/pharmacodynamic studies also inform dosing and decision-making by complex networks in these stages, particularly in antibacterial drugs (Jorda et al., 2020).

4.1.5. Role of Pharmaceutical Companies

Pharmaceutical companies are the driving force behind drug discovery and clinical trials, promoting innovation in the form of substantial investment and research efforts. Drug corporations work with Contract Research Organizations (CROs) to improve the efficiency and professionalism of clinical research, even as they take on the important and expensive responsibility of introducing new medications to the market. As suggested, there has been rapid growth in outsourcing clinical research with the facilitation of the ability of pharmaceutical firms to tap into specialized competencies and technologies with CROs, a key determinant in navigating the involved territory of modern drug development (Fokunang et al., 2025). Besides, in the aftermath of acute health emergencies like the COVID-19 pandemic, pharmaceutical industries have made forays into new therapeutic classes, characterized by clinical trials for anti-inflammatory drugs that mitigate significant disease effects (Park et al., 2022). Thus, the operations of pharmaceutical companies extend beyond drug manufacturing; they are central to propelling innovations that affect public health (Figure 4.4).

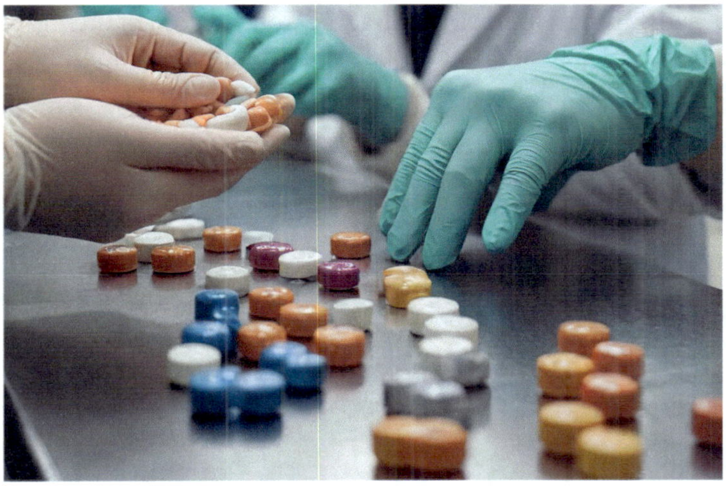

Figure 4.4. Pharmaceutical companies serve as the cornerstone of drug development and clinical trials, driving innovation through substantial investment and research efforts.

Source: https://synergbiopharma.com/wp-content/uploads/2024/09/drug-development.jpg.

4.1.6. Collaboration with Academic Institutions

Integrating academic institutions into the drug development and clinical trials process is vital for optimizing research output and driving innovation. Academic-industry collaboration among pharmaceutical companies and academia leverages domain knowledge, resources, and technology, and can potentially speed up the drug discovery process. For instance, the increasing number of clinical trials with a boost from collaborative networks demonstrates the effectiveness of collaborations in addressing public health problems such as tuberculosis, particularly in disease-endemic regions, since Brazil's input so heavily confirms (da Santos et al., 2024). Additionally, research indicates that positive relationships in interdisciplinary cooperation are frequently linked to successful clinical trials, suggesting that trial success is ensured by diversity in partnerships between big pharmaceutical companies, academic institutions, and other organizations (Lin et al., 2020). Through leading these cooperative systems, stakeholders can all collaborate to navigate the complexities of drug development better, ultimately toward accessible and effective therapeutic interventions for disadvantaged populations.

4.1.7. Funding and Investment in Drug Development

The investment and funding environment for drug development is complex, with numerous both public and private stakeholders affecting it. The federal government is the largest public financier, especially for diseases with no cure or effective treatments, such as Alzheimer's disease, where institutes like the National Institute on Aging and the National Institute of Mental Health play an important role in financing research activities (Cummings et al., 2018). This public investment is essential, as vaccine development demonstrates; firms are not willing to invest heavily because the costs are substantial and the risk of failure high, necessitating substantial public investment to offset such hindrances (Veugelers et al., 2020). Moreover, charity programs and pressure groups significantly complement public investment, bridging the gap usually encountered in drug discovery phases. Therefore, the overlap between these diverse sources of financing produces a spread but vital economy, all in service of advancing drug development and enabling more extensive access to beneficial treatments (Figure 4.5).

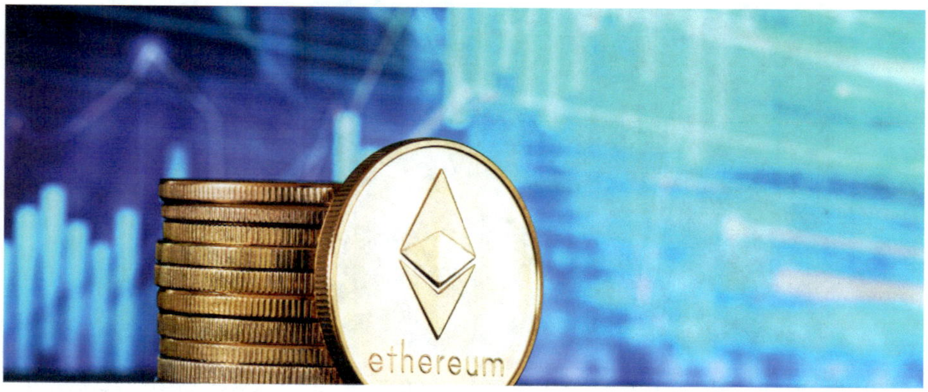

Figure 4.5. The landscape of funding and investment in drug development is intricate, shaped by a multitude of public and private stakeholders.

Source: https://www.epw.in/sites/default/files/images/2024/10/24/DeFI_MI.png.

4.1.8. Challenges Faced During Development

The drug development process is full of numerous challenges, particularly at the clinical trial phases that can hinder progress and drive costs up manifold. The poor recruitment and participant retention are one of the key challenges that can prolong trials unnecessarily. As stated, failure to address these issues means it will take longer and be more expensive to make drugs, and results from trials may not accurately represent drug effectiveness or may not be transportable beyond the study (Grill et al., 2010). Moreover, the globalization of clinical trials has also introduced regulatory compliance and ethical oversight issues, especially in developing countries with inadequate infrastructure. Mexico and other developing countries face unique challenges in complying with strict international standards for clinical trials, highlighting the delicate balance between local infrastructure and international requirements (Santiago-Rodriguez et al.). The barriers underscore the imperative for creative solutions to optimize trial efficiency and subject engagement in drug development.

4.1.9. Success Rates and Timelines

Success rates and times associated with drug development are the most important determinants that technically characterize the pharmaceutical industry. Historically, the process has been bedeviled with issues, as evidenced by the mind-boggling prices that are over $2 billion per medication, and the protracted timeline that usually takes longer than a decade, with success rates having been less than 10% for new compounds. The integration of advanced technologies such as machine learning (ML) and artificial intelligence (AI) renders this pipeline significantly more effective by streamlining essential processes. For instance, ML facilitates the identification and validation of therapeutic targets and predictive toxicology that can significantly reduce patient stratification in clinical trials. Meanwhile, AI models such as AlphaFold offer precise protein structure predictions to assist drug design and enhance discovery. Despite these advances, the industry must overcome regulatory and data quality challenges, thus emphasizing the need for multidisciplinary collaboration to optimize the utilization of these advancements towards maximal improvements in success rates and minimum timeline optimization (Aña et al., 2025; Gurung et al., 2025) (Figure 4.6).

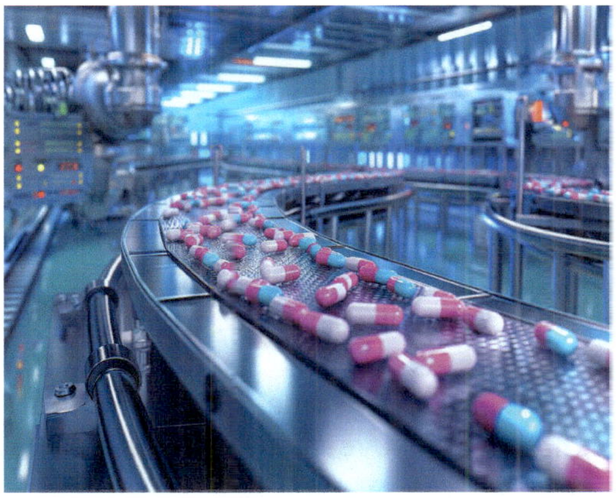

Figure 4.6. The success rates and timelines associated with drug development are critical factors that fundamentally shape the pharmaceutical landscape.

Source: https://assets.isu.pub/document-structure/240919084917-1f45a338045f10714276d667da549c5f/v1/7622ab371f43f3f9c9adea18e95609ce.jpeg

Test Your Knowledge

1. How do researchers determine the appropriate dosage of a new drug?
2. How is the safety of a drug ensured during early development?

4.2. Clinical Trial Design

Learning Outcome

1. Understand types of clinical trials
2. Explain randomized controlled trials (RCTs)
3. Learn observational studies
4. Focus on blinding and placebo effects
5. Perform sample size determination
6. Discuss inclusion and exclusion criteria
7. Explain data collection methods
8. Describe statistical analysis in clinical trials
9. Know the importance of trial design in outcomes

A strong trial design is crucial for the success of developing new treatments, especially in diseases like glioblastoma, which present unique challenges due to the blood-brain barrier (BBB) and tumor microenvironment. Newer innovations in clinical trial designs, such as adaptive platform trials and basket trials, are being explored to optimize therapeutic benefit while streamlining patient recruitment. These newer designs facilitate simultaneous assessment of several treatments against specific biomarkers and thus a more sensitive, more responsive method of assessing treatment effects (Narsinh et al., 2024). Moreover, the inclusion of patient engagement strategies has grown in vogue, describing a shift towards a patient-valued approach of recognizing patients lived experiences and patient needs in clinical studies. This patient-centric approach, alongside the exploitation of the use of technology for monitoring health outcomes, is restructuring trial protocols to become more patient-centered and patient-sensitive (Faulkner et al., 2023). The development of clinical trial design is thus crucial to surpass complex medical conditions and improve drug development results.

4.2.1. Types of Clinical Trials

Clinical trials are essential to the advancement of medical science and to assessing the safety and efficacy of new treatments. Divided broadly into interventional and observational trials, the latter includes randomized controlled trials (RCTs), which are considered to be the gold standard due to their ability to exclude bias. These trials compare the impact of specific interventions on patient outcomes and allow for the creation of personalized treatments, particularly in cancer, where precision medicine is becoming more prevalent. Observational trials, conversely, provide real-world efficacy and are valuable for examining long-term outcomes outside clinical settings. As detailed in recent studies, the establishment of community-based motivations at the time of trial planning is key to ensuring maximum cooperation and enrollment in drug development initiatives, especially in settings of global health (Brown et al., 2009). Moreover, harmonization of clinical trial strategies with the employment of molecular profiling will maximize therapeutic benefits while overcoming related challenges in drug discovery (Hollebecque et al., 2015) (Figure 4.7).

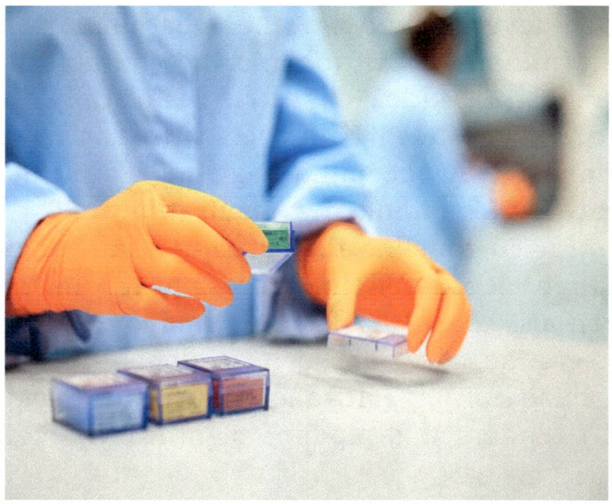

Figure 4.7. Clinical trials are essential for advancing medical knowledge and evaluating the safety and efficacy of new therapies.

Source: https://assets.roche.com/f/176343/1920x1281/5aaa43e309/roche_35952.png.

4.2.2. Randomized Controlled Trials (RCTs)

RCTs are part of drug development, providing a systematic method for establishing the efficacy and safety of potential treatments. RCTs are the gold standard for clinical trials due to their ability to minimize bias through random allocation of study subjects to the control and treatment arms. This is particularly relevant in specialties such as oncology, where new therapies for low-prognosis cancers are put through rigorous testing to secure regulatory and reimbursement approval. Stakeholder controversy more recently has highlighted the need for RCT design, which is not only fulfilling its scientific requirements but also respects patient opinion so that a patient-focused initiative is maintained (Bird et al., 2024). Moreover, RCTs can identify the best treatment strategies through a comparison of new treatments with existing ones and addressing issues of safety, particularly when standard practices are not yielding results (Bu et al., 2025). Overall, RCTs are at the center of realizing therapeutic advances and improving patients' outcomes.

4.2.3. Observational Studies

The contribution of observational studies in drug development and clinical trials cannot be overstated, as they provide informative information supplementing RCTs. The study is designed to measure the real-life impact of treatments in a broad spectrum of patient populations, thereby providing enhanced knowledge of drug efficacy and safety in real-life practice.

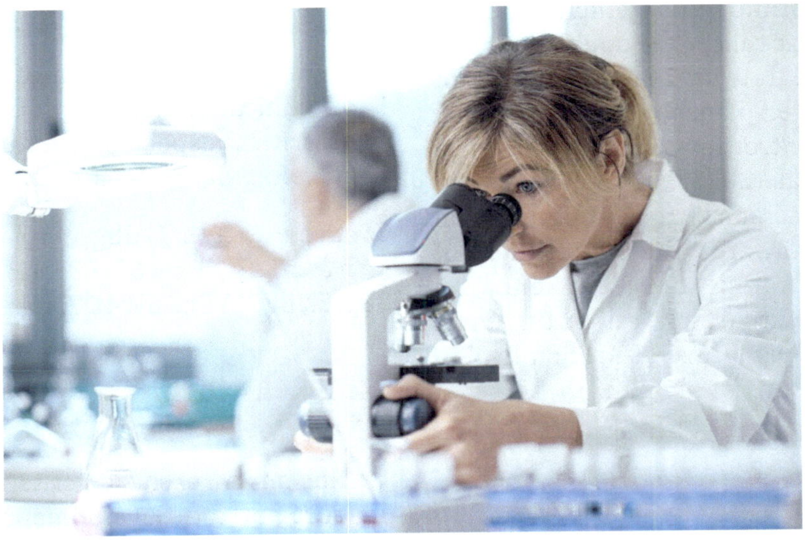

Figure 4.8. The significance of observational studies in drug development and clinical trials cannot be overstated, as they provide essential insights that complement randomized controlled trials.

Source: https://clinicaltrial.be/storage/media/14/iStock-1410783230.jpg.

Notably, observational data have sanctioned the application of regimens like the EXTREME regimen in recurrent and/or metastatic head and neck squamous cell carcinoma with significant survival benefits that are credited to randomized trials as well as follow-up observational research (Castro et al., 2017). Further, the advancement of distributed pharmacoepidemiology networks has enhanced the strength of observational studies by allowing data analysis on a large scale without sacrificing patient confidentiality (Brown et al., 2020). Together, all these aspects emphasize the significance of observational studies in the direction of clinical decision-making and regulatory practice and, ultimately, in improving patient outcomes (Figure 4.8).

4.2.4. Blinding and Placebo Effects

In drug development and clinical trials, blinding and the use of placebos are necessary to reduce bias and achieve credible study outcomes. Blinding, particularly in RCTs, contributes to result quality by making participants and researchers unaware of which treatment they receive and hence ruling out expectations that may bias reported effects. Moreover, placebo effects can profoundly skew outcomes by causing treatment responses in patients who believe they are on active therapy. For instance, in a study of erlotinib plus gemcitabine for metastatic pancreatic cancer, the double-blinding was able to demonstrate statistically significant survival benefit over placebo, underlining the need to strictly control for such psychological factors (Moore et al., 2023). In the same vein, research using transcranial magnetic stimulation has also pointed towards the significance of placebos in determining drug efficiency on cortical excitability accurately, reiterating their relevance in building proof-of-mechanism in phase-one trials (Ruijs et al., 2022).

4.2.5. Sample Size Determination

In clinical trials and drug development, sample size determination is a critical step that determines the reliability and validity of trial outcomes. Proper sample size determination enables the trial to pick up on an existing effect, balanced against participant exposure ethics. For instance, in trials of new treatments vs. active control and in randomized trials, statistical methods grapple with the complexity of non-inferiority margins and assumptions about study design (Liu et al., 2014). Second, endpoint selection at trials—i.e., overall survival—should be planned in advance; a cure proportion model can handle necessary event counts and times positively, increasing trial power (Heinzmann et al., 2019). Last, correct estimation of sample size for good sound is not only required statistically but also to perform trials ethically and thus constitutes a cornerstone block of the drug development process (Figure 4.9).

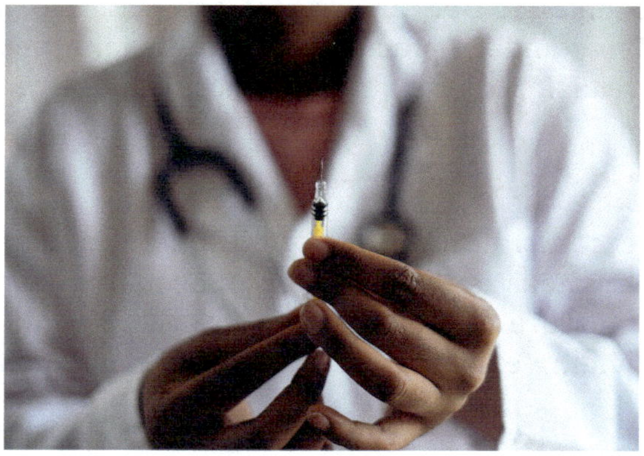

Figure 4.9. In the realm of drug development and clinical trials, sample size determination is a critical aspect that influences the validity and reliability of trial outcomes.

Source: https://dbgp98ysvt3y0.cloudfront.net/blog/Fz96773kIHig755f8h5k7oSpIuNEvOeYGxOuW4D7.jpg.

4.2.6. Inclusion and Exclusion Criteria

Inclusion and exclusion criteria are fundamental aspects of the development of clinical trials, guiding participant recruitment to ensure the validity and reliability of study outcomes. These criteria determine who can be included in the study, thus influencing the generalizability of outcomes to wider populations. For instance, in Alzheimer's disease research, the establishment of well-set staging criteria has led to more consistent inclusion and exclusion parameters, which are vital to identify treatment effects accurately, as highlighted in the recent debates by the Alzheimer's Association Research Roundtable (AARR) during their Fall 2021 meeting (Petersen et al., 2025). Similarly, in type 1 diabetes clinical trials, the application of personalized inclusion and exclusion criteria along with advanced simulation tools enhances the ability to predict disease course and optimize trial efficiency, thus facilitating better drug development strategies (Morales et al., 2024). Hence, proper consideration of these criteria is required for scientific integrity and ethical responsibility in clinical studies.

4.2.7. Data Collection Methods

Effective drug development and clinical trials are partly contingent on successful data collection methods, as such data inform efficacy and safety determination over time.

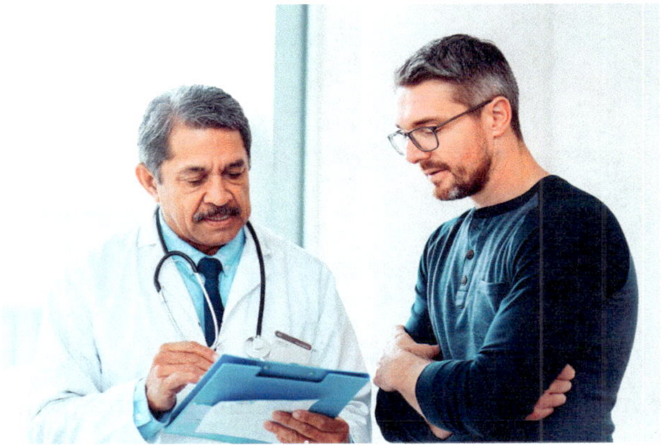

Figure 4.10. Effective data collection methods are integral to the success of drug development and clinical trials, as they inform the evaluation of efficacy and safety over time.

Source: https://www.allucent.com/wp-content/uploads/2020/02/What-are-Adaptive-Clin-Trial-Designs.webp.

One such sophisticated approach is data extraction from clinical trial registries, the outcomes of which can yield informative data on neurological disease treatment pathways. Use of such tools like NeuroTrialNER, where a through annotated corpus of clinical trials' summaries is used, has enhanced named entity recognition and helps researchers investigate complex data scenarios (Doneva et al., 2024). ECAs also offer a robust alternative to estimate the drug efficacy, especially when RCTs are faced with either practical or ethical limitations. Applying rigorous statistical matching techniques to historical clinical trial data, researchers can build ECAs with similarly reliable relative efficacy estimates as those attainable employing RCTs, thus improving drug evaluation and possibly reducing the therapeutic development time (Yin et al., 2023) (Figure 4.10).

4.2.8. Statistical Analysis in Clinical Trials

Statistical analysis forms the basis of clinical trials and drug development, in assessing new treatments' safety profiles and efficacy. Through the application of appropriate statistical procedures, researchers can draw correct conclusions from complex data, with direct implications to clinical decision-making. Traditional statistical techniques, although prevalent, do not take into consideration the intricacies surrounding patient-reported outcomes (PRO) due to inherent heterogeneity and missing data issues.

For instance, the application of population modeling techniques can enhance the analytical framework to address such challenges effectively and support better estimation of the treatment effect on patients' quality of life (Zhou et al., 2025). Furthermore, the use of statistical estimates such as relative risk and confidence intervals is unavoidable in the interpretation of findings in RCTs, as exemplified in combination regimen meta-analyses such as bevacizumab combined with platinum-based chemotherapy in advanced non-small cell lung cancer (Han et al., 2024). Therefore, sound statistical analysis not only aids in regulatory compliance but also guarantees that the therapeutic value of new pharmaceuticals is well conveyed to clinicians and stakeholders.

4.2.9. Importance of Trial Design in Outcomes

Good trial design is a key to the definition of drug development and clinical trials' success, as it directly affects the validity and reliability of the findings. A well-structured trial not only ensures that the research question relates to the matter at hand, but also enhances the applicability of the findings to bigger patient populations. For instance, the emergence of PRO measures for drugs, such as *omecamtiv mecarbil* used in heart failure studies, illustrates the necessity of developing studies that account for the patient's own experience. Qualitative research conducted in this environment, such as cognitive interviews and focus groups, identified determinative symptoms like shortness of breath and fatigue, which led to the development of corresponding measurement tools (Anatchkova et al., 2016). Therefore, the integration of stakeholder engagement and iterative feedback into trial design is paramount to effectively capture patient experience, finally informing regulatory decision-making and the therapeutic application of novel drugs (Ford et al., 2016) (Figure 4.11).

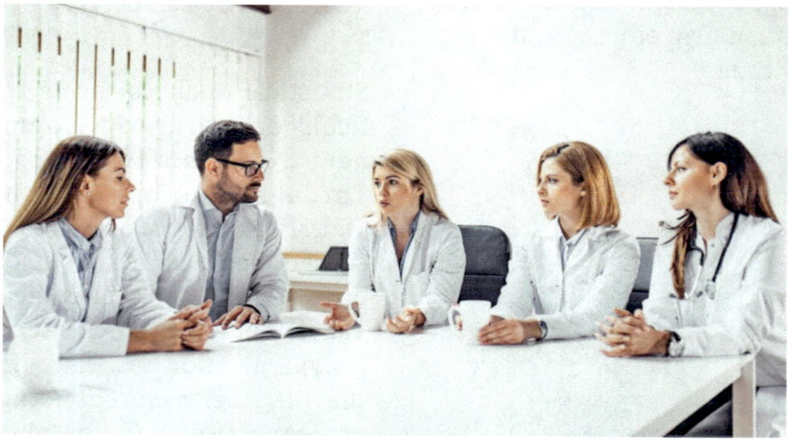

Figure 4.11. Effective trial design is pivotal in determining the outcomes of drug development and clinical trials, as it ultimately shapes the validity and reliability of the results.

Source: https://images.squarespace-cdn.com/content/v1/56a042fb25981d9326c9bbdb/e979c5e3-d10a-4be4-a314-016286ed8c4a/Clinical+Trials+Team.jpg.

Test Your Knowledge

1. How is patient safety monitored during clinical trials?
2. What does informed consent entail in clinical trials?

4.3. Regulatory Framework

Learning Outcome

1. Know role of the FDA in drug approval;
2. Understand international regulations and guidelines;
3. Explain good clinical practice (GCP);
4. Focus on ethical review boards and their functions;
5. Discuss post-marketing surveillance;
6. Learn adverse event reporting;
7. Describe fast track and breakthrough therapy designations;
8. Explain global harmonization of regulations;
9. Know impact of regulations on drug development timelines.

The drug development and clinical trial regulation system is an entity for providing assurance of the safety, efficacy, and ethical conduct of medical research. Developed by agencies such as the United States' FDA, these regulations mandate pharmaceutical companies to strictly follow approved protocols in their entire drug development process. This system not only addresses the scientific needs of drug testing but also includes provisions for patient enrollment since the success of clinical trials greatly relies on the compliance of healthcare providers to assist and recruit patients. As acknowledged by the latest research, there are barriers to effective patient recruitment into phase III trials, e.g., insufficiency of focus on clinical trial study in medical education and a gap in principal investigators' and drug representatives' trust (Dane et al., 2022). An adaptive and open regulatory framework is hence crucial in overcoming these barriers, encouraging collaboration and ultimately improving patient access to cutting-edge therapy (Khalid, 2025).

4.3.1. Role of the FDA in Drug Approval

The FDA function of approving drugs lies at the core of ensuring new drugs' safety and effectiveness. After exhaustive preclinical testing, drugs undergo an arduous process of testing by going through numerous phases of clinical trials that can last 7 to 12 years and cost between $2 to $3 billion, attributing the complexity of drug development (Gooneratne, 2019). The FDA also has the responsibility of reviewing New Drug Applications (NDAs), assessing data from trials to make well-informed decisions about approval. Recent developments, particularly in oncology, have also involved debate on refining the approval process to react more rapidly to emergent needs in healthcare, according to Dr. Richard Pazdur at JADPRO Live 2020 (Pazdur, 2021). Therefore, the FDAs new role not only enhances public safety but also drives innovation in the pharmaceutical industry, while making available effective treatments to patients in a timely manner (Figure 4.12).

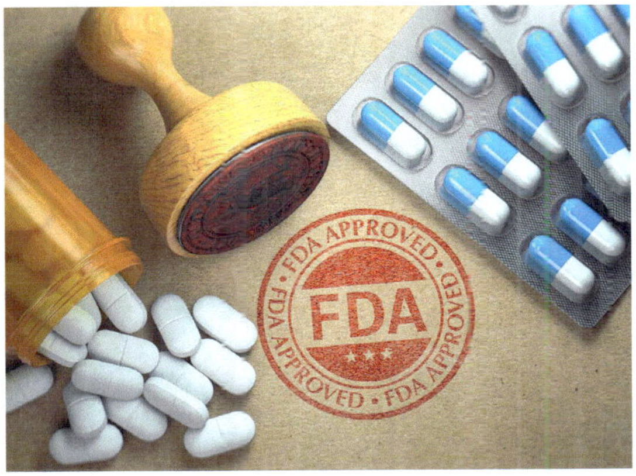

Figure 4.12. The role of the Food and Drug Administration (FDA) in drug approval is pivotal in ensuring the safety and efficacy of new pharmaceuticals.

Source: https://www.investopedia.com/thmb/QYVCaLVatqlV1UTgZUZNJel_cEg=/1500x0/filters:no_upscale():max_bytes(150000):strip_icc()/GettyImages-1188568920-056f66c163fc46a19d817eef55d14933.jpg.

4.3.2. International Regulations and Guidelines

The clinical trial and drug development environment is primarily influenced by international regulatory guidelines and regulations, which offer guidelines for maintaining the scientific and ethical integrity of the conduct of research practices worldwide. The International Council for Harmonization of Technical Requirements for Pharmaceuticals for Human Use E6(R2) Good Clinical Practice (GCP) and the Declaration of Helsinki are two of the most significant documents that offer fundamental ethical principles to be employed while performing clinical trials. These guidelines emphasize the need for informed consent, which, while vital, is often marred by readability and completeness shortcomings. Studies indicate that most informed consent forms are incomplete regarding experimental procedures and post-trial procedures (Dukaew et al., 2023). Moreover, regulatory affairs experts handle the complexities of drug legislation, which also differ across countries like the USA, Europe, and India, finally impacting the quality, safety, and effectiveness of candidate drugs (Ramya et al., 2023). Thus, adhering to these global guidelines is essential in ensuring participant well-being as well as encouraging innovative drug development.

4.3.3. Good Clinical Practice (GCP)

GCP offers the basis for ensuring ethical and scientific quality throughout drug development, including clinical trials. Intended to protect the rights, safety, and well-being of trial participants, GCP guidelines require the standards of designing, conducting, and reporting clinical studies.

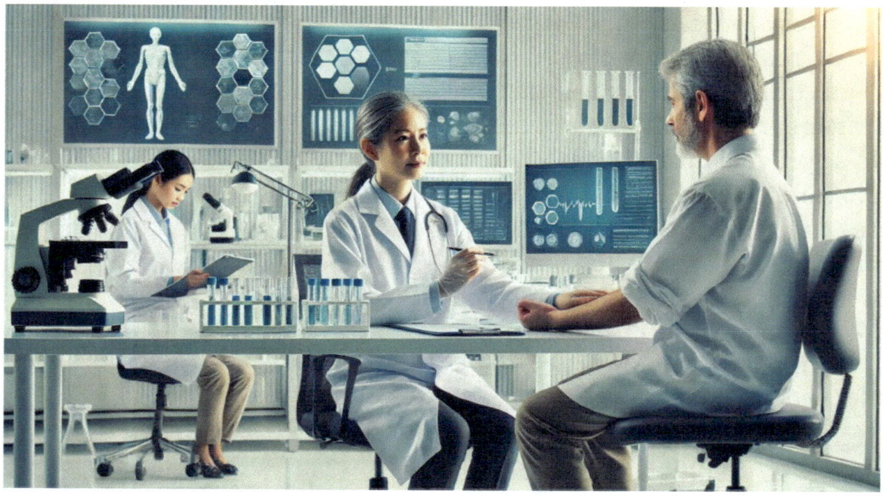

Figure 4.13. Good Clinical Practice (GCP) serves as the backbone for ensuring ethical and scientific integrity in drug development and clinical trials.

Source: https://media.licdn.com/dms/image/v2/D5612AQHmpRjI1eIbsA/article-cover_image-shrink_720_1280/B56ZVucQoGHoAI-/0/1741314659447?e=2147483647&v=beta&t=rCP7AssuaRgXOZzchEElKUfejxCD8qhOn22EbhmcZ68.

Although adherence to the guidelines is obligatory, their day-to-day use is more a matter of striking a balance between compliance with the rules and practice realities in clinical trials. As noted, implementation of GCP diminishes risk in addition to enhancing the validity of study outcomes, justifying the reliance on clinical study results (Diamant et al., 2014). The issue, however, is accompanied by guidelines having primarily expert opinion rather than high-quality evidence, particularly in specialist fields like management of rheumatoid arthritis through the foot and ankle (Williams et al., 2016). Consequently, while GCP is an essential guideline, ongoing review and research are the ways of enhancing the quality and appropriateness of drug development clinical practice guidelines overall (Figure 4.13).

4.3.4. Ethical Review Boards and their Functions

Ethical review boards (ERBs) are the watchful guardians of participant welfare throughout drug development and clinical trials, enrolling with keen attention to ethical factors throughout the research process. ERBs attentively review trial protocols for consideration on whether or not the proposed studies honor the principles of beneficence, respect for persons, and justice. Their function involves assessing risk factors of participant enrollment, as highlighted by the requirement for proper screening criteria to prevent unethical practices such as misleading participants (Moore et al., 2022). Further, ERBs play a significant role in facilitating the integration of sophisticated biomarker analysis in studies and thus informing appropriate patient populations for new treatments (Edsj et al., 2024). Through the application of strict scrutiny, ERBs promote ethical transparency in clinical trials and thereby create trust between experimenters and subjects, which is imperative to the validity and success of drug development projects.

4.3.5. Post-Marketing Surveillance

The role of post-marketing surveillance in drug development cannot be overemphasized, since it is a vital tool for ongoing safety assessment of medicines once they are marketed. It offers a chance to keep an ongoing watch on drugs in the field and, therefore, allows for the detection of side effects that were not evident in clinical studies. The integration of electronic health records (EHRs) provides a valuable asset to this surveillance, enabling researchers to take advantage of existing data to enhance patient safety with reduced capturing of health outcomes data over time (Blomster et al., 2016). Furthermore, the analogy between non-active implantable medical devices' safety evaluation methods and other fields highlights the growing need for effective systems to monitor safety profiles throughout a product's life cycle (Coloma et al., 2017). Apart from affirming regulatory authority, such methodologies guarantee harmony between long-term safety and efficacy and evolving patient needs (Figure 4.14).

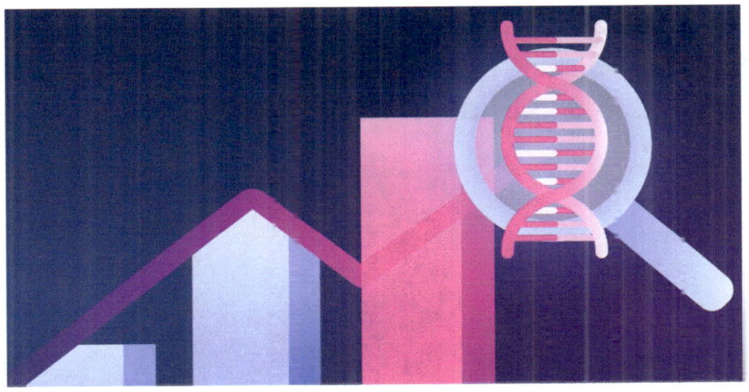

Figure 4.14. The significance of post-marketing surveillance in the drug development process cannot be overstated, as it serves as a critical mechanism for ongoing safety assessment of pharmaceuticals once they reach the market.

Source: https://blog.drugbank.com/content/images/2024/09/20240708-Q3-Biosimilars-Blog-Headerlrg_1200x627-2x-.png.

4.3.6. Adverse Event Reporting

Reporting of adverse events (AEs) is a critical part of drug development and clinical trials as a patient safety guarantee and an efficacy evaluation tool. The advanced character of accurately collecting and documenting AEs is especially salient in susceptible populations, such as neonates, who undergo multiple health complications and stages of advancement. Recent debates have highlighted the need for regulators to emphasize the importance of complete AE documentation in neonates within clinical settings, alongside calls for methodologies that are specifically tailored to meet trial objectives, thereby avoiding undue burdens on trial sites (Hill et al., 2025). Secondly, age-specific variations in AEs require a nuanced understanding to optimize therapeutic outcomes in children, as evidenced by the analysis of the American FDA Adverse Event Reporting System data (Ogura et al., 2024). Last but not least, robust AEs reporting is essential for drug safety and therapeutic efficacy optimization in varying populations.

4.3.7. Fast Track and Breakthrough Therapy Designations

The Fast Track and Breakthrough Therapy designations have significantly changed drug development and clinical trials, particularly for serious conditions with no satisfactory treatments. The FDA gives these designations with the motive of facilitating expedited review of drugs that have demonstrated potential for fulfilling unmet medical needs. For instance, Breakthrough Therapy Designation allows for greater dialogue with the FDA and a faster development process, which can be crucial for innovative therapies. As supported by the recent approval of *Nadofaragene firadenovec*, which was designated both Breakthrough and Fast Track status, these designations facilitate faster access to potentially life-altering therapy treatment for patients with non-muscle invasive bladder cancer (Steinmetz et al., 2025). Furthermore, a review of FDA authorized drugs verifies that Breakthrough and Fast Track designation is linked with timely market approval in markets like China, and this emphasizes the importance of their accessibility globally (Zhu et al., 2024) (Figure 4.15).

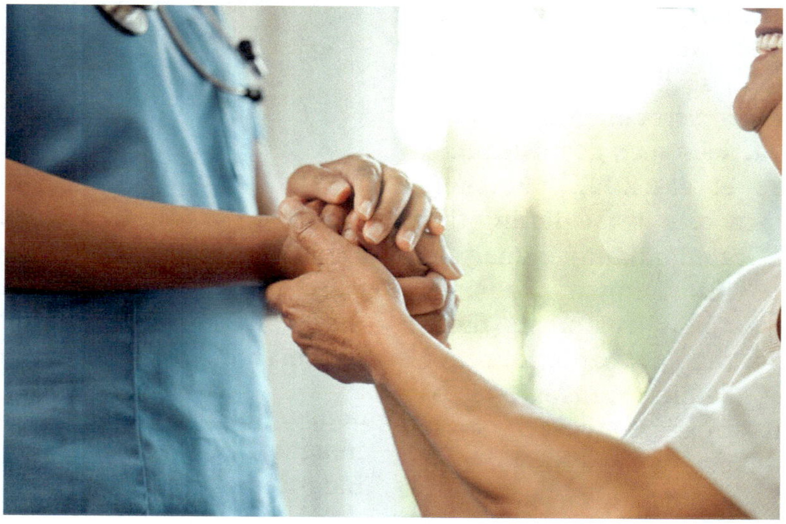

Figure 4.15. The implementation of Fast Track and Breakthrough Therapy designations has significantly transformed drug development and clinical trials, particularly for serious conditions that lack effective treatments.

Source: https://synergbiopharma.com/wp-content/uploads/2025/03/patient-and-doctor.jpg.

4.3.8. Global Harmonization of Regulations

Global harmonization of standards is essential to simplify the process of drug development and clinical trials in different countries. As the world becomes more integrated, the necessity for single standards becomes even more evident, especially concerning public health and safety. The move towards reconciling standards can reduce many of the discrepancies that have previously stalled global collaboration, as in efforts to standardize U.S. standards with those from other countries. Harmonization of this sort not only serves the interests of efficiency in bringing new treatments to market but can even reduce the cost of expensive, redundant testing and approval procedures. Industry-controlled groups' influence on forging such global standards is a huge challenge, however, and one that potentially could subvert health and safety regulation in place to protect public interests. Thus, global sharing of data and developing cooperative frameworks is needed to provide fair access to healthcare innovations (Augustine et al., 2019) (Figure 4.16).

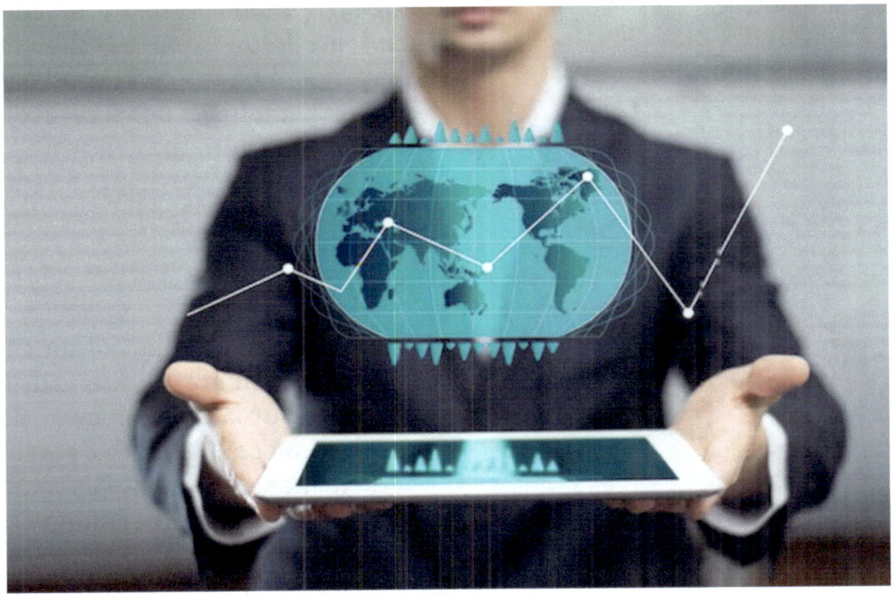

Figure 4.16. The global harmonization of regulations is crucial for streamlining the drug development and clinical trial processes across various countries.

Source: https://www.freyrsolutions.com/sites/default/files/blog-thumbnails/The%20Impact%20of%20Global%20Regulatory%20Harmonization%20on%20Streamlining%20Medici_Thmb-Wt.webp.

4.3.9. Impact of Regulations on Drug Development Timelines

The regulatory framework is critical in deciding drug development timelines and is a double-edged sword in the majority of circumstances. Regulation is essential for guaranteeing patient safety and drug efficacy, but also adds time to bring new treatments to market. For example, the current COVID-19 pandemic led to stakeholders embracing novel trial designs and decentralized approaches, which are capable of accelerating patient access to innovative treatments; such a paradigm shift demonstrates that adaptable regulations can enable quicker approval processes, as reported by an international panel of oncology leaders in Sessa et al. (2021). Conversely, rigid compliance requirements can hinder progress, particularly on first-stage studies, as attested in the limited success of the ARRIVE guidelines for enhancing reporting transparency in animal studies and experimental design (Sert et al., 2020). Addressing the demand for surveillance without compromising quick drug approval remains a top stumbling block in the acceleration of drug development processes.

Test Your Knowledge

1. What are the key regulatory agencies involved in drug development?
2. What are the steps involved in obtaining regulatory approval for a drug after clinical trials?

4.4. Ethical Considerations in Drug Trials

Learning Outcome

1. Understand the informed consent process
2. Explain risks vs. benefits analysis
3. Focus on vulnerable populations in clinical trials
4. Learn about placebo use and ethical implications
5. Focus on transparency and data sharing
6. Describe conflicts of interest
7. Know the role of ethics committees
8. Explain historical abuses in clinical trials
9. Know current ethical standards and practices

The ethical concerns surrounding drug trials are central to the validity and safety of clinical research. Fundamental to these concerns is the principle of informed consent, which mandates participants to distinctly recognize the potential risks and benefits before joining. Additionally, protection of vulnerable populations typically poses a significant challenge; there must be careful consideration to avoid exploitation while ensuring equal access to new treatments. The emergence of artificial intelligence (AI) in drug development, unveiled by the examination of the ethical issues, aggravates these challenges, especially algorithmic bias and data privacy, which must be addressed so that trust can be maintained in the process (Warokar et al., 2024). Furthermore, with changing clinical trial methods such as the development of adaptive designs and decentralized trials, ethical guidelines need to evolve accordingly to keep pace with these novel approaches while also protecting participant rights and welfare (Parveen et al., 2024).

4.4.1. Informed Consent Process

Informed consent is a foundation of moral standards in clinical trials and drug development, which ensures participants understand the nature and stakes of the research before the participant's agreement. The traditional informed consent procedure demands that researchers present elaborate descriptions of the purpose, risks, and advantages of trials, making provision for an environment of candor and trust. However, the virtual clinical trial presents both issues and possibilities in this regard. Whereas virtual trials make it easier for people to take part as they can do so from anywhere, they might render it more difficult to get informed consent because essential subtleties may be lost online (Andrews et al., 2017). Furthermore, clinicians also attribute difficulties in the process of informed consent as a significant barrier in recruiting participants, emphasizing the necessity for better communication strategies (Abe et al., 2017). Therefore, it is necessary to refine the process of informed consent to weigh ethics concerns against new research techniques (Figure 4.17).

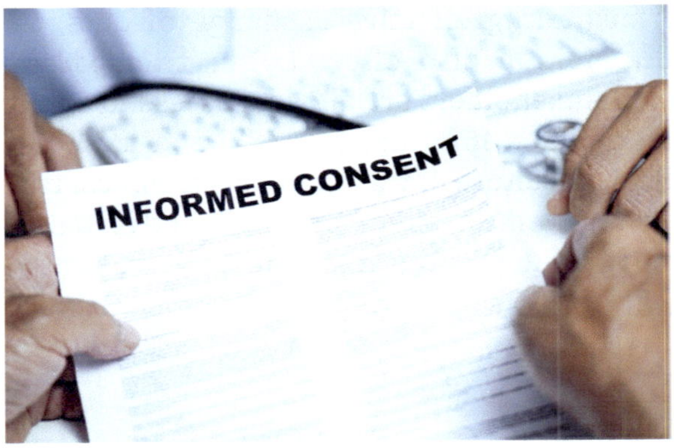

Figure 4.17. Informed consent is a cornerstone of ethical standards in drug development and clinical trials, ensuring that participants are fully aware of the research's nature and implications before agreeing to participate.

Source: https://clinicaltrial.be/storage/media/10/iStock-1144982329.jpg.

4.4.2. Risks vs. Benefits Analysis

In drug discovery and clinical trials, an exhaustive benefits vs risk evaluation is crucial to determine the promise of novel therapies. This assessment is often confounded by the demands of trial design and previous findings, typically reflected in the pattern of bypassing or avoiding phase 2 trials in favor of going straight to phase 3. Research has indicated that nearly half of the phase 3 trials reviewed for neurologic diseases were initiated with no affirmative phase 2 trial, with statistically significantly lower probabilities of achieving primary efficacy outcomes compared with trials adhering to the conventional protocol (Moyer et al., 2024). Also, while patients in substance use disorder studies can experience reductions in drug use, these decreases concomitantly with improvement in clinical outcomes and thus may represent an essential outcome alongside abstinence (Aminesmaeili et al., 2024). Consequently, establishing a firm framework for balancing possible harm against clinical benefit remains at the forefront of protecting clinical trial integrity and effectiveness.

4.4.3. Vulnerable Populations in Clinical Trials

Their inclusion in clinical trials is essential to realizing equitable access to new therapeutics and better evaluation of treatment outcomes in diverse populations. The groups traditionally underrepresented in clinical trials have included racial and ethnic minorities and economically disadvantaged groups. They have only seen a tiny fraction, 2.5–9%, of potentially eligible cancer patients enroll for trials, as the evidence provided in Burke et al. (2014) explained. This underrepresentation leaves a broad disparity in the efficacy and safety information that is relevant to these populations, threatening the creation of treatments specifically tailored to their health needs. Also, the development of virtual clinical trials poses a possible solution to bridging this disparity through online recruitment, potentially democratizing access to clinical trials. However, challenges remain, since digital methods must satisfy requirements of informed consent and confidentiality no differently than more traditional approaches, as outlined in Andrews et al. (2017) (Figure 4.18).

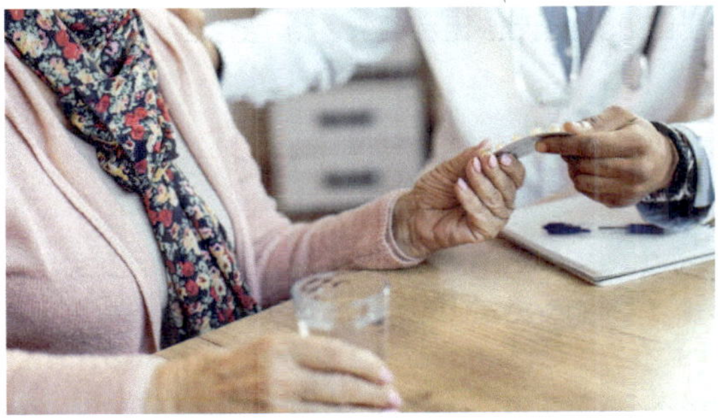

Figure 4.18. The inclusion of vulnerable populations in clinical trials is paramount to ensuring equitable access to new therapeutics and a better understanding of treatment effects across diverse demographics.

Source: https://exeltis.com/sumtrial/wp-content/uploads/2023/11/IMAGEN_BLOG_1200X700_Vulnerable-groups-and-inclusion-in-clinical-trials-04-1024x597.webp.

4.4.4. Placebo Use and Ethical Implications

The use of placebos in clinical trials has significant ethical implications that are very controversial to medical practitioners. To some extent, placebos can contribute to the power of drug development by providing a valid control against which active intervention effects can be contrasted and then assist in establishing actual therapeutic effects. However, ethical considerations arise when the use of placebos may lead to deception of the patients or the exclusion of participants from receiving treatment, particularly for life-threatening conditions. The concern is even greater in adaptive platform trials where multiple drugs are tested simultaneously against a common control, i.e., a placebo arm, raising concerns around informed consent and the participant's well-being (Sasaki et al., 2024). Moreover, while the majority of well-informed consent forms attempt to include sufficient ethical standards, they are incomplete and vague, which can hide crucial details concerning experimental research status (Dukaew et al., 2023). It is thus vital to scrutinize these ethical factors closely so that clinical research integrity is not compromised.

4.4.5. Transparency and Data Sharing

The value of transparency and data sharing in clinical trials and drug development cannot be overstated, particularly in regard to optimizing research outcomes and enhancing the public's confidence. The COVID-19 pandemic has placed a spotlight on collaboration among stakeholders, where flaws in data sharing practices have been revealed, reinforcing the position of transparency in clinical trial management (Kumar et al., 2024). With the use of the latest technologies such as blockchain and smart contracts, scientists can better secure data and effectively exchange critical information between various stakeholders in drug development. In addition to facilitating effective exchange of data, this new method also offers better transparency since stakeholders are allowed access to correct and updated information (Nabila et al., 2024). Finally, a culture of transparency in clinical trials can result in stronger findings, better patient safety, and greater trust in new treatments (Figure 4.19).

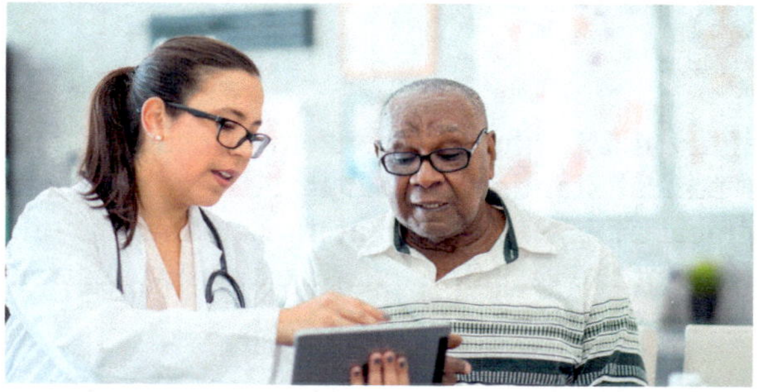

Figure 4.19. The significance of transparency and data sharing in drug development and clinical trials cannot be overstated, particularly in the context of optimizing research outcomes and enhancing public trust.

Source: https://www.allucent.com/wp-content/uploads/2020/08/Importance-of-Clinical-Trial-Transparency-in-Drug-Dev.webp.

4.4.6. Conflicts of Interest

It has a path through the complex process of drug development and clinical trials, which necessarily raises serious issues of conflict of interest. The conflict tends to occur where clinical decisions and guideline development are being driven by financial relationships between pharmaceutical firms and health practitioners. A recent study indicates that of 16 guidelines analyzed, 10 advised changes that broadened disease definitions, showing an increase in diagnoses without sufficient consideration of harms (Bero et al., 2013). Also, under the umbrella of international research collaborations, research and development internationalization has led to multinational enterprises outsourcing clinical trials to developing nations, thus raising ethical oversight concerns (Santiago-Rodriguez et al.). Such circumstances underscore the need for openness and robust regulatory systems to minimize conflicts of interest and maximize decision-making processes' focus on giving utmost weight to patient benefit over financial gains. Resolution of these kinds of disputes is crucial in maintaining the integrity of clinical research and public trust in medical advances.

4.4.7. Role of Ethics Committees

In the intricate drug development and clinical trial process, ethics committees are vigilant watchdogs in safeguarding participant welfare and research integrity. Ethics committees serve as gatekeepers, examining the ethical foundations of trial protocols and risks and benefits to participants.

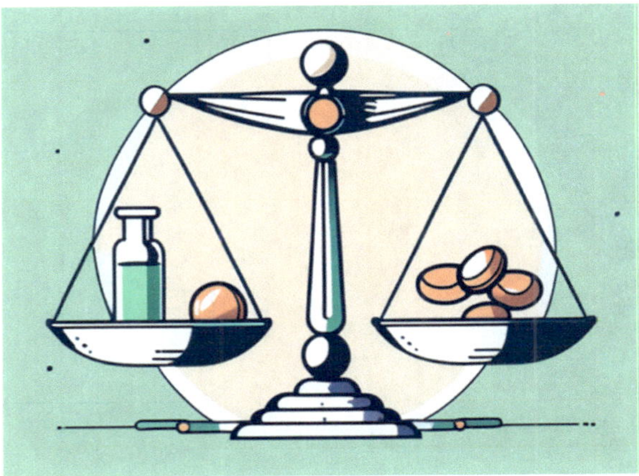

Figure 4.20. In the complex landscape of drug development and clinical trials, ethics committees play a pivotal role in safeguarding participant welfare and ensuring research integrity.

Source: https://www.laboratoriosrubio.com/wp-content/uploads/2024/03/pharma-ethics-3.png.

Due to the heterogeneity of membership, rigorous peer review is facilitated, convening the perspectives of multiple stakeholders such as drug firms, regulatory agencies, and patients. Of special concern, with clinical trials increasingly likely to employ digital health technology, ethics committees are faced by new data protection and privacy issues (Avigdor, 2024). They are also faced by the need to harmonize disparate privacy legislations insofar as they interpret conflicting perspectives informing application of the research (Jiang et al., 2025). Thus, ethics committees have a significant role not only in supplementing participant protections but also in ensuring ethically sound and scientifically acceptable drug development methods (Figure 4.20).

4.4.8. Historical Abuses in Clinical Trials

The issue of clinical trials is tainted by numerous abuses that have had a profound impact on modern moral values. Forensic to everyone were the atrocities committed by the Nazi doctors during World War II, which led to the creation of the Nuremberg Code, which brought about a sea change in the application of informed consent and human rights consideration in medical studies.

This evolution highlighted the stark need for ethical regulation, even in the face of heinous cases of abuse, such as the Tuskegee Syphilis Study, where patients were lied to and denied treatment so the disease could be examined. These abuses throughout history indicated not only the vulnerability of certain groups but also the reforms of regulation that promised patients' rights and protection in research. Today, as evident from the recent controversy over the marketing of new drugs, the ethical concerns arising due to drug promotion and susceptibility to manipulation underscore the presence of a persistent need to maintain high ethical standards for clinical trials (Vărăstoae et al., 2024; Malshy et al., 2025).

4.4.9. Current Ethical Standards and Practices

Compliance with modern ethical practice and principles is mandatory in drug development and clinical trials to provide safeguards for the volunteers' rights and safety. Regulatory authorities like the FDA and EMA focus, therefore, on the employment of sound approaches, such as Physiologically Based Biopharmaceutics Modeling (PBBM), in drug development procedures. This approach not only progresses drug behavior understanding within biologic systems but also guides safety evaluation and regulatory applications, facilitating ethical study approaches (Tannergren et al., 2024). Second, employing adaptive trial designs that offer real-time dosing and participant adaptation is a step toward more effective and ethical clinical studies. These trial designs minimize risk to participants and maximize the scientific yield from trials, as per the moral principle of do-no-harm, specifically for dose-finding (Nasrollahzadeh et al., 2021). It is essential in this new environment that ethics standards be maintained upholding public confidence and advancing the progress of medical science (Figure 4.21).

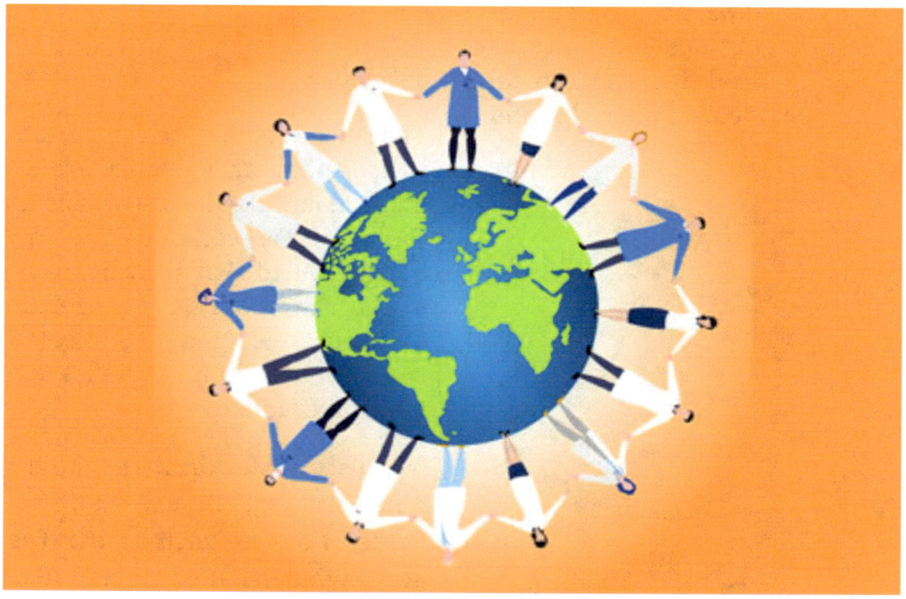

Figure 4.21. In the realm of drug development and clinical trials, adherence to current ethical standards and practices is paramount to ensure the safety and rights of participants.

Source: https://vertassets.blob.core.windows.net/image/59808fc6/59808fc6-f9cf-477b-97af-fed1b6ef5dfd/doctos_nurses_aroound_world_gettyimages_1224540891.jpg.

Test Your Knowledge

1. Why is participant confidentiality important in clinical trials?
2. What is the ethical guideline for conducting trials involving vulnerable populations, such as children or pregnant women?

Summary

The environment of drug development and clinical trials is changing rapidly, marked by both landmark achievements and ongoing challenges. The formation of early-phase clinical trial (EFCT) consortia is a prime example of collaboration as a means to promote research efficiency as well as treatment options centered on the patient. As has been observed, such consortia have appeared worldwide, tackling patient enrollment problems as well as optimizing procedural processes to bypass inefficiencies associated with conventional trial approaches (Liu et al., 2025). Furthermore, incorporating artificial intelligence into the drug development environment is a paradigm shift, enabling the discovery of new therapeutic targets and expediting the R&D process. Although issues such as algorithmic bias and explainability of AI models remain, no one can deny the revolutionary ability of AI to transform pharmaceutical innovation (Niazi et al., 2025). Thus, the confluence of collaboration and technological revolution opens up a new era in clinical research, promising improved prospects for effective therapies and improved patient outcomes.

Through the examination of the complexity of drug development and clinical trials, several important takeaways can be noted to show the merit of foresighted approaches. One such approach is model-informed drug development (MIDD) to enable data-driven dose practices through the use of deep pharmacological evaluation, as with the ZENITH trials involving zibotentan and dapagliflozin (Mercier A-et al., 2024). To achieve optimum efficacy and safety, especially in high-risk populations, the trials underscored the importance of appropriate dose selection. Additionally, new scientific and regulatory technologies in rare pediatric disease drug development highlight another critical area, where poor patient recruitment and response heterogeneity to the drug require robust quantitative integration (Krishna et al., 2024). Together, these discoveries reveal mechanisms through which strategic methods and collaborative frameworks can amplify the efficacy and success of drug development processes, particularly for multicomponent therapeutic scenarios.

KEY TERMS FROM THIS CHAPTER

- Molecular profiling
- Patient engagement strategies
- Pharmaceutical industries
- Preclinical models
- Public health
- Randomized controlled trials (RCTs)
- Resources
- Stakeholders
- Therapeutic targets
- New Drug Applications (NDAs)
- Patient-reported outcomes (PRO)
- Preclinical efficacy
- Predictive toxicology
- Quantum computing
- Recruitment
- Sample size determination
- Technology
- Tumor microenvironment (TME)

Critical Thinking Questions

1. **What is the primary goal of preclinical testing in drug development?**
   a. To determine the drug's market price
   b. To test the drug on human subjects
   c. To assess the safety and biological activity of the drug in non-human models
   d. To register the drug with regulatory bodies
2. **In which phase of clinical trials is the safety of a drug tested on the smallest group of healthy volunteers?**
   a. Phase I
   b. Phase II
   c. Phase III
   d. Phase IV
3. **Which of the following is the primary purpose of Phase III clinical trials?**
   a. To test the drug in animals
   b. To evaluate the drug's long-term safety and effectiveness in a larger group of patients
   c. To determine the drug's market price
   d. To test the drug in a small group of healthy volunteers
4. **Which regulatory agency is responsible for approving new drugs in the United States?**
   a. World Health Organization (WHO)
   b. Food and Drug Administration (FDA)
   c. European Medicines Agency (EMA)
   d. Centers for Disease Control and Prevention (CDC)
5. **Which of the following is NOT typically an inclusion criterion for clinical trial participants?**
   a. Age
   b. Pre-existing medical conditions
   c. Gender
   d. Geographical location of participants

Answers to Critical Thinking Questions

1. (c); 2. (a); 3. (b); 4. (b); 5. (d).

Short Answer Questions

1. What are the phases of drug development?
2. How do you identify potential drug candidates?
3. What preclinical studies are necessary before clinical trials can begin?
4. What are the different phases of clinical trials?
5. How are participants selected for clinical trials?
6. What is the role of randomization in clinical trials?

References

1. Yanagawa, H., Nishiya, M., Miyamoto, T., Shikishima, M., Imura, M., Nakanishi, R., Ariuchi, K., Akaishi, A., Takai, S., Abe, S., Kisyuku, M., Kageyama, C., Sato, C., Yamagami, M., Urakawa, N., Sone, S., & Irahara, M. (2006). Clinical trials for drug approval: a pilot study of the view of doctors at Tokushima University Hospital. *The Journal of Medical Investigation*, *53*(3–4), 292–296. https://doi.org/10.2152/jmi.53.292Ali, S., Freedman, S. B., Hickes, S., Jong, et al. (2019). Innovative approaches to investigator-initiated, multicenter pediatric clinical trials in Canada. https://core.ac.uk/download/534388837.pdf (accessed on 10th June 2025).

2. Aminesmaeili, M., Farokhnia, M., Susukida, R., Leggio, L., Johnson, R. M., Crum, R., & Mojtabai, R. (2024). Reduced drug use as an alternative valid outcome in individuals with stimulant use disorders: Findings from 13 multisite randomized clinical trials. *Addiction*. https://www.semanticscholar.org/paper/a79fe94574decf2611486ece0fbd7646b6a32601 (accessed on 10th June 2025).

3. Anatchkova, M., Chau, D., Malik, F. I., et al. (2016). Incorporating development of a patient-reported outcome instrument in a clinical drug development program: Examples from a heart failure program. https://core.ac.uk/download/323063368.pdf (accessed on 10th June 2025).

4. Andrews, L., Franco, A., Kostelecky, K., et al. (2017). Virtual clinical trials: One step forward, two steps back. https://core.ac.uk/download/128127841.pdf (accessed on 10th June 2025).

5. Arora, A., Gambardella, A., Pammolli, F., et al. (2025). The nature and the extent of the market for technology in biopharmaceuticals. https://core.ac.uk/download/pdf/6381764.pdf (accessed on 10th June 2025).

6. Astărăstoae, V., Rogozea, L. M., Leaşu, F., & Roşca, S. (2024). Drug promotions between ethics, regulations, and financial interests. *American Journal of Therapeutics, 31*, e268–e279. https://www.semanticscholar.org/paper/372b1120e14744b7abc5dea3fdb0a15bd3ec6a91 (accessed on 10th June 2025).

7. Augustine, E., Austin, C., Chase, M., et al. (2019). The global academic research organization network: Data sharing to cure diseases and enable learning health systems. https://core.ac.uk/download/323072711.pdf (accessed on 10th June 2025).

8. Avigdor, G. (2024). Balancing the legal, ethical, and practical aspects of using digital health technologies in clinical research. *Regulatory Affairs Watch*. https://www.semanticscholar.org/paper/ecb4dbc0a24480adb0dcd43e868ecbd0a389edb5 (accessed on 10th June 2025).

9. Balogh, E. P., Bindman, A. B., Eckhardt, S. G., et al. (2019). Challenges and opportunities to updating prescribing information for longstanding oncology drugs. https://core.ac.uk/download/286362252.pdf (accessed on 10th June 2025).

10. Banerjee, R., Murugesan, D., & Ramesh Kumar, G. (2016). Clinical data management: Importance in clinical research. https://core.ac.uk/download/477852233.pdf (accessed on 10th June 2025).

11. Bannister, J. B. (2018). Regulating rare disease: Safely facilitating access to orphan drugs. https://core.ac.uk/download/216957566.pdf (accessed on 10th June 2025).

12. Bero, L., Cooke, G. P. E., Doust, J. A., et al. (2013). Expanding disease definitions in guidelines and expert panel ties to industry: A cross-sectional study of common conditions in the United States. https://core.ac.uk/download/196601152.pdf (accessed on 10th June 2025).

13. Bigelow, R., Burns, S., Dickerson, S., Hafley, G., et al. (2013). *Methodology of a Reevaluation of Cardiovascular Outcomes in The Record Trial: Study Design and Conduct*. https://core.ac.uk/download/42359786.pdf (accessed on 10th June 2025).

14. Bird, N., Scobie, N., Berlanga, P., Blanc, P., Buenger, V., Campbell-Hewson, Q., Casanova, M., et al. (2024). Stakeholder perspectives on randomized clinical trials for children with poor-prognosis cancers. *JAMA Network Open, 7*(12), e2449239. https://www.semanticscholar.org/paper/07c12eccf270bb9f26a7847d1d00c423ae9f98da (accessed on 10th June 2025).

15. Blomster, J. I., Cowie, M. R., Curtis, L. H., Duclaux, S., et al. (2016). *Electronic Health Records to Facilitate Clinical Research*. https://core.ac.uk/download/46559266.pdf (accessed on 10th June 2025).

16. Bourgeois, J., Goodman, M. S., & Braga, C. (2025). Navigating oncology clinical trials: From drug development to delivery. *Clinical Journal of Oncology Nursing, 29*(1), 91–95. https://www.semanticscholar.org/paper/1497a404029e17b10227f44e9131b7aa272f2961 (accessed on 10th June 2025).

17. Brown, C. J., & Frame, P. (2009). *Communities of Practice in The Public-Private-Partnership Sector for Neglected Diseases Drug Development: The Importance of Mindset Mapping*. https://core.ac.uk/download/1639972.pdf (accessed on 10th June 2025).

18. Brown, J. S., Henry, D. A., Klungel, O. H., Platt, R., et al. (2020). *How Pharmacoepidemiology Networks Can Manage Distributed Analyses to Improve Replicability and Transparency and Minimize Bias*. https://core.ac.uk/download/196607041.pdf (accessed on 10th June 2025).

19. Bu, X. J., Li, Z. R., Wang, W. Y., Liu, R., Ren, J. Y., Xu, L., Liao, X., et al. (2025). [Oral Chinese patent medicines in treatment of dysmenorrhea and clinical research status: A scoping review]. *Zhongguo Zhong Yao Za Zhi, 50*(3), 787–797. https://www.semanticscholar.org/paper/ee229bf4574cfd3003246189e1d24f9075d5e6aa (accessed on 10th June 2025).

20. Burke, N. J. (2014). *Rethinking the Therapeutic Misconception: Social Justice, Patient Advocacy, and Cancer Clinical Trial Recruitment in the US Safety Net*. https://core.ac.uk/download/323063825.pdf (accessed on 10th June 2025).

21. Castro, A. F., Argiris, A., Schulten, J., Harrington, K. J., Licitra, L., Tahara, M., et al. (2017). Evidence-based treatment options in recurrent and/or metastatic squamous cell carcinoma of the head and neck. https://core.ac.uk/download/129191057.pdf (accessed on 10th June 2025).

22. Cimiano, P., Collins, B., De Vuono, M. C., Escudier, T., Gottowik, J., Hartung, M., Leddin, M., et al. (2024). Patient listening on social media for patient-focused drug development: A synthesis of considerations from patients, industry and regulators. *Frontiers in Medicine, 11*. https://www.semanticscholar.org/paper/68b7a02886de2366bda163abb5642e8e1850e47c (accessed on 10th June 2025).

23. Coloma, P. M., Pane, J., Rebollo, I., Sturkenboom, M., et al. (2017). *Evaluating The Safety Profile of Non-Active Implantable Medical Devices Compared with Medicines*. https://core.ac.uk/download/154417147.pdf (accessed on 10th June 2025).

24. Cox, M. C., Mendes, R., Halwachs, K. N., Domenici, G., Brito, C., & Boghaert, E. (2023). Tackling the tumor microenvironment–how can complex tumor models *in vitro* aid oncology drug development? *Expert Opinion on Drug Discovery, 18*, 753–768. https://www.semanticscholar.org/paper/80e292720a8f948dcfe3b4e044670abc1622f796 (accessed on 10th June 2025).

25. Cummings, J., Kumar, P., & Reiber, C. (2018). *The Price of Progress: Funding and Financing Alzheimer's Disease Drug Development*. https://core.ac.uk/download/215451781.pdf (accessed on 10th June 2025).

26. Dane, A., Ashraf, S., Timmis, J., Bos, M., Uyl-de Groot, C. U., & van der Kuy, P. M. (2022). Barriers to patient enrolment in phase III cancer clinical trials: Interviews with clinicians and pharmaceutical industry representatives. *BMJ Open, 12*. https://www.semanticscholar.org/paper/0251e3ad0d2c194fdf0806c18d55a87d02166498 (accessed on 10th June 2025).

27. Danese, S., Solitano, V., Jairath, V., & Peyrin-Biroulet, L. (2022). The future of drug development for inflammatory bowel disease: The need to ACT (advanced combination treatment). *Gut, 71*, 2380–2387. https://www.semanticscholar.org/paper/f19b6d33d19bea6a432cbb43a4e44c29d86f858c (accessed on 10th June 2025).

28. Dekker, M., de Vries, S. T., Versantvoort, C. H., Drost-van Velze, E. G. E., Bhatt, M., van Meer, P., Havinga, I. K., et al. (2021). Sex proportionality in pre-clinical and clinical trials: An evaluation of 22 marketing authorization application dossiers submitted to the European Medicines Agency. *Frontiers in Medicine, 8*. https://www.semanticscholar.org/paper/24989db299774da23744f190b764cd873fcf07a5 (accessed on 10th June 2025).

29. Diamant, Z., & Pieterse, H. (2014). *Good Clinical Practice in Clinical Interventional Studies*. https://core.ac.uk/download/55803925.pdf (accessed on 10th June 2025).

30. Domingo-Fernández, D., Gadiya, Y., Preto, A. J., Krettler, C. A., Mubeen, S., Allen, A., Healey, D., et al. (2024). Natural products have increased rates of clinical trial success throughout the drug development process. *Journal of Natural Products, 87*, 1844–1851. https://www.semanticscholar.org/paper/9ba13119f41d89a37b2e09b75b256444e49dca6b (accessed on 10th June 2025).

31. Doneva, S., Ellendorff, T., Sick, B., Goldman, J. P., Cannon, A., Schneider, G., & Ineichen, B. (2024). NeuroTrialNER: An annotated corpus for neurological diseases and therapies in clinical trial registries. https://www.semanticscholar.org/paper/56eef417c3b24678963de6478e7a3e46cdf15a77 (accessed on 10th June 2025).

32. Dukaew, N., Na Takuathung, M., Sakuludomkan, W., Chairaksa, K., Klinjan, P., Morakote, N., & Koonrungsesomboon, N. (2023). Regulatory compliance and readability of informed consent forms in industry-sponsored drug development clinical trials. *Clinical Trials, 20*, 517–527 https://www.semanticscholar.org/paper/d2e827351900fe535fc72bcbe35655cff87b3583 (accessed on 10th June 2025).

33. Edsjö, A., Russnes, H., Lehtiö, J., Tamborero, D., Hovig, E., Stenzinger, A., & Rosenquist, R. (2024). High-throughput molecular assays for inclusion in personalized oncology trials–State-of-the-art and beyond. *Journal of Internal Medicine, 295*, 785–803. https://www.semanticscholar.org/paper/ba7432dcd8b7c3e67b55a6e51e739bcac8fa5085 (accessed on 10th June 2025).

34. Faulkner, S., Somers, F., Boudes, M., Nafria, B., & Robinson, P. (2023). Using patient perspectives to inform better clinical trial design and conduct: Current trends and future directions. *Pharmaceutical Medicine, 37*, 129–138. https://www.semanticscholar.org/paper/b20ace539c697d52aaf34da7bed9b11eb1e17f44 (accessed on 10th June 2025).

35. Fokunang, C., Tembe-Fokunang, E., Djuidje Ngounou, M., Ngono, B., Mantsana, I., Duclaire, P. S. J., Etoundi, J., et al. (2025). Ethical and regulatory challenges for contract research organizations conducting (outsourced) clinical research in Sub-Saharan Africa with a case

study of Cameroon. *Journal of Advances in Medical and Pharmaceutical Sciences.* https://www.semanticscholar.org/paper/23eb7343a954013f7e7c8297e558c3b28eef769a (accessed on 10th June 2025).

36. Ford, I., & Norrie, J. (2016). *Pragmatic Trials.* https://core.ac.uk/download/46558805.pdf (accessed on 10th June 2025).

37. Gazerani, P. (2024). *Human Brain Organoids in The Preclinical Phase of Drug Development for Migraine.* https://core.ac.uk/download/636678994.pdf (accessed on 10th June 2025).

38. Gooneratne, N. (2019). *Overview of Drug Development.* https://core.ac.uk/download/231833988.pdf (accessed on 10th June 2025).

39. Gooneratne, N. S. (2019). Overview of drug development. *Academic Entrepreneurship for Medical and Health Sciences.* https://www.semanticscholar.org/paper/4512344054b1ced08624c573c1c57db6550400ea (accessed on 10th June 2025).

40. Grill, J. D., & Karlawish, J. (2010). Addressing the challenges to successful recruitment and retention in Alzheimer's disease clinical trials. https://core.ac.uk/download/pdf/8521880.pdf (accessed on 10th June 2025).

41. Gurung, M., & Shrestha, S. (2025). Machine learning in modern drug discovery: Applications, advances, and future horizons. *KEC Journal of Science and Engineering.* https://www.semanticscholar.org/paper/394239ed4ed122e9d608e6dc1de10533f2e008c8 (accessed on 10th June 2025).

42. Han, G., Li, C., & Yi, P. (2024). The efficacy of bevacizumab combined with platinum-containing chemotherapy in the treatment of advanced non-small cell lung cancer in China: A systematic review and meta-analysis of randomized clinical trials. *Frontiers in Pharmacology, 15.* https://www.semanticscholar.org/paper/7a43fd9f4e9247305bfb54edbad267d5bf98a1fe (accessed on 10th June 2025).

43. Hassan, A., & Ibrahim, A. (2023). *The Coming Quantum Computing Evolution in The Pharmaceutical Industry and Drug R&D.* https://core.ac.uk/download/596254333.pdf (accessed on 10th June 2025).

44. Heinzmann, D., Monnet, A., & Rufibach, K. (2019). Integrating Phase 2 into Phase 3 based on an intermediate endpoint while accounting for a cure proportion: With an application to the design of a clinical trial in acute myeloid leukemia. *arXiv.* http://arxiv.org/abs/1901.01308 (accessed on 10th June 2025).

45. Hill, L. F., Obiero, C., Bekker, A., Walker, A. S., Bielicki, J., Sharland, M., & Schiavone, F. (2025). Safety reporting in neonatal clinical trials: Reflections towards optimal, globally relevant approaches. *Trials, 26.* https://www.semanticscholar.org/paper/7201282d1963e9c4fb52174ee803020ba7c09c53 (accessed on 10th June 2025).

46. Hoffmann, G. F., Mechler, K., Mountford, W. K., Ries, M., et al. (2015). Pressure for drug development in lysosomal storage disorders: A quantitative analysis thirty years beyond the US Orphan Drug Act. https://core.ac.uk/download/32585968.pdf (accessed on 10th June 2025).

47. Hollebecque, A., Tsimberidou, A. M., Barker, A. D., Tam, A. L., Biankin, A. V., Shaw, A. T., Biankin, A. V., et al. (2015). Patient-centric trials for therapeutic development in precision oncology. https://core.ac.uk/download/42364362.pdf (accessed on 10th June 2025).

48. Jiang, C., Beji, C., Zebachi, S., Hayek, G. Y., Cetinyurek-Yavuz, A., Fayyad, M. B. N., Rodwell, L., et

al. (2025). Decision-making criteria and methods for initiating late-stage clinical trials in drug development from a multi-stakeholder perspective: A scoping review. *Clinical Pharmacology and Therapeutics, 117*, 978–988. https://www.semanticscholar.org/paper/1a812a8fc4be0acb04b1f23937465024c89be59 (accessed on 10th June 2025).

49. Jorda, A., & Zeitlinger, M. (2020). Preclinical pharmacokinetic/pharmacodynamic studies and clinical trials in the drug development process of EMA-approved antibacterial agents: A review. *Clinical Pharmacokinetics, 59*, 1071–1084. https://www.semanticscholar.org/paper/31fc67d0a5cd7d24d4ce6512820c082c7519be9c (accessed on 10th June 2025).

50. Khalid, S. (2025). Optimization of pharmaceutical processes using artificial intelligence. *Clinical Medicine and Health Research Journal*. https://www.semanticscholar.org/paper/c98f55d63fdccaae9204143d61e93c09c0a56416 (accessed on 10th June 2025).

51. Krishna, R., Sebastien, B., Corriol-Rohou, S., Cheung, S. Y. A., Liu, J., & Suryawanshi, S. (2024). Pediatric rare diseases development in the pharmaceutical industry: An international consortium whitepaper. *Clinical Pharmacology & Therapeutics, 116*. https://www.semanticscholar.org/paper/9311217e05e626b49345b81d37f3e11a2db2ffce (accessed on 10th June 2025).

52. Kumar, S., Kumar, H., Lahon, J., & Saikia, D. (2024). A brief review on the lessons learned from COVID-19 on drug discovery and research. *Medicine and Pharmacy Reports, 97*, 243–248. https://www.semanticscholar.org/paper/126e5967520a8c0c2bfbcc2d6f3c673abbd184ba (accessed on 10th June 2025).

53. Lin, G., Siddiqui, S., Bernstein, J., Martínez, D., Gardner, L., Albright, T., & Igusa, T. (2020). Examining association between cohesion and diversity in collaboration networks of pharmaceutical clinical trials with drug approvals. *Journal of the American Medical Informatics Association: JAMIA*. https://www.semanticscholar.org/paper/671f0ba6539bd3f0e59f441085980c375c27d469 (accessed on 10th June 2025).

54. Liu, J. T., Tsou, H. H., & Tzeng, C. S. (2014). Establishing non-inferiority of a new treatment in a three-arm trial: Apply a step-down hierarchical model in a papulopustular acne study and an oral prophylactic antibiotics study. https://core.ac.uk/download/493036859.pdf (accessed on 10th June 2025).

55. Liu, J., Farrow, M., Seymour, L., Desai, J., Loong, H., Ivy, P., Koyoma, T., et al. (2025). Accelerating the future of oncology drug development: The role of consortia in the delivery of precision oncology early phase clinical trials. *Journal of Clinical Oncology, 43*, 735–747. https://www.semanticscholar.org/paper/acb3c8dbc611aa504de494ddec9b443b05973f32 (accessed on 10th June 2025).

56. Malshy, K., Steinmetz, A. R., Yuen, K. M., Bandari, J., & Rabinowitz, R. (2025). Military influences on the evolution of clinical trials throughout history. *Clinical Trials*. https://www.semanticscholar.org/paper/1457f9d54129621daa48ffb7680954961ef06580 (accessed on 10th June 2025).

57. Martin-Kerry, J., Taylor, J., Scott, S., Patel, M., Wright, D., Clark, A., Turner, D., et al. (2023). 509 Developing a core outcome set for hospital deprescribing trials with older people under the care of a geriatrician. *International Journal of Pharmacy Practice*. https://www.semanticscholar.org/paper/6777d6e7db95ef11093b5b11237c1cf4dee0562d (accessed on 10th June 2025).

58. Mercier, A. K., Ueckert, S., Sunnåker, M., Hamrén, B., Ambery, P., Greasley, P. J., & Åstrand, M.

(2024). From plan to pivot: How model-informed drug development shaped the dose strategy of the Zibotentan/Dapagliflozin ZENITH trials. *Clinical Pharmacology & Therapeutics, 116*. https://www.semanticscholar.org/paper/ff13935e1be3d9d1b98eb7c9f0272ca35d99c867 (accessed on 10th June 2025).

59. Moore, K., Fossler, M., & Younis, I. (2022). The importance of participant tracking when conducting clinical pharmacology drug trials. *The Journal of Clinical Pharmacology, 62*. https://www.semanticscholar.org/paper/9ce549a0bbfcbdaf9289cc05b5fe49319bb78d2f (accessed on 10th June 2025).

60. Moore, M., Goldstein, D., Hamm, J., Figer, A., Hecht, J., Gallinger, S., Au, H., et al. (2023). Erlotinib plus gemcitabine compared with gemcitabine alone in patients with advanced pancreatic cancer: A Phase III trial of the National Cancer Institute of Canada Clinical Trials Group. *Journal of Clinical Oncology, 41*, 4714–4720. https://www.semanticscholar.org/paper/1a6ab5ded3face432eed101b9a694517562403bb (accessed on 10th June 2025).

61. Morales, J. F., Klose, M., Hoffert, Y., Podichetty, J. T., Burton, J., Schmidt, S., Romero, K., et al. (2024). Type 1 diabetes prevention clinical trial simulator: Case reports of model-informed drug development tool. *CPT: Pharmacometrics & Systems Pharmacology, 13*, 1309–1316. https://www.semanticscholar.org/paper/08c64777bd2f7b57247cbfbba576dae29c0973b1 (accessed on 10th June 2025).

62. Moyer, H., Mellett, R., Vigneault, K., McKeown, M., Karlawish, J., Augustine, E., Schneider, L., et al. (2024). Prevalence and impact of bypassing or overriding phase 2 trials in neurologic drug development. *Neurology, 103*. https://www.semanticscholar.org/paper/e457a1ac8988f1d68dcb18f1c32a14166a61c490 (accessed on 10th June 2025).

63. Nabila, A., Wulandari, E., & Purwono, P. (2024). Smart contracts for data sharing in drug development: A systematic review of security and transparent measurement. *Journal of Advanced Health Informatics Research*. https://www.semanticscholar.org/paper/947c305c048360f99b86a0a5a66e55ae38a7504e (accessed on 10th June 2025).

64. Nagarajan, V., Juul, A., Backeljauw, P., Kawai, M., Linglart, A., Zuckerman-Levin, N., Horikawa, R., et al. (2022). Abstract 102: Once-weekly somapacitan versus daily growth hormone in children born small for gestational age: 1-year results from a randomized phase 2 trial. *Indian Journal of Endocrinology and Metabolism, 26*, 44. https://www.semanticscholar.org/paper/c0efa54d6b4ae4fe4e0f0ab374eaa73d010d5b67 (accessed on 10th June 2025).

65. Narsinh, K., Perez, E., Haddad, A. F., Young, J. S., Savastano, L., Villanueva-Meyer, J., Winkler, E., et al. (2024). Strategies to improve drug delivery across the blood–brain barrier for glioblastoma. *Current Neurology and Neuroscience Reports, 24*, 123–139. https://www.semanticscholar.org/paper/7f1c73502ebb5e6e9026f5c216e1fff63e380f8a (accessed on 10th June 2025).

66. Nasrollahzadeh, A. A., & Khademi, A. (2021). Dynamic programming for response-adaptive dose-finding clinical trials. *INFORMS Journal on Computing, 34*, 1176–1190. https://www.semanticscholar.org/paper/183d7b7201d41907b32fcda210d99a094f343be4 (accessed on 10th June 2025).

67. Niazi, S. K., & Mariam, Z. (2025). Artificial intelligence in drug development: Reshaping the therapeutic landscape. *Therapeutic Advances in Drug Safety, 16*. https://www.semanticscholar.org/paper/b84e4d9fa836057fcba1883406d13a4d5bea2b42 (accessed on 10th June 2025).

68. Ocaña, A., Pandiella, A., Privat, C., Bravo, I., Luengo-Oroz, M. A., Amir, E., & Győrffy, B.

(2025). Integrating artificial intelligence in drug discovery and early drug development: A transformative approach. *Biomarker Research, 13*. https://www.semanticscholar.org/paper/34cae377aed3d2719465e8ab8803fb38d968a632 (accessed on 10th June 2025).

69. Ogura, T., & Shiraishi, C. (2024). Analysis of adverse events following phenobarbital administration for pediatric patients categorized by one-year age increments using the U.S. Food and Drug Administration Adverse Event Reporting System. *Cureus, 16*. https://www.semanticscholar.org/paper/19abca64f015c3e111aa0412f2a065569ad71f67 (accessed on 10th June 2025).

70. Park, Y., Na, J. Y., Cho, J. Y., Oh, J., & Rhee, S. J. (2022). Key considerations for phase 2 or 3 clinical study design of anti-inflammatory agent for COVID-19 treatment. *Frontiers in Pharmacology, 13*. https://www.semanticscholar.org/paper/82b20431169e4115bd9b595d61d8070d67e0622d (accessed on 10th June 2025).

71. Parveen, A., Khalid, M., Singh, S. P., Gupta, M., & Kumar, A. (2024). Clinical trials of drugs: A comprehensive review of methodologies, challenges, and advances. *International Journal of Research Publication and Reviews*. https://www.semanticscholar.org/paper/d28c74920c4cb9b36cf9ef3f657b99a1a090bcad (accessed on 10th June 2025).

72. Pazdur, R. (2021). FDA and its role in drug development. *Journal of the Advanced Practitioner in Oncology, 12*, 293–295. https://www.semanticscholar.org/paper/c4070d44538f7027b76f326e05fea642ab54e18e (accessed on 10th June 2025).

73. Percie du Sert, N., Ahluwalia, A., Alam, S., Avey, M. T., Baker, M., Browne, W. J., Clark, A., et al. (2020). Reporting animal research: Explanation and elaboration for the ARRIVE guidelines 2.0. *PLOS Biology, 18*, e3000411. https://doi.org/10.1371/journal.pbio.3000411.

74. Petersen, R. C., Graf, A., Brady, C., De Santi, S., Florian, H., Landen, J., Pontecorvo, M. J., et al. (2025). Operationalizing selection criteria for clinical trials in Alzheimer's disease: Biomarker and clinical considerations. *Alzheimer's & Dementia: Translational Research & Clinical Interventions, 11*. https://www.semanticscholar.org/paper/02b8dfc312c9355269d13ac44b4614b6942c8131 (accessed on 10th June 2025).

75. Ramya, M., & Subamoorthy, U. (2023). Risk and opportunities in development of new drug. *International Journal of Allied Medical Sciences and Clinical Research*. https://www.semanticscholar.org/paper/fab7fd1798cc23cb3216f6d5d41f46036d8098fb (accessed on 10th June 2025).

76. Ruijs, T., Heuberger, J., de Goede, A. A., Ziagkos, D., Otto, M. E., Doll, R., van Putten, M. V., et al. (2022). Transcranial magnetic stimulation as biomarker of excitability in drug development: A randomized, double-blind, placebo-controlled, cross-over study. *British Journal of Clinical Pharmacology, 88*, 2926–2937. https://www.semanticscholar.org/paper/9352b77c3cd3b6b02e77c6a88c5cb21b2db7c3f2 (accessed on 10th June 2025).

77. Santiago-Rodriguez, F. (2025). Facing the trial of internationalizing clinical trials to developing countries: Some evidence from Mexico. https://core.ac.uk/download/pdf/6941422.pdf (accessed on 10th June 2025).

78. Santos, S. P. da S., Mendes, F. M. L., & Borges Gouvea Barroso, W. B. (2024). Panorama dos principals estudos clínicos sobre medicamentos contra tuberculose no Brasil e no mundo. *Vigilância Sanitária em Debate*. https://www.semanticscholar.org/paper/a4543df4f82bfe8202cdcd7bbdf59982198766f4 (accessed on 10th June 2025).

79. Sasaki, M., Sato, H., Uemura, Y., Mikami, A., Ichihara, N., Fujitani, S., Kondo, M., et al. (2024). How much more efficient are adaptive platform trials than multiple stand-alone trials? A comprehensive simulation study for streamlining drug development during a pandemic. *Clinical Pharmacology & Therapeutics, 115*. https://www.semanticscholar.org/paper/0f39a275a4d12f6a3bcfecb4b1e129b58dae1b36 (accessed on 10th June 2025).

80. Sessa, C., Cortés, J., Conté, P., Cardoso, F., Choueiri, T. K., Dummer, R., LoRusso, P., et al. (2021). The impact of COVID-19 on cancer care and oncology clinical research: An experts' perspective. *ESMO Open, 7*, 100339. https://doi.org/10.1016/j.esmoop.2021.100339.

81. Sikora, J. P. (2008). Providing hope: Developing a viable regulatory framework for providing terminally ill patients with adequate access to investigational drugs. https://core.ac.uk/download/12214773.pdf (accessed on 10th June 2025).

82. Steinmetz, A. R., Jazayeri, B., Pierce, M., Mokkapati, S., McConkey, D., Li, R., & Dinney, C. P. N. (2025). Integrating gene therapy into the treatment paradigm for non-muscle invasive bladder cancer. *Expert Opinion on Biological Therapy, 25*, 149–159. https://www.semanticscholar.org/paper/07f11b9830b89d6db2fd607b741e8aabf3b50815 (accessed on 10th June 2025).

83. Tannergren, C., Arora, S., Babiskin, A., Borges, L., Chatterjee, P., Cheng, Y. H., Dallmann, A., et al. (2024). Current state and new horizons in applications of physiologically based biopharmaceutics modeling (PBBM): A workshop report. *Molecular Pharmaceutics, 22*, 5–27. https://www.semanticscholar.org/paper/bdcaf477795ea797a915089f85542323a8e58f28 (accessed on 10th June 2025).

84. Veugelers, R., & Zachmann, G. (2020). Racing against COVID-19: A vaccines strategy for Europe. *Bruegel Policy Contribution*, Issue 7. https://core.ac.uk/download/322353892.pdf (accessed on 10th June 2025).

85. Warokar, P., & Lote, S. B. (2024). Ethical and regulatory consideration in AI-assisted drug development. *2024 2nd DMIHER International Conference on Artificial Intelligence in Healthcare, Education and Industry (IDICAIEI)*. https://www.semanticscholar.org/paper/bc73bc4dad21e3b65cf5cde0380a4e1d777cbb24 (accessed on 10th June 2025).

86. Williams, A. E., Wickman, A. M., Colebatch, A. N., Combe, B., et al. (2016). Clinical practice guidelines for the foot and ankle in rheumatoid arthritis: A critical appraisal. https://core.ac.uk/download/293883527.pdf (accessed on 10th June 2025).

87. Yin, X., Stuart, E., Burcu, M., Stewart, M., Lamont, E., & Davi, R. C. (2023). The validity of a synthetic control arm derived from historical multiple myeloma clinical trials. *Blood*. https://www.semanticscholar.org/paper/4afa02c44b1db5979e447d7775b9f50954c699c5 (accessed on 10th June 2025).

88. Yu, X., Zhao, H., Wang, R., Chen, Y., Ouyang, X., Li, W., Sun, Y., et al. (2024). Cancer epigenetics: From laboratory studies and clinical trials to precision medicine. *Cell Death Discovery, 10*. https://www.semanticscholar.org/paper/c76b08674da1f1a7930def1a27acc1c219216e39 (accessed on 10th June 2025).

89. Zhou, J., Muluneh, B., Li, Q., & Hughes, J. H. (2025). Revolutionizing patient-reported outcomes analysis for oncology drug development using population models. *Clinical Cancer Research, 31*, 1580–1586. https://www.semanticscholar.org/paper/f935129be2ffd42e7ec65d59d1ecd72d99dd04ee (accessed on 10th June 2025).

90. Zhu, X., & Chen, Y. (2024). Bridging the new drug access gap between China and the United States and its related policies. *Frontiers in Pharmacology, 14*. https://www.semanticscholar.org/paper/8bc05578ceefec4caa08a19f6b85b0479bb1f8bc (accessed on 10th June 2025).

THERAPEUTIC DRUG MONITORING (TDM)

5

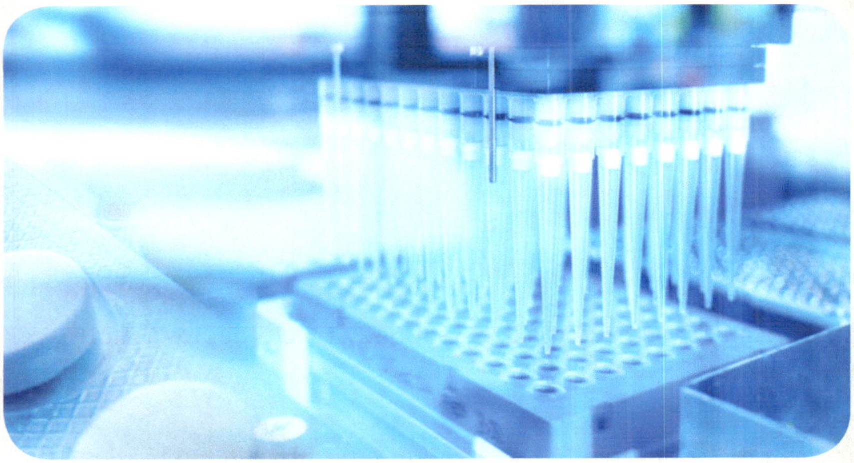

LEARNING OBJECTIVES

After studying this chapter, you will be able to:

1. Understand principles of therapeutic drug monitoring
2. Know the applications of therapeutic drug monitoring
3. Identify challenges and controversies in TDM

Introduction

Therapeutic Drug Monitoring (TDM) is a key approach to personalized medicine, most notably in the management of severe diseases like inflammatory bowel disease (IBD). Through systematic monitoring of drug levels, TDM seeks to maximize therapeutic success while reducing unwanted side effects, tailoring treatment to individual patients. With the evolving therapy landscape of IBD, particularly after the advent of biologics and novel small molecules, the significance of TDM becomes more vital. It mirrors the necessity of precise dosing being tailored to some therapy targets, disease phenotypes, and inflammatory load. Recent reports underscore the heterogeneity of optimal drug concentrations, pointing out that increased levels most frequently are associated with better clinical outcomes and, therefore, with potential benefits of a proactive TDM strategy in optimizing treatment effectiveness (Irving et al., 2022). Besides that, the persistent challenges in the area of study, e.g., drug resistance and metabolic heterogeneity, warrant continuous innovation and improvement in TDM protocols to ensure they facilitate effective patient-centered care (Arastehfar et al., 2021) (Figure 5.1).

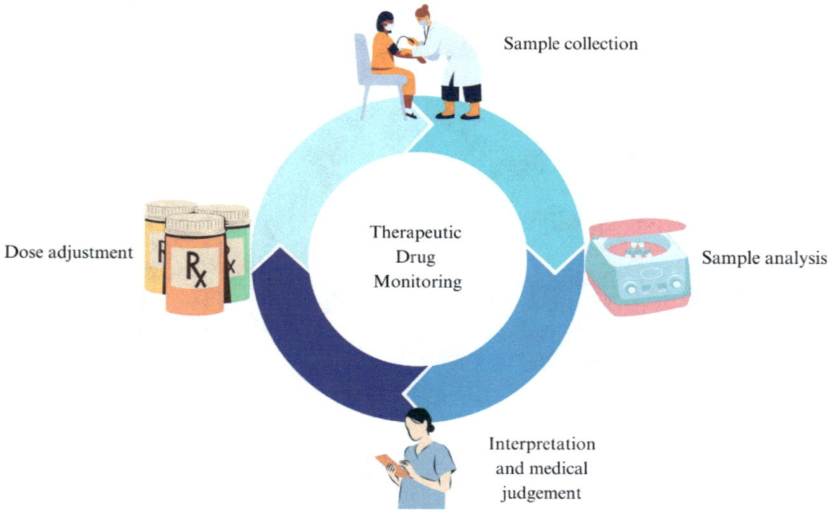

Figure 5.1. Therapeutic drug monitoring (TDM).

Source: https://www.mdpi.com/pharmaceuticals/pharmaceuticals-17-00642/article_deploy/html/images/pharmaceuticals-17-00642-g001.png.

5.1. Principles of Therapeutic Drug Monitoring

Learning Outcome

1. Understand pharmacokinetics and its role in TDM
2. Explain pharmacodynamics and drug response
3. Know the therapeutic range and its significance
4. Identify factors influencing drug levels
5. Describe sampling methods for TDM
6. Know the timing of drug level measurements
7. Discuss interpretation of TDM results
8. Focus on clinical decision-making based on TDM
9. Learn the limitations of TDM

In pharmacotherapy, TDM practices are crucial to maximize patient outcomes and promote drug safety. TDM is fundamentally interested in individualizing drug dosing based on empirical data related to pharmacokinetics, which explores the mechanisms by which drugs become absorbed, distributed, metabolized, and excreted. Population variability is central because it can potentially have drastically negative impacts on dose-exposure-response relationships. For instance, physiological variations in patients' phenotypes necessitate the application of modeling and simulation platforms to provide correct prediction of pharmacokinetic profiles (Bailey et al., 2018). Besides, in some patient groups, e.g., patients on extracorporeal membrane oxygenation (ECMO), pharmacokinetic alterations lead to decreased drug effect or enhanced side effects, meaning careful monitoring and dose adjustment based on the individual patient response (Aebi et al., 2017). Therefore, TDM is a key approach for therapy optimization to achieve maximum favorable effects and minimize adverse outcomes.

5.1.1. Pharmacokinetics and Its Role in TDM

Pharmacokinetics plays a pivotal role in the field of TDM by providing vital information regarding how drugs get absorbed, distributed, metabolized, and eliminated in the body. This is significant, particularly in critically ill patients who may have their pharmacokinetic profiles changed due to conditions like organ dysfunction or through the use of invasive therapies such as ECMO (Castro et al., 2024). For instance, variation in drug clearance can lead to inadequate therapeutic outcomes unless dosing regimens are suitably adjusted. Further, TDM gains added importance in antifungal treatment, particularly with triazoles, where variability in pharmacokinetics can directly affect the efficacy and safety of the treatment (Boyer et al., 2024). Therefore, through the use of TDM, health professionals can attain optimal drug dosing, enhance therapeutic efficacy, and decrease the possibility of unwanted side effects, thus improving patient outcome in complex clinical settings (Figure 5.2).

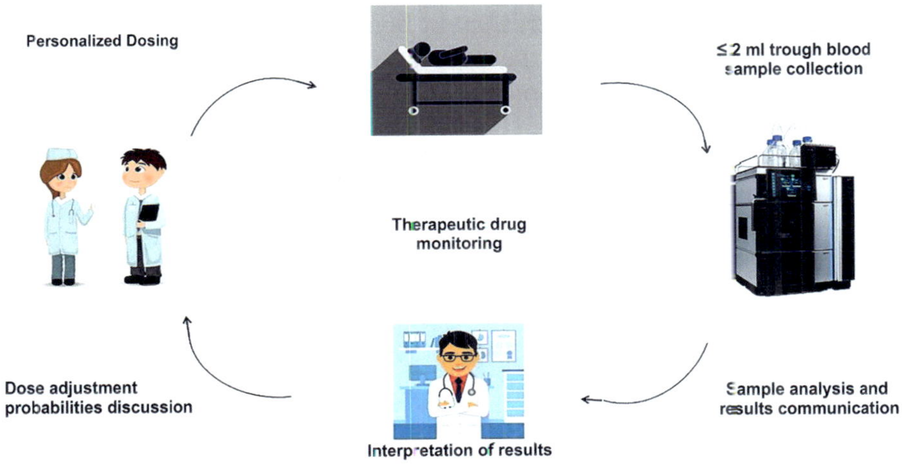

Figure 5.2. Pharmacokinetics plays a pivotal role in the context of Therapeutic Drug Monitoring (TDM) by providing essential insights into how drugs are absorbed, distributed, metabolized, and excreted in the body.

Source: https://www.frontiersin.org/files/Articles/1015200/fonc-12-1015200-HTML/image_m/fonc-12-1015200-g001.jpg.

5.1.2. Pharmacodynamics and Drug Response

Pharmacodynamics is critical in the context of TDM since it directly influences the way drugs operate against the body and yield a therapeutic response. Pharmacodynamics entails how drugs influence biological processes, yielding desired therapeutic responses as well as unwanted side effects. For instance, the introduction of cenobamate, an antiseizure medication, is a classic case of how vital it is to take into account pharmacokinetic and pharmacodynamic principles in patient management. A clear monitoring during the titration of cenobamate is essential due to potential DDI, especially among patients who could be being treated concomitantly with several antiseizure medications (Steinhoff et al., 2024). In addition, it should be observed that tolerance—the decreased body response to chronic drug exposure—can complicate dose adjustment and therapeutic effect, which underscores the need to observe drug concentrations and their pharmacodynamic effect still (Labay et al., 2024). Thus, TDM is a necessary method to optimize therapy and enhance the outcome of a patient in pharmacological treatment.

5.1.3. Therapeutic Range and Its Significance

Therapeutic range is the foundation of TDM because it determines the effective and safe levels of medication dosing. The therapeutic range for a drug is the range in which the drug has the desired therapeutic effect with no toxicity. This range is crucial, especially among high-risk groups, such as the elderly, where inappropriately given doses can result in high morbidity and mortality, as seen with the high sedation rates for gastroenterological procedures reported among elderly patients (Bell et al., 2006). Effective TDM relies on accurate data regarding therapeutic and toxic plasma concentration ranges, allowing practitioners to tailor drug regimens according to individualized patient needs (Andresen et al., 2012). By continuous monitoring of drug concentration within the therapeutic range, clinicians can optimize treatment benefits and prevent excessive adverse effects, resulting in improved patient safety and success in pharmacotherapy. And the awareness and appreciation of these ranges are a part of improving clinical practice and patient care (Figure 5.3).

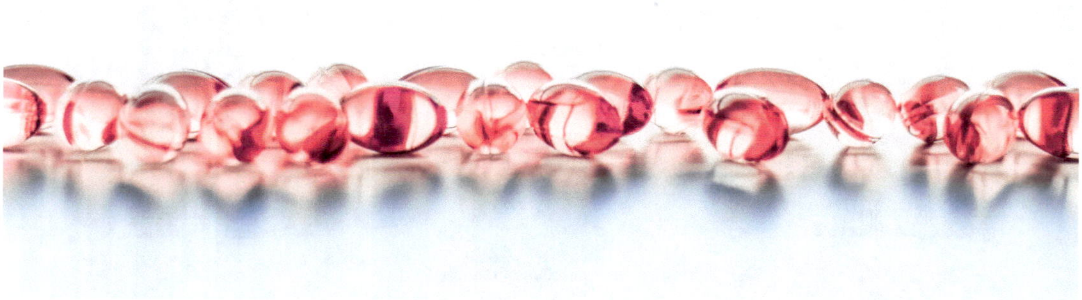

Figure 5.3. A drugs therapeutic range is the concentration within which it yields the desired therapeutic effect without producing toxicity.

Source: https://www.allucent.com/wp-content/uploads/2020/04/What-is-Toxicokinetics-TK_.webp.

5.1.4. Factors Influencing Drug Levels

It is crucial to have an understanding of factors influencing drug levels to ensure successful TDM, particularly in pediatric patients. Drug clearance and metabolism vary greatly depending on physiological factors like age, weight, and organ function. For instance, for children on voriconazole, a study established that the doses required to achieve therapeutic plasma levels were typically greater than the recommended dosages, particularly in children below the age of eight years, warranting individualized dosing regimens (Carabante et al., 2021). In addition, patient-specific factors such as clinical hypoalbuminemia and elevated C-reactive protein were found to be linked with suboptimal plasma levels, affecting the efficacy and safety of treatment (Carabante et al., 2021). Thus, TDM emerges as an essential instrument for drug dosage adjustment based on these determinants, subsequently optimizing therapeutic responses and avoiding potential adverse effects in pediatric patients.

5.1.5. Sampling Methods for TDM

Efficient TDM is based on efficient sampling methods that will provide appropriate drug concentration to be measured in order to obtain the optimal management of the patient. Various methods can be used, such as serum sampling representing drug levels after therapeutic application or whole blood measurement providing a more accurate pharmacokinetic representation. Emergence of innovative technologies, such as the D-SERS device, improves sampling efficiency in the rapid quantitation of antimicrobial content, thus cutting the time gap of dose adaptation of critically ill ICU patients (Pytlarz et al., 2025). Moreover, advanced analytical techniques like high-performance liquid chromatography-mass spectrometry have been validated for the determination of different tyrosine kinase inhibitors (KIs) from plasma, justifying the necessity for accurate sampling protocols that cater to changing drug properties and patient demands (Hirasawa et al., 2021). Lastly, the selection of proper sampling protocols is essential to maximizing TDM in diverse clinical scenarios (Figure 5.4).

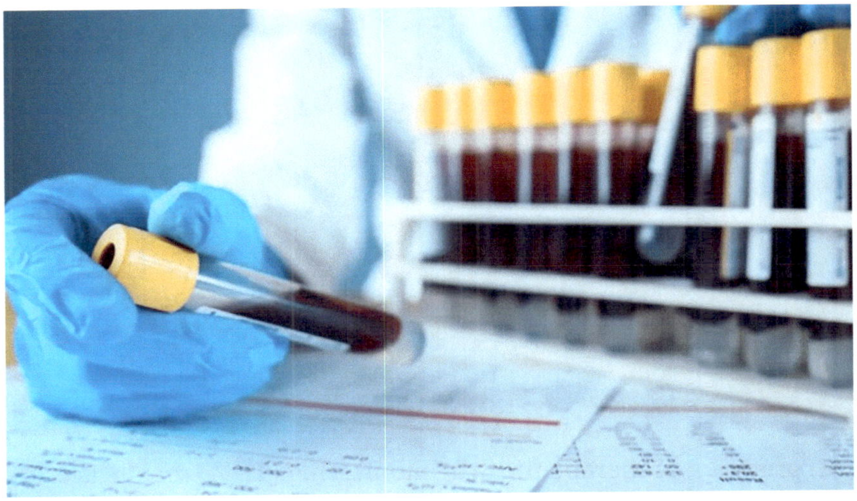

Figure 5.4. Effective sampling methods are crucial for the success of Therapeutic Drug Monitoring (TDM).

Source: https://utak.com/wp-content/uploads/2023/07/Untitled-design-96.png.

5.1.6. Timing of Drug Level Measurements

The timing of drug level measurements plays a pivotal role in the effectiveness of TDM, as it directly influences the accuracy of interpreting a patient's response to medication. It is essential to give the drug at the right time to check if the levels in the body are therapeutic. For instance, the measurement of vancomycin levels necessitates strict adherence to timing protocols due to its narrow therapeutic index, underscoring the importance of precise timing in avoiding toxicity and ensuring efficacy (Bandere et al., 2022). Moreover, TDM seeks to optimize dosing regimens based on individual patient characteristics, including their metabolic response and concurrent medications (Aronson et al., 2009). Therefore, incorporating systematic timing into TDM protocols helps patients by using drug doses that match the drug's changing levels in the body, which improves the management of complicated medical conditions.

5.1.7. Interpretation of TDM Results

The interpretation of TDM results is crucial for optimizing pharmacotherapy, particularly for drugs with narrow therapeutic windows, such as phenytoin and clozapine. For instance, phenytoin exhibits non-linear kinetics and high protein binding, which complicates its dosing and necessitates frequent monitoring to maintain effective serum concentrations (Tobler-Giger et al., 2016). Likewise, the pharmacokinetics of clozapine reveal significant gender differences, with women often presenting higher plasma concentrations than men, despite receiving similar dosing (Anderson et al., 2015). This difference is significant in clinical situations because it shows why doctors should use individualized dosing plans. As a result, the correct interpretation of TDM outcomes depends on knowing the drug's characteristics and also being aware of the patient's age, gender, and other diseases, so that the therapy can be adjusted to suit them (Figure 5.5).

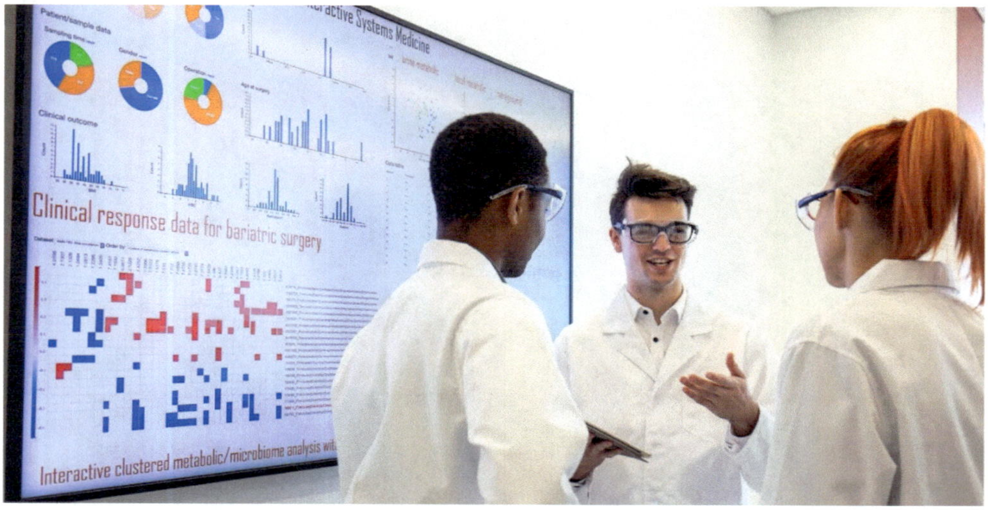

Figure 5.5. The interpretation of therapeutic drug monitoring (TDM) results is crucial for optimizing pharmacotherapy, particularly for drugs with narrow therapeutic windows, such as phenytoin and clozapine.

Source: https://eu-images.contentstack.com/v3/assets/blt485767b4a9c4cef5/blt85fe72d241b3a536/673f6eaa637c6813750beaea/Pharmacology.webp?width=1280&auto=webp&quality=95&format=jpg&disable=upscale.

5.1.8. Clinical Decision-Making Based on TDM

One of the key roles for TDM is to aid in clinical decision-making through optimization of treatment outcomes. By adjusting the dosages of drugs based on individual patient response, TDM enables healthcare professionals to cope with the complexity of pharmacotherapy. For instance, in the treatment of acute myeloid leukemia (AML), measurable residual disease (MRD) is a critical factor in informing the strategy of treatment. Clinicians utilize MRD tests to determine the requirement of stem cell transplants and other maintenance therapies, indicating how TDM has direct clinical implications for patient-specific therapies (Short et al., 2024). Additionally, the application of TDM among seriously ill patients receiving beta-lactams has been proven to enhance clinical efficacy, resulting in enhanced treatment success and microbiological eradication (Guly Eás et al., 2024). Therefore, TDM incorporation in clinical practice not only maximizes therapeutic outcomes but also signifies a move towards personalized medicine, solving for the unique pharmacokinetic characteristics of every patient.

5.1.9. Limitations of TDM

Although it has a very crucial function of optimizing patient care, TDM suffers from several limitations that can act against it in both clinical and forensic scenarios. The most significant problem is the intraindividual pharmacokinetic variability among individuals, which can lead to variable drug levels at the site of action and, consequently, make it difficult to optimize dosages. Such heterogeneity is often further modulated by external factors such as diet and adjunctive therapy, highlighted in the need for more extensive studies to account for confounding variables (Ingelman-Sundberg et al., 2024). Additionally, the efficacy of TDMs also depends on the sensitivity and specificity of the utilized assays, which are potentially limited by technical constraints (Jena et al., 2024). Thus, drug levels can be interpreted with difficulty in atypical matrices of biology. All these challenges call for ongoing research and method development for maximizing TDMs potential to optimize therapeutic efficacy as well as patient safety (Figure 5.6).

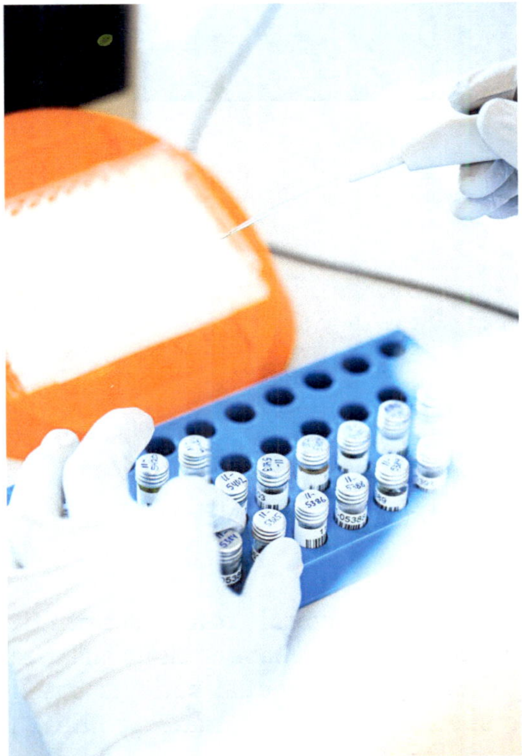

Figure 5.6. One primary challenge is the inherent variability in pharmacokinetics among individuals, which can lead to inconsistent drug levels at the site of action, complicating dosage adjustments.

Source: https://www.svarlifescience.com/hubfs/Imagebank/Close-ups/Svar-Life-Science-gloved-hand-placing-test-tubes-in-blue-rack-and-using-a-pipette.jpg.

Test Your Knowledge

1. What is the impact of TDM in personalized medicine?
2. Why is timing critical when performing TDM?

5.2. Applications of Therapeutic Drug Monitoring

Learning Outcome

1. Understand TDM in chronic disease management, psychiatric medications
2. Explain the role of TDM in antibiotics and infectious diseases
3. Focus on TDM in oncology
4. Describe TDM in pediatric populations and geriatric patients
5. Discuss TDM in patients with renal impairment.
6. Focus on TDM in polypharmacy scenarios
7. Explain emerging applications of TDM

TDM plays a pivotal role in optimizing pharmacotherapy by enabling clinicians to tailor drug dosages to individual patients based on their specific pharmacokinetic profiles. This way of prescribing medicine makes drugs more effective and reduces the chances of harmful reactions, especially among those who use many drugs or have different body functions. Moreover, TDM is increasingly being integrated into traditional healthcare frameworks, notably in settings where African Traditional Medicine (ATM) coexists with modern practices. It is clear that the challenge of joining these systems is high because many cultures use different medicinal plants and practices, so it is vital for practitioners to exchange knowledge. As such, applying sophisticated modeling techniques, including those mentioned in Diallo et al. (2013), can systematically compile and formalize the extensive traditional knowledge, fostering safer and more effective treatment protocols while supporting patient safety through vigilant drug monitoring (Capiau et al., 2016).

5.2.1. TDM in Chronic Disease Management

TDM is essential in the management of chronic disease as it offers a practice of enhancing therapeutic effects while minimizing adverse reactions. Through the synergy of TDM, healthcare professionals can adjust drug dosages based on a patient's unique features and responses, thereby initiating precision medicine. It is particularly relevant in chronic disease when treatment regimens are complex and patients respond differently to drugs. For instance, proteomics has emerged as a valuable tool that helps detect biomarkers that enable better stratification and monitoring of treatment response, as demonstrated in recent research (Frantzi et al., 2017). Additionally, rising spending for specialty medications highlights the need to optimize therapy interventions with TDM, considering that health plans are increasingly attempting to control costs while sustaining patient safety and successful therapy (Samuel et al., 2012). Thus, TDM not only advantages personalized medicine but also addresses economic factors in the treatment of chronic illnesses (Figure 5.7).

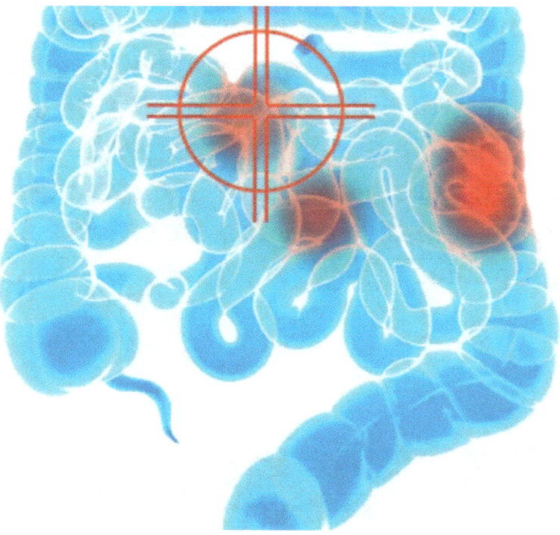

Figure 5.7. Therapeutic Drug Monitoring (TDM) plays a pivotal role in the management of chronic diseases, offering a strategy that enhances therapeutic efficacy while minimizing adverse effects.

Source: https://biohithealthcare.co.uk/wp-content/uploads/2021/06/TDM-edit.png.webp.

5.2.2. TDM in Psychiatric Medications

Application of TDM with psychiatric drugs has increasingly taken center stage in optimizing treatment efficacy and outcomes. As psychiatric disease is characteristically complex, e.g., BD, where response to treatment can be significantly variant across patients, TDM represents a key means of maximizing pharmacological therapies. By tailoring the doses of drugs to achieve target plasma levels of drugs, TDM reduces the risk of drug toxicity and optimizes the rate of successful therapy. The tailoring is illustrated by research proving that consideration must be given to the genetic determinants of drug response, as in the case of BD, to improve treatment strategies (Berghofer et al., 2014). In addition, managing psychological distress of chronic illnesses, such as cystic fibrosis, prioritizes the use of an interdisciplinary collaborative care model that integrates psychological intervention with pharmacologic therapy to manage comorbidities effectively (Abbott et al., 2015). Lastly, TDM results in more rational clinical decisions and improved quality of life.

5.2.3. TDM in Antibiotics and Infectious Diseases

The imperative role of TDM in controlling the use of antibiotics in infectious disease cannot be overemphasized, as it resolves the major issues of subtherapeutic dosing and drug resistance. By a kind of application of simple pharmacokinetic and pharmacodynamic principles, TDM attempts to optimize dosing of antibiotics for efficacy with an acceptable degree of toxicity, an issue of special concern with rising drug-resistant infections. This requirement for proper dosage is reaffirmed in studies correlating subtherapeutic dosing with adverse clinical outcomes and increased resistance (Brock et al., 2015). Additionally, the problem of AMR is complex and calls for comprehensive policy frameworks involving prudent use and proper surveillance in various sectors (Aarestrup et al., 2015). Thus, the application of TDM in clinical practice not only advances the interests of individual patient outcomes but also promotes the overall goals of preventing antibiotic resistance within health care systems (Figure 5.8).

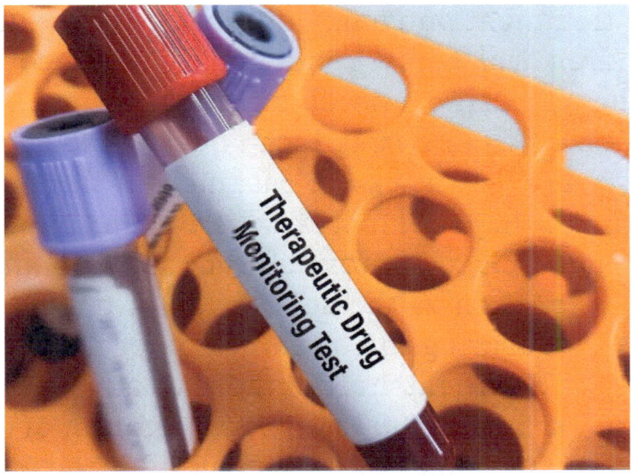

Figure 5.8. TDM in antibiotics and infectious diseases.

Source: https://d10lvax23vl53t.cloudfront.net/images/Article_Images/ImageForArticle_3064_17199662093188389.jpg.

5.2.4. TDM in Oncology

Application of TDM for oncology has emerged as a crucial strategy to maximize cancer therapy, particularly for KIs. Based on the wide interpatient variability of drug response and associated risks of standard dosing regimens, TDM offers the benefit of individualized dose adjustment based on real-time pharmacokinetic data. Exposure-response and exposure-toxicity relationships have been shown in studies for the majority of KIs, highlighting the requirement for TDM to maximize therapeutic impact and minimize toxicity. Additionally, precision medicine, enabled by the advances in –omics technologies, offers further scope for personalization. Of special interest is proteomics, which has applications in oncology by shaping dynamic molecular phenotypes, which in turn reflect better patient stratification and targeted interventions. Oncology can advance toward a more customized therapeutic culture by combining proteomics and pharmacokinetic monitoring, particularly in complicated illnesses like bladder cancer where therapy is severely limited (Frantzi et al., 2017; Guchelaar et al., 2023).

5.2.5. TDM in Pediatric Populations

For treatment outcome improvement in children, the employment of TDM is extremely promising. Children will possess individual pharmacokinetic and pharmacodynamic profiles due to varying body composition, developmental age, and maturation of organ function. These make conventional one-size-fits-all dosing techniques ineffective and require cautious dosing to avoid subtherapeutic response or toxicity. For instance, in the treatment of tuberculosis, TDM has gained prominence, especially in patients with severe comorbidities like HIV and diabetes, since it enables maximization of drug levels to improve efficacy and minimize side effects (Ivanova et al., 2025). Moreover, specific therapies such as the application of tyrosine KIs in children's cancer highlight the importance of TDM in ensuring the optimization of pharmacokinetics and tailoring treatment protocols towards enhanced patient needs, thereby advocating for improved management strategies in children (Bellouard et al., 2023). The integration of TDM into children's treatment can hence significantly provide for enhanced therapeutic outcomes as a means of guaranteeing treatment schedules are both practical and safe (Figure 5.9).

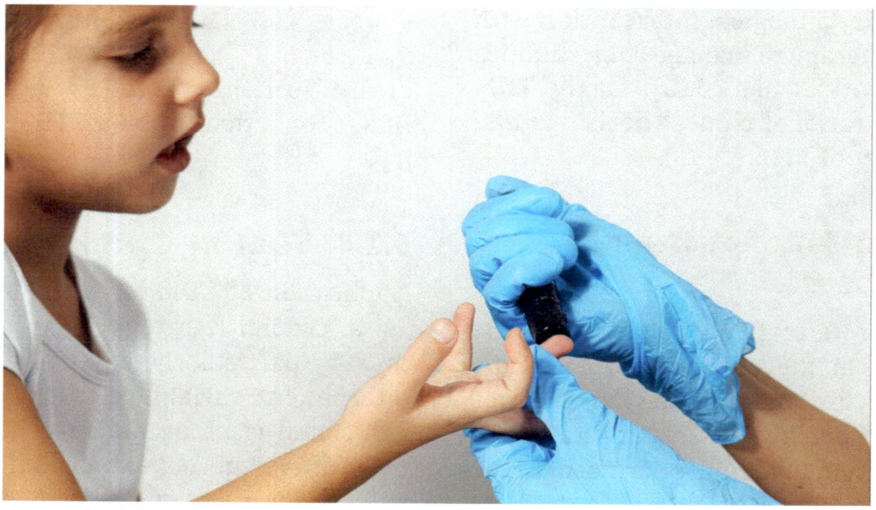

Figure 5.9. In pediatric populations, the application of Therapeutic Drug Monitoring (TDM) holds significant promise for enhancing treatment outcomes.

Source: https://www.neoteryx.com/hubfs/child-finger-stick-sampling-iStock-1343557535.jpeg.

5.2.6. TDM in Geriatric Patients

As elderly patients usually have multiple comorbidities and polypharmacy, the application of TDM is essential in ensuring maximum pharmacotherapy effect. A well-designed TDM will be able to neutralize the risk of increased adverse drug events, which are pretty prevalent in the elderly due to the physiological changes and multiple drug regimens. To reduce such risks, measures such as medication evaluation tools and interprofessional working have been developed to support good prescribing habits (Corsonello et al., 2016). Additionally, in the field of oncology practice, the treatment of polypharmacy is essential because older patients with cancer experience high rates of complex drug interactions based on their cancer treatment and comorbid conditions. Having clinical pharmacists as part of the healthcare team will enhance drug management through the identification of risk and optimization of drug safety (Khanal et al., 2019). TDM is therefore not only a means to optimize drug efficacy but also a way of avoiding potential risks involved in prescribing drugs in older patients.

5.2.7. TDM in Patients with Renal Impairment

The necessity of TDM in renally compromised patients is underscored by the complex pharmacokinetics of fluctuating renal function. Subtherapeutic drug levels or toxic accumulation may arise from interindividual variations in drug clearance in this patient population, necessitating careful monitoring to ensure effective and safe therapeutic outcomes. For instance, plazomicin, approved for complicated urinary tract infections, shows the relevance of TDM; patients with varying degrees of renal impairment require dose-adjusted dosing to minimize nephrotoxicity without loss of activity (Zhuang et al., 2022). There is also evidence that trough monitoring maximizes therapy but that a quantitative advantage from peak concentration data is uncertain (Kim et al., 2023). Thus, establishing a TDM protocol based on renal function is essential in avoiding risks and reaching therapeutic levels, setting the stage for the central role of TDM in optimizing patient safety and therapeutic efficacy (Figure 5.10).

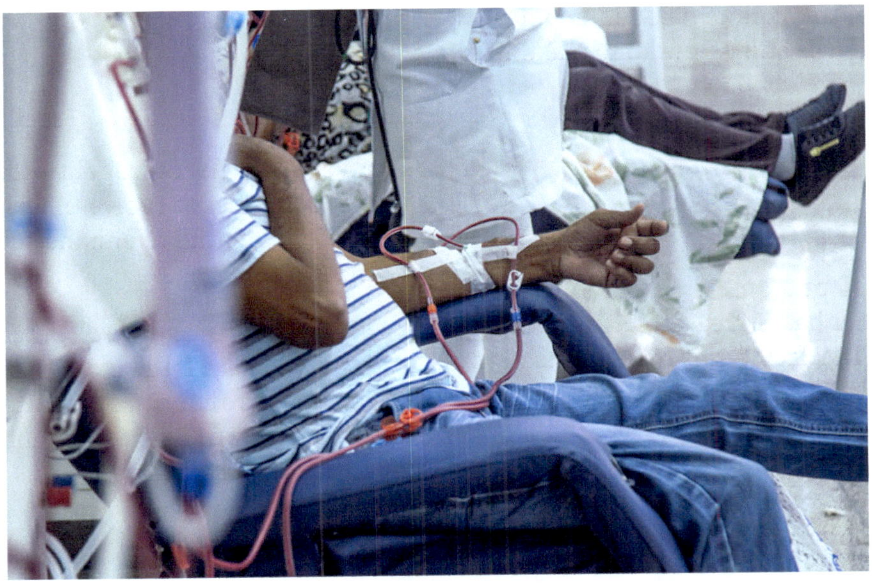

Figure 5.10. The necessity for therapeutic drug monitoring (TDM) in patients with renal impairment is underscored by the complex pharmacokinetics associated with altered renal function.

Source: https://pharmaceutical-journal.com/wp-content/uploads/2023/02/person-on-dialysis-927x617.jpg.

5.2.8. TDM in Polypharmacy Scenarios

Concerning polypharmacy, TDM becomes pivotal to ensuring the utmost safety of patients and treatment efficacy. As drug regimens become more complicated, particularly among patient populations such as cancer patients, the potential for harmful drug interactions is greatly enhanced. For example, a report quoted the severe side effects of co-administration between dapsone and methylene blue, leading to serotonin syndrome due to other serotonin-acting drugs (Zhu et al., 2024). Such a scenario emphasizes the need for thorough medication assessment during conditions of polypharmacy. In addition, with the development of wearable and sensor technology, real-time TDM is also increasingly becoming possible. TDM can tailor drug dosing and improve clinical outcomes according to differences in the metabolism of drugs among individuals and thereby pave the way for precision medicine that can solve the problems induced by polypharmacy (Liang et al., 2024). Hence, the role of TDM in advanced therapeutic practice is still essential to maximize patient care.

5.2.9. Emerging Applications of TDM

With growing advances in TDM, emerging applications hold great promise for enhanced clinical outcomes. In recent years, pharmacogenomics has increased its integration into the work of TDM, facilitating the dispensation of drugs according to individual genetic profiles. The personalized medicine approach not only optimizes drug treatment effectiveness but also minimizes adverse drug reactions—a concern especially crucial to minimize in polypharmacy scenarios. Additionally, the use of sophisticated analytical methods, such as high-performance liquid chromatography and mass spectrometry, has improved the precision and accuracy of drug level measurements, enabling prompt therapy modification. Recent research has established that a streamlined regulatory review process, as highlighted in Cone et al., (2018), can accelerate approval for new TDM applications, thereby enhancing patient treatment. As these applications expand, future TDM protocols will incorporate real-time monitoring systems and further improve therapeutic interventions in clinics (FitzGerald et al., 2013) (Figure 5.11).

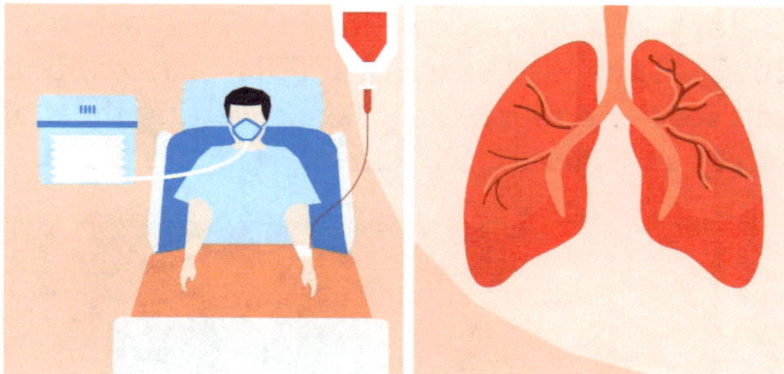

Figure 5.11. As therapeutic drug monitoring (TDM) continues to evolve, emerging applications reveal its potential to enhance clinical outcomes significantly.

Source: https://roche.scene7.com/is/image/RocheDiaProd/hero-benefits-of-mass-spectrometry-in-monitoring-immunosuppressive-drugs-for-organ-transplants?scl=1.

Test Your Knowledge

1. How is TDM used in the management of patients with renal or hepatic impairment?
2. Why is TDM important in the management of patients receiving anticancer therapy?

5.3. Challenges and Controversies in TDM

Learning Outcome

1. Understand variability in individual responses to drugs
2. Explain the cost-effectiveness of TDM
3. Know ethical considerations in TDM
4. Focus on standardization of TDM protocols
5. Discuss integration of TDM into clinical guidelines
6. Identify patient adherence and compliance issues
7. Explain technological advancements and their impact
8. Know the misinterpretation of TDM results
9. Explain future directions and research needs

TDM is fraught with dangers and controversies, which are mostly a reflection of the complexity of varied patient responses to therapy. Among the concerns on the table is the varying effect of antidepressants on neuroplasticity, such that long-term therapy has an initially beneficial neurogenic impact but finally leads to irreversible fixation of brain flexibility, challenging the efficacy of future therapy (Varela et al., 2024).

Furthermore, controversy over the optimal resuscitation fluid in critically ill patients has similar issues in TDM. The SAFE trial provided evidence that albumin may lead to higher mortality than saline in traumatic brain injury, contrary to earlier expectations of fluid resuscitation (Colen et al., 2019). These differences underscore the requirement for continuous monitoring and individualized adjustments in TDM approaches, as the clinician functions at the intersection of deep-rooted treatment algorithms and novel evidence obtained through serial investigation.

5.3.1. Variability in Individual Responses to Drugs

Variability in drug response in individuals is a significant challenge in clinical practice, particularly for psychiatric and neurological conditions. The pharmacokinetics of certain drugs, including second-generation antipsychotics, vary significantly among individuals due to genetics, metabolism, and concomitant drugs. This heterogeneity often leads to suboptimal therapeutic outcomes, since patients may experience suboptimal symptom control or side effects of uniform dosing schedules (Včí et al., 2024). Similarly, the effectiveness of Parkinson's disease therapy is dependent upon intricate pharmacological interactions and drug compliance, and is influenced by multidimensional pharmacological interactions and drug compliance issues, leading to more complicated dosing regimens (Müller et al., 2024).

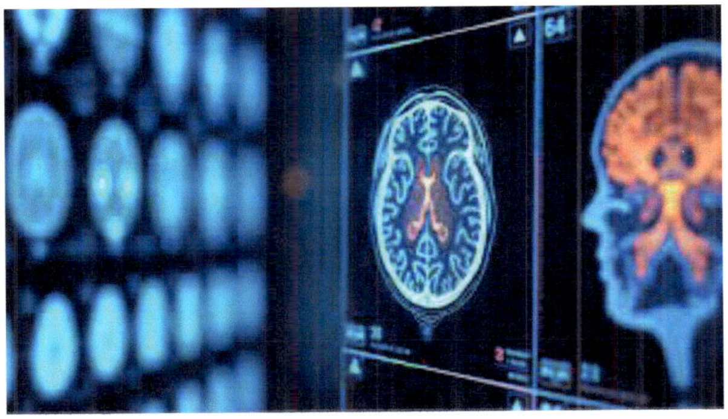

Figure 5.12. Variability in individual responses to drugs poses a significant challenge in clinical practice, particularly in the realms of psychiatric and neurological disorders.

Source: https://encrypted-tbn0.gstatic.com/images?q=tbn:ANd9GcQeRTN6exc1sI_FXqPls_m_8OH72rdW-TR7of3pveNLzosN83vzZQ9QW1PRBfTrHQIo1gc&usqp=CAU.

Therefore, TDM emerges as an essential strategy in individualizing drug management. Through the individualization of doses based on distinctive pharmacokinetic profiles, TDM holds the potential to optimize drug efficacy, promote patient compliance, and minimize the risk of adverse effects, thus leading to enhanced and individualized treatment regimens (Figure 5.12).

5.3.2. Cost-Effectiveness of TDM

The cost-effectiveness of TDM is presently an issue of focal interest, particularly in the optimization of disease drug therapy for conditions such as breast cancer and IBD. In tamoxifen-directed research, TDM-directed dosing not only improved clinical benefit, providing increased life years and QALYs, but also reduced treatment expenditures across the board, with a dominant effect being seen for TDM compared to routine dosing algorithms (Braal et al., 2022). Similarly, in anti-TNF biologic drugs like infliximab and adalimumab, TDM strategies have time and again been found to be economically viable and helpful in maximizing patient outcomes and minimizing immunogenicity (Márquez-Megías et al., 2022). The robust evidence of the cost-effectiveness of TDMs indicates that it can extend an innovative approach toward optimizing therapeutic efficacy at the same time by minimizing the financial burden on healthcare systems, ultimately leading to more sustainable treatment regimens.

5.3.3. Ethical Considerations in TDM

As TDM technologies become increasingly integrated, a complex chain of ethical concerns emerges that must be critically examined. Ethical considerations are prone to focus on patient autonomy, informed consent, and clinical interpretation of information. For instance, the transition from traditional monitoring mechanisms to real-time data analysis challenges the clarity of information provided to patients, particularly its relevance to therapeutic choices (Pedada, 2025). In addition, the success of home monitoring, for instance, finger-prick self-testing of immunosuppressants in post-transplant subjects, necessitates careful examination of the potential risks and benefits of such activities (Vethe et al., 2024). Such equity of access to these advanced monitoring tools must be ensured lest disparities in technology exacerbate existing healthcare inequalities. Resolving these ethical considerations is thus critical to guarantee equitable use of TDM in clinical practice (Figure 5.13).

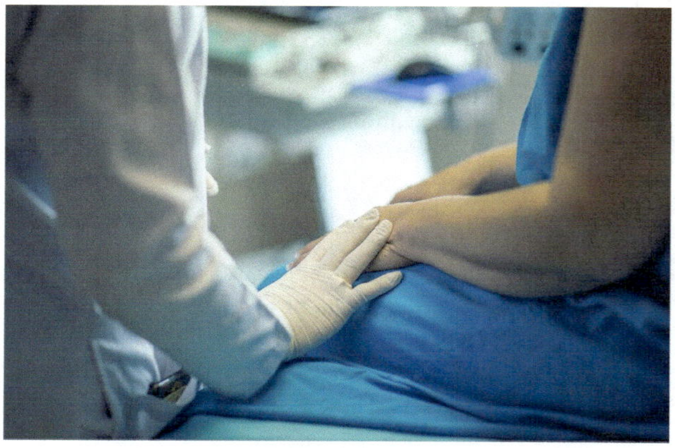

Figure 5.13. Ethical concerns often revolve around patient autonomy, informed consent, and the interpretation of data in clinical settings.

Source: https://studypages.com/blog/content/images/2024/06/image4.jpg.

5.3.4. Standardization of TDM Protocols

Standardization of TDM practices is crucial in optimizing patient outcomes, particularly for those on complex therapies like asparaginase in pediatric Acute Lymphoblastic Leukemia (ALL) and targeted metabolic regimens in glioblastoma (GBM). High institutional variability in practice has been evidenced, especially in monitoring methods and administration protocols (Morgan et al., 2024). A consensus framework can enhance the precision in monitoring patient response to such treatment, and as a result, safety and effectiveness. The application of standardized guidelines will also facilitate easier comparisons of data among studies, which is required to conduct a thorough evaluation of outcomes of treatment and side effects (Duraj et al., 2024). With the use of stable TDM regimens, clinicians not only strengthen drug treatment efficacy but also contribute to generalized education in drug metabolism and its implications in clinical oncology. Eventually, a standardized method implies commitment to precision medicine and working towards smarter treatment management.

5.3.5. Integration of TDM Into Clinical Guidelines

The integration of TDM in clinical practice guidelines is necessary for maximizing patient outcomes, particularly with the treatment of conditions such as IBD with anti-tumor necrosis factor agents such as infliximab.

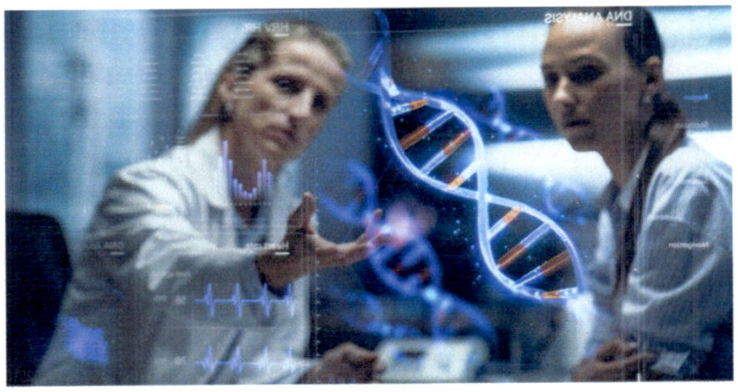

Figure 5.14. The integration of Therapeutic Drug Monitoring (TDM) into clinical guidelines is crucial for enhancing patient outcomes.

Source: https://www.laboratoriosrubio.com/wp-content/uploads/2025/02/personalized-medicine-scaled.jpeg.

Although growing amounts of evidence recommend that TDM is effective and associated with improved clinical outcomes and reduced surgical needs, there remain significant barriers to routine implementation. Among the issues are the lack of an agreement among healthcare providers regarding its application in practice and uncertainty regarding the cost-effectiveness of TDM uses (Shubow et al., 2025). According to the American Association of Pharmaceutical Scientists, establishing consensus among healthcare stakeholders—such as payers, patients, and legislators—about the benefits of TDM is crucial to its practical application (Shim et al., 2024). Overcoming these challenges will allow for greater standardization in TDM, ultimately enhancing patient care by optimizing dosing and management regimens (Figure 5.14).

5.3.6. Patient Adherence and Compliance Issues

Patient compliance and adherence are crucial elements of the success of treatment, particularly concerning TDM. One significant issue is when patients do not follow prescribed drug regimens, leading to suboptimal therapeutic effects. For instance, in hydroxychloroquine (HCQ) level testing, non-adherence problems were identified in approximately 10.5% of the samples, with some patients having undetectable or virtually undetectable levels of drugs, which can serve as a barrier to the effectiveness of treatment as well as be associated with risks of side effects such as retinopathy (Yang et al., 2024). Similar findings were observed in vancomycin treatment studies among children, whereby the requests by healthcare providers for 54% of patients only initiated therapeutic monitoring requests, although adherence to treatment protocols was noted at a high rate of 91.7% (Mohamed et al., 2024). The implications of these statistics suggest the need for stronger measures of patient education and compliance by healthcare providers to achieve the TDMs' effect on patient outcomes.

5.3.7. Technological Advancements and Their Impact

The integration of technology advances has had a remarkable influence on TDM, increasing the precision and efficacy of patient treatment. As medical advancements are revealed, particularly with HIV drugs, standards in treatment become more complex and still necessary to optimize patient outcomes (Bonaccorsi et al., 2025). These advances not only make treatments more effective but also lead to a reorientation of clinical practice guidelines to integrate new therapies. Furthermore, augmented 5G technology, in tandem with technological progress in artificial intelligence and big data, will revolutionize the provision of healthcare through real-time data analysis and greater patient connectivity (Farooq et al., 2017). The tech environment supports informed decision-making by healthcare providers in drug dosing and monitoring, thus ensuring enhanced therapeutic regimen compliance. Hence, as TDM develops with these improvements, it will help reduce past inefficiencies, creating a more responsive and equitable health system (Figure 5.15).

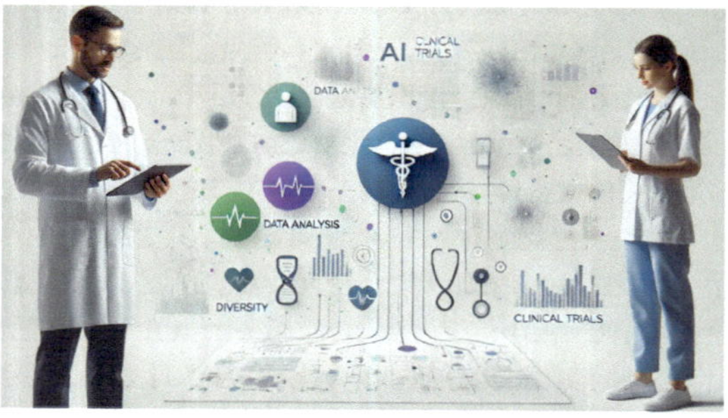

Figure 5.15. The integration of technological advancements has significantly transformed therapeutic drug monitoring (TDM), enhancing the precision and effectiveness of patient care.

Source: https://www.clinicaltrialvanguard.com/wp-content/uploads/2024/06/DALLE-2024-06-14-114754-A-simple-minimalist-image-with-a-lot-of-white-space-The-background-is-predominantly-white-with-subtle-accents-of-the-colors-from-the-attached-file--1250x715.webp.

5.3.8. Misinterpretation of TDM Results

Misinterpretation of TDM results is one of the significant barriers to the optimization of patient treatment outcomes. Variability in drug metabolism, drug dosage, and genetic pharmacokinetic polymorphisms are some of the causes of this limitation. For instance, voriconazole management has exhibited a vexing level of heterogeneity, in which 45% only of pediatric patients were documented to reach therapeutic concentration levels, illustrating the complexity of interpreting TDM data within multigroup populations (Resztak et al., 2024). Furthermore, while empirical TDM methods may enhance standardization of exposure, they remain secondary to model-informed precision dosing (MIPD), which utilizes population pharmacokinetic data even better to personalize treatments (Haefliger et al., 2025). Unless such advanced methodologies are incorporated, clinicians risk biased estimations, leading to inadequate therapeutic responses as well as reduced effectiveness of treatments. Therefore, enhancing the accuracy of TDM interpretation is crucial to ensure enhanced patient care and therapy outcomes.

5.3.9. Future Directions and Research Needs

With the advancement in TDM, guidelines and requirements for future research are more critical than ever before to optimize patient care and therapeutic efficiency. At the center of this should be the integration of innovative technologies such as pharmacogenomics and artificial intelligence that would significantly enhance personalized medication regimens by adjusting dosing based on genetic profile and predictive insights. Further, new strategies like nanoparticle therapy, which have been recognized with encouraging potential for the overcoming of the problem of drug delivery and reducing the toxicity, must be researched further in TDM (since the process of the disease is difficult to monitor to detect the advanced phase of the diseases, cytotoxicity induced by drugs, and problems related to drug delivery;

nanoparticle therapy has also impressed the researchers) (Kanwar et al., 2015). More interactions between researchers and clinicians will also be significant to identify the knowledge gaps and to develop uniform protocols that would facilitate the practical application of TDM practices in different fields of therapy (Capiau et al., 2016) (Figure 5.16).

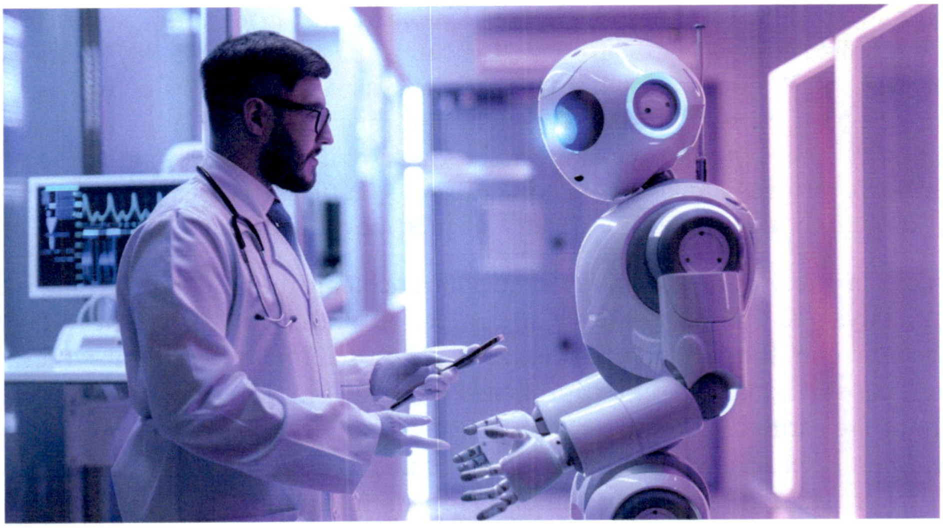

Figure 5.16. An essential focus is the integration of advanced technologies such as pharmacogenomics and artificial intelligence, which could significantly refine personal medication regimens by individualizing dosing based on genetic profiles and predictive analytics.

Source: https://cdn.sanity.io/images/0mnqm898/production/447e5a773392e549b12c80c4cdff7499fe162bec-2240x1260.png.

Test Your Knowledge

1. Why is the timing of blood sample collection a significant challenge in TDM?
2. What is the controversy surrounding the application of TDM in outpatient care?

Summary

TDM serves the primary purpose of optimizing patient care through keeping drug levels within therapeutic ranges. The research on pharmacists' knowledge and attitudes towards antimicrobial TDM revealed limited knowledge, with a median score of 5 out of 10, as indicated in recent studies in Qatar (Alkhiyami et al., 2024). Besides, the patient parameter interaction, such as renal function, affects drug metabolism to a large degree, highlighting the intricacy of TDM data interpretation (El-Khateeb et al., 2023). Since pharmacists have demonstrated positive attitudes towards TDM, there is a clear need for more educational activities in bridging knowledge gaps. By establishing a higher level of awareness of pharmacokinetics, especially in the case of patients with conditions like CKD, healthcare professionals can maximize therapeutic outcomes and tailor interventions more suitably, ultimately advancing the quality of pharmaceutical care.

TDM is crucial in maximizing patient-specific pharmacologic therapy, highlighting the importance of precise data analysis to optimize efficacy and safety of treatment. A key aspect of TDM is its use of Bayesian predictive methods, which maximize decision-making by predicting therapy outcomes based on individual variation. Current approaches typically employ maximum a-posteriori (MAP) estimates without the estimation of uncertainty, but Bayesian DA methods remove these limitations and thus provide more precise clinical decisions. Besides, the imaging biomarker role of [18F]FLT uptake is also emphasized in assessing tumor response to therapy. This PET tracer can quantify cell proliferation in a non-invasive fashion and is a potential response assessment marker in the clinic. However, understanding the determinants of [18F]FLT retention, as determined in past research, is vital for successful integration into TDM paradigms, thus leading to better therapeutic performance under varying interventions (Aboagye et al., 2016; de Wiljes et al., 2020).

KEY TERMS FROM THIS CHAPTER

- Acute myeloid leukemia (AML)
- Adjunctive therapy
- Adverse effects
- African Traditional Medicine (ATM)
- Antifungal treatment
- Antiseizure medication
- Biologics
- Cenobamate
- Clozapine
- Continuous monitoring
- C-reactive protein
- Critically ill patients
- Cultures
- Cystic fibrosis
- Diet
- Drug resistance
- D-SERS device

Critical Thinking Questions

1. **What is the primary purpose of Therapeutic Drug Monitoring (TDM)?**
   a. To monitor the patient's blood pressure
   b. To adjust drug doses based on blood levels to ensure efficacy and avoid toxicity
   c. To test the patient's genetic response to medications
   d. To determine the drug's market price
2. **Which of the following drugs is most likely to require Therapeutic Drug Monitoring (TDM)?**
   a. Acetaminophen
   b. Ibuprofen
   c. Warfarin
   d. Paracetamol
3. **When should blood samples be taken for Therapeutic Drug Monitoring (TDM) to ensure accurate results?**
   a. Immediately after drug administration
   b. Just before the next dose (trough level) or after peak concentration
   c. Only when the patient reports symptoms
   d. 24 hours after the last dose
4. **Which of the following is a key factor influencing the need for Therapeutic Drug Monitoring (TDM)?**
   a. The drug's pharmacokinetics, such as half-life and therapeutic range
   b. The patient's age and weight
   c. The color of the blood sample
   d. The cost of the drug
5. **What is considered a "narrow therapeutic index" in drug monitoring?**
   a. A large range between effective and toxic drug levels
   b. A small range between effective and toxic drug levels
   c. The range between the drug's peak and trough levels
   d. A slight difference between the drug's price and market demand

Answers to Critical Thinking Questions

1. (b); 2. (c); 3. (b); 4. (a); 5. (b).

Short Answer Questions

1. What is therapeutic drug monitoring (TDM)?
2. When is therapeutic drug monitoring (TDM) most commonly used?
3. What type of drugs typically require therapeutic drug monitoring (TDM)?
4. What is the most common biological sample used for therapeutic drug monitoring (TDM)?
5. How can therapeutic drug monitoring (TDM) improve patient outcomes?

References

1. Dar, O. A., Hasan, R., Schlundt, J., Harbarth, S., Caleo, G., Dar, F. K., Littmann, J., Rweyemamu, M., Buckley, E. J., Shahid, M., Kock, R., Li, H. L., Giha, H., Khan, M., So, A. D., Bindayna, K. M., Kessel, A., Pedersen, H. B., Permanand, G., . . . Heymann, D. L. (2015). Exploring the evidence base for national and regional policy interventions to combat resistance. *The Lancet, 387*(10015), 285–295. https://doi.org/10.1016/s0140-6736(15)00520-6Abanibhusan Jena, A., Pati, R. N., Mahajan, S., & Yadav, S. (2024). The significance of therapeutic drug monitoring: Investigating clinical and forensic toxicology. *Journal of Applied Bioanalysis*. https://www.semanticscholar.org/paper/15bd036534bcb37766a5d054d34b22246a621799 (accessed on 10th June 2025).
2. Abbott, J., Elborn, S., Georgiopoulos, A. M., Goldbeck, L., et al. (2015). *International Committee on Mental Health in Cystic Fibrosis: Cystic Fibrosis Foundation and European Cystic Fibrosis Society Consensus Statements for Screening and Treating Depression and Anxiety*. https://core.ac.uk/download/42137601.pdf (accessed on 10th June 2025).
3. Abboudi, H., & Macphee, I. A. (2012). *Individualized Immunosuppression in Transplant Patients: Potential Role of Pharmacogenetics*. https://core.ac.uk/download/17297975.pdf (accessed on 10th June 2025).
4. Aboagye, E., Bollineni, V. R., Heinzmann, K., Jacobs, M. A., et al. (2016). *Preclinical Applications of 3'-deoxy-3'-[18F]fluorothymidine in Oncology–A Systematic Review*. https://core.ac.uk/download/77021482.pdf (accessed on 10th June 2025).
5. Acharya, T., & Deedwania, P. (2015). *An Evidence-Based Review of Edogawa and Its Role in Stroke Prevention in Patients with Nonvalvular Atrial Fibrillation*. https://core.ac.uk/download/323310727.pdf (accessed on 10th June 2025).
6. Aebi, M. E., Shah, A. G., Anderson, C., Arlt, W., Barr, R., et al. (2017). *Medication Complications in Extracorporeal Membrane Oxygenation*. https://core.ac.uk/download/129191716.pdf (accessed on 10th June 2025).
7. Agabiti-Rosei, E., Cruickshank, J. K., Dominiczak, A., Erdine, S., et al. (2016). *2016 European Society of Hypertension Guidelines for The Management of High Blood Pressure in Children and Adolescents*. https://core.ac.uk/download/46165193.pdf (accessed on 10th June 2025).
8. Akkerman, O. W., Alffenaar, J. W. C., Bolhuis, M. S., Hofman, M., et al. (2015). *Role of Therapeutic Drug Monitoring in Pulmonary Infections: Use and Potential for Expanded Use of Dried Blood Spot Samples*. https://core.ac.uk/download/55746955.pdf (accessed on 10th June 2025).
9. Alkhiyami, D., Higazy, A. S., & Saad, M. (2024). A survey on the knowledge and attitudes of pharmacists towards the application of antimicrobial therapeutic drug monitoring and its challenges in Qatar. *PLOS ONE, 19*. https://www.semanticscholar.org/paper/94c9239137bf60faa37317424aae910ba07c84e0 (accessed on 10th June 2025).
10. Anderson, S. G., Connolly, M., Couchman, L., Flanagan, R. J., et al. (2015). Sex differences in plasma clozapine and norclozapine concentrations in clinical practice and in relation to body mass index and plasma glucose concentrations: A retrospective survey. https://core.ac.uk/download/42367102.pdf (accessed on 10th June 2025).
11. Andresen, H., Iwersen-Bergmann, S., Schmoldt, A., Schulz, K., et al. (2012). Therapeutic and toxic blood concentrations of nearly 1,000 drugs and other xenobiotics. https://core.ac.uk/download/14525457.pdf (accessed on 10th June 2025).

12. Arastehfar, A., Carvalho, A., Houbraken, J., Lombardi, L., Garcia-Rubio, R., Jenks, J. D., Rivero-Menéndez, O., et al. (2021). *Aspergillus fumigatus* and aspergillosis: From basics to clinics. *Studies in Mycology, 100*, 100115. https://doi.org/10.1016/j.simyco.2021.100115.

13. Aronson, J. K., Atkinson, A. J., Barr, J. T., Birkett, D. J., Bochner, F., Bootman, J. L., et al. (2009). Overview of therapeutic drug monitoring. https://core.ac.uk/download/pdf/8291262.pdf (accessed on 10th June 2025).

14. Attarbaschi, A., Barzilai, S., Escherich, G., Frandsen, B., et al. (2016). Consensus definitions of 14 severe acute toxic effects for childhood lymphoblastic leukemia treatment: A Delphi consensus. https://core.ac.uk/download/42370388.pdf (accessed on 10th June 2025).

15. Bailey, D., Bon, C., Cox, E., Darwich, A., Dorey, G., Duwal, S., Ette, E., et al. (2018). Population variability in animal health: Influence on dose-exposure-response relationships. Part II: Modelling and simulation. https://core.ac.uk/download/159992803.pdf (accessed on 10th June 2025).

16. Bandere, D., Darbiniece, K., Erts, R., Krūmiņa, A., et al. (2022). Experience of Vancomycin therapeutic drug monitoring in two multidisciplinary hospitals in Latvia. https://core.ac.uk/download/543079144.pdf (accessed on 10th June 2025).

17. Barber, N., Franklin, B. D., Gallivan, S., Taxis, K., et al. (2006). Can the Heinrich ratio be used to predict harm from medication errors? https://core.ac.uk/download/1747122.pdf (accessed on 10th June 2025).

18. Barone, R., Conti, M., Giorgi, B., Gatti, M., Cojutti, P., Viale, P., & Pea, F. (2023). Fast and sensitive analysis of fosfomycin in human plasma microsamples using liquid chromatography–tandem mass spectrometry for therapeutic drug monitoring. *Therapeutic Drug Monitoring, 46*, 384–390. https://www.semanticscholar.org/paper/648413f56d46bd03646148548855dad34ab66acb9 (accessed on 10th June 2025).

19. Bell, G. D., Bowles, J., De La Iglesia, B., Gray, J., et al. (2006). Sedation for gastrointestinal endoscopic procedures in the elderly: Getting safer but still not nearly safe enough. https://core.ac.uk/download/16428378.pdf (accessed on 10th June 2025).

20. Bellouard, M., Donadieu, J., Thiebot, P., Giroux Leprieur, E., Saiag, P., Etting, I., Dugues, P., et al. (2023). Validation of liquid chromatography coupled with tandem mass spectrometry for the determination of 12 tyrosine kinase inhibitors (TKIs) and their application to therapeutic drug monitoring in adult and pediatric populations. *Pharmaceutics, 16*. https://www.semanticscholar.org/paper/98145ac365da720419befb582640707fa01b367e (accessed on 10th June 2025).

21. Benítez Carabante, M. I., Díaz de Heredia, C., Martin-Gomez, M. T., Mendoza-Palomar, N., et al. (2021). Voriconazole use in children: Therapeutic drug monitoring and control of inflammation as key points for optimal treatment. https://core.ac.uk/download/477979226.pdf; https://core.ac.uk/download/521159119.pdf (accessed on 10th June 2025).

22. Berghofer, A., Heils, A., Koski, A., Serretti, A., Szczepankiewicz, A., et al. (2014). *Towards The Clinical Implementation of Pharmacogenetics in Bipolar Disorder*. https://core.ac.uk/download/323064927.pdf (accessed on 10th June 2025).

23. Bonaccorsi, A., & Merito, M. (2025). Innovation and standards in clinical practice: The case of HIV treatments. https://core.ac.uk/download/pdf/6964419.pdf (accessed on 10th June 2025).

24. Bowers, R., & Asbill, C. S. (2022). Traditional lecture versus case-based learning in a therapeutic drug monitoring course within an integrated pharmacy curriculum. *Innovations in Pharmacy, 13*. https://www.semanticscholar.org/paper/4ad25d234840be14215b8701d7593fb2b57c63b2 (accessed on 10th June 2025).

25. Boyer, J., Hoenigl, M., & Kriegl, L. (2024). Therapeutic drug monitoring of antifungal therapies: Do we really need it and what are the best practices? *Expert Review of Clinical Pharmacology, 17*, 309–321. https://www.semanticscholar.org/paper/653b899334d2451018d7431c8229c896b2316ea8 (accessed on 10th June 2025).

26. Braal, C. L., Kleijburg, A., Jager, A., Koolen, S., Mathijssen, R., Corro Ramos, I., Wetzelaer, P., et al. (2022). Therapeutic drug monitoring-guided adjuvant tamoxifen dosing in patients with early breast cancer: A cost-effectiveness analysis from the prospective TOTAM trial. *Clinical Drug Investigation, 42*, 163–175. https://www.semanticscholar.org/paper/78d2043529f2b78f594b0d6e9692a70e35429ece (accessed on 10th June 2025).

27. Brock, T. P., Le, P. V., Njuguna, B., Pastakia, S., et al. (2015). To address emerging infections, we must invest in enduring systems: The kinetics and dynamics of health systems strengthening. https://core.ac.uk/download/46964053.pdf (accessed on 10th June 2025).

28. Brocks, D., & Wang, M. (2023). Use of a common spreadsheet program to demonstrate the ability of Bayesian forecasting to estimate the pharmacokinetic parameters of antibiotics. *The Journal of Pharmacy and Pharmacology*. https://www.semanticscholar.org/paper/15183deca4eb73e0574ea05e4e134b196f8d38a6 (accessed on 10th June 2025).

29. Bunch, S. E., Cheuk, D. K., Cunningham, J. G., Dayrell-Hart, B., Durkes, T. E., Dyer, K. R., et al. (2016). 2015 ACVIM small animal consensus statement on seizure management in dogs. https://core.ac.uk/download/45467849.pdf (accessed on 10th June 2025).

30. Capiau, S., Stove, C., & Velghe, S. (2016). Opening the toolbox of alternative sampling strategies in clinical routine: A key-role for (LC-)MS/MS. https://core.ac.uk/download/84043363.pdf (accessed on 10th June 2025).

31. Colen, T. W., Wang, L. C., Ghodke, B., Cohen, W. A., Hollingworth, W., & Anzai, Y. (2019). Pakistan of Neurological Sciences (PJNS) neuroradiology. https://www.semanticscholar.org/paper/f10d1c94f704ed0243cdd0a85eb6f6941b9f8641 (accessed on 10th June 2025).

32. Cone, M., Cone, M., McAuslane, N., Al-Essa, R., & Ratanawijitrasin, S. (2018). The regulatory review process in South Africa: Challenges and opportunities for a new improved system. https://core.ac.uk/download/287581237.pdf (accessed on 10th June 2025).

33. Corsonello, A., Jha, A., Leendertse, A., Somers, A., Spinewine, A., et al. (2016). *Geriatric Pharmacotherapy: Optimization Through Integrated Approach in The Hospital Setting*. https://core.ac.uk/download/55809733.pdf (accessed on 10th June 2025).

34. Costa, A. R. C. e C., Gomes, A., Varejão, E. V. V., Brunes, R., Tavares, W., Santana, L. A., & Siqueira-Batista, R. (2024). Piperacillin-tazobactam: An update for clinical use. *Brazilian Journal of Health and Biomedical Sciences*. https://www.semanticscholar.org/paper/3be7eaa48882303e529624cfdb14940444babb66 (accessed on 10th June 2025).

35. de Wiljes, J., Hartung, N., Huisinga, W., & Kloft, C. (2020). Bayesian data assimilation to support informed decision-making in individualized chemotherapy. https://core.ac.uk/download/286352833.pdf (accessed on 10th June 2025).

36. Dekkers, A., Vander Laenen, F., Vanderplasschen, W., Wittouck, C. et al. (2014). Psychosocial functioning of drug treatment court clients: A study of the prosecutor's files in Ghent. https://core.ac.uk/download/55800675.pdf (accessed on 10th June 2025).

37. Diallo, G., Foguem, C., & Kamsu-Foguem, B. (2013). Conceptual graph-based knowledge representation for supporting reasoning in African traditional medicine. https://core.ac.uk/download/12044019.pdf (accessed on 10th June 2025).

38. do Valle Varela, J. P., da Silva Costa, V. R., Vaz, N. S., de Melo Almeida, T. H., Bernardes, G. S. O., de Almeida, L. R., & Caetano, A. L. F. M. (2024). Impact of prolonged use of antidepressants on neuroplasticity. *Health and Society*. https://www.semanticscholar.org/paper/06dcc40ec8c480e38cca4840a8d5fd8fdf273fd1 (accessed on 10th June 2025).

39. Du Bruyn, E., Morris, T., Rockwood, N., Wilkinson, R. J., et al. (2016). Assessment of treatment response in tuberculosis. https://core.ac.uk/download/77015882.pdf (accessed on 10th June 2025).

40. Duraj, T., Kalamian, M., Zuccoli, G., Maroon, J. C., D'Agostino, D. P., Scheck, A. C., Poff, A., et al. (2024). Clinical research framework proposal for ketogenic metabolic therapy in glioblastoma. *BMC Medicine, 22*. https://www.semanticscholar.org/paper/09ca12ede124e38fcf53d6bddb7edded4dda0adf (accessed on 10th June 2025).

41. El-Khateeb, E., Chinnadurai, R., Al Qassabi, J., Scotcher, D., Darwich, A., Kalra, P., & Rostami-Hodjegan, A. (2023). Using prior knowledge on systems through PBPK to gain further insight into routine clinical data on trough concentrations: The case of tacrolimus in chronic kidney disease. *Therapeutic Drug Monitoring, 45*, 743–753. https://www.semanticscholar.org/paper/070f0939c53a517cdf6787a2ceac795c704adb12 (accessed on 10th June 2025).

42. Farooq, S., Imran, M. A., Latif, S., Qadir, M. I., et al. (2017). How 5G wireless (and concomitant technologies) will revolutionize healthcare? https://core.ac.uk/download/143476480.pdf (accessed on 10th June 2025).

43. FitzGerald, O. R., Stephen, S., Opeyemi, A., Staunton, B., et al. (2013). Biomarkers of inflammatory arthritis and proteomics. https://core.ac.uk/download/288637789.pdf (accessed on 10th June 2025).

44. Forsythe, L. (2013). Measuring mental health in criminology research: Lessons from the Drug Use Monitoring in Australia program. https://core.ac.uk/download/pdf/30577468.pdf (accessed on 10th June 2025).

45. Frantzi, M., Latosinska, A., Merseburger, A. S., Mischak, H., et al. (2017). Clinical proteomics for precision medicine: The bladder cancer case. https://core.ac.uk/download/111557430.pdf (accessed on 10th June 2025).

46. Gerhardtová, I., Čižmárová, I., Jankech, T., Olešová, D., Jampílek, J., Parrak, V., Nemergutova, K., et al. (2024). Implementation of modern therapeutic drug monitoring and lipidomic approaches in clinical practice: A case study with colistin treatment. *Pharmaceuticals, 17*. https://www.semanticscholar.org/paper/cd81b39edf6a216dd9a82f2b7bb8e96b81c0c98c (accessed on 10th June 2025).

47. Guchelaar, N. A. D., Huitema, A. D. R., Koolen, S. L. W., Mathijssen, R. H. J., et al. (2023). Therapeutic drug monitoring of kinase inhibitors in oncology. https://core.ac.uk/download/588746890.pdf (accessed on 10th June 2025).

48. Gulyás, E., Horváth, I. L., Engh, M., Bunduc, S., Dembrovszky, F., Fehérvári, P., Bánvölgyi, A., et al. (2024). Assessment of the practical impact of adjusting beta-lactam dosages based on therapeutic drug monitoring in critically ill adult patients: A systematic review and meta-analysis of randomized clinical trials and observational studies. *Scientific Reports, 14*. https://www.semanticscholar.org/paper/4bef1c4dc51fb0fa43843876ea0ded280ab83011 (accessed on 10th June 2025).

49. Haefliger, D., Mina, L., Guidi, M., Marzolini, C., Thoueille, P., Rothuizen, L., Thoma, Y., et al. (2025). Individualization of piperacillin dosage based on therapeutic drug monitoring with or without model-informed precision dosing: A scenario analysis. *The Journal of Antimicrobial Chemotherapy*. https://www.semanticscholar.org/paper/d530f4d114e3cfec0c74501b525dee9cfebdd173 (accessed on 10th June 2025).

50. Hanžel, J., & Drobne, D. (2023). Editorial: Golimumab dosing intensification effective in ulcerative colitis with no need for therapeutic drug monitoring. *Alimentary Pharmacology & Therapeutics, 57*. https://www.semanticscholar.org/paper/1605a367d5235dc4e5c05d2d8b937395bcea5d36 (accessed on 10th June 2025).

51. Harshitha, K. B., Lakshmi, G. A., & Gaddam, R. (2024). Navigating complex comorbidities: A case of Behcet's syndrome with lumbar disc bulging and cardiovascular disease. *International Journal of Science and Research (IJSR)*. https://www.semanticscholar.org/paper/02abe8d2b40e9d69041a36cabd9c5f627d323794 (accessed on 10th June 2025).

52. Hirasawa, T., Kikuchi, M., Shigeta, K., Takasaki, S., Sato, Y., Sato, T., Ogura, J., et al. (2021). High-throughput liquid chromatography/electrospray ionization tandem mass spectrometry method using in-source collision-induced dissociation for simultaneous quantification of imatinib, dasatinib, bosutinib, nilotinib, and ibrutinib in human plasma. *Biomedical Chromatography: BMC*. https://www.semanticscholar.org/paper/c175faf2fe0b48b83ecd4fda2f3248dc9028d517 (accessed on 10th June 2025).

53. Horie, T., Oga, E. F., Sekine, S., Shitara, Y., et al. (2015). Pharmacokinetic herb-drug interactions: Insight into mechanisms and consequences. https://core.ac.uk/download/42138675.pdf (accessed on 10th June 2025).

54. Ingelman-Sundberg, M., & Molden, E. (2024). Therapeutic drug monitoring, liquid biopsies or pharmacogenomics for prediction of human drug metabolism and response. *British Journal of Clinical Pharmacology*. https://www.semanticscholar.org/paper/b3ba5f81045bc59517b08aeba30ba70424b4c16d (accessed on 10th June 2025).

55. Irving, P. M., & Gecse, K. (2022). Optimizing therapies using therapeutic drug monitoring: Current strategies and future perspectives. *Gastroenterology, 162*, 1512–1524. https://doi.org/10.1053/j.gastro.2022.02.014.

56. Ivanova, D. A., Litvinova, N. V., Yurovskaya, E. I., Kubrakova, E. P., & Mitrofanova, Y. Y. (2025). Therapeutic drug monitoring in the treatment of tuberculosis patients. *Tuberculosis and Socially Significant Diseases*. https://www.semanticscholar.org/paper/9524b526c05f2fe50b2d30a9cefd35e2bfab932e (accessed on 10th June 2025).

57. Kanwar, J. R., Kanwar, R. K., & Roy, K. (2015). Molecular targets in arthritis and recent trends in nano therapy. http://hdl.handle.net/10536/DRO/DU:30079045 (accessed on 10th June 2025).

58. Kawano-Dourado, L., Kristianslund, E. K., Zeraatkar, D., Jani, M., Makharia, G., Hazlewood,

G. S., Smith, C., et al. (2024). Proactive therapeutic drug monitoring of biologic drugs in adult patients with inflammatory bowel disease, inflammatory arthritis, or psoriasis: A clinical practice guideline. *BMJ, 387*. https://www.semanticscholar.org/paper/a9bcad8b4cff326489d5b2910e30be8dbf9e91dd (accessed on 10th June 2025).

59. Khanal, S., Shrestha, S., & Shrestha, S. (2019). Polypharmacy in elderly cancer patients: Challenges and the way clinical pharmacists can contribute in resource-limited settings. https://core.ac.uk/download/287605655.pdf (accessed on 10th June 2025).

60. Kim, H. K., & Jeong, T. D. (2023). Evaluation of vancomycin area under the concentration–time curve predictive performance using Bayesian modeling software with and without peak concentration: An academic hospital experience for adult patients without renal impairment. *Annals of Laboratory Medicine, 43*, 554–564. https://www.semanticscholar.org/paper/c9b8db7a88a6e00654dce6180d24b03b717c9ba4 (accessed on 10th June 2025).

61. Kodyvaur, K., Murthy, K., Kirupa, P., Pandian, G., & Goel, P. (2024). The role of digital innovation in modernizing railway networks: Case studies and lessons learned. *International Journal for Research Publication and Seminar*. https://www.semanticscholar.org/paper/6283e7782678f0530761a3f546e7b57b78d12643 (accessed on 10th June 2025).

62. Krejčí, V., Murínová, I., Slanař, O., & Šíma, M. (2024). Evidence for therapeutic drug monitoring of atypical antipsychotics. *Prague Medical Report, 125*(2), 101–129. https://www.semanticscholar.org/paper/0d71ab5101dffebe80c1448920c9d62df9429ef9 (accessed on 10th June 2025).

63. Labay, L., Kacinko, S. L., Casey, B. K., & Brower, J. O. (2024). Tolerant or intolerant? Learning from studying drug concentrations in the living and the dead. *The American Journal of Forensic Medicine and Pathology, 45*, 292–296. https://www.semanticscholar.org/paper/b5e0d3d12d9fb7de8fd1c2151ce4ee1e2e1a819f (accessed on 10th June 2025).

64. Liang, W. S., Beaulieu-Jones, B., Smalley, S., Snyder, M., Goetz, L. H., & Schork, N. J. (2024). Emerging therapeutic drug monitoring technologies: Considerations and opportunities in precision medicine. *Frontiers in Pharmacology, 15*. https://www.semanticscholar.org/paper/7ca0d051c229715ec2e3325d70f73c524f2218da (accessed on 10th June 2025).

65. López Pérez, J., Inda-Landaluce, M., Nocito-Colón, M., & Martínez-Lostao, L. (2025). Comparative analysis of 2 commercially available assays for therapeutic drug monitoring of infliximab and adalimumab. *Therapeutic Drug Monitoring, 47*, 433–437. https://www.semanticscholar.org/paper/0ab9611845eabbd00b46238e73d06b4227d9e115 (accessed on 10th June 2025).

66. Márquez-Megías, S., Nalda-Molina, R., Sanz-Valero, J., Más-Serrano, P., Díaz-González, M., Candela-Boix, M. R., & Ramon-Lopez, A. (2022). Cost-effectiveness of therapeutic drug monitoring of anti-TNF therapy in inflammatory bowel disease: A systematic review. *Pharmaceutics, 14*. https://www.semanticscholar.org/paper/c7af11c3d4415a4ba430c94dbeaa5ba44dedd991 (accessed on 10th June 2025).

67. Mohamed, R. G., Saber, R., Hussein, M. A., Shalaby, A., Yasser, N., Kamal, S., Shalaby, L., et al. (2024). Optimizing vancomycin therapeutic drug monitoring compliance in pediatric oncology: Towards personalized medication management. *Personalized Medicine*. https://www.semanticscholar.org/paper/f66253c400c47e033b6b49bd72355b009dc80661 (accessed on 10th June 2025).

68. Morales Castro, D., Granton, J. T., & Fan, E. (2024). Ceftobiprole and cefetecol for patients on extracorporeal membrane oxygenation: The role of therapeutic drug

monitoring. *Current Drug Metabolism*. https://www.semanticscholar.org/paper/e52f7235fb597ede24af40f28ea46d8684f7849a (accessed on 10th June 2025).

69. Morgan, L. E., Raybin, J. L., Chang, B. H., & Stork, L. C. (2024). Survey on institutional practices of calaspargase administration. *Blood*. https://www.semanticscholar.org/paper/b49ff640d75b5d24b5e38b77e03b10854bb449aa (accessed on 10th June 2025).

70. Müller, T., Gerlach, M., Hefner, G., Hiemke, C., Jost, W., & Riederer, P. (2024). Therapeutic drug monitoring in Parkinson's disease. *Journal of Neural Transmission, 131*, 1247–1262. https://www.semanticscholar.org/paper/f458e2df1e6f3e7da02b117369643a413813cd6e (accessed on 10th June 2025).

71. Pedada, N. K. (2025). Advancements in real-time data processing in medical research. *International Journal of Scientific Research in Computer Science, Engineering and Information Technology*. https://www.semanticscholar.org/paper/c60941e5110aa4d39070662d372883b5cac2929d (accessed on 10th June 2025).

72. Pytlarz, M. A., Soufi, G., Badillo-Ramírez, I., Serioli, L., Slipets, R., Perner, A., & Boisen, A. (2025). Improving meropenem quantification in a compact SERS-based centrifugal microfluidic platform: Toward TDM of antibiotics in ICU. *Analytical Chemistry, 97*, 7888–7896. https://www.semanticscholar.org/paper/e1474497e4ff95dd1ced04106d79ce0a8cd3a88a (accessed on 10th June 2025).

73. Resztak, M., Zalewska, P., Wachowiak, J., Sobkowiak-Sobierajska, A., & Główka, F. (2024). Voriconazole therapeutic drug monitoring including analysis of CYP2C19 phenotype in immunocompromised pediatric patients with invasive fungal infections. *European Journal of Clinical Pharmacology, 80*, 1829–1840. https://www.semanticscholar.org/paper/57f3f2b19b144328904a9c0147e7ae9355856945 (accessed on 10th June 2025).

74. Samuel, D. R., & Tu, H. T. (2012). Limited options to manage specialty drug spending. https://core.ac.uk/download/71358608.pdf (accessed on 10th June 2025).

75. Shim, A., Han, P., Young, K., St. Jacque, S., Sabban, A., Eisdorfer, R., & Rosenberg, S. (2024). Comparing real-world outcomes, measured as 12 and 24-month IBD-related surgeries, between infliximab dose optimized patients using therapeutic drug monitoring (TDM) vs an unoptimized control group, in a large US community-based gastroenterology practice. *Gastroenterology*. https://www.semanticscholar.org/paper/bfa1fddd0ea6d51e42a7370ff003ab7ffff63ba1 (accessed on 10th June 2025).

76. Short, N., & Dillon, R. (2024). Measurable residual disease monitoring in AML: Prospects for therapeutic decision-making and new drug development. *American Journal of Hematology, 100*, 15–5. https://www.semanticscholar.org/paper/78e494893361a0b2002a4dbe6d0e7a3917aa4dd4 (accessed on 10th June 2025).

77. Shubow, S., Gunsior, M., Rosenberg, A. S., Wang, Y. M. C., Altepeter, T., Guinn, D., Rajabiabhari, M., et al. (2025). Therapeutic drug monitoring of biologics: Current practice, challenges and opportunities–A workshop report. *The AAPS Journal, 27*(2), 62. https://www.semanticscholar.org/paper/7dc8fdb73772550930f7c7eebc519eaf6860114b (accessed on 10th June 2025).

78. Steinhoff, B. J., Ben-Menachem, E., Klein, P., Peltola, J., Schmitz, B., Thomas, R. H., & Villanueva, V. (2024). Therapeutic strategies during cenobamate treatment initiation: Delphi panel recommendations. *Therapeutic Advances in Neurological Disorders, 17*, Article 565c3bbefdd3e28604699a6262cadddc48686588. https://www.semanticscholar.org/paper/

565c3bbefdd3e28604699a6262cadddc48686588 (accessed on 10th June 2025).

79. Tobler-Giger, A. (2016). *Contributions to an Improved Phenytoin Monitoring and Dosing in Hospitalized Patients*. https://core.ac.uk/download/46605133.pdf (accessed on 10th June 2025).

80. Vethe, N. T., Åsberg, A., Bergan, S., Robertsen, I., & Midtvedt, K. (2024). Implementation of volumetric finger-prick self-sampling for therapeutic drug monitoring of immunosuppressants after kidney transplantation: Lessons learned from the practice. *Therapeutic Drug Monitoring, 47*, 98–104. https://www.semanticscholar.org/paper/09456abc575ed7a835882dd4a0cb4a53d7483026 (accessed on 10th June 2025).

81. Vlasceanu, A., Balalau, C., Tuchila, C., Pirvu, C., Baconi, D., Balalau, D., Stan, M., et al. (2017). Therapeutic drug monitoring and methods of quantitation for carbamazepine. https://core.ac.uk/download/144553870.pdf (accessed on 10th June 2025).

82. von Hentig, N. (2012). Personalizing HIV therapy, mission impossible? https://core.ac.uk/download/17028337.pdf (accessed on 10th June 2025).

83. Yang, J., Holmquist, B., & Chun, K. (2024). B-302 therapeutic drug monitoring (TDM) of hydroxychloroquine in whole blood: Analysis of over 10,000 patient results. *Clinical Chemistry*. https://www.semanticscholar.org/paper/890cb7685ae9b7578013006b91e0ff8ac02c9cb6 (accessed on 10th June 2025).

84. Zhu, A., Kuhnly, N., Chen, L., & Dulu, A. O. (2024). A case study of polypharmacy-induced serotonin syndrome in a cancer patient. *Journal of the American Association of Nurse Practitioners, 36*, 728–732. https://www.semanticscholar.org/paper/d9e600ed242d774f4839faa3a30d0c9dcc519346 (accessed on 10th June 2025).

85. Zhuang, L., Wu, K., Jang, S., Reynolds, K., Mishra, S., & Iarikov, D. (2022). Application of population pharmacokinetic modeling, exposure-response analysis, and classification and regression tree analysis to support dosage regimen and therapeutic drug monitoring of plazomicin in complicated urinary tract infection patients with renal impairment. *Antimicrobial Agents and Chemotherapy, 66*. https://www.semanticscholar.org/paper/72b459bdaee84da26c769a76399d5c04590dd990 (accessed on 10th June 2025).

ADVERSE DRUG REACTIONS (ADRS)

6

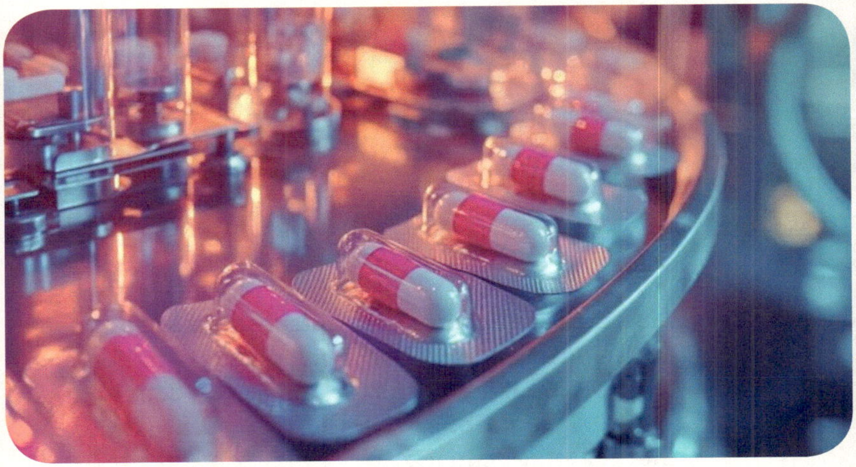

LEARNING OBJECTIVES

After studying this chapter, you will be able to:

1. Identify types of adverse drug reactions
2. Explain mechanisms of adverse drug reactions
3. Focus on risk factors for adverse drug reactions
4. Discuss management and prevention of adverse drug reactions

Introduction

The increasing reliance on drug therapies in practice is raising critical concerns regarding adverse drug reactions (ADRs), a substantial public health issue. ADRs may lead to various types of complications, like prolonged hospital stays and even death, highlighting the need for rigorous pharmacovigilance. Despite advancements in drug safety testing, the complexity of causative factors for ADR episodes, such as gender differences and polypharmacy, renders medication safety complicated (Abate et al., 2024). Of particular interest are vulnerable populations like neonates, who are most susceptible to ADRs according to the scarcity of specific drug trials conducted on this population (Byskov et al., 2024). Thus, spontaneous reporting and critical appraisal of ADR information are crucial to identify trends and enhance drug safety protocols. Thus, understanding the intricate nature of ADRs is significant to and improve patient outcomes and rationalize therapeutic interventions in different patient populations (Figure 6.1).

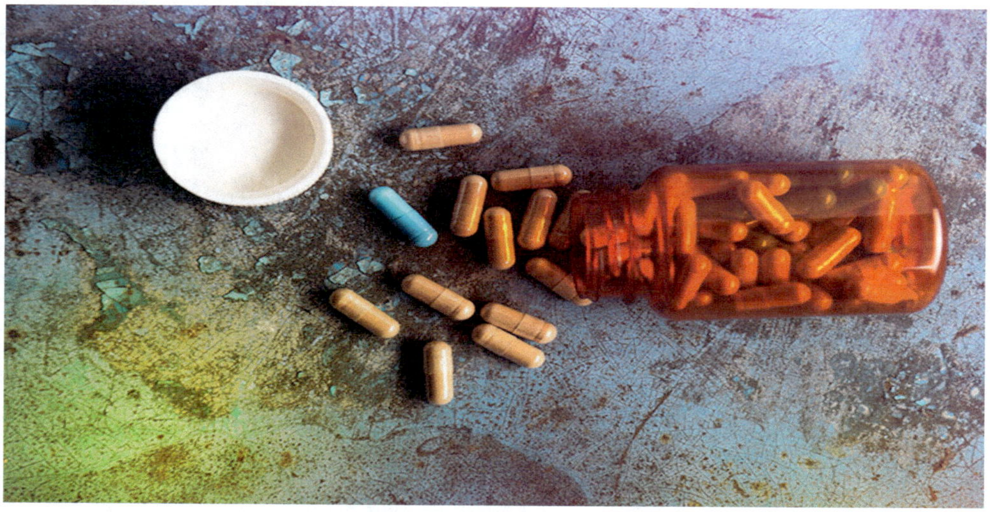

Figure 6.1. Adverse drug reactions (ADRs).

Source: https://hospitalpharmacyeurope.com/wp-content/uploads/2004/03/ADR-1.jpg.

6.1. Types of Adverse Drug Reactions

Learning Outcome

1. Explain type A (augmented), type B (bizarre), type C (chronic), type D (delayed), type E (end of use), and type F (failure) reactions
2. Learn classification based on severity
3. Know classification based on onset
4. Give examples of common ADRs

It is essential to recognize the various categories of ADRs for effective pharmacovigilance and patient safety. ADRs are usually classified into two large categories: Type A (predictable) and Type B (unpredictable) reactions. Type A reactions are dose-related and are related to the drug's pharmacological action and constitute the bulk of reported ADRs. Examples of common Type A reactions include gastrointestinal disturbance caused by nonsteroidal anti-inflammatory drugs. Conversely, Type B reactions are idiosyncratic and dose-independent, usually immunologically mediated, and cause a surprise effect. Research has demonstrated that a high percentage of ADRs, particularly hospital ADRs, are preventable, e.g., in research where 75.9% of patients experienced temporary harm from predictable ADRs (Chandra et al., 2023) and where the majority of pediatric ADRs were certainly preventable (Mathur et al., 2022). Individuals identifying these categories can enhance the initiatives to counter the risks of medication use (Figure 6.2).

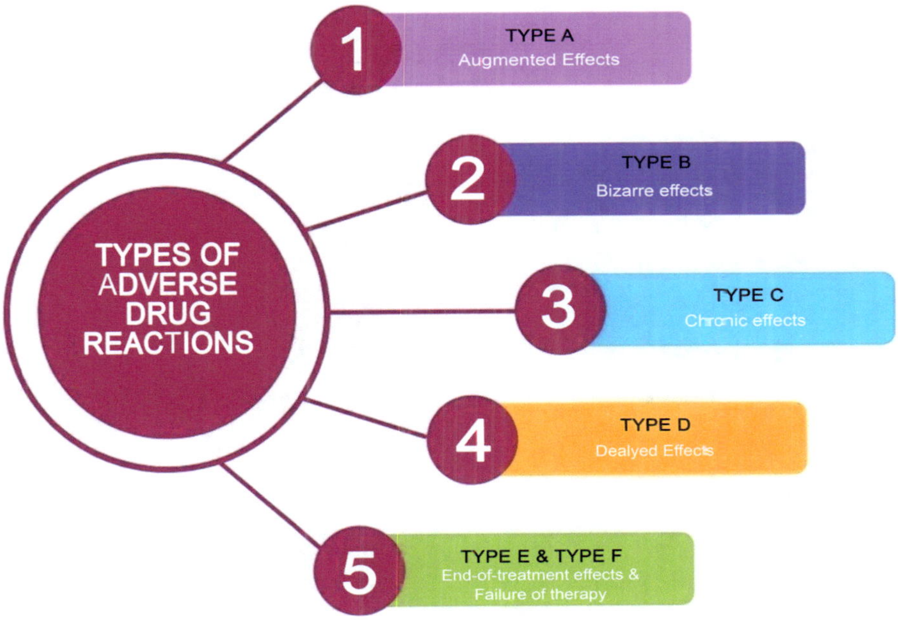

Figure 6.2. Various types of adverse drug reactions (ADRs).

Source: https://lh5.googleusercontent.com/u_xvKgpYqMmEyFb4Oi0T_13-mz-keUHVyVxpwKCvos4GU2Z71I6FsddZ8v73as--86rzjEuYKCzKtAAYJtpQyF0PMZUhxIhLmKnAn9J2gK5zn8yoxvRoW1gW0Jnn_9s1R2LB4j_8gGR9Ue0R-w=s1600-rw.

6.1.1. Type A (Augmented) Reactions

Type A (Augmented) reactions constitute an interesting class of ADRs that are both predictable and dose-proportional. They are generally not severe but can produce significant morbidity if left untreated. According to the World Health Organization (WHO), Type A reactions are normal and are caused by the drug's pharmacologic effect at therapeutic doses of treatment; thus, they are very predictable and controllable (Vín et al., 2018).

In clinical practice, an extremely high percentage of patients experience Type A reactions, as reported in a study of 1,250 inpatients, where 42.4% of the reported ADRs were due to antimicrobial agents, with many cases having to be brought to medical attention (Adhikari et al., 2009). Identification and monitoring of Type A reactions play a critical role in modifying therapeutic approaches, minimizing detrimental effects, and ensuring maximum patient protection through careful pharmacovigilance practices (Figure 6.3).

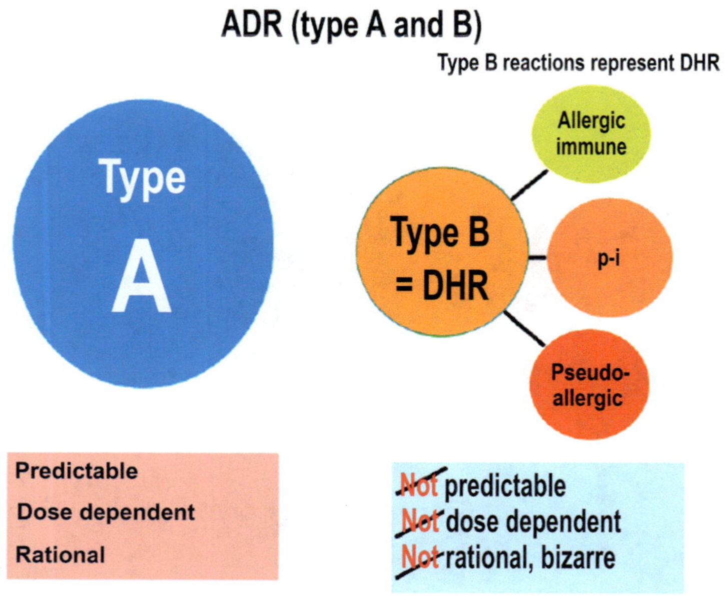

Figure 6.3. Type A (Augmented) reactions.

Source: https://www.researchgate.net/publication/278646475/figure/fig2/AS:523002732978176@1501704976690/ADR-are-subclassified-as-type-A-and-B-reactions-Type-B-reactions-correspond-to-DHR.png.

6.1.2. Type B (Bizarre) Reactions

Type B (Bizarre) reactions are a critical group of drug reactions (ADRs) characterized by their being unusual and unpredictable, as opposed to more common Type A reactions. Unlike dose-related and usually predictable Type A reactions, Type B reactions result from pathological reactivity on the patient's side, i.e., idiosyncrasy or hypersensitivity. They therefore can appear without warning, often with hazardous consequences. For instance, aplastic anemia induced by chloramphenicol is one such response, which happens at a rate of 1 in 30,000 and demonstrates the inherent risk associated with seemingly innocuous drugs (Vín et al., 2018). The clinical implications of Type B reactions necessitate vigilant monitoring and reporting, as evidence by study findings that among hospitalized patients, a significant percentage of ADRs are attributed to combined drugs, which illustrates the unpredictable nature of drug interactions and the final imperative for heightened vigilance in ADR monitoring to prevent morbidity and mortality (Adhikari et al., 2009).

6.1.3. Type C (Chronic) Reactions

Type C (Chronic) reactions constitute a significant category of drug reaction (ADRs), characterized by their chronic duration and capacity for long-term impact. Unlike immediate or acute reactions, Type C reactions tend to emerge very late following chronic treatment with a medication, typically resulting in the type of cumulative effect that seriously compromises health. For instance, from research, it has been established that aged individuals, who are usually on more than one medication, are most susceptible to these long-term effects. In the majority of instances, severe health outcomes such as gastrointestinal diseases and cardiovascular diseases, leading to increased morbidity and mortality rates (Chiumia et al., 2024). Moreover, systematic reviews have indicated that interventions aimed at preventing general and severe ADRs, especially by pharmacists, can significantly reduce their incidence, which underscores the importance of active medication management in averting the sequelae of chronic drug reactions (Gray et al., 2023). Type C reaction management is required for assurance of better patient outcomes as well as for assurance of better medication safety overall (Figure 6.4).

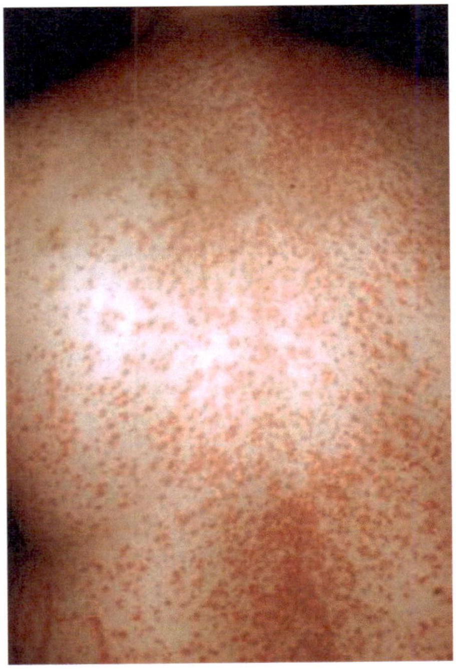

Figure 6.4. Drug eruptions.

Source: https://img.medscapestatic.com/pi/meds/ckb/56/27456tn.jpg.

6.1.4. Type D (Delayed) Reactions

Type D (Delayed) reactions are a significant subset of the range of ADRs, and are often seen after a protracted period of drug exposure. They will tend to pose challenges in early diagnosis and control, as onset can occur well after initial dosing of the drug. The delayed nature of such reactions makes it harder for the work of pharmacovigilance, leading to underreporting and loss of alertness about possible risks from certain drugs. Research emphasizes the need to increase awareness and knowledge of healthcare professionals in identifying and managing delayed ADRs since training interventions improve reporting rates and attitudes toward pharmacovigilance (Cervantes-Arellano et al., 2024). Moreover, some classes of drugs, such as anticancer drugs, are particularly notorious for D-type reactions, necessitating vigilant monitoring to prevent the hazards of moderate to serious toxicities and enhance patient safety (Pilla et al., 2022).

6.1.5. Type E (End of Use) Reactions

Among ADRs, Type E reactions, or end-of-use reactions as otherwise generally referred to, are a particular challenge for healthcare providers. Such reactions usually appear when a drug is being withdrawn, either through withdrawal symptoms or through the recurrence of the underlying condition being treated by the drug. For example, patients who discontinue treatment for immunotherapeutic drugs like atezolizumab will not only face a relapse of the underlying disease but also the other sequelae of rapid withdrawal from therapy, highlighting the significant interplay between the efficacy of the drug and the stability of the patient (Finn et al., 2020). While healthcare professionals navigate such complexities, responsibility remains in ensuring that the decisions are made under well-established guidelines, concerning every patient's unique circumstances (Mach et al., 2019). Hence, understanding Type E reactions is essential to clinicians who wish to balance cessation techniques with patient safety in managing drug therapy (Figure 6.5).

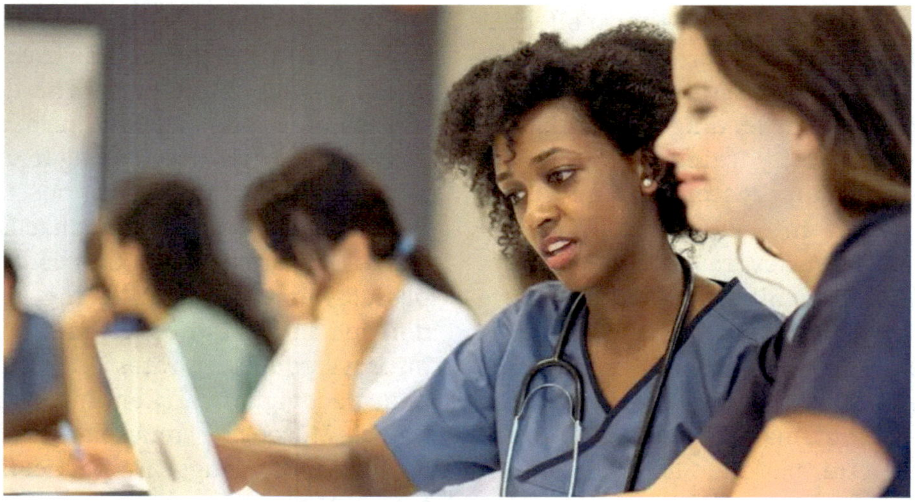

Figure 6.5. As health professionals navigate these complexities, the responsibility remains to ensure that decisions are informed by comprehensive guidelines while considering each patient's unique circumstances.

Source: https://sollers.college/wp-content/uploads/2021/03/Evaluation-Adverse-Drug-Reactions.jpg.

6.1.6. Type F (Failure) Reactions

Type F (Failure) reactions are a significant category of drug adverse reactions (ADRs) that happen primarily due to therapeutic failures rather than through direct toxicity. Such reactions tend to occur when a drug is not effective in managing the target disease, and quite often, it leads to unjustified continued therapy or, conversely, sudden withdrawal, both processes with deleterious effects on patient outcome. For example, in the elderly, these failures will be fueled by the complications of polypharmacy and pharmacokinetic changes that come with age, which will increase morbidity and mortality from ADRs (Onder et al., 2012). In research that pointed out the impact of such reactions, therapeutic failures were mainly due to issues like suboptimal dosing or DDI, which are particularly prevalent among patients who use multiple medications (Adhikari et al., 2009). Hence, recognition and management of Type F reactions are necessary for optimum achievement of treatment effects and overall improvement of patient safety in clinical practice.

6.1.7. Classification Based on Severity

The severity-based classification of ADRs is essential for the effective clinical management and safety of patients. ADRs are usually classified into three categories: mild, moderate, and severe. Mild reactions, though uncomfortable, do not need cessation of the drug and may resolve on their own. Moderate reactions, however, require dose changes or short-term interruption of the drug, and complicate the patient's treatment regimen. Serious ADRs entail serious health threats, the likelihood of which could result in hospitalization or irreversible harm, and this explains why systematic observation is essential. Academic research shows that it is vital to identify and classify these reactions to help recognize medication mistakes and their effects on patient safety in different health contexts. For example, a study noted the lack of serious damage associated with drug errors and suggested the existence of a Heinrich ratio that would facilitate ADR assessment across varying environments (Barber et al., 2006). Further, systematic reviews have reported that a high percentage of such errors could be preventable and have therefore necessitated strict means of reporting ADRs and the implementation of necessary reforms (Yassin et al., 2018) (Figure 6.6).

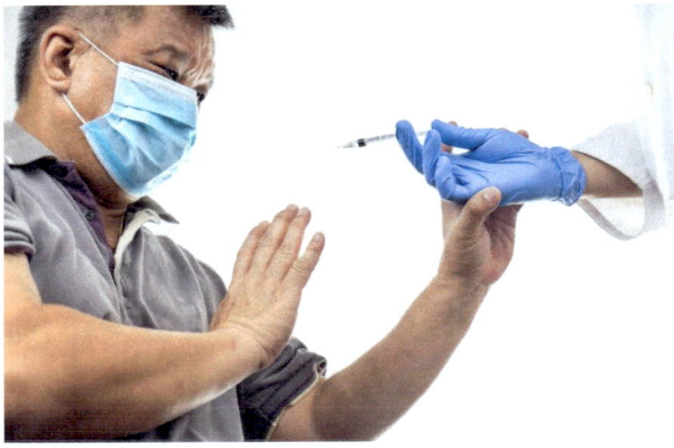

Figure 6.6. The classification of adverse drug reactions (ADRs) based on severity is crucial for effective clinical management and patient safety.

Source: https://pharmuni.com/wp-content/uploads/2024/07/fearful-worried-middle-age-man-reacting-to-medical-practitioner-holding-syringe-loaded-with-covid-19-768x512.jpg.

6.1.8. Classification Based on Onset

The on-set based categorization of ADRs holds significance in understanding their meaning in clinical practice. ADRs are categorized into immediate, early, and delayed onset reactions, which offer information about their pathophysiologic mechanisms and risk factors. Acute reactions are prompt in onset, typically occurring minutes to hours after exposure, and may be of profound effect, particularly in susceptible populations such as the elderly, who can manifest with atypical presentations secondary to alterations in pharmacokinetics and pharmacodynamics (Onder et al., 2012). Onset reactions typically occur within days and can be associated with cumulative drug exposure, highlighting the need for vigilant monitoring. Delayed onset reactions, which occur weeks or even months after the start of treatment, can complicate therapy, particularly in conditions of a chronic nature. The understanding of these classifications enables one to conduct risk assessment and management strategies, which ultimately enhance patient care in the complex nature of medication therapy (Neligan et al., 2015).

6.1.9. Examples of Common ADRs

ADRs are a wide range of unwanted effects caused by drugs that are likely to complicate treatment regimens. Some common ADRs are gastrointestinal reactions, nausea, and diarrhea, which often follow the use of antibiotics and NSAIDs. Neurological adverse effects, such as dizziness and somnolence, will tend to accompany antidepressants and antihistamines, compromising patient compliance and general health. Some drugs have the potential to cause more serious side effects, such as anaphylaxis or organ poisoning, which must be closely watched and treated right away. As Dr. Wiener indicates, there can be an evolution towards an interdependent paradigm for healthcare that allows for improved understanding and handling of such ADRs, and yet keeps public health objectives and patient safety as priorities (Wiener et al., 1998). To this end, effective risk communication strategies need to be integrated so that better regulatory control and improved patient education on potential ADRs are attained (Vertinsky et al., 1991) (Figure 6.7).

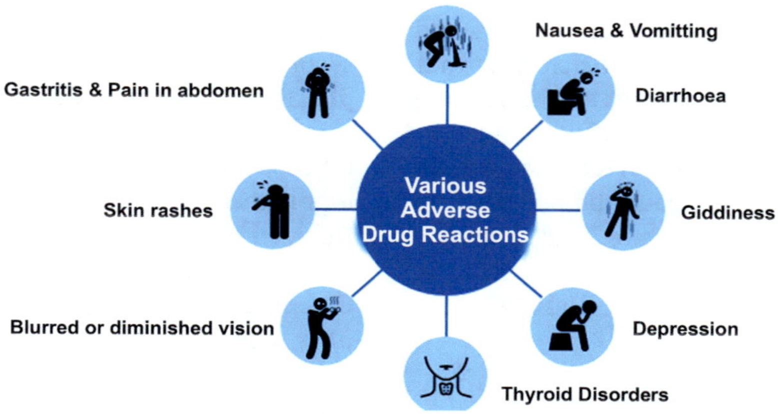

Figure 6.7. Common ADRs examples.

Source: https://ntep.in/sites/default/files/h5p/content/15912/images/file-642136d535e30.png.

Test Your Knowledge

1. How do Type A and Type B ADRs differ in terms of their causes and characteristics?
2. What are the characteristics of Type C ADRs, and how do they typically manifest?

6.2. Mechanisms of Adverse Drug Reactions

Learning Outcome

1. Understand pharmacological mechanisms
2. Explain immunological mechanisms
3. Identify genetic factors influencing ADRs
4. Explain drug interactions and their role in ADRs
5. Know environmental factors contributing to ADRs
6. Focus on the role of metabolism in ADRs
7. Know the influence of age and gender on ADRs
8. Discuss mechanisms of idiosyncratic reactions

The mechanisms of ADRs are complex and multifactorial, with a tendency to highlight the interaction between drug metabolism and patient factors as complex. Of special concern is the neuropsychiatric effect of certain drugs, such as statins, which have been associated with mood and behavior changes. Reports also indicate that statin-treated patients experienced symptoms ranging from irritability to severe depression. In a few instances, suicidality, suggesting a cause-and-effect correlation that needs to be investigated (Cham et al., 2015). Pharmacovigilance centers like those in Tanzania also play an essential role in monitoring drug safety as well as finding ADRs of antiretroviral drugs. Despite this, training and reporting deficiencies impede efficient detection and handling of ADRs in such systems, and the need for strengthened guidelines and professional education for healthcare providers has been emphasized (Baraka et al., 2013). Understanding these mechanisms is essential to minimize risks and ensure patient safety.

6.2.1. Pharmacological Mechanisms

Pharmacological mechanisms are significant in managing ADRs, since they illustrate the mechanisms whereby drugs act within the body and may lead to unforeseen side effects. Heightened sensitivity about such pathways is particularly relevant in the geriatric population, who most commonly express atypical ADRs due to pharmacokinetic and pharmacodynamic changes associated with advancing age. The identification of high-risk patients through tools like the GerontoNet ADR Risk Score can justify intervention to minimize untoward outcomes, bringing into focus the need to adopt judicious prescribing practices. Additionally, the complexity of herbal preparations, widely utilized in the African setting, again underscores the need for widespread understanding of pharmacological interactions as the majority of indigenous treatments are related to unrecognized ADRs resulting from inadvertent usage or handling. Therefore, it is imperative to strengthen the relationship between healthcare professionals and traditional practitioners to realize effective pharmacovigilance and enhance patient safety (Onder et al., 2012; Foguem et al., 2014) (Figure 6.8).

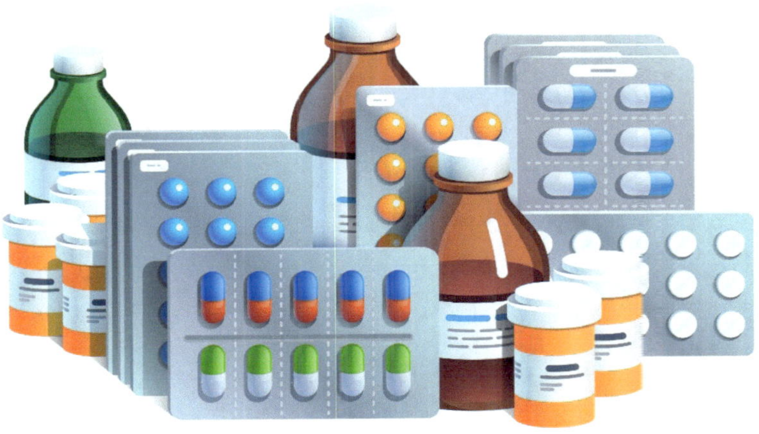

Figure 6.8. The understanding of pharmacological mechanisms is crucial in addressing Adverse Drug Reactions (ADRs), as these mechanisms reveal how drugs interact within the body and can lead to unintended side effects.

Source: https://d2jx2rerrg6sh3.cloudfront.net/images/news/ImageForNews_727564_16654984405829814.jpg.

6.2.2. Immunological Mechanisms

Elucidating immunological mechanisms of ADRs is essential to maximize therapeutic efficacy and guarantee patient safety. Immune-mediated ADRs typically arise as a consequence of the body's hypersensitivity responses against drugs, in which genetic polymorphisms, particularly within drug-metabolizing enzymes like glutathione S-transferases (GSTs), play an essential role in individual susceptibility. For instance, GST gene polymorphisms have been linked with variability in the frequencies of ADRs between different categories of drugs, i.e., antiepileptic and immunosuppressants, suggesting a polyfactorial interaction of genes and drug response (Ettoury et al., 2024). Moreover, pharmacovigilance (PV) activities reveal that a significant percentage of hospitalizations is due to ADRs, suggesting the need for enhanced monitoring systems that account for such immunological mechanisms (Sulakhiya et al., 2023). By enhancing such mechanisms, researchers can develop improved methods for anticipating and preventing ADRs, ultimately leading to better patient care.

6.2.3. Genetic Factors Influencing ADRs

Expression of drug adverse effects (ADRs) is also largely genetics-based, in that they can alter the response of an individual to a drug. Genetic polymorphism of drug-metabolizing enzymes is likely to impose variability in drugs regarding efficacy and toxicity on both the therapeutic effect and the likelihood of ADRs. For instance, certain genetic variants have been found to enhance drug-protein adduct formation, a mechanism of key importance for immunological recognition in drug hypersensitivity reactions, providing evidence of the multifactorial etiology of such responses (Aldini et al., 2016). Furthermore, the diversity of drug-induced diseases, including nephrotoxicity, calls for a multidisciplinary approach to genetic predispositions, as exemplified by phenotypes established in recent years to analyze drug-induced kidney disease (Awdishu et al., 2015). These findings underscore the necessity of integrating genetic data into clinical practice to facilitate personalized medication and, therefore, reduce the frequency of ADRs through tailored therapeutic strategies (Figure 6.9).

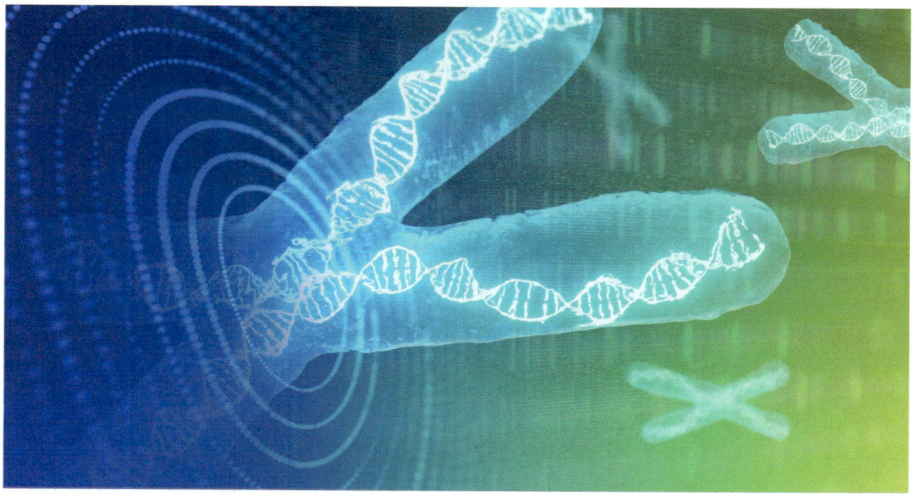

Figure 6.9. Genetic polymorphisms, particularly in drug-metabolizing enzymes, can lead to variations in drug efficacy and toxicity, affecting both the therapeutic outcomes and the risk of ADRs.

Source: https://incitehealth.com/wp-content/uploads/2024/03/The-Synergy-of-Pharmacogenomics.jpg.

6.2.4. Drug Interactions and Their Role in ADRs

The drug interaction complexity is one of the primary causes of ADRs, often complicating the patients' treatment regimens. Since drugs are more and more targeting specific biological pathways, the risk of these drugs interacting with one another increases, leading to altered pharmacokinetics or pharmacodynamics and thus unforeseen side effects. For example, bioinformatics makes a significant contribution to understanding these interactions by analyzing large biological data and predicting how drugs will affect each other so that patients are made safer (Arthur et al., 2023). Furthermore, integrating network pharmacology concepts with personalized medicine presents a significant opportunity to overcome such threats. Understanding the intricate network of drug interactions may lead to more individualized therapeutic measures that enhance efficacy while reducing ADRs (Marsh et al., 2010). Identification and prevention of drug interactions are thus of utmost relevance in the ongoing pursuit of enhanced patient care and outcomes in drug therapy

6.2.5. Environmental Factors Contributing to ADRs

The occurrence of ADRs is closely linked with environmental conditions, which may significantly influence the vulnerability of patients to such adverse effects. The genetic make-up of individuals, for instance, can interact with the environment to cause uneven drug metabolism and response to pharmacologic intervention. In addition, exposure to toxins or nutrients can also increase the likelihood of ADRs through the influence of liver enzyme activity for drug metabolism. Moreover, socioeconomic status in terms of health service availability and educational institution availability is also a key factor in how individuals adhere to their medication, hence the reporting rate of ADRs and management. Existing research also suggested the underreporting of ADR cases, particularly in the developing world, like Ethiopia, where only 0.5 cases of ADR per million population per year were reported, on average, between 2002 and 2007 (Ermias et al., 2012). This implies that there is a need for more stringent environmental and system interventions to curb the impact of ADRs globally and ensure safe drug practice (Cham et al., 2015) (Figure 6.10).

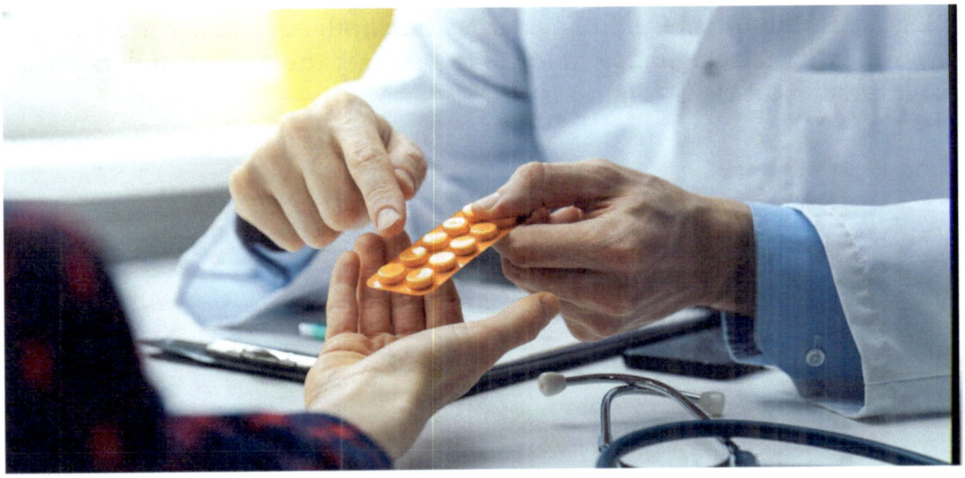

Figure 6.10. The genetic makeup of individuals can interact with the environment, leading to differential drug metabolism and varying responses to pharmacological treatments.

Source: https://images.theconversation.com/files/424091/original/file-20210930-20-1cwddsq.jpg?ixlib=rb-4.1.0&rect=19%2C244%2C2121%2C1060&q=45&auto=format&w=1356&h=668&fit=crop.

6.2.6. Role of Metabolism in ADRs

The metabolic contribution to drug-induced ADRs is significant, as metabolism plays a crucial role in determining the pharmacokinetics and pharmacodynamics of drugs extensively. Interestingly, variations in metabolizing pathways can potentially generate reactive metabolites, which lead to hypersensitivity reactions or other types of toxicity. In older persons, for instance, age-related physiological alterations can influence drug metabolism, increasing vulnerability to

ADRs and complicating their clinical presentation (Onder et al., 2012). Certain drug groups, such as antiepileptics, show how metabolic interactions can induce severe clinical cutaneous reactions. Clinical Presentation. Studies have determined that hypersensitivity syndromes caused by antiepileptic medications are more often associated with certain genetic markers such as the HLA-B*1502 allele, further substantiating the contribution of metabolic processes to ADRs (Cohen et al., 2011). Clarification of these metabolic underpinnings can optimize drug safety and inform interventions aimed at reducing ADR risk across patient populations.

6.2.7. Influence of Age and Gender on ADRs

The influence of age and gender on drug adverse reactions (ADRs) is a critical area of study, which has identified significant differences in susceptibility among different groups of the population. For example, physiological factors such as reduced metabolic capacity and the existence of comorbidities make older people more prone to have higher ADR rates. A study noted that drug-induced liver injury (DILI) patients were 59.27 years old on average, a vast proportion of them being male, and how gender and age might correlate with heightened risk (Arrang et al., 2018). Further, in the pediatric age group, age-related reactions were observed with inhaled corticosteroids (ICS), with boys being more frequently reported in suspected ADRs such as growth retardation and behavioral changes (den Berg et al., 2006). These findings prove that both sex and age are fundamental factors to be considered in pharmacovigilance, informing better patient care and tailored therapeutic strategies to counteract ADR risks (Figure 6.11).

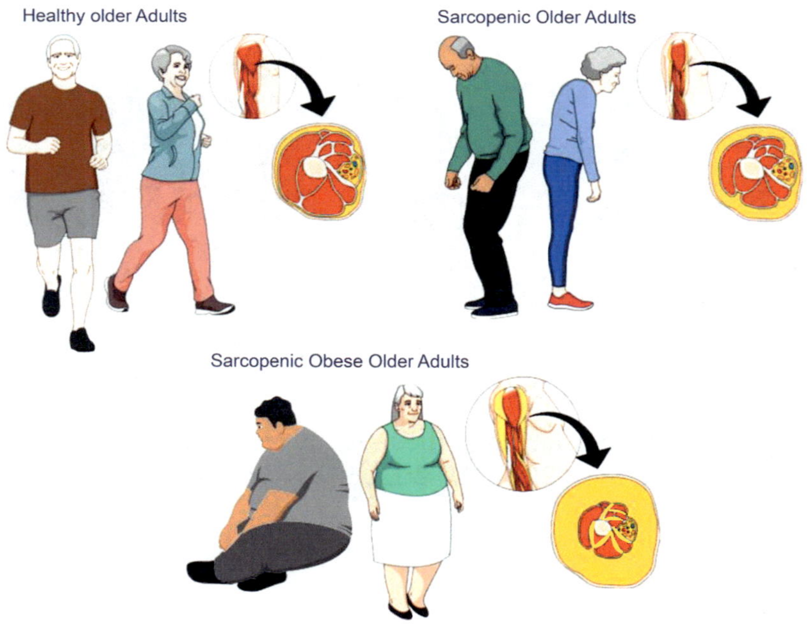

Figure 6.11. Older adults often experience higher incidences of ADRs due to physiological changes including diminished metabolic capacity and the presence of comorbid conditions.

Source: https://www.endo.theclinics.com/cms/10.1016/j.ecl.2022.10.001/asset/270c9579-66e5-4a04-93d6-fd3b1dc3aabb/main.assets/gr2_lrg.jpg.

6.2.8. Mechanisms of Idiosyncratic Reactions

Idiosyncratic drug reactions are a big challenge for pharmacology since they are unanticipated and may result in horrific damage. As opposed to dose-dependent reactions, in which one may anticipate the manifestation of a reaction by a drug's pharmacological properties, idiosyncratic reactions most frequently arise due to complex interactions at the genetic level. For instance, HLA allele association with hypersensitivity reactions demonstrates the genetic underpinning of such occurrences as seen in the case of abacavir, whereby modification of the HLA-B*57:01 specificity by the drug triggers cytotoxic T cell activation that results in severe adverse effects (Lucas et al., 2012). Likewise, drug-induced kidney disease classification underscores the value of understanding the associated underlying biological mechanisms because recognition of such distinctions can aid in treatment and diagnosis (Awdishu et al., 2015). Through continued research efforts, elucidation of such mechanisms will be critical in maximizing drug safety and minimizing idiosyncratic reactions in the clinic.

Test Your Knowledge

1. How do immune-mediated mechanisms contribute to Type B (idiosyncratic) ADRs?
2. What are the roles of drug metabolism and enzyme interactions in the occurrence of ADRs?

6.3. Risk Factors for Adverse Drug Reactions

Learning Outcome

1. Identify patient-related risk factors
2. Explain drug-related risk factors
3. Discuss disease-related risk factors
4. Understand polypharmacy and its implications
5. Learn age-related considerations
6. Focus on gender differences in ADR susceptibility
7. Discuss socioeconomic factors affecting ADRs
8. Know the role of healthcare provider in risk assessment
9. Describe strategies for identifying at-risk patients

Detection of risk factors for ADRs plays a crucial role in improving patient safety and therapeutic efficacy. Research has demonstrated that certain populations, such as age and gender, are significant, with individuals above 60 years being extremely prone to ADRs due to physiological changes and development of comorbidities like diabetes and chronic liver disease (Zhang et al., 2025). Besides, some drug groups, such as target drugs and first-line antitubercular drugs, have individual ADR profiles and therefore should be monitored cautiously at the onset of treatment (Oh et al., 2024; Zhang et al., 2025). Further, illnesses such as alcohol and drug abuse may pose an increased risk of dangerous reactions and call for discontinuation of therapy as well as dose modification. Clarification of such risk factors not only provides hints towards the mechanistic pathways for ADRs but also enables predictive models to be formulated, which can enhance patient management interventions in a clinical setting.

6.3.1. Patient-Related Risk Factors

ADRs often are the result of a complex interaction of patient-related risk factors with significant impacts on the safety and efficacy of pharmacotherapy. The most important risk factors are advanced age, comorbidities, and polypharmacy. Elderly patients, for instance, possess a heightened sensitivity to drugs owing to age-related physiological changes as well as the concomitant administration of many drugs, which increase the risk of AEs (Benard-Laribiere et al., 2016). In addition, some conditions, such as deranged renal function, may contribute to the risk of toxicity further, particularly with high-risk medicines such as anticoagulants (Aljadhey et al., 2018). Additionally, pharmacogenetic variations may influence the response to drugs in individuals, thus necessitating personalized approaches to management. All this emphasizes the importance of exercising vigilance in medication management and close monitoring in susceptible populations to minimize the occurrence of ADRs and improve patient outcomes. Thus, the integration of customized patient assessment into clinical practice can substantially enhance drug safety (Figure 6.12).

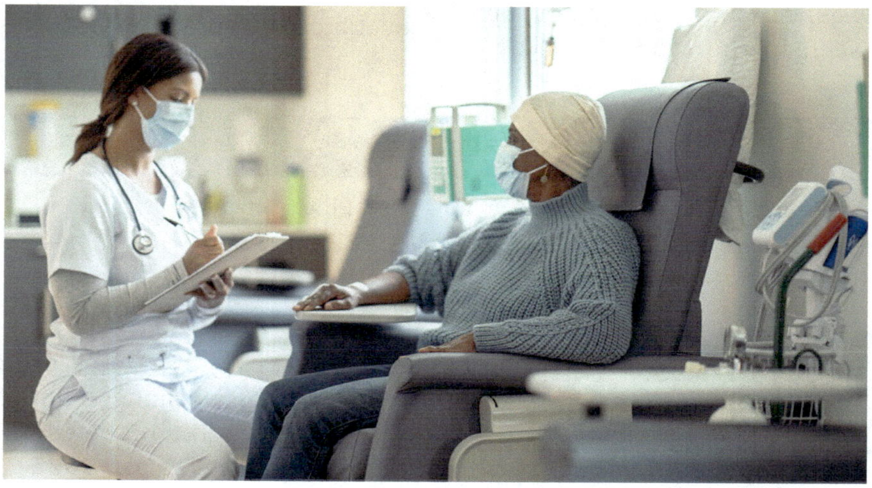

Figure 6.12. Adverse drug reactions (ADRs) often result from a complex interplay of patient-related risk factors, significantly impacting the safety and efficacy of pharmacotherapy.

Source: https://www.cdc.gov/covid/media/images/2024/11/GettyImages-1384528178_1200x675.jpg.

6.3.2. Drug-Related Risk Factors

The risk factors for drugs are a significant aspect of the understanding and prevention of drug-related ADRs in clinical settings. Nine significant risk factors, such as age, treatment modality, and cancer types, were identified as affecting the incidence of ADRs with targeted therapies by a current study (Zhang et al., 2025). Similarly, another research on the first-line antitubercular drugs identified that age, sex, and comorbid diseases were important variables that significantly increased the risk of ADR development, with cutaneous reactions being strongly prevalent (Oh et al., 2024). These findings emphasize the need for patient-specific treatment strategies to enhance treatment outcomes with minimal side effects. By recognizing these risk factors, health care providers can utilize enhanced monitoring and intervention strategies, eventually minimizing patient morbidity and maintaining the quality of life throughout complex treatment regimens. Awareness of the multi-dimensionality of drug-associated risks is imperative in the ongoing quest to optimize patient care in diverse clinical situations.

6.3.3. Disease-Related Risk Factors

Disease-related risk factors are crucial in the assessment of drug-related adverse reactions (ADRs) in patients with chronic diseases. The research has identified certain pre-existing conditions, such as CKD, as well as inflammatory diseases, which significantly increase the risk of experiencing ADRs when on pharmacotherapy. For instance, in a study comparing prophylactic sulfamethoxazole-trimethoprim (SMX/TMP) in musculoskeletal and rheumatic disease patients, 18.7% had ADRs, and older age and conditions like adult-onset Still's disease were independent risk factors for such ADRs (Hiramoto et al., 2024). Further, drug metabolism also depends on genetic predispositions, thereby determining drug efficacy along with safety. Genetic alterations in drug metabolism enzymes or drug transporters have the potential to influence pharmacokinetics and pharmacodynamics and yield adverse effects (Sychev et al., 2022). Clinicians should therefore consider both genetic susceptibility and related illness while prescribing medications to prevent ADRs (Figure 6.13) effectively.

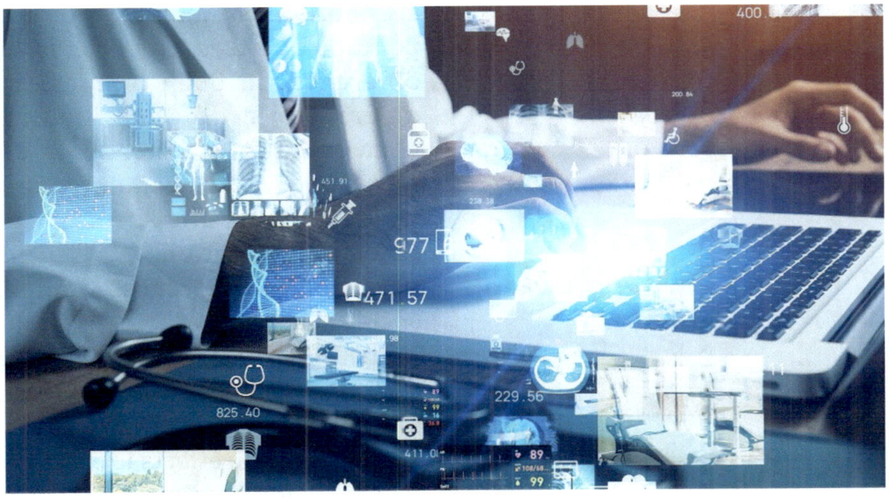

Figure 6.13. Disease-related risk factors is critical in the assessment of adverse drug reactions (ADRs).

Source: https://news.harvard.edu/wp-content/uploads/2025/04/Illustrating-doctor-looking-computer.jpg?resize=1680%2C945.

6.3.4. Polypharmacy and Its Implications

The course of polypharmacy in elderly patients carries a severe risk for ADRs that can lead to harmful clinical outcomes. As older patients develop several chronic illnesses, drug therapies are more likely to expand into numerous prescriptions, consequently increasing the likelihood of DDIs. Research has indicated that a staggering 45% of high-risk DDIs are expected to cause serious complications, such as gastrointestinal bleeding and cognitive impairment, highlighting the urgent need for better pharmacovigilance in such patients (Khan et al., 2025). Adding fuel to the fire, a study conducted among elderly Egyptian adults documented a 30.5% incidence of medication-related harm (MRH) post-discharge, inappropriate prescribing sharing a high correlation with AEs (Jamil et al., 2024). These findings demonstrate that polypharmacy not only adds complexity to treatment regimens but also deserves a reconsideration of prescribing practices for enhancing patient safety and minimizing the risk of ADRs.

6.3.5. Age-Related Considerations

The influence of age on drug adverse reactions (ADRs) is a critical concept in pharmacology since the elderly are typically susceptible to higher rates of ADRs due to physiological changes and polypharmacy. The pharmacokinetic and pharmacodynamic variables of an individual alter significantly with advancing age, affecting the absorption, distribution, metabolism, and excretion of drugs.

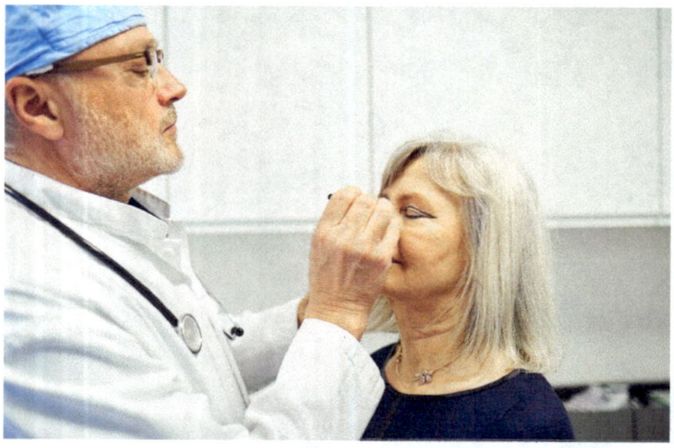

Figure 6.14. Age-related considerations.

Source: https://www.asthmaallergydoctors.com/wp-content/uploads/2023/07/Allergy-Doctors-Nasal-Polyps-in-Seniors_-Age-Related-Factors-and-Treatment-Considerations-min-scaled.jpg.

In particular, as people age, functional changes in the kidneys and liver may result in impaired drug clearance and the buildup of medications that may be more hazardous. Additionally, geriatric patients usually suffer from comorbidities such as dementia that not only complicate drug management but also enhance the risk of side effects, e.g., delirium and decreased cognitive performance (Livingston et al., 2020). Besides, age-adjusted changes need to be taken into consideration when treatment regimens are being planned, particularly in the case of emerging health issues like COVID-19, where the older groups have had less desirable outcomes and higher risk factors associated with viral infections and concerning drug therapy (AUTHOR_ID et al., 2020) (Figure 6.14).

6.3.6. Gender Differences in ADR Susceptibility

Gender differences affect the susceptibility to ADRs by the complex interaction of pharmacological, biological, and sociocultural determinants. It has been shown that women are more likely than men to experience ADRs, perhaps due to differences in hormone levels, differences in body composition, and genetic differences in drug metabolism. For instance, females have a higher ratio of body fat and lower body water content compared to males, which in turn affects drug distribution and excretion. Additionally, the impact of these physiological differences is amplified by varying social roles and access to healthcare, as seen in the disproportionate effects of certain drugs among women in most societies (Murray et al., 2022). Understanding these drug-induced gender-specific effects is essential for modifying pharmacologic therapy and promoting patient safety, particularly in the context of growing health disparities due to structural elements (Bentley, 2020).

6.3.7. Socioeconomic Factors Affecting ADRs

Socioeconomic determinants have a significant contribution to the occurrence and management of ADRs, and this underscores the core significance of access to healthcare and compliance with drugs. The lower socioeconomic status is more susceptible to ADRs because of health disparities and restricted access to drug care. These populations can also face barriers such as inadequate health education, which leads to drug misuse and increased risks of side effects (Atif et al., 2022). Patients from poorer populations can also receive less tailored treatment, with new lifestyle or genetic determinants of drug metabolism and safety remaining undiagnosed (Wée et al., 2023). Hence, integration of socioeconomic variables into pharmacogenomics and personalized medicine is vital in improving patient outcomes. Awareness of these underlying conditions can assist healthcare providers in designing interventions that minimize the risk of ADRs, ultimately promoting health equity among diverse populations. (Figure 6.15).

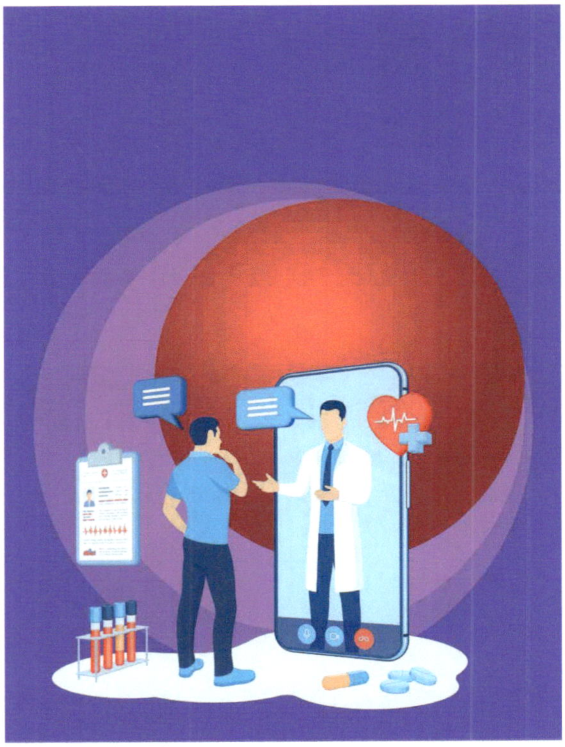

Figure 6.15. Socioeconomic factors significantly influence the incidence and management of adverse drug reactions (ADRs), underscoring the pivotal role of access to healthcare and medication adherence.

Source: https://assets.isu.pub/document-structure/230509110145-e022872f38647a4c3d655586e49c8fb9/v1/8d85d473d957bd2a28ddc644a7d8b970.jpeg.

6.3.8. Role of Healthcare Provider in Risk Assessment

The role of the healthcare provider in risk assessment, particularly in ADRs, is intricate and crucial. Experts are responsible for carrying out patient history assessment, current medicines, and potential drug interactions to identify those who may be at greater risk for ADRs. This dynamic response includes embracing the use of advanced technologies such as EHRs and predictive analytics, which can be employed to enhance risk analysis accuracy. By incorporating these technologies, healthcare providers can develop personalized treatment plans that reduce the risk of side effects, thereby enhancing patient outcomes. Furthermore, ongoing pharmacovigilance activities initiated by providers create a feedback loop that informs public health policies and improves medication safety measures. Collaboration between healthcare providers and regulatory agencies, as underscored by the literature, is key to the facilitation of an overarching framework for surveillance and prevention of pharmacotherapy-related risks, thereby promoting patient health and safety (Wagh et al., 2024).

6.3.9. Strategies for Identifying at-Risk Patients

The most critical region of avoiding harmful drug reactions (ADRs) is the identification of susceptible patients, and that has to be a multidimensional one that converges clinical, demographic, and pharmacological data. Health professionals may use patient history screening and risk stratification tools to be able to anticipate potential ADRs more reliably. For instance, one approach comparing the use of proton pump inhibitors (PPIs) and histamine-2 receptor blockers (H2RBs) has demonstrated differing results among ICU patients, demonstrating the necessity for individualized medication choices determined by distinctive risk profiles (Young et al., 2020). Besides, a review of recent trials involving drugs, such as hydroxychloroquine for post-exposure prophylaxis, shows that a high proportion of side effects were not related to drug efficacy, which stresses the need for careful observation of high-risk individuals (Casamitjana et al., 2020). In general, an integrated strategy that systematically evaluates and ranks risk factors can make drug treatments significantly safer and more effective (Figure 6.16).

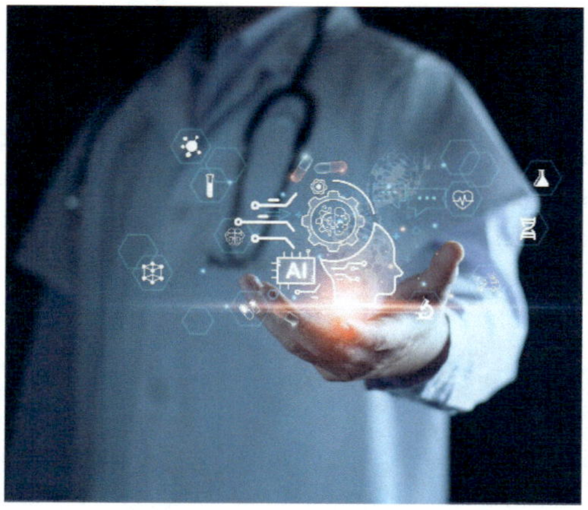

Figure 6.16. Healthcare providers can employ patient history assessments alongside risk stratification tools to better anticipate potential ADRs.

Source: https://healthsnap.io/wp-content/uploads/2023/09/c8544029-c7ed-4dea-8f12-8be26ca1133f.png.

Test Your Knowledge

1. How do underlying medical conditions, such as liver or kidney disease, contribute to ADR risks?
2. Why are pregnant women considered a high-risk group for ADRs, and what precautions should be taken?

6.4. Management and Prevention of Adverse Drug Reactions

Learning Outcome

1. Understand monitoring and reporting ADRs
2. Explain the role of healthcare professionals in prevention
3. Discuss patient education and awareness
4. Learn guidelines for safe prescribing
5. Describe pharmacovigilance systems
6. Explain risk minimization strategies
7. Focus on the use of technology in ADR management
8. Know the importance of clinical trials in ADR understanding
9. Understand future directions in ADR prevention

Accurate management and ADR prevention are critical aspects of pharmacotherapy, particularly in complex treatment regimens such as TB. ADR detection requires an extensive understanding of their clinical presentation and risk factors, as discussed in recent research that provides insight into the determinants of ADRs in African contexts (Irá et al., 2021). Healthcare professionals are tasked with careful observation of the patients and assessment of the benefit-risk profile of medicines to reduce the incidence of ADR. Practical methods such as implementing efficient pharmacovigilance systems and enhancing healthcare professional communication can significantly improve the identification and control of adverse effects (Choudhary et al., 2023). Additionally, patient education regarding potential side effects and adherence to prescribed medications can foster better outcomes. Finally, an integrated approach incorporating systematic surveillance, sound communication, and patient participation is warranted to maximize drug safety and efficacy in clinical practice.

6.4.1. Monitoring and Reporting ADRs

Effective monitoring and reporting of drug adverse reactions (ADRs) are critical for the safety of the patient as well as the overall efficacy of pharmacotherapy. Despite its significance, a number of studies show a sizable practice gap among medical professionals. For instance, a study conducted in a teaching hospital in Kano, Nigeria, revealed that only 42.7% of the healthcare professionals had ever reported an ADR and over 75% were reported verbally and not formally by means of the standard yellow reporting form, which was known to only 35.9% of the respondents (Afolabi et al., 2011). Similarly, research emphasizes the need to have active participation of pharmacists in ADR monitoring, with recurring training and sensitization being required to address knowledge gaps and improve reporting strategies (Amin et al., 2016).

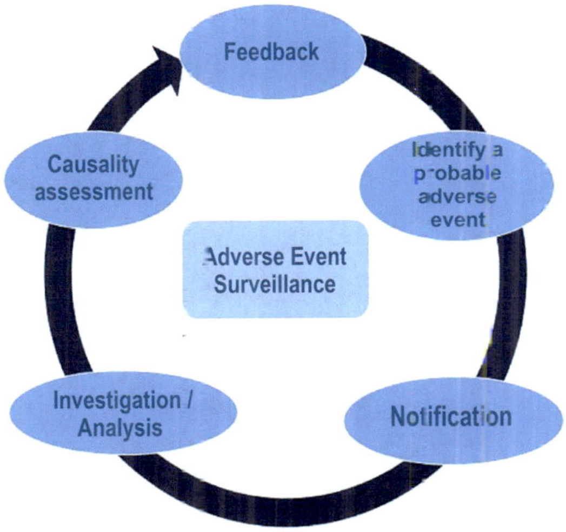
Feedback
Identify a probable adverse event
Notification
Investigation / Analysis
Causality assessment
Adverse Event Surveillance

Figure 6.17. Effective monitoring and reporting of adverse drug reactions (ADRs) are critical for patient safety and the overall efficacy of pharmacotherapy.

Source: https://assets.cureus.com/uploads/figure/file/445503/article_river_5281fac0296111ed869fd1a2e7bad300-Untitled44qwer.png.

In the absence of a robust ADR reporting framework, the healthcare system risks losing the effort associated with pharmacovigilance, jeopardizing patient safety and therapeutic outcomes (Figure 6.17).

6.4.2. Role of Healthcare Professionals in Prevention

Prevention of ADRs is a challenging endeavor that falls mainly in the hands of healthcare professionals, whose roles are more as prescribers and drug dispensers. Active patient assessment and patient education by healthcare professionals can most effectively decrease the risk of ADRs. For instance, ADR reporting systematically not only aids pharmacovigilance activity but also enhances medication safety awareness among healthcare providers (Nabi et al., 2023). Additionally, information exchange among healthcare providers creates a platform on which present risks can be identified and rectified at early stages (Choudhary et al., 2023). This cross-disciplinary approach, with the capacity to enable patients to report side effects, generates a more robust safety system. This is why healthcare practitioners have a significant function not only for curing disease but also for optimizing the therapeutic impact of medications at the least possible cost in side effects.

6.4.3. Patient Education and Awareness

For instance, drug adverse reactions (ADRs), patient education and sensitization play a central role in minimizing ensuing health dangers. The majority of the patients were not aware of the possible side effects of the drugs, as evidenced in a systematic review where 81% of patients receiving bisphosphonates and other medications did not know that they had a risk for medication-related osteonecrosis of the jaw (MRONJ) (Mauceri et al., 2024).

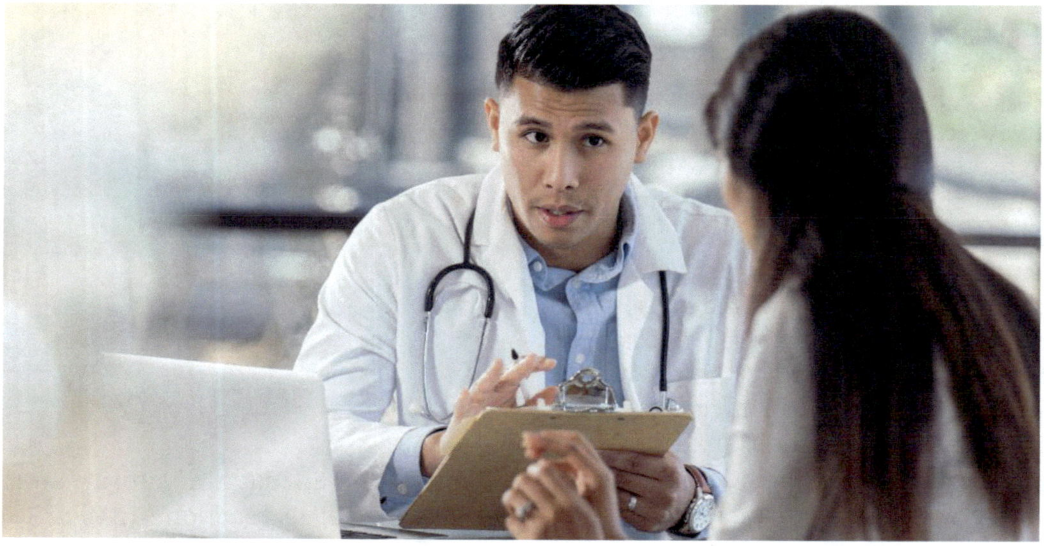

Figure 6.18. In the context of adverse drug reactions (ADRs), patient education and awareness play a pivotal role in mitigating potential health risks.

Source: https://therapybrands.com/wp-content/uploads/2024/02/Preventing-Adverse-Drug-Reactions-During-Healthcare.jpg.

This lack of awareness indicates the necessity for broad-reaching education programs for all healthcare facilities. Strong provider-patient communication can also foster a culture of safety, whereby patients are asked and queried regarding being vigilant for their treatment regimens and reporting any suspicious symptoms. Moreover, incorporation of systematic patient education programs detailing the importance of ADR detection can empower individuals, thereby encouraging their active engagement and participation in their healthcare process (Khan et al., 2024). Hence, an educational focus at a strategic level is necessary to improve patient outcomes regarding ADRs (Figure 6.18).

6.4.4. Guidelines for Safe Prescribing

Good prescribing guidelines for safe prescribing are key to reducing the occurrence of ADRs, a worldwide issue that affects patient safety and healthcare quality. Most central to these guidelines is the recognition of balance between patient well-being and transparency, as highlighted by Lassman, who condemns the FDA's proposed Drug Watch site for the risk that it carries of disrupting this balance in distributing safety information more rapidly (Lassman et al., 2006). Strict adherence to prescribing recommendations, e.g., complete medication reconciliation and focus on high prescription error rates of up to 91% in specific researches, can help diminish risks from ADRs to a great extent (Yassin et al., 2018). In addition, understanding the complexities of patient adherence and the numerous contextual variables contributing to drug-related problems is critical for health workers. Such concerted efforts ensure that prescriptions not only take into account effectiveness but also safeguard patients against the dangers of medication therapy.

6.4.5. Pharmacovigilance Systems

Effective handling of ADRs demands robust pharmacovigilance systems with the ability to monitor and analyze drug safety data systematically.

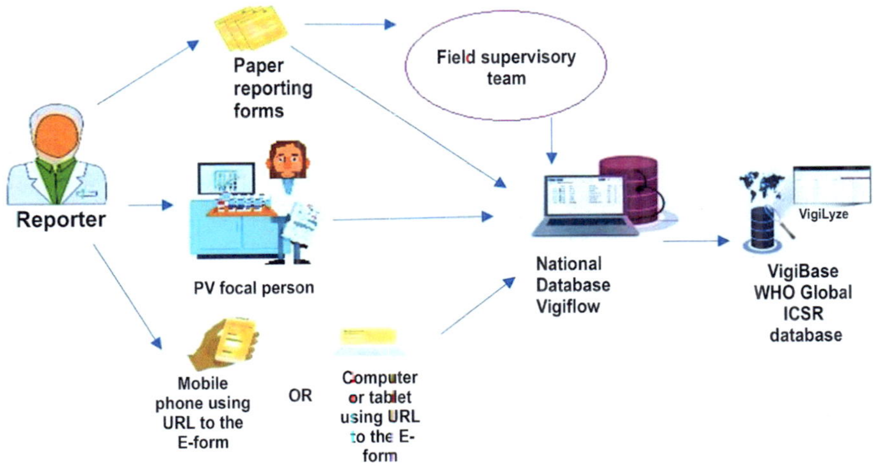

Figure 6.19. The effective management of adverse drug reactions (ADRs) necessitates robust pharmacovigilance systems that can systematically monitor and analyze drug safety data.

Source: https://www.mdpi.com/ijerph/ijerph-19-03264/article_deploy/html/images/ijerph-19-03264-g001.png.

According to recent studies, pharmacovigilance is critical for the detection of etio-clinical profiles of ADRs, particularly in vulnerable patients such as the elderly, who possess unique physiological reactions to drugs (James et al., 2025). By applying techniques such as causality judgments and severity scores, health professionals can assess the impact of ADRs and subsequently implement targeted measures for prevention.

Moreover, the integration of emerging technologies such as Artificial Intelligence (AI) and Machine Learning (ML) in pharmacovigilance frameworks has been promising regarding the efficient and accurate detection of ADRs. These new approaches enable computer-assisted prioritization and classification of ADR reports, facilitating the implementation of timely interventions and ultimately improving patient outcomes (Jasphin et al., 2024). Therefore, it is essential to augment pharmacovigilance frameworks to optimize drug safety and therapeutic efficacy in clinical practice (Figure 6.19).

6.4.6. Risk Minimization Strategies

Implementation of risk reduction measures is most crucial in the management of ADRs associated with pharmacotherapy. In keeping with the realization that discontinuation of antiseizure drugs (ASMs) due to ADRs is a key issue, individualized measures for managing these risks need to be studied. For instance, identification of clinical presentation of cutaneous adverse drug reactions (cADRs) from mild rashes to life-threatening conditions like Stevens-Johnson syndrome (SJS) and toxic epidermal necrolysis (TEN) enhances diagnostic accuracy and timely treatment (R-Romo et al., 2024).

Additionally, analysis of pharmacovigilance databases to detect likely risk factors for ADRs facilitates early detection of safety signals that affect clinical decision-making (Attelind et al., 2023). By integrating genetic factors, for instance, the existence of specific human leucocyte antigens, and applying evidence-based interventions in drug withdrawal and control, clinicians can essentially minimize the adverse impact of ADRs on patient outcomes.

6.4.7. Use of Technology in ADR Management

In recent years, the application of technology in managing ADRs has been a vital strategy to enhance the safety of the patient, particularly among the elderly. Utilization of EHR and advanced clinical decision support (CDS) systems enables healthcare professionals to monitor medication histories systematically and identify suspected ADRs before their occurrence. Tools such as the GerontoNet ADR Risk Score illustrate how technology can be employed for identifying at-risk patients to provide targeted intervention and reduce the risk of harmful outcomes among the elderly, who have multiple medication therapies (Onder et al., 2012).

Additionally, healthcare organizations, including the National Health Service (NHS), have recognized the importance of establishing a culture of safety by the use of wide-scale reporting and learning systems to inform clinical practice (Bourne et al., 2005). Technology, thus, not only enables the detection and handling of ADRs but also promotes proactive patient safety in drug management (Figure 6.20).

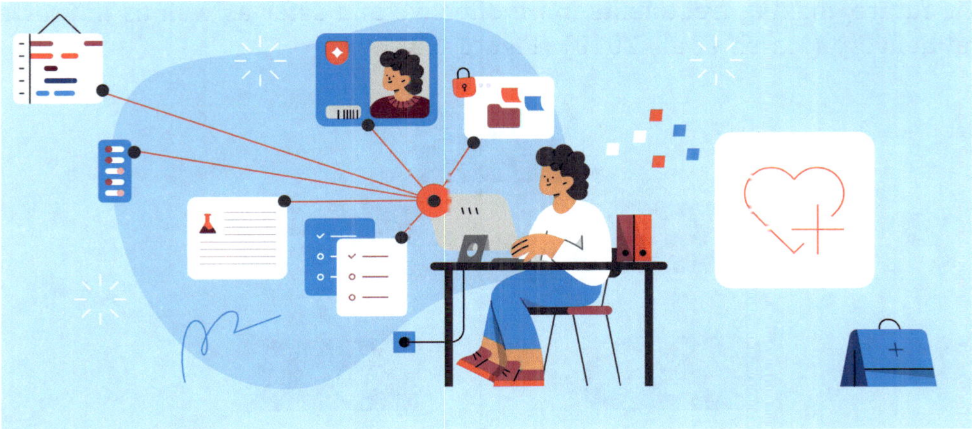

Figure 6.20. The utilization of electronic health records (EHR) and advanced clinical decision support systems enables healthcare providers to systematically track medication histories and identify potential ADRs before they occur.

Source: https://www.iso.org/files/live/sites/isoorg/files/news/insights/healthcare/Healthcare_Evergreen%20-%20Electronic%20Health%20Records.svg.

6.4.8. Importance of Clinical Trials in ADR Understanding

An understanding of ADRs is at the core of ensuring patient safety and the effectiveness of therapeutic regimens. Clinical trials play a pivotal role to this understanding through systematic assessment of the mode of action of drugs with various body systems and deciding potential adverse effects before drugs are released into the market. For instance, the Daclizumab (DAC) situation emphasizes the subtlety of drug safety;. However, it had the potential to cause immune responses, it was also found to cause severe adverse effects, including autoimmune hepatitis and DRESS syndrome, resulting in its market withdrawal (Cohan et al., 2019). This points to the necessity of adequate investigation in clinical settings that can reveal both expected and rare ADRs, ultimately translating to recommendations for safer therapeutic processes. Moreover, as stated in the ESC guidelines, the inclusion of clinical trial data is critical in ensuring appropriate clinical decision-making regarding drug use (Mach et al., 2019).

6.4.9. Future Directions in ADR Prevention

With the evolving landscape of medicine, future directions in the prevention of ADR rely on innovative strategies that integrate personalized medicine and complete medication management. One of the major strategies is the use of medication evaluation tools and interventions to enhance prescribing practice, particularly in vulnerable populations such as the elderly. These interventions are aimed at minimizing misuse-related issues and optimizing outcomes of drug therapy with systematic reviews of medication and intervention by pharmacists, which have yielded positive outcomes in increasing appropriateness of prescribing (Corsonello et al., 2016). Moreover, personalized medicine offers a promising avenue to improve the prevention of ADRs by tailoring therapies according to individual patient profiles, resulting in reduced risks of drug interactions and side effects. The coordination of network pharmacology with personalized medicine can determine the course of therapy in the future, making treatments more effective and safer as well as improving the drug discovery and delivery (Marsh et al., 2010) (Figure 6.21).

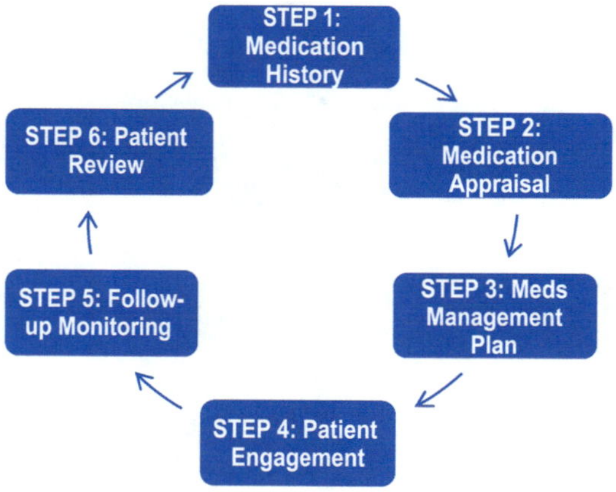

Figure 6.21. Implementation of medication assessment tools and interventions designed to enhance prescribing practices, particularly among vulnerable populations such as the elderly.

Source: https://media.springernature.com/lw1200/springer-static/image/art%3A10.1186%2Fs40814-024-01484-6/MediaObjects/40814_2024_1484_Fig2_HTML.png.

Test Your Knowledge

1. How do healthcare professionals determine whether an ADR is dose-dependent or idiosyncratic?
2. What role do patient education and counseling play in preventing ADRs, especially for individuals with known drug allergies?

Summary

Observations on ADRs bring into focus their prevalence in therapeutic practice, particularly when antibiotics and anti-tuberculosis drugs are involved. Studies show that a significant proportion of ADRs reported are concerning antibiotics and reflect their extensive use and the imperative need for enhanced monitoring within healthcare systems (Moyo et al., 2015). Moreover, the association of anti-TB drug ADRs and treatment defaults indicates how ADRs pose a risk to patient compliance and health outcomes (Ascob et al., 2019). This suggests a necessity for health care professionals to prioritize ADR reporting and intervention choices to neutralize threats. Ultimately, through the development of a culture of wariness and surveillance for ADRs, health systems can improve patient safety, optimize curative outcomes, and enhance overall therapeutic pathways, thereby driving enhanced healthcare outcomes on a larger scale.

In analyzing ADRs, certain fundamental factors were noted that reflect the complexities of pharmacovigilance. The need for uniform guidelines of reporting, as established by the Reporting of A Disproportionality analysis for Drug Safety signal detection using individual case safety reports in PharmacoVigilance (READUS-PV), reflects the significance of comprehensive data interpretation to ensure spurious conclusions in safety evaluation are not made (Fusaroli et al., 2024). Apart from that, the inclusion of novel technologies, i.e., attention-based models, in drug development processes has shown significant promise to enhance data analysis and predictive precision of drug safety profiles (Zhang et al., 2023). Such debates reflect on a twin strategy: the need for rigorous reporting criteria and application of new techniques to clarify further and minimize ADRs. Lastly, addressing these factors is paramount to facilitating safe medication practices and improving patient outcomes within healthcare environments.

KEY TERMS FROM THIS CHAPTER

- Anaphylaxis
- Drug-induced liver injury (DILI)
- Genetic polymorphisms
- Hypersensitivity
- Inhaled corticosteroids (ICS)
- Mild reactions
- Organ poisoning
- Antiepileptics
- Gastrointestinal diseases
- Genetic predispositions
- Idiosyncrasy
- Irritability
- Nausea
- Drug safety testing
- Gender differences
- Glutathione S-transferases
- Inflammatory drugs
- Medication safety
- Neuropsychiatric effect

Critical Thinking Questions

1. **What is an Adverse Drug Reaction (ADR)?**
   a. A beneficial effect of a drug
   b. A harmful and unintended response to a drug at normal therapeutic doses
   c. A side effect that is desired by the patient
   d. A reaction that only occurs with overdose
2. **Which of the following is an example of a Type A (dose-dependent) ADR?**
   a. Anaphylaxis from penicillin
   b. Nausea and vomiting from chemotherapy
   c. Skin rash from a sulfonamide
   d. Liver failure from acetaminophen overdose
3. **Which of the following ADR types is also known as "idiosyncratic"?**
   a. Type A
   b. Type B
   c. Type C
   d. Type D
4. **What is the most common cause of ADRs in elderly patients?**
   a. Polypharmacy (taking multiple medications)
   b. Genetic differences in drug metabolism
   c. Drug allergies
   d. High body weight
5. **What is a common risk factor for adverse drug reactions?**
   a. Age (especially extremes of age like very young and elderly)
   b. A healthy immune system
   c. A sedentary lifestyle
   d. Low cholesterol levels

Answers to Critical Thinking Questions

1. (b); 2. (b); 3. (b); 4. (a); 5. (a).

Short Answer Questions

1. What is the primary goal of pharmacovigilance?
2. What is an example of a serious Type B (idiosyncratic) ADR?
3. What is the best strategy for preventing ADRs in a patient taking multiple medications?
4. How can healthcare professionals reduce the risk of ADRs related to drug allergies?
5. What is the primary risk factor for ADRs in pediatric patients?

References

1. Aagaard, L. (2015). Off-Label and Unlicensed prescribing of medicines in paediatric populations: Occurrence and safety aspects. *Basic & Clinical Pharmacology & Toxicology*, 117(4), 215–218. https://doi.org/10.1111/bcpt.12445Abate, A., Rossini, E., Tamburello, M., Paganotti, D., Cinquini, M., Sigala, S., & Lodi Rizzini, F. (2024). Retrospective analysis of patient-reported adverse drug reactions in an Italian allergy unit: ALLERG-RAF study. *Pharmacology, 109*, 129–137. https://www.semanticscholar.org/paper/5448df0350abe115ac957e9a4f00baec3b215508 (accessed on 10th June 2025).
2. Adhikari, P., Padmaja, U., & Pereira, P. (2009). A prospective analysis of adverse drug reactions in a South Indian hospital. https://core.ac.uk/download/pdf/87416.pdf (accessed on 10th June 2025).
3. Afolabi, A. O., Chedi, B. A. Z., Enwere, O. O., Fadare, J. O., et al. (2011). Knowledge, attitude and practice of adverse drug reaction reporting among healthcare workers in a tertiary center in Northern Nigeria. https://core.ac.uk/download/478318560.pdf (accessed on 10th June 2025).
4. Aldini, G., González-Morena, J. M., Montañez, M. I., Pérez-Sala, D., et al. (2016). Proteomics in drug hypersensitivity. https://core.ac.uk/download/80866841.pdf (accessed on 10th June 2025).
5. Aljadhey, H., Aloudah, N., Assiri, G., Grant, E., et al. (2018). What is the epidemiology of medication errors, error-related adverse events and risk factors for errors in adults managed in community care contexts? A systematic review of the international literature. https://core.ac.uk/download/287581034.pdf (accessed on 10th June 2025).
6. Amin, A., Hussain, A., & Malik, M. (2016). Evolving trends and future prospects of ADR monitoring and reporting: A literature review. https://core.ac.uk/download/477852064.pdf (accessed on 10th June 2025).
7. Arrang, S. T., & Widyati, W. (2018). The incidence and risk factor analysis of drug induced liver injury (DILI) in a Surabaya hospital. https://media.neliti.com/media/publications/295807-the-incidence-and-risk-factor-analysis-o-684c196c.pdf (accessed on 10th June 2025).
8. Arthur, V., Elbasyouni, A., Jerpkorir, M., Kamau, R., et al. (2023) The role of bioinformatics in drug discovery: A comprehensive overview. https://core.ac.uk/download/595554929.pdf (accessed on 10th June 2025).
9. Atif, M., Munir, K., Malik, I., Al-Worafi, Y. M., Mushtaq, I., & Ahmad, N. (2022). Perceptions of healthcare professionals and patients on the role of the pharmacist in TB management in Pakistan: A qualitative study. *Frontiers in Pharmacology, 13*. https://doi.org/10.3389/fphar.2022.965806.
10. Attelind, S., Eriksson, N., Sundström, A., Wadelius, M., & Hallberg, P. (2023). Identification of risk factors for adverse drug reactions in a pharmacovigilance database. *Pharmacoepidemiology and Drug Safety, 32*, 1431–1438. https://www.semanticscholar.org/paper/5e20c4bcb9dedf878ad57274b6161edf275f3132 (accessed on 10th June 2025).
11. Awdishu, L., Cerda, J., Chakaravarthi, R., Davenport, A., et al. (2015). Phenotype standardization for drug-induced kidney disease. https://core.ac.uk/download/323065889.pdf (accessed on 10th June 2025).
12. Baraka, V., Fakih, B., Francis, F., Filbert, E., Kabanywanyi, A., et al. (2013). Strengthening

pharmacovigilance system to capture safety data from HIV clients on ART in Tanzania: Identification of gaps in safety reporting system. https://core.ac.uk/download/pdf/19726103.pdf (accessed on 10th June 2025).

13. Barber, N., Franklin, B. D., Gallivan, S., Taxis, K., et al. (2006). Can the Heinrich ratio be used to predict harm from medication errors? https://core.ac.uk/download/1747122.pdf (accessed on 10th June 2025).

14. Benard-Laribiere, A., Mangoni, A. A., Leendertse, A. J., Leuchs, A. K., Giusti, B., Violan, C., et al. (2016). Individualized versus standardized risk assessment in patients at high risk for adverse drug reactions (IDrug)–Study protocol for a pragmatic randomized controlled trial. https://core.ac.uk/download/618219416.pdf (accessed on 10th June 2025).

15. Bentley, G. R. (2020). Don't blame the BAME: Ethnic and structural inequalities in susceptibilities to COVID-19. *American Journal of Human Biology, 32*. https://doi.org/10.1002/ajhb.23478.

16. Bond, C. M., Francis, J. J., Haughney, J., Helms, P. J., et al. (2014). Linked health data for pharmacovigilance in children: Perceived legal and ethical issues for stakeholders and data guardians. https://core.ac.uk/download/19888923.pdf (accessed on 10th June 2025).

17. Bond, C., Francis, J., Haughney, J., Helms, P. J., et al. (2013). Views of healthcare professionals to linkage of routinely collected healthcare data: A systematic review. https://core.ac.uk/download/19968082.pdf (accessed on 10th June 2025).

18. Bourne, J., Firman, E., Mottram, C., Round, A., et al. (2005). A safer place for patients: Learning to improve patient safety. https://core.ac.uk/download/105328.pdf (accessed on 10th June 2025).

19. Byskov, P. K., Baden, C. S., Andersen, J. T., Jimenez-Solem, E., Olsen, R. H., Gade, C., & Lausten-Thomsen, U. (2024). Adverse drug reactions in neonates: A brief analysis of the FDA adverse event reporting system. *Frontiers in Pharmacology, 15.* https://www.semanticscholar.org/paper/f83e550931368a1cb4a864d8ec04181f26a03c2b (accessed on 10th June 2025).

20. Casamitjana, N., Corbacho-Monné, M., Ubals, M., Alemany, A., Suñer, C., Tebé, C., Tobías, A., et al. (2020). A cluster-randomized trial of hydroxychloroquine for prevention of COVID-19. *New England Journal of Medicine, 384*, 417–427. https://doi.org/10.1056/nejmoa2021801.

21. Cervantes-Arellano, M. J., Castelán-Martínez, O., Marín-Campos, Y., Chávez-Pacheco, J., Morales-Ríos, O., & Ubaldo-Reyes, L. M. (2024). Educational interventions in pharmacovigilance to improve the knowledge, attitude and the report of adverse drug reactions in healthcare professionals: Systematic review and meta-analysis. *DARU Journal of Pharmaceutical Sciences, 32*, 421–434. https://www.semanticscholar.org/paper/d5f0be0eecb8ed6c4804dda601c721c1b5af9991 (accessed on 10th June 2025).

22. Cham, S., Golomb, B. A., & Koslik, H. J. (2015). Mood, personality, and behavior changes during treatment with statins: A case series. https://core.ac.uk/download/323064248.pdf (accessed on 10th June 2025).

23. Chandra, S., Jaybhaye, D. J., Kaur, S., & Ubale, A. (2023). Pharmacovigilance: Study of pattern of adverse drug reactions at a tertiary care teaching hospital, Aurangabad, and Maharashtra, India: A prospective study and forthcoming challenge for the future. *National Journal of Physiology, Pharmacy and Pharmacology.* https://www.semanticscholar.org/paper/c83ca33ee09609659bb3d9588acd3dfd5bfa97de (accessed on 10th June 2025).

24. Chiumia, F., Chimimba, F., Nyirongo, H., Kampira, E., Muula, A., & Khuluza, F. (2024). Adverse drug reactions related with antibiotic medicines in Malawi: A retrospective analysis of prevalence and associated factors. *Drug, Healthcare and Patient Safety, 16*, 89–101. https://www.semanticscholar.org/paper/c9482d653330a829a8e018baccc688054ef5de71 (accessed on 10th June 2025).

25. Choudhary, E., Jain, S., Mahto, S., & Ahuja, D. (2023). Adverse drug reactions: Identification, prevention and management. *International Journal for Multidisciplinary Research*. https://www.semanticscholar.org/paper/c835120d9f3f5f0880190b0977200d217de15b2c (accessed on 10th June 2025).

26. Cohan, S., Lucassen, E. B., Romba, M., & Linch, S. N. (2019). Daclizumab: Mechanisms of action, therapeutic efficacy, adverse events and it's uncovering the potential role of innate immune system recruitment as a treatment strategy for relapsing multiple sclerosis. *Biomedicines, 7*, 18. https://doi.org/10.3390/biomedicines7010018.

27. Cohen, L., Neuman, M. G., Hwang, P. A., & Nanau, R. M. (2011). Genetic and immune predictors for hypersensitivity syndrome to antiepileptic drugs. https://core.ac.uk/download/pdf/290366.pdf (accessed on 10th June 2025).

28. Corsonello, A., Jha, A., Leendertse, A., Somers, A., Spinewine, A., et al. (2016). Geriatric pharmacotherapy: Optimisation through integrated approach in the hospital setting. https://core.ac.uk/download/55809733.pdf (accessed on 10th June 2025).

29. de Jong-van den Berg, L. T. W., de Vries, T. W., Duiverman, E. J., Langen-Wouterse, et al. (2006). Reported adverse drug reactions during the use of inhaled steroids in children with asthma in the Netherlands. https://core.ac.uk/download/pdf/12920067.pdf (accessed on 10th June 2025).

30. De Pretis, F., van Gils, M., & Forsberg, M. (2022). A smart hospital-driven approach to precision pharmacovigilance. *Trends in Pharmacological Sciences, 43*, 473–481. https://doi.org/10.1016/j.tips.2022.03.009.

31. Dehury, S., Sahoo, S., Maharana, D., & Mohapatra, N. (2023). Metabolic adverse drug reactions in geriatric patients in Odisha. *National Journal of Physiology, Pharmacy and Pharmacology.* https://www.semanticscholar.org/paper/b355648f69be5a3965ae83fc4ad16109a9629bc3 (accessed on 10th June 2025).

32. Dil, S. (2024). Evaluation of adverse drug reactions associated with Monocef (ceftriaxone) in a 65-year-old male with hypertension and COPD: A case study. *International Journal of Clinical Case Reports and Reviews.* https://www.semanticscholar.org/paper/0b92f6717a3af9901e9d9ad3d6d4a4eeb8fb0bd5 (accessed on 10th June 2025).

33. Ermias, A., Gurmesa, G., Mengistu, A., et al. (2012). Adverse drug reaction monitoring in Ethiopia: Analysis of case reports, 2002–2007. https://core.ac.uk/download/478298334.pdf (accessed on 10th June 2025).

34. Ettoury, S., Louati, S., Saad, I., Bentayebi, K., Zarrik, O., Bourkadi, J., Daali, Y., et al. (2024). Association of GST polymorphism with adverse drug reactions: An analysis across multiple drug categories. *Expert Opinion on Drug Metabolism & Toxicology, 21*, 191–201. https://www.semanticscholar.org/paper/68a4c3be1d3d550ccd15e0a94cb67710d1c83a88 (accessed on 10th June 2025).

35. Finn, R. S., Qin, S., Ikeda, M., Galle, P. R., Ducreux, M., Kim, T. Y., Kudo, M., et al. (2020).

Atezolizumab plus bevacizumab in unresectable hepatocellular carcinoma. *New England Journal of Medicine, 382*, 1894–1905. https://doi.org/10.1056/nejmoa1915745.

36. Foguem, C., & Kamsu-Foguem, B. (2014). Adverse drug reactions in some African herbal medicine: Literature review and stakeholders' interview. https://core.ac.uk/download/33663740.pdf (accessed on 10th June 2025).

37. Fusaroli, M., Salvo, F., Bégaud, B., Alshammari, T. M., Bate, A., Battini, V., Brueckner, A., et al. (2024). The REporting of A Disproportionality Analysis for Drug Safety Signal Detection Using Individual Case Safety Reports in Pharmacovigilance (READUS-PV): Explanation and elaboration. *Drug Safety, 47*, 585–599. https://doi.org/10.1007/s40264-024-01423-7.

38. G. A., S. G., Vijay, J. J., & Mohanakrishnan, K. (2024). A novel pharmacovigilance strategy for detecting adverse drug reactions in healthcare using machine learning and blockchain. In *2024 Second International Conference on Intelligent Cyber Physical Systems and Internet of Things (ICoICI).* https://www.semanticscholar.org/paper/39e6ff5f57fb76998bc358930b89c4d15ad5ef78 (accessed on 10th June 2025).

39. González, D., Rao, G. G., Bailey, S. C., Brouwer, K. L. R., Cao, Y., Crona, D. J., Kashuba, A. D. M., et al. (2017). Precision dosing: Public health need, proposed framework, and anticipated impact. *Clinical and Translational Science, 10*, 443–454. https://doi.org/10.1111/cts.12490.

40. Götzinger, F., Reichrath, J., Millenaar, D., Lauder, L., Meyer, M. R., Böhm, M., & Mahfoud, F. (2022). Photo-induced skin reactions of cardiovascular drugs–A systematic review. *European Heart Journal–Cardiovascular Pharmacotherapy*. https://www.semanticscholar.org/paper/0aba7d9c0c985049539291a76da84a409ae5bc2c (accessed on 10th June 2025).

41. Gray, S. L., Perera, S., Soverns, T., & Hanlon, J. T. (2023). Systematic review and meta-analysis of interventions to reduce adverse drug reactions in older adults: An update. *Drugs & Aging, 40*, 965–979. https://www.semanticscholar.org/paper/3d683d60ef74d818f6d2ba1df12420aff98aac5f (accessed on 10th June 2025).

42. Hassan, E., & Omenogor, C. E. (2025). AI-powered predictive healthcare: Deep learning for early diagnosis, personalized treatment, and disease prevention. *International Journal of Science and Research Archive*. https://www.semanticscholar.org/paper/ec0c261ebd56d77ad5be886a09cde32ac9ff051d (accessed on 10th June 2025).

43. Hiramoto, K., Akiyama, M., & Kaneko, Y. (2024). Risk factors for adverse drug reactions to sulfamethoxazole-trimethoprim prophylaxis in patients with rheumatic and musculoskeletal diseases. *Modern Rheumatology*. https://www.semanticscholar.org/paper/8fb920af5f9fd08e8ae5bafb0aa5d439f263779c (accessed on 10th June 2025).

44. Irá, T., Tovela, N. T., Varela, E., Laljeeth, P. D., Beharilal, R., & Ojewole, E. (2021). Determinants of adverse drug reactions due to tuberculosis therapy in African countries: A systematic scoping review protocol. https://www.semanticscholar.org/paper/4fc770fc5518bd65cfa1a51733f8d11587ae3384 (accessed on 10th June 2025).

45. James, J., Gowtham, B., Kala, P., Jamuna Rani, S. V. (2025). Pharmacovigilance in geriatrics: Exploration of etio-clinical profile and severity of adverse drug reactions at a tertiary hospital in South India. *Current Drug Safety*. https://www.semanticscholar.org/paper/c81063d653bc29019a8d37b6b12e4db56b44f448 (accessed on 10th June 2025).

46. Jamil, M., Sweed, H., Abou-Hashem, R., Shaltoot, H., & Ali, K. (2024). Medication-related harm (MRH) in Egyptian older adults' post-hospital discharge: A health-care challenge. *Quality in*

Ageing and Older Adults. https://www.semanticscholar.org/paper/86ccc56a3c8ce290c99b3941bde51057feed3c02 (accessed on 10th June 2025).

47. Khan, E., Ijaz, A., Jan, F., Rashid, S., & Mercado Mercado, G. (2025). Investigating specific drug-drug interactions and their clinical implications in polypharmacy, particularly in elderly patients. *Journal of Medical & Health Sciences Review*. https://www.semanticscholar.org/paper/dd62153842c39c65f32b46d753442d68f8c62567 (accessed on 10th June 2025).

48. Khan, M. S., Mishra, A., Giri, I. C., & Pujari, N. M. (2024). Role of ADR reporting culture in advancing patient safety: A review of challenges and solutions. *Journal of Drug Discovery and Health Sciences*. https://www.semanticscholar.org/paper/a6169ca6fced2285d676b3441046365ea71344ea (accessed on 10th June 2025).

49. Lassman, S. M. (2006). Transparency and innuendo: An alternative to reactive over-disclosure. https://core.ac.uk/download/62553444.pdf (accessed on 10th June 2025).

50. Livingston, G., Huntley, J., Sommerlad, A., Ames, D., Ballard, C., Banerjee, S., Brayne, C., et al. (2020). Dementia prevention, intervention, and care: 2020 report of the Lancet Commission. *The Lancet, 396*, 413–446. https://doi.org/10.1016/s0140-6736(20)30367-6.

51. Lucas, A., English, A. M., Sette, A., Wriston, A., Grant, B. J., Peters, B., de Oliveira, C. A. F., et al. (2012). Drug hypersensitivity caused by alteration of the MHC-presented self-peptide repertoire. https://core.ac.uk/download/11239743.pdf (accessed on 10th June 2025).

52. Mach, F., Baigent, C., Catapano, A. L., Koskinas, K. C., Casula, M., Badimón, L., Chapman, M. J., et al. (2019). 2019 ESC/EAS guidelines for the management of dyslipidemias: Lipid modification to reduce cardiovascular risk. *European Heart Journal, 41*, 111–188. https://doi.org/10.1093/eurheartj/ehz455.

53. Marsh, A., Singer, D. R. J., Taylor, P. C., et al. (2010). Personalized medicine: The impact on chemistry. https://core.ac.uk/download/45676.pdf (accessed on 10th June 2025).

54. Mathur, S., Jain, S., & Mishra, A. (2022). A retrospective study: Analysis of adverse drug reaction in pediatric patients in a tertiary care hospital. *Asian Journal of Pharmaceutical and Clinical Research*. https://www.semanticscholar.org/paper/ffa8c495a4f502a510517f332869f3b5c8b43ebe (accessed on 10th June 2025).

55. Mauceri, R., Arduini, S., Coppini, M., Bazzano, M., Trujillo, I., & Campisi, G. (2024). Drug assumption and awareness about adverse drug reactions. The right to know. The case of the bone-modifying agents: A systematic review. *Frontiers in Oral Health, 5*. https://www.semanticscholar.org/paper/b6ad139c1b06c161089eb9f219f34428cfcb54d9 (accessed on 10th June 2025).

56. Moyo, N. S. (2016). Evaluating adverse drug reactions associated with antibiotic use in a public sector hospital. https://core.ac.uk/download/304374820.pdf (accessed on 10th June 2025).

57. Murray, C. J. L., Ikuta, K. S., Sharara, F., Swetschinski, L. R., Robles Aguilar, G., Gray, A. P., Han, C., et al. (2022). Global burden of bacterial antimicrobial resistance in 2019: A systematic analysis. *The Lancet, 399*, 629–655. https://doi.org/10.1016/s0140-6736(21)02724-0.

58. Nabi, F., Malik, A. B., & Dar, M. A. (2023). Safeguarding health: The impact of pharmacovigilance practices in community pharmacies. *Journal of Community Pharmacy Practice*. https://www.semanticscholar.org/paper/4b208e7bb3cba7399f41cd6247b975abddfe318e (accessed on 10th June 2025).

59. Neligan, A., Tipold, A., Wessmann, A., Pakozdy, Á., Fischer, A., Callaghan, B., et al. (2015). International Veterinary Epilepsy Task Force Consensus Proposal: Outcome of therapeutic interventions in canine and feline epilepsy. https://core.ac.uk/download/36778777.pdf (accessed on 10th June 2025). (accessed on 10th June 2025).

60. Oh, A., Makmor-Bakry, M., Islahudin, F., Ting, C., Chan, S. K., & Tie, S. T. (2024). Adverse drug reactions of first-line antitubercular drugs: A retrospective study on characteristics, management, factors, and impacts. *Asian Pacific Journal of Tropical Medicine*. https://www.semanticscholar.org/paper/8ea5cf9d736a662d55d906e9151e7877fb297ea8 (accessed on 10th June 2025).

61. Onder, G., Petrovic, M., & van der Cammen, T. (2012). Adverse drug reactions in older people: Detection and prevention. https://core.ac.uk/download/55848564.pdf (accessed on 10th June 2025).

62. Palafox-Romo, R., & Méndez-Flores, S. (2024). Cutaneous adverse drug reactions to antiseizure medications. *Journal of Epilepsy Research, 14*, 53–58. https://www.semanticscholar.org/paper/f8ecfcbb7506836fc41cb4225b07f69c10760199 (accessed on 10th June 2025).

63. Pandey, A. R., Dubey, D., Marchande, S., Gaikwad, V. S., & Gadhave, N. S. (2024). The significance of real-world evidence in pharmacovigilance: Enhancing the drug safety monitoring. *International Journal of Pharmaceutical Research and Applications*. https://www.semanticscholar.org/paper/36b027970d203820e4e753b03475e3c2b1b487d5 (accessed on 10th June 2025).

64. Pilla, S., Konda, V., Bhargavi, D., R., S., & Umamaheswara, K. (2022). Retrospective analysis of adverse drug reactions to anticancer drugs at a tertiary care hospital in South India. *National Journal of Physiology, Pharmacy and Pharmacology*. https://www.semanticscholar.org/paper/9a0b236c2230c97da27df21046a8b0b5b75f8560 (accessed on 10th June 2025).

65. Sadée, W., Wang, D., Hartmann, K. E., & Toland, A. E. (2023). Pharmacogenomics: Driving personalized medicine. *Pharmacological Reviews, 75*, 789–814. https://doi.org/10.1124/pharmrev.122.000810.

66. Sethi, N. (2014). The promotion of data sharing in pharmacoepidemiology. https://core.ac.uk/download/28977826.pdf (accessed on 10th June 2025).

67. Setiawan, S. I., & Ascobat, P. (2019). Adverse reactions to first-line anti-tuberculosis drugs as a risk factor of pulmonary tuberculosis treatment default in Jakarta, Indonesia. https://core.ac.uk/download/482243303.pdf (accessed on 10th June 2025).

68. Silva, M., Fernandes, J., Ribeiro Parracha, E., Gamboa, A., & Lima Alves, C. (2024). Adverse drug reactions to β-lactam antibiotics: A Portuguese pharmacovigilance database analysis. *The European Journal of Public Health, 34*. https://www.semanticscholar.org/paper/e15f7b7f4314c48e7e432b3e614b8ffee65cea6f (accessed on 10th June 2025).

69. Sulakhiya, K., Shukla, S., Sharma, P., Gupta, P., Pandey, S., Agrawal, R., Rathour, D., et al. (2023). Current scenario and future prospects of adverse drug reactions (ADRs) monitoring and reporting mechanisms in the rural areas of India. *Current Drug Safety*. https://www.semanticscholar.org/paper/1e29c6cd32328cf9f5a6c6685a374e6c54f49d12 (accessed on 10th June 2025).

70. Sychev, D., Chernyaeva, M. S., & Ostroumova, O. (2022). Genetic risk factors for adverse drug reactions. *Safety and Risk of Pharmacotherapy*. https://www.semanticscholar.org/paper/c7189a9784631e895f6abc4674af380a1d21850a (accessed on 10th June 2025).

71. Turner, R. M., Magavern, E., & Pirmohamed, M. (2022). Pharmacogenomics: Relevance and opportunities for clinical pharmacology. *British Journal of Clinical Pharmacology, 88*, 3943–3946. https://doi.org/10.1111/bcp.15329.

72. Ufuah, U. F., Ikwuka, A. O., Oli, A., & Ogbonna, B. (2024). Adverse drug reactions in Nigeria's geriatric population and its prevalence, etiologies, implications: A systematic review. *American Journal of Chemistry and Pharmacy.* https://www.semanticscholar.org/paper/be2bc5a6633521adce55def2bb76f3a1acaf5bae (accessed on 10th June 2025).

73. Velasco Martín, A., & Velasco Sendra, M. (2018). Reacciones adversas medicamentosas (RAM). https://core.ac.uk/download/364251092.pdf (accessed on 10th June 2025).

74. Vertinsky, I. B., & Wehrung, D. A. (1991). Risk perception and drug safety evaluation. https://core.ac.uk/download/72057000.pdf (accessed on 10th June 2025).

75. Wagh, S. C., & Kadbhane, S. (2024). A review on pharmacovigilance. *International Journal of Advanced Research in Science, Communication and Technology.* https://www.semanticscholar.org/paper/16fe0ed08770beb3cf32367c044ea3e3d56076e1 (accessed on 10th June 2025).

76. Wallace, R. (2003). Structured psychosocial stress and therapeutic intervention: Toward a realistic biological medicine. https://core.ac.uk/download/pdf/35483.pdf (accessed on 10th June 2025).

77. Wei, P. F. (2020). Diagnosis and treatment protocol for novel coronavirus pneumonia (Trial version 7). *Chinese Medical Journal, 133*, 1087–1095. https://doi.org/10.1097/cm9.0000000000000819.

78. Wiener, J. B. (1998). Managing the iatrogenic risks of risk management. https://core.ac.uk/download/72056418.pdf (accessed on 10th June 2025).

79. Yassin, A., Abushaiqa, A., Ackroyd-Stolarz, S., Al Anany, M., Al Anazi, M., Al Hamid, A., Al Khaja, K., et al. (2018). Systematic review of the safety of medication uses in inpatient, outpatient and primary care settings in the Gulf Cooperation Council countries. https://core.ac.uk/download/287581298.pdf (accessed on 10th June 2025).

80. Young, P. J., Bagshaw, S. M., Forbes, A., Nichol, A., Wright, S. E., Bailey, M., Bellomo, R., et al. (2020). Effect of stress ulcer prophylaxis with proton pump inhibitors vs histamine-2 receptor blockers on in-hospital mortality among ICU patients receiving invasive mechanical ventilation. *JAMA, 323*, 616. https://doi.org/10.1001/jama.2019.22190.

81. Zhang, Y., Liu, C., Liu, M., Liu, T., Lin, H., Cheng-Bing, H., & Ning, L. (2023). Attention is all you need: Utilizing attention in AI-enabled drug discovery. *Briefings in Bioinformatics, 25.* https://doi.org/10.1093/bib/bbad467 (accessed on 10th June 2025).

82. Zhang, Z., Zhu, M., & Jiang, W. (2025). Risk factors analysis of cutaneous adverse drug reactions caused by targeted therapy and immunotherapy drugs for oncology and establishment of a prediction model. *Clinical and Translational Science, 18.* https://www.semanticscholar.org/paper/58e69796dfc12a873d832e4114cbd4115be50cbd (accessed on 10th June 2025).

DRUG INTERACTIONS

7

LEARNING OBJECTIVES

After studying this chapter, you will be able to:

1. Identify types of drug interactions
2. Understand mechanisms of drug interactions
3. Explain the clinical implications of drug interactions
4. Discuss strategies for managing drug interactions

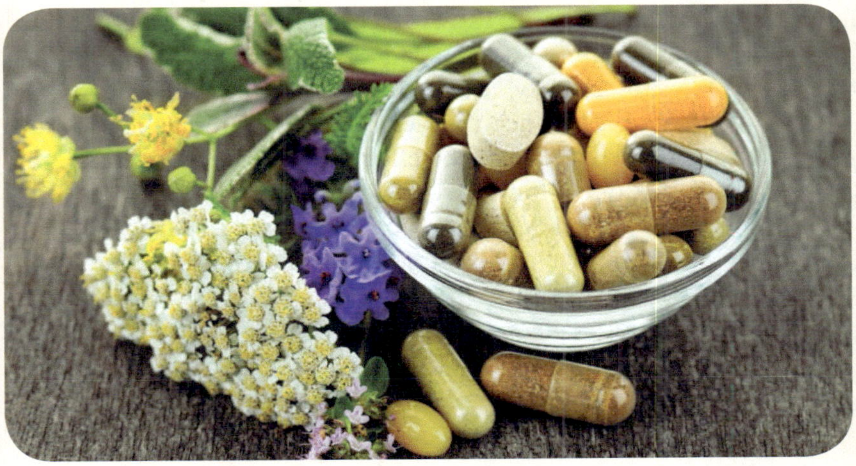

Introduction

In the pharmacological context, drug interaction is an area of concern in terms of therapeutic efficacy and patient safety. With increasingly large numbers of drugs being prescribed, knowledge regarding drug interactions helps in optimizing treatment regimens. Drug interaction leads to alterations in pharmacokinetic and pharmacodynamic parameters, typically causing undesirable side effects or failure of treatment. According to (Strilchuk et al., 2019), these interactions are particularly worrisome if urate-lowering drugs are included because their safety profiles require special attention to reduce the frequency of adverse reactions. The new European Medicines Agency guidelines also lay a great emphasis on evaluating pharmacological interactions with different populations and thus require increased caution at an early period in clinical trials (Gerven et al., 2018). An extensive understanding of drug interactions is and vital in the avoidance of dangers and affirmation that therapeutic interventions are safe and effective for patients.

7.1. Types of Drug Interactions

Learning Outcome

1. Understand pharmacokinetic interactions
2. Explain pharmacodynamic interactions
3. Discuss drug-drug interactions
4. Focus on drug-food interactions
5. Describe drug-alcohol interactions
6. Define drug-herbal interactions
7. Learn drug-disease interactions
8. Know synergistic interactions
9. Discuss antagonistic interactions

Understanding the nature of interactions among drugs is critical in the practice of medicine because the interactions have a powerful impact on treatment. Pharmacokinetic and pharmacodynamic forms of interactions among drugs are broad categorizations. Pharmacokinetic interactions arise from alteration by one drug in the absorption, distribution, metabolism, or excretion of another, which typically causes altered levels of drugs in the body. On the other hand, pharmacodynamic interactions entail alterations in the effect of the drugs without affecting their concentration, which may yield additive, synergistic, or antagonistic effects. Synergistic interactions, for instance, can increase therapy efficacy but also toxicity, making treatment more complex, especially in combination treatments for purposes of targeting pathogens or tumors (Weinstein et al., 2018). Additionally, drug-protein interactions are essential since they can determine therapeutic as well as toxic side effects, hence necessitating the need for thorough comprehension in the process of drug development (Wang et al., 2018). Therefore, understanding of these interactions is of utmost importance in ensuring maximal patient safety and efficacy of treatment (Figure 7.1).

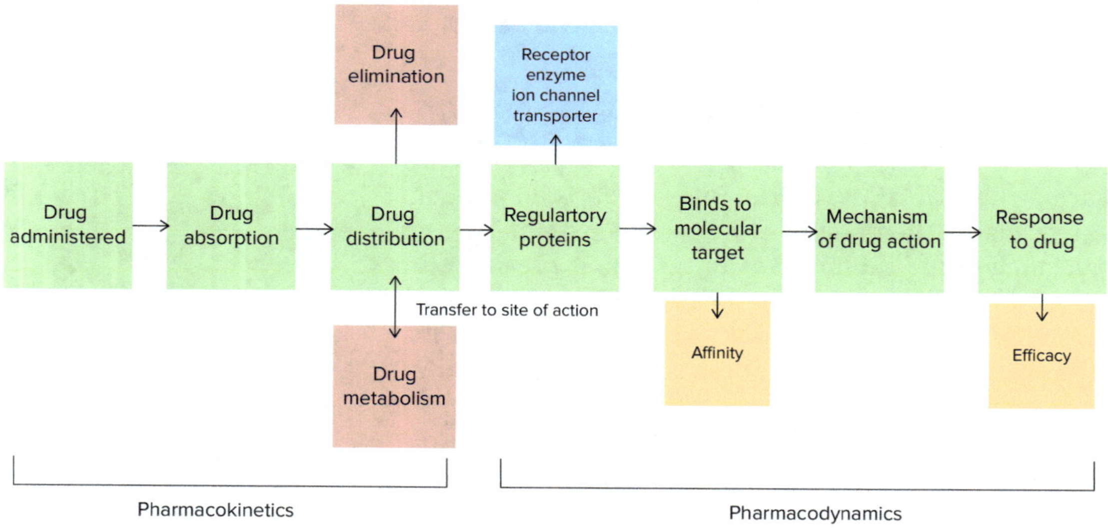

Figure 7.1. Drug interactions can be broadly categorized into pharmacokinetic and pharmacodynamic types.

Source: https://cdn.lecturio.com/assets/Pharmacokinetics-and-pharmacodynamics.png.

7.1.1. Pharmacokinetic Interactions

Pharmacokinetic drug interactions, which involve the alteration of drug distribution, excretion, metabolism, or absorption by the action of a second drug, represent a crucial essential challenge to clinical practice. For instance, opioids, which are extensively used for analgesia, are prone to sophisticated pharmacokinetic drug interactions that can lead to severe toxicity, primarily as a result of enzyme inhibition or induction by other medications (Coates et al., 2023). Similarly, conventional herbal medicines like Jingyin granules, frequently co-prescribed with conventional drugs, have been shown to significantly affect the pharmacokinetics of these drugs by inhibiting crucial drug-metabolizing enzymes, thereby altering their therapeutic profiles (Zhang et al., 2021). Such interactions will need vigilant monitoring from doctors to ensure patients' safety as well as optimal therapeutic effects. It is essential to understand the pharmacokinetic interactions in their totality since they have the potential to influence how drugs interact with one another in the body, as well as result in enhanced side effects or reduced efficacy.

7.1.2. Pharmacodynamic Interactions

Pharmacodynamic interaction is relevant to understand how different drugs affect the therapeutic effect and safety of one another. These interactions can lead to enhanced efficacy or toxicity based on the pair of drugs. For instance, simultaneous administration of sedatives and analgesics can produce synergism leading to over-sedation and respiratory depression. Conversely, certain interactions are sure to disrupt therapeutic action, rendering complicated regimens of treatment. The elderly and other susceptible groups are probably more likely to experience altered physiological reactions and heightened sensitivity due to polypharmacy, which calls for close observation and patient-specific care strategies. Moreover, ongoing education for medical practitioners on such interactions is of paramount significance, like information discussed in research on antibiotic-drug interaction and food–drug interaction, to optimize the benefits of patients and minimize risks of side effects (Radu et al., 2024; Bukić et al., 2024) (Figure 7.2).

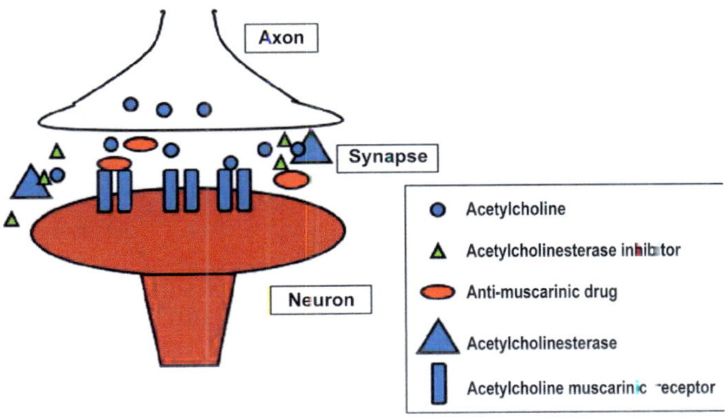

Figure 7.2. The study of pharmacodynamic interactions is crucial for understanding how different drugs affect each other's therapeutic effects and safety profiles.

Source: https://www.researchgate.net/publication/282131255/figure/fig1/AS:614236883533824@1523456893503/Pharmacodynamic-drug-drug-interaction-in-a-cholinergic-synapse-acetylcholinesterase.png.

7.1.3. Drug-Drug Interactions

Understanding DDIs is essential in keeping patients safe, particularly within the hospital setting where polypharmacy is routine. DDIs can lead to drug-related adverse effects that significantly impact a patient's health and well-being, particularly for inpatients who might be put at risk with their illness. Research indicates that the prevalence of clinically evident adverse drug events due to DDIs has the potential to be extremely high, and thus the need for close monitoring and treatment in clinical practice (Aksoy et al., 2023). The patients also unknowingly bear responsibility for the risk of DDIs by using drugs that they self-prescribe without proper knowledge of their potential interactions (Juhi et al., 2023). With increasingly complicated drug regimens, healthcare professionals must educate patients and perform intensive medication assessment. Finally, early identification and prevention of DDIs are vital to foster better patient care and prevent adverse health consequences.

7.1.4. Drug-Food Interactions

The drug-diet interaction has the potential to influence therapeutic outcomes significantly and needs careful attention within the clinical setting. Some foods are capable of inhibiting the absorption, metabolism, or excretion of certain drugs, which can ultimately affect their efficacy and safety profiles. For instance, the effect of some antibiotics can be affected by the ingestion of dairy foods, which complex the drug and reduce its bioavailability. In addition, medications like grapefruit juice are metabolic enzyme inhibitors like CYP3A4, leading to higher drug concentrations and enhanced potential for side effects; this is of concern with narrow therapeutic index drugs.

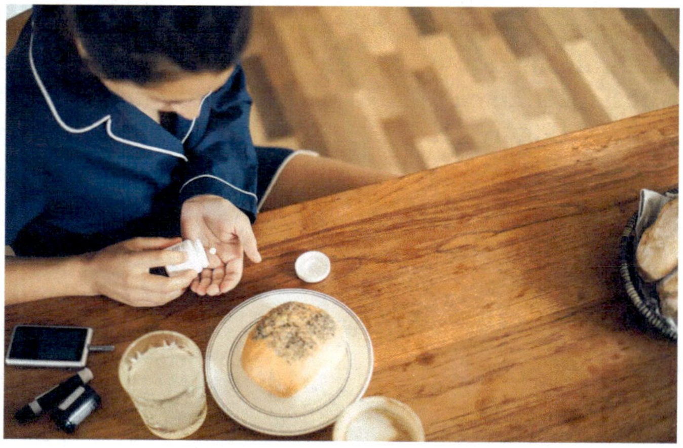

Figure 7.3. The interplay between drugs and food can significantly influence therapeutic outcomes, necessitating careful consideration in clinical settings.

Source: https://cdn-assets-eu.frontify.com/s3/frontify-enterprise-files-eu/eyJvYXV0aCI6eyJjbGllbn RfaWQiOiJmcm9udGlmeS1 maW5kZXIifSwicGF0a CI6ImloaC1oZWFsdGhjYXJ lLWJlcmhhZFwvZmlsZVwvcUs2QVlCT VB6UUNzYnFoRkhxWEMuanBnIn0: ihh-healthcare-berhad:D_ ONA-SpCO5oHnQ7zQQ7BhFHJ2H mIwvyzOzcnIcy2DU?format=webp.

In this case, drug-food interaction enters the scene, underlining the need for clinicians to inform patients about potential dietary influences to guarantee maximum effectiveness of the treatment and to prevent unwanted effects, especially when dealing with complex illnesses like pulmonary infection or migraines, as highlighted in respective studies (Akkerman et al., 2015; Capi et al., 2016) (Figure 7.3).

7.1.5. Drug-Alcohol Interactions

The interaction between drug interactions and alcohol is a significant clinical concern, both about therapeutic impact as well as patient safety. Alcohol's ability to influence the metabolism of most drugs tends to yield negative consequences, particularly because most drugs are metabolized by the same liver enzymes utilized in the metabolism of alcohol. Such a common pathway in metabolism can lead to potentiation of toxicity or drug failure. For instance, persons engaged in drug abuse, such as alcohol and illicit drugs, tend to be at a higher risk of suffering from drug effects, as in studies highlighting the correlation between drug misuse and compromised liver function (Tarantino et al., 2022). Moreover, HIV/AIDS patients have an increased incidence of substance use disorders and are therefore at a high risk of adverse drug-alcohol interactions that undermine adherence to essential therapies (Desai et al., 2020). Thus, awareness of the same is extremely vital for optimizing therapeutic interventions and promoting healthy outcomes in at-risk populations.

7.1.6. Drug-Herbal Interactions

The increasing use of herbal supplements alongside prescribed drugs raises serious drug-herbal interaction issues that can lead to altered therapeutic response or adverse effects. The reason for such interactions is the complex processes by which herbal agents can affect the metabolism of conventional drugs, primarily through the cytochrome P450 enzyme system. For instance, certain herbs like St. John's Wort have been reported to induce CYP enzymes, thereby diminishing the effectiveness of drugs metabolized by way of these pathways (Steffel et al., 2021). Furthermore, herbal supplements are also known to influence blood coagulability, hence complicating patient management on anticoagulant therapy. This area was especially brought to the forefront when it came to managing COVID-19 patients, who have heightened risks of venous thromboembolism (Wichmann, 2020). Therefore, healthcare professionals must exercise care and adequately educate the patient on the potential risks associated with concomitant use of herbs and drugs to offer efficient and safe treatment regimens (Figure 7.4).

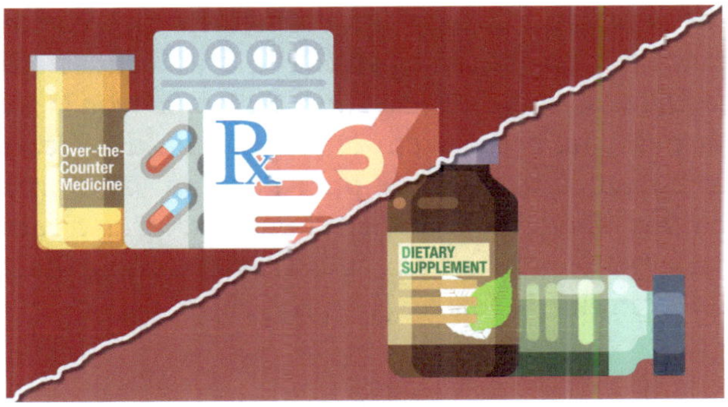

Figure 7.4. The increasingly widespread use of herbal supplements alongside prescribed medications raises significant concerns regarding drug-herbal interactions, which can lead to altered therapeutic outcomes or adverse effects.

Source: https://www.fda.gov/files/Mixing%20Medications%20and%20Dietary%20Supplements%20May%20Endanger%20Your%20Health_1600x900.png.

7.1.7. Drug-Disease Interactions

The principle of drug-disease interaction emphasizes the complexity of pharmacotherapy, particularly for patients with an underlying disease or health. The interaction occurs if the underlying disease of the patient alters the drug's pharmacokinetics or pharmacodynamics, leading to a therapeutic failure or toxicity. For instance, patients with non-alcoholic fatty liver disease (NAFLD) often experience changes in drug metabolism through liver dysfunction, necessitating dosage adjustments of drugs to prevent toxicity or suboptimal therapeutic effects (Rinella et al., 2023). Similarly, there has been mounting evidence that viral infections, as in the case of COVID-19 patients, contribute to damage to the liver, hence complicating the management of conditions of liver dysfunction. Thorough knowledge of such drug interactions is necessary for clinicians to optimize treatment regimens and ensure patient safety, and reflects the necessity of careful patient assessment in clinical practice.

7.1.8. Synergistic Interactions

Pharmacological synergistic drug interaction theory describes the potential for multiple drugs to interact with each other to produce effects greater than would be made if they acted separately. As an example, ketamine—a drug traditionally associated with NMDA receptor antagonism—has been shown to interact synergistically with opioid receptors, thereby offering a multipurpose therapeutic strategy for refractory depression and related disorders (Levinstein et al., 2025). Similarly, in ischemic stroke, a study illustrated that triple oral medication combination against individual risk genes generated improved results in the reduction of infarct size and prevention of complications even at subthreshold doses (Casas et al., 2025). These instances highlight the importance of network pharmacology and promote an integrative approach to drug development, emphasizing the necessity of multifactorial treatment regimens. Ultimately, recognizing and leveraging synergistic interactions could revolutionize therapeutic strategies, yielding more effective treatments for complex diseases (Figure 7.5).

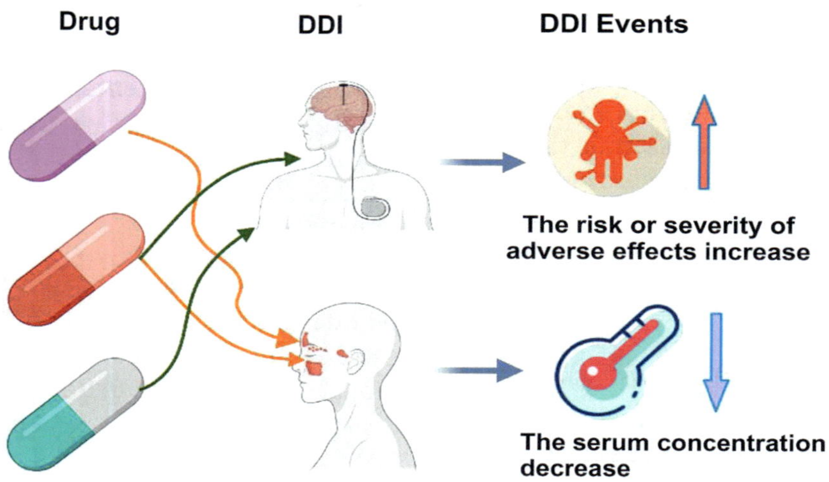

Figure 7.5. The concept of synergistic interactions in pharmacology highlights the potential for multiple drugs to work together in ways that enhance their therapeutic effects beyond what could be achieved individually.

Source: https://www.mdpi.com/electronics/electronics-13-02935/article_deploy/html/images/electronics-13-02935-g001.png.

7.1.9. Antagonistic Interactions

Antagonistic interactions are a big category in the broad category of drug interactions, involving one drug in effect diminishing or countering the activity of another. It could have several different forms, such as competing with the same receptor sites or interfering with drug metabolism pathways. A case involving antagonistic pharmacodynamics in therapeutic settings, where two drugs are used simultaneously, results in unanticipated reductions in efficacy, potentially making treatment more challenging. Furthermore, such potential is strengthened in herbal medicine, where herbal supplements are commonly consumed with orthodox drugs, and this also comes with the issues of herb-drug interactions (HDIs). Notably, some of the HDIs have been found to possess antagonistic effects, whereby orthodox drug therapeutic benefits are jeopardized by the effects of the herbal supplements (Fasinu et al., 2012). As highlighted before, it is critical to enhance understanding of these interactions by mechanistic modeling and simulation so that safe pharmacotherapy may be optimized (Niu et al., 2019).

Test Your Knowledge

1. How do pharmacokinetic drug interactions differ from pharmacodynamic drug interactions?
2. What is the difference between drug-drug interactions, drug-food interactions, and drug-disease interactions?

7.2. Mechanisms of Drug Interactions

Learning Outcome

1. Understand absorption mechanisms
2. Explain distribution mechanisms
3. Focus on metabolism mechanisms
4. Discuss excretion mechanisms
5. Learn enzyme induction
6. Focus on enzyme inhibition
7. Describe transporter interactions
8. Explain receptor interactions
9. Identify genetic factors influencing interactions

Drug interaction processes are multifaceted and complex, affecting both pharmacokinetics and pharmacodynamics. On a pharmacokinetic ground, drug interaction can alter the absorption, distribution, metabolism, or excretion of a drug, which is often responsible for undesirable therapeutic failures or toxicities. For example, some drugs can induce or inhibit metabolic enzymes, significantly affecting the plasma concentrations of co-administered medications. In addition, the drug interaction may extend beyond pharmacological properties to include cellular microenvironments that can become resistant to pharmacological modalities. This has even been observed in cancer treatment, where resistance due to stroma can arise through mechanisms such as hepatocyte growth factor secretion, which initiates crucial signaling events, resulting in lowered drug efficacy (Barzily-Rokni et al., 2012). Furthermore, literature mining methods can help broaden our understanding of such interactions by offering pertinent information to enhance our understanding of such complex mechanisms (Kolchinsky et al., 2012).

7.2.1. Absorption Mechanisms

The mechanisms of absorption for drugs are responsible for establishing their pharmacokinetics and overall therapeutic effect, particularly regarding possible drug interactions. pH, gastrointestinal motility, and food ingestion are factors that can significantly affect the absorption rates of many pharmaceuticals. Besides, the gut microbiome's role here cannot be overstated; its composition can alter drug metabolic activity and bioavailability, leading to wide variations in absorption and effectiveness. For instance, particular bacterial species may enhance or inhibit the bioactivation of drugs, showing the delicate link between the microbiome and pharmacology. In addition, physiological differences among critical patients will further complicate processes of absorption, necessitating stringent control and moderation of medication plans for maximal efficacy (Verdegaal et al., 2024; Via et al., 2025). Finally, understanding such absorption processes is crucial to effectively manage interactions and improve patient care (Figure 7.6).

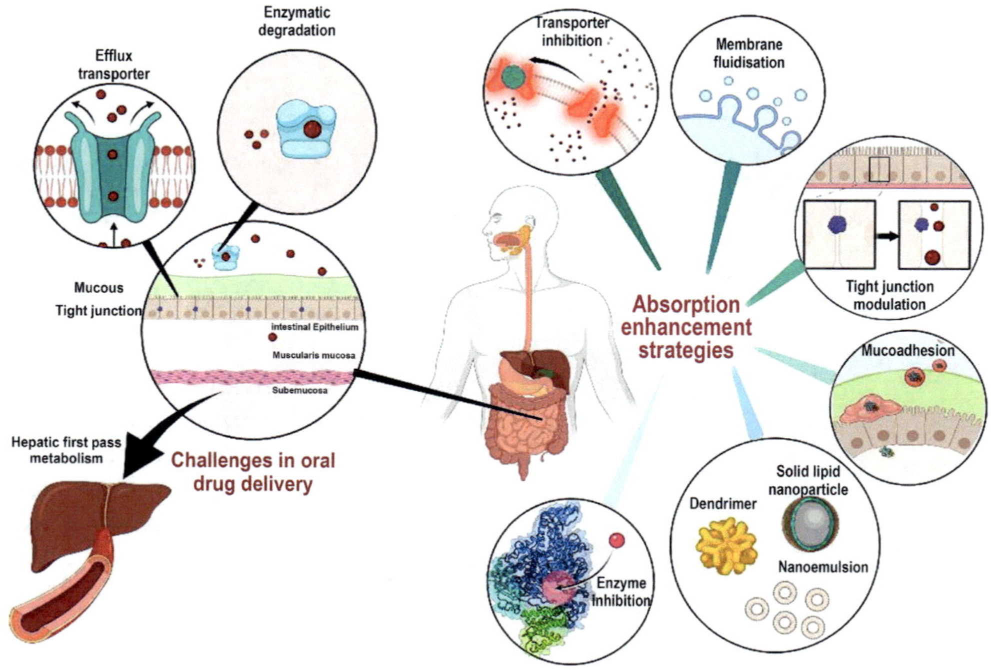

Figure 7.6. The absorption mechanisms of drugs play a critical role in determining their pharmacokinetics and overall therapeutic efficacy, especially when considering potential drug interactions.

Source: https://pub.mdpi-res.com/pharmaceuticals/pharmaceuticals-15-00975/article_deploy/html/images/pharmaceuticals-15-00975-ag.png?1659933267.

7.2.2. Distribution Mechanisms

Distribution mechanisms are a requirement in demystifying the complexity of drug interactions. Distribution refers to how a drug distributes itself throughout compartments of the body once administered, influencing its effectiveness and safety as a whole. The process is influenced by multiple factors, including drug formulation, chemical properties, and physiological conditions. For instance, antisense oligonucleotides (ASOs) are an example of modifying the chemical structure of a drug so that it is distributed and works better by binding more favorably to target proteins and influencing gene expression, as elaborated in Crooke et al., (2020). Distribution kinetics can also be significantly affected by food by modifications in gastrointestinal tract physiological conditions, which in turn influences the absorption and distribution of drugs in the body. It is crucial to identify such interactions when making the most of pharmacotherapy, particularly given the potential effect of food components such as milk or grapefruit juice on drug effectiveness and metabolism, as cited in Koziolek et al., (2019).

7.2.3. Metabolism Mechanisms

Understanding the mechanisms of metabolism is relevant to explaining drug interactions, particularly pharmacokinetic drug–drug interactions (DDIs). Drug metabolism through enzymes, primarily the cytochrome P450 (CYP) enzymes, can have a significant influence on the efficacy and safety of drugs when multiple drugs are taken concomitantly. Here, inhibition or induction of the enzymes can lead to monumental variations in drug concentration and trigger adverse effects or failure of treatment. Research has established that the evaluation of DDI potential usually begins with *in vitro* tests of kinetic parameters of co-medicines and guides subsequent clinical studies (Lee et al., 2024). Moreover, modeling with physiologically based pharmacokinetic (PBPK) models enables simulation of DDIs through incorporating respective *in vitro* data to scale up *in vivo* outcomes (Peng et al., 2021). Therefore, an extensive understanding of metabolic pathways holds the secret to predicting and managing drug interactions successfully (Figure 7.7).

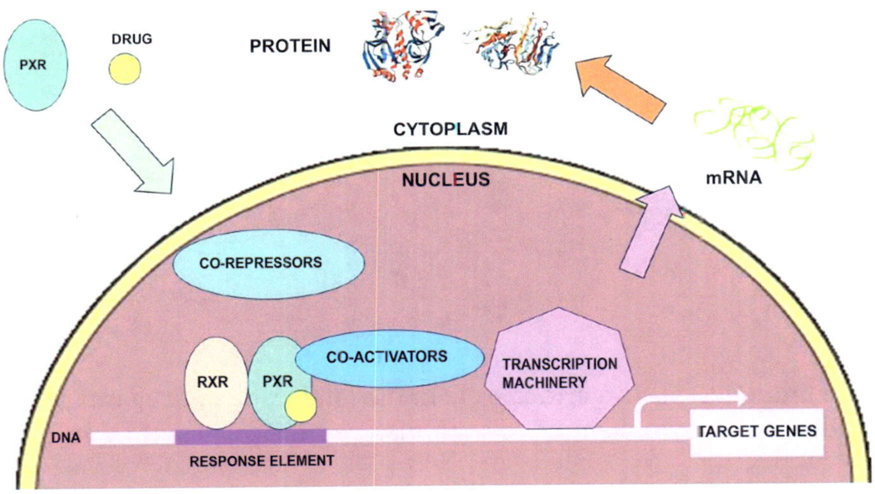

Figure 7.7. Understanding metabolism mechanisms is crucial for elucidating drug interactions, particularly in relation to pharmacokinetic drug–drug interactions (DDIs).

Source: https://www.mdpi.com/jcm/jcm-12-07120/article_deploy/html/images/jcm-12-07120-g001.png.

7.2.4. Excretion Mechanisms

Excretion mechanisms are a prominent characteristic of pharmacokinetics, which influence the efficacy and safety of drugs in the treatment process. After metabolism, drug elimination from the body is primarily in renal and hepatic form, and various factors including organ impairment and drug interaction can influence their modes. For instance, critical illness may decrease renal function and hepatic metabolism and lead to increased plasma drug levels and toxicity (Via et al., 2025). Secondly, the gut microbiome is in close association with drug metabolism and drug elimination; bacterial populations may modify drug bioavailability and promote or inhibit metabolic activity on drug clearance (Verdegaal et al., 2024). These episodes underscore the complexities of drug interactions, with great need for vigilant monitoring of drug concentration and pharmacologic effect, particularly in patients with varying levels of organ function. An understanding of excretion mechanisms is central to the rational tailoring of drug therapy and the prevention of adverse reactions in clinical settings.

7.2.5. Enzyme Induction

Enzyme induction plays a central role in the domain of drug interactions, particularly because of its capacity for modifying co-administered drugs' metabolism with ensuing changed therapeutic effects.

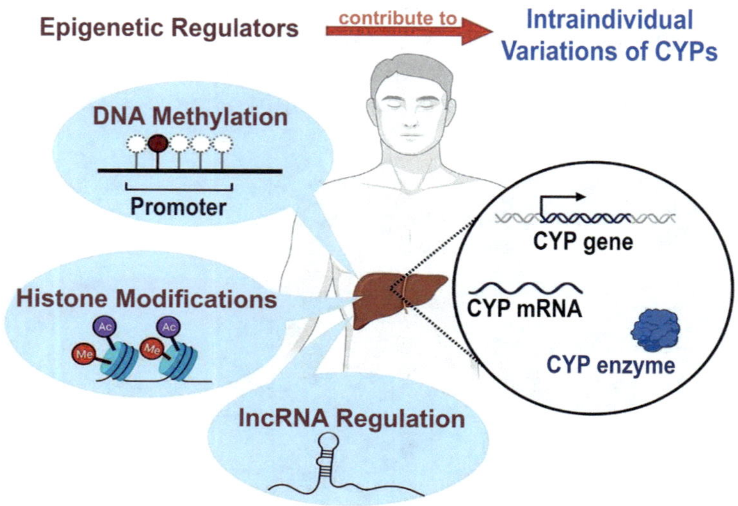

Figure 7.8. Enzyme induction plays a critical role in the landscape of drug interactions, particularly because it can modify the metabolism of co-administered drugs, resulting in altered therapeutic outcomes.

Source: https://dmd.aspetjournals.org/cms/10.1124/dmd.122.001007/asset/4d0f5326-9109-436c-b0b1-686fe41e212a/main.assets/fx1_lrg.jpg.

It is associated with increased activity of enzymes, primarily from the cytochrome P450 family, resulting in enhanced clearance of certain drugs and diminished effectiveness. For instance, protease inhibitors and non-nucleoside reverse transcriptase inhibitors are particularly engaged in such interactions, generally complicating the treatment of patients under combination therapy for conditions like HIV and cancer. The outcome of such dynamic pharmacokinetics is not just enhanced risk of treatment failure, but also the possibility of toxicity due to therapeutic drugs if the dosage is delayed (Branch et al., 2024). Furthermore, the case of polypharmacy in vulnerable populations may enhance these risks, further highlighting the need for careful monitoring and interprofessional communication to ensure optimal patient safety and efficacy in medication regimens (AlJassas et al., 2024) (Figure 7.8).

7.2.6. Enzyme Inhibition

Enzyme inhibition is a process of crucial significance in drug interactions that significantly affects both therapeutic response and side effects. Enzyme inhibitors can alter the metabolism of concurrently administered drugs and lead to increased toxicity or diminished therapeutic efficacy. For instance, nonsteroidal anti-inflammatory drugs (NSAIDs) show how enzyme inhibition manifests clinically. The main way that NSAIDs work is by blocking cyclooxygenase isozymes, which reduces pain but may also have gastrointestinal and cardiovascular side effects because different people react differently to these drugs (Maseda et al., 2020). Besides, DDI is complicated by the interaction of transporters and metabolic enzymes, which warrants cautious evaluation during the development of drugs to prevent the risk of enzyme inhibition (Lu et al., 2019). It is thus essential to comprehend enzyme inhibition for optimal pharmacotherapy and prevention of undesired effects in clinical practice.

7.2.7. Transporter Interactions

The drug transporter interaction is highly critical in the pharmacodynamics and pharmacokinetics of drugs, which dictates their absorption, distribution, metabolism, and excretion.

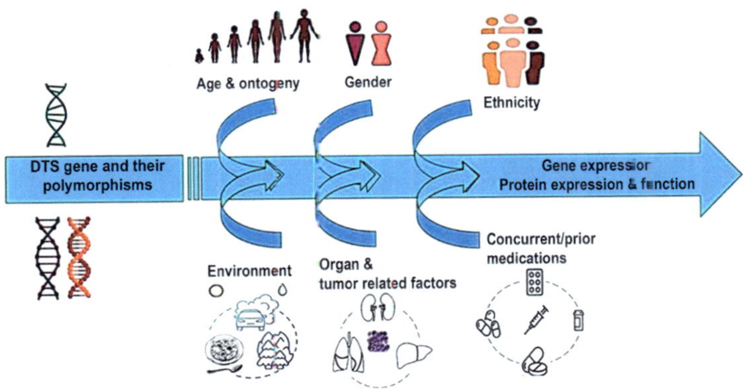

Figure 7.9. The interactions between drug transporters play a critical role in the pharmacokinetics and pharmacodynamics of therapeutic agents, influencing their absorption, distribution, metabolism, and excretion.

Source: https://pub.mdpi-res.com/pharmaceuticals/pharmaceuticals-15-00990/article_deploy/html/images/pharmaceuticals-15-00990-g001.png?1660732528.

For example, in individuals with type 2 diabetes who also have cardiovascular disorders, SGLT2 inhibitors are frequently administered in addition to statins. Recent case reports show toxicity, which calls for further investigation of this combination medication even though pharmacokinetic studies have not shown clinically significant changes in statin levels when taken concurrently with SGLT2 inhibitors (Lalagkas et al., 2021). Similarly, the variability among species for transporter interactions highlights the challenge of extrapolating human effects from animal models. Research examining human organic cation transporter (hOCT1) interactions demonstrates differential drug response, with the majority of compounds showing strong inhibitory effects on transporter activity (Floerl et al., 2020). Elucidating such interactions is vital for optimizing therapeutic regimens and minimizing side effects (Figure 7.9).

7.2.8. Receptor Interactions

Understanding receptor interactions is key to understanding drug interactions, as receptor interactions determine the pharmacological activity and therapeutic action of various compounds. For instance, padsevonil, which is a new-generation antiepileptic, possesses selective binding profiles, interacting primarily with synaptic vesicle 2 (SV2) proteins and showing partial agonism on GABAA receptors. Its unique pharmacological characteristics, including binding affinity and kinetics, illustrate the manner through which receptor interactions might influence drug action and safety profiles (Wood et al., 2019). Secondly, the GPCR domain exhibits complex extracellular and transcellular interactions that significantly impact its function, contributing to the regulation of physiological processes like synaptic adhesion and cellular signaling (Dunn et al., 2019). These figures emphasize the intricate relationship of receptor interactions, noting their significance in drug interaction design and targeted pharmacologic treatment formulation.

7.2.9. Genetic Factors Influencing Interactions

The dialogue between drug efficacy and genetic influences is crucial for understanding personal reactions to medications, as it significantly impacts clinical outcomes. Genetic differences, especially among metabolizing enzymes, may modify drug pharmacokinetics and pharmacodynamics, enhancing toxicity or diminishing therapeutic responses.

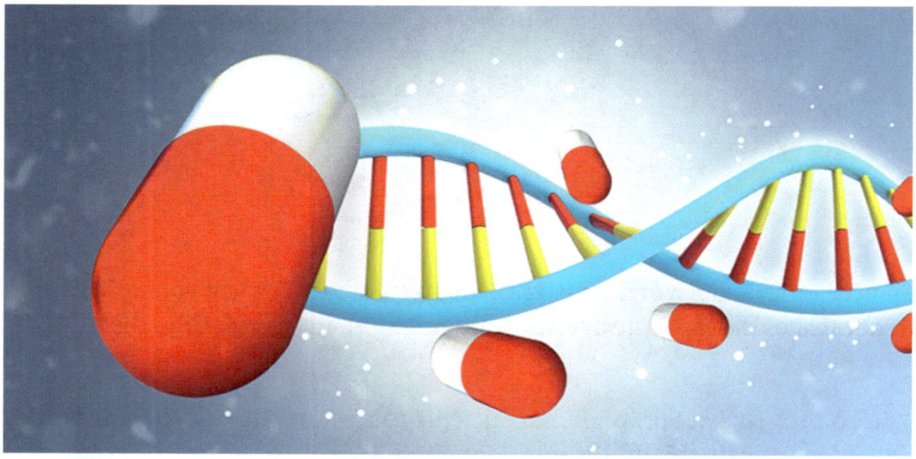

Figure 7.10. Genetic variations, particularly in metabolizing enzymes, can alter the pharmacokinetics and pharmacodynamics of various drugs, leading to increased toxicity or reduced therapeutic effects.

Source: https://amudim.org/wp-content/uploads/2022/09/Genetics-and-Epigenetics-of-Addiction-DrugFacts-.jpg.

For instance, mutations in the gene for nudix hydrolase 15 (NUDT15 have been found to influence the metabolism of thiopurine drugs as well as drug response and risk of severe side effects, including myelosuppression (Jarrar et al., 2025). Similarly, genetic factors such as SLCO1B1 polymorphisms can play a highly significant role in response to statins, affecting cholesterol control and the risk of adverse effects (Maheta et al., 2025). As pharmacogenomics advances, understanding these genetic factors not only enhances personalized treatment strategies but also aims to minimize harmful drug interactions, resulting in overall patient safety and effectiveness of the treatment in clinical scenarios (Figure 7.10).

Test Your Knowledge

1. How do enzyme inhibition and enzyme induction lead to drug interactions in the body?
2. How do genetic variations in drug-metabolizing enzymes contribute to the likelihood of drug interactions in different individuals?

7.3. Clinical Implications of Drug Interactions

Learning Outcome

1. Understand adverse drug reactions
2. Explain therapeutic failures
3. Focus on increased healthcare costs
4. Know the importance of medication reconciliation
5. Discuss the role of pharmacists in managing interactions
6. Learn patient education and awareness
7. Discuss monitoring and follow-up strategies
8. Explain case studies illustrating clinical implications
9. Understand guidelines for preventing drug interactions

The clinical significance of drug interaction is significant as it has a profound effect on patient safety and treatment outcome. This is especially so for drugs like sodium-glucose co-transporter-2 inhibitors, which tend to cause an immediate reduction in estimated glomerular filtration rate (eGFR) upon administration. In one trial involving participants of the EMPA-REG OUTCOME trial, there was a transient decrease in eGFR in over a quarter of patients on empagliflozin, raising concern for AKI, particularly with underlying renal impairment or diuretic use (Kraus et al., 2020). Close monitoring and readjustment of treatments are indicated in such interactions, testifying to the importance of personalized evaluation of patients to minimize risks. Moreover, under new stressors like the COVID-19 pandemic, individuals with substance use disorders are at increased vulnerability due to health inequalities and limitations in treatment access, for which increased awareness is paramount to address drug interactions in this population (Volkow, 2020).

7.3.1. Adverse Drug Reactions

Adverse drug reactions (ADRs) are a significant issue under the ambit of drug interactions, especially among older patients who tend to be involved in polypharmacy. A study reports that 50% of older patients had ADRs, with severe ADRs reported in 20% of patients, reflecting the clinician's significance of side effects related to medications (Bharti et al., 2025). These types of interactions often occur due to concurrent therapeutic effects or pharmacokinetic changes that enhance drug toxicity. Further, a recent study used strict methodologies to discover underreported serious ADRs caused by DDI and found 111 significant signals, such as dangerous threats including respiratory depression and acute kidney injury (Jeong et al., 2024). All this indicates the need for heightened surveillance in pharmacotherapy, particularly when dealing with drugs in susceptible populations. By understanding the scope of ADRs and how they correlate with drug interactions, healthcare workers will be in a better position to implement more effective monitoring and prevention strategies, hence improving patient outcomes (Figure 7.11).

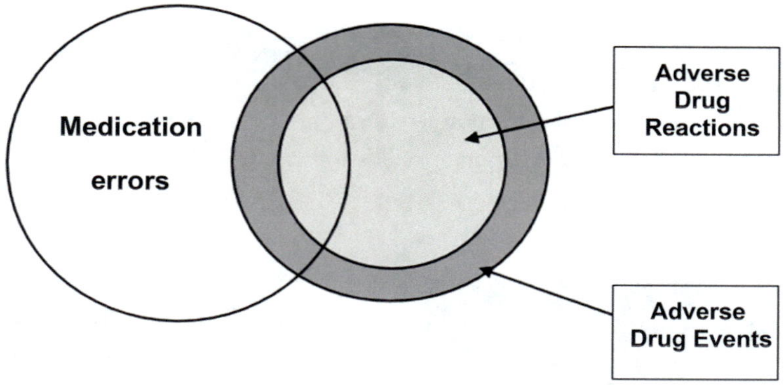

Figure 7.11. Adverse drug reactions (ADRs) represent a significant concern within the framework of drug interactions, particularly among elderly patients who often engage in polypharmacy.

Source: https://www.mdpi.com/pharmacoepidemiology/pharmacoepidemiology-03-00013/article_deploy/html/images/pharmacoepidemiology-03-00013-g001.png.

7.3.2. Therapeutic Failures

The status of therapeutic failure is typically triggered by complex drug interactions that compromise the effectiveness of treatments. In diseases such as nonalcoholic fatty liver disease (NAFLD), therapeutic interventions may be blunted by superimposed pharmacological profiles regulating drug metabolism. For instance, NAFLD patients can experience elevated levels of toxicity from impaired hepatic function, affecting the safety and effectiveness of co-administered drugs (Mary E Rinella et al., 2023). Moreover, in the context of novel therapeutic agents like microRNA (miRNA) therapies, their flexibility renders them challenging to quantify, as a single miRNA is directly or indirectly associated with multiple pathways and can bring about adverse effects (Diener et al., 2022). This multidimensional interaction calls for personalized treatment regimens to take into account potential drug interactions and variable patient response, which in turn aims to avoid therapeutic failures and optimize clinical results in complicated disease states.

7.3.3. Increased Healthcare Costs

The mounting cost of healthcare delivery has become a critical concern in current medical practice, particularly with the case of drug interactions. As patients typically receive multiple different medications to manage comorbidities, opportunities for drug interaction increase, complicating treatment and, in turn, raising overall healthcare costs. Health care providers must navigate these complexities while adhering to specific guidelines; however, the guidelines set in the ESC guidelines are a helpful guide to making therapeutic approaches secure to establish. Notably, the ESC emphasizes the need for health professionals to employ clinical judgment since they are not exempted from considering relevant public health authorities' guidelines in dealing with individual cases (Visseren et al., 2021). Consequently, with rising healthcare costs, drug interaction education remains necessary because effective management not only improves patient care but also helps in averting ever-growing expenses in the healthcare system (Mach et al., 2019) (Figure 7.12).

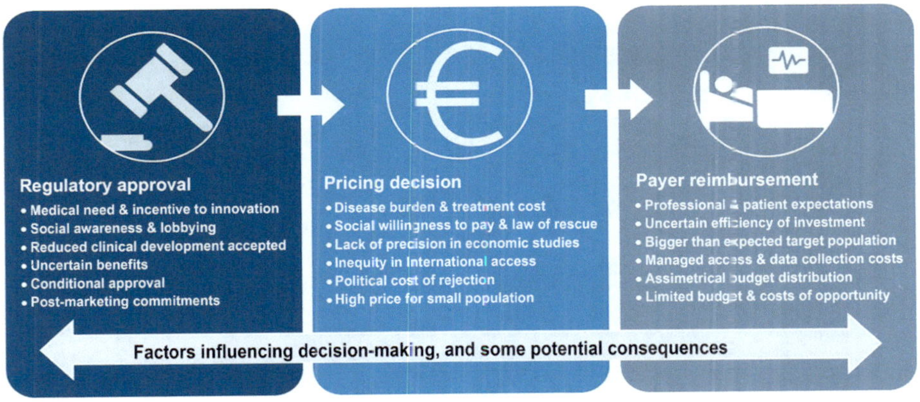

Figure 7.12. The rising costs of healthcare services have become a pressing concern in contemporary medical practice, particularly in the context of drug interactions.

Source: https://www.frontiersin.org/files/Articles/1449707/fpubh-12-1449707-HTML/image_m/fpubh-12-1449707-g001.jpg.

7.3.4. Importance of Medication Reconciliation

Medication reconciliation is a critical process that ensures that patients' medication lists are accurately and comprehensively reconciled in care transitions and minimize drug interactions. As patients move from one care setting to another, such as from inpatient to outpatient settings, there can be unintended discrepancies that expose individuals to drug-related adverse reactions. The power of medication reconciliation is brought to the fore in polypharmacy, where multiple prescriptions amplify the potential for life-threatening DDI. For instance, in QTc prolongation, active medication reconciliation by pharmacists can identify and mitigate the risks of medications like dovetailed, which can trigger cardiac conditions if not carefully monitored (Zhu et al., 2021). Finally, an effective medication reconciliation process not only enhances patient safety but also improves health results, demonstrating the value of interprofessional collaboration in being able to efficiently deal with complicated medication regimens (Kleinpell et al., 2021).

7.3.5. Role of Pharmacists in Managing Interactions

In the evolving healthcare setting, pharmacists become key players as drug interaction managers, ultimately enhancing patient safety and therapeutic efficacy. Their role extends beyond that of a mere dispenser, encompassing exhaustive patient counseling and proactive identification of potential adverse effects. A study clarifies that while pharmacists in the UAE possess a superb understanding of their profession, their influence is likely to be disrupted by limitations such as inadequate patient awareness and time constraints (Kharaba et al., 2022). Furthermore, front-line health workers have emphasized the need for firm expectations from pharmacists, highlighting the importance of including these professionals in the clinical decision-making process. This includes drug interaction management, for which pharmacists should be drug therapy specialists capable of traversing complex medication regimens (Jia et al., 2021). Ultimately, increasing the inclusion of pharmacists in healthcare teams can lead to better drug interaction management, pointing out their essential role in contemporary pharmaceutics (Figure 7.13).

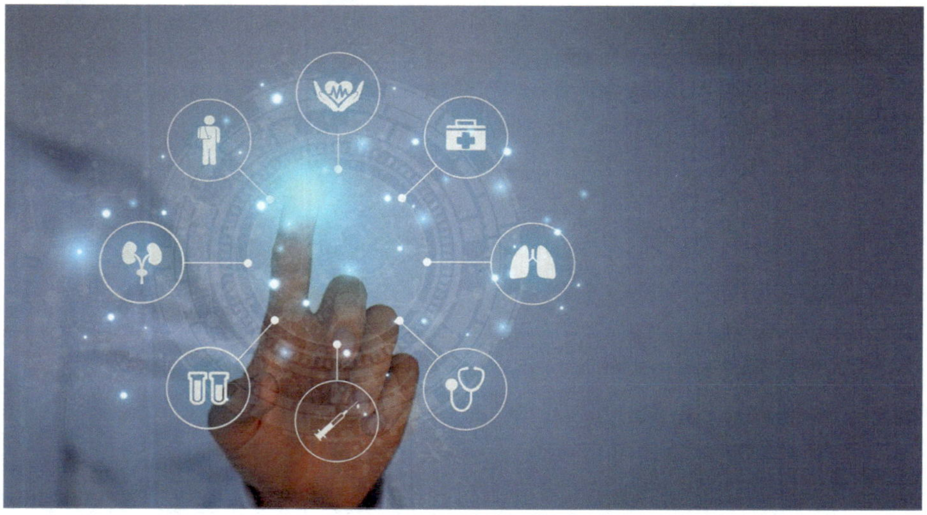

Figure 7.13. In the evolving landscape of healthcare, pharmacists serve as critical intermediaries in managing drug interactions, ultimately enhancing patient safety and therapeutic efficacy.

Source: https://www.tigahealth.com/wp-content/uploads/2024/05/what-is-digital-healthcare-ecosystem5.jpg.

7.3.6. Patient Education and Awareness

Effective patient education and knowledge are crucial factors in the management of drug interactions because they allow patients to become active players in their health. With a solid knowledge base of drug interactions, patients can avoid adverse effects and enhance therapeutic gains. The increasing complexity of drug regimens requires medical practitioners to properly report on potential interactions, emphasizing adherence to prescribed regimens and clarity in communication with patients. For instance, the way health professionals, as per the ESC/EAS Guidelines, must ensure their clinical experience accounts for the guidelines as well as individual patient requirements, thereby ensuring informed decisions (Mach et al., 2019). Besides, utilizing AI technologies like ChatGPT can assist in making educational material more personalized and patient interaction more augmented. However, it remains crucial that this technology supports, but does not replace, the depth of expertise healthcare professionals can provide (Xue et al., 2023). Thus, enhancing patient education and awareness can do much to reduce the risks of drug interactions.

7.3.7. Monitoring and Follow-Up Strategies

Good follow-up and monitoring are most crucial in pharmacology to regulate patient safety and drug interactions. It is estimated that 70% of patients have more than one prescription, and this makes them more susceptible to adverse interactions. Detailed follow-up mechanisms, such as frequent patient assessment and lab tests, help practitioners monitor the effectiveness of drugs and detect any toxic effects earlier. This is crucial not only in regard to medication regimen changes but also in regard to assistance with patient adherence to prescribed treatment. Furthermore, guidelines like those published by the ESC highlight the collaborative responsibility of healthcare providers in reaching rational decisions based on each patient's unique medical history and medications (Visseren et al., 2021). The emergence of drug resistance and new challenges, such as the challenges of new pathogens like SARS-CoV-2, emphasize the need for ongoing research on drug interactions and the identification of successful therapy that may involve multidisciplinary approaches (Gordon et al., 2020) (Figure 7.14).

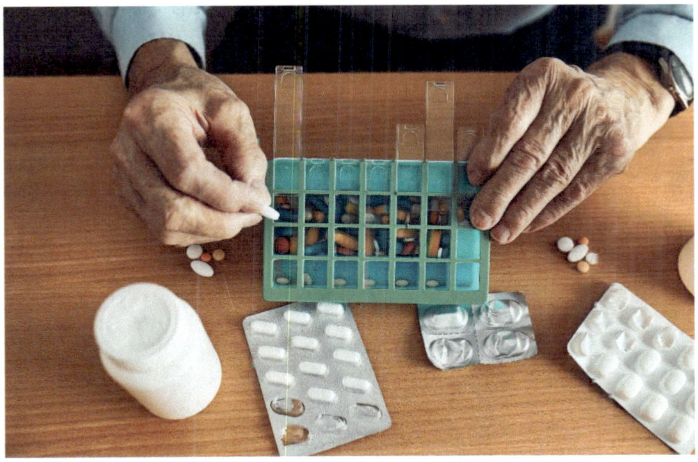

Figure 7.14. Approximately 70% of patients receive multiple prescriptions, increasing the potential for adverse interactions.

Source: https://reverehealth.com/_next/image/?url=https%3A%2F%2Frevere-health.hqdemo.app%2Fwp-content%2Fuploads%2F2023%2F09%2FManaging-prescriptions-scaled.jpeg&w=2048&q=75.

7.3.8. Case Studies Illustrating Clinical Implications

Case study analysis is particularly insightful in the matter of clinical relevance of DDI, particularly for patients with complex medical history. For instance, COVID-19 patients have shown heightened susceptibility to venous thromboembolism, traditionally compounded by the concurrent use of anticoagulants and other medications, necessitating scrutiny of their therapeutic regimens. A case report by Wichmann et al. illustrates the fatal outcome of pulmonary embolism in critically ill patients with COVID-19, which calls for critical consideration of prophylactic measures and dosing strategies (Wichmann, 2020). Furthermore, Volkow's research on drug abuse disorders during the pandemic shed light on the possible danger posed by opioid or stimulant users whose interactions with antiviral drugs could make treatment more difficult and ultimately result in unfavorable clinical outcomes. (Volkow, 2020). These case reports highlight the need for close monitoring and individualized treatment protocols to avoid drug interaction side effects.

7.3.9. Guidelines for Preventing Drug-Drug Interactions

Drug-drug interactions must be avoided in ensuring patient safety and optimization of the effectiveness of drug therapy. Adherence to guidelines can significantly minimize polypharmacy risks, particularly for those patient populations prone to chronic disease. Clinicians should seek to avoid adverse interactions by performing thorough drug reviews, including the determination of the pharmacokinetics and pharmacodynamics of all prescribed medicines. Additionally, after strict patient education protocols regarding potential interactions, it is required so that patients know why taking medication is necessary and the risks of self-medication. The need for close monitoring becomes even more essential in acute settings, e.g., in hospitalized patients with an admission of illness such as COVID-19, whose drug interactions of antiviral and anticoagulants lead to complex interactions that need close monitoring (Group TW on Guidelines for et al., 2023). Use of extensive worldwide and country-specific standards enhances the ability to deal with these challenges efficiently, thereby giving top priority to drug safety in practice (Bogachev et al., 2025) (Figure 7.15).

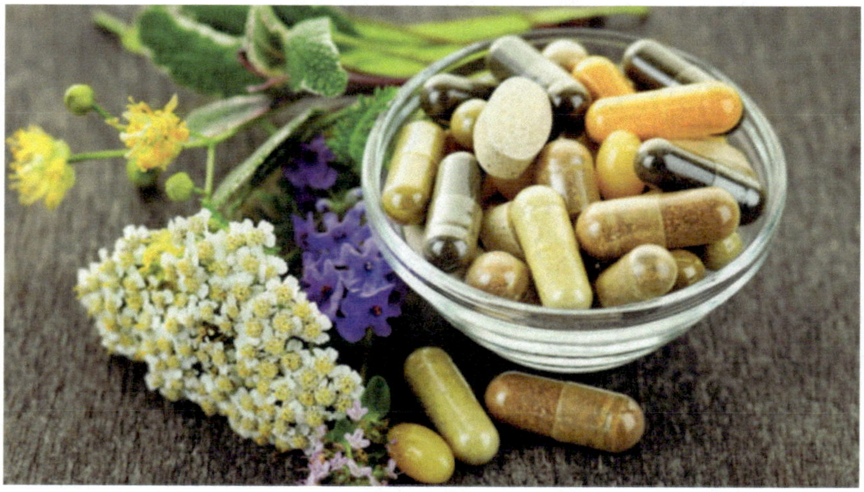

Figure 7.15. To avoid adverse interactions, healthcare providers are encouraged to conduct thorough medication reviews, which encompass evaluating the pharmacokinetics and pharmacodynamics of all prescribed drugs.

Source: https://decisionsindentistry.com/wp-content/uploads/2020/02/featured-drug-interactions-750x430.jpg.

Test Your Knowledge

1. How do drug interactions affect the treatment of chronic conditions such as hypertension or diabetes?
2. How do drug interactions impact pediatric or geriatric populations differently from the general adult population?

7.4. Strategies for Managing Drug Interactions

Learning Outcome

1. Understand comprehensive medication review
2. Know the use of drug interaction databases
3. Focus on patient-centered care approaches
4. Discuss collaboration among healthcare providers
5. Describe adjusting dosages and schedules
6. Focus on alternative therapies and options
7. Perform regular monitoring of drug levels
8. Focus on educating patients on potential interactions
9. Utilizing technology in managing interactions

Effective management of drug interactions is critical to enhancing patient safety and the effectiveness of therapy. One of the key strategies involves the conduct of thorough reviews of medications to screen for potential interactions, especially in patients on multiple drugs, a condition commonly found in postoperative practice. For instance, implementation of an active practice through hiring tried risk-scoring algorithms enables individualized pharmacologic treatment, practically decreasing the incidence of postoperative nausea and vomiting (PONV) and post-discharge nausea and vomiting (PDNV) (Elvir-Lazo et al., 2020). Moreover, the use of multimodal analgesic approaches can decrease opioid intake and its attendant risk of drug interactions. This strategy is particularly applicable to cancer pain treatment, where patients are likely to develop chronic pain compounded by complex drug treatment regimens (Fallon et al., 2018). Patient education about the importance of informing the healthcare provider of all medications, both prescription and over-the-counter (OTC) medications, can also enhance treatment safety and efficacy, thereby enhancing the health outcomes of patients.

7.4.1. Comprehensive Medication Review

In drug interaction practice, it is obligatory to conduct a comprehensive review of medication in order to identify and avoid potential side effects resulting from polypharmacy. Reviews are particularly crucial among vulnerable populations, including older patients, who may become more exposed to the abuse of medicines that lead to drug-related problems (DRPs), including DDI and ADRs (Murali et al., 2024). By employing tools such as the Screening Tool of Older Persons Prescriptions (STOPP) and the Screening Tool to Alert Doctors to the Right Treatment (START), clinicians are able to systematically evaluate appropriateness, thereby maximizing prescription regimes. Moreover, administration of bioenhancers, for example, piperine, is also known to significantly contribute to the pharmacokinetic profile of various drugs by enhancing bioavailability and further reducing required doses, and in the process, minimizing side effects (Najar et al., 2024). Thus, comprehensive medication reviews are an integral part of the practice of drug effectiveness and safety (Figure 7.16).

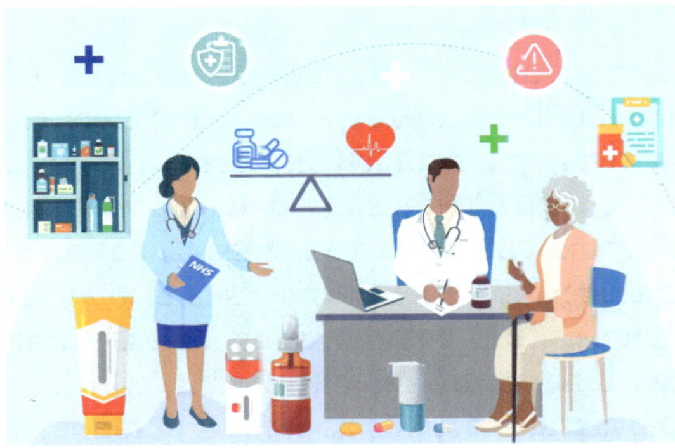

Figure 7.16. In the context of drug interactions, a comprehensive medication review is essential for identifying and mitigating potential adverse effects that may arise from polypharmacy.

Source: https://coreprescribingsolutions.co.uk/wp-content/uploads/2024/01/MANAGING-POLYPHARMACY-IN-ELDERLY-CARE-scaled.jpg

7.4.2. Use of Drug Interaction Databases

Drug interaction database usage is at the heart of contemporary pharmacotherapy, guaranteeing patient safety and peak treatment outcomes. Such databases, which collect enormous volumes of DDI information together with the related risk, are critical resources for healthcare providers. By providing evidence-based facts, they help clinicians identify potential adverse reactions not evident during pre-marketing clinical trials, therefore raising awareness for serious adverse drug reactions (SADRs) as highlighted in recent studies (Jeong et al., 2024). Moreover, drug interaction databases provide an easy understanding of intricate pharmacokinetic phenomena, thereby enabling clinicians to develop strategies minimizing risk with polypharmacy, particularly in highly comorbid patients. Further, cross-referencing of EHRs and literature enhances the reliability of these databases, where clinicians can access updated and accurate data for making informed prescribing choices (Tiwari et al., 2025).

7.4.3. Patient-Centered Care Approaches

Among strategies of patient-centered care, identifying discrete patient needs and preferences is critical, particularly in drug interaction management. With shared decision-making, healthcare clinicians can engage patients in discussing the benefits and risks of their drug regimens. This collaboration is essential in prescribing medicines like statins, which have cardiovascular actions as well as potential side effects like drug interactions making treatment more difficult (Maheta et al., 2025). Moreover, technological advancements like Large Language Models (LLMs) have the potential to enhance patient education around drug management significantly. Such computerized tools provide patients with easily accessible information regarding drug interactions, thereby empowering them to make well-informed decisions regarding their health (Aydin et al., 2025). Lastly, the integration of patient-centered care practices not only increases treatment compliance but also improves safety and efficacy, minimizing the risk for harmful drug interactions in diverse patient populations (Figure 7.17).

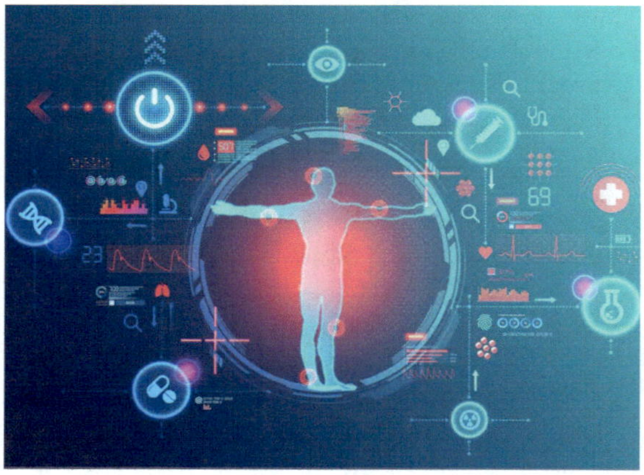

Figure 7.17. By emphasizing shared decision-making, healthcare providers can engage patients in discussions about the risks and benefits associated with their medication regimens.

Source: https://chcm.com/wp-content/uploads/2023/12/better-health-outcomes-and-patient-preferences-chcm.webp.

7.4.4. Collaboration Among Healthcare Providers

In the complex healthcare setting, provider collaboration becomes imperative for minimizing the risks of drug interactions. With the prevalence of polypharmacy on the rise, particularly in older patients as well as patients with a comorbid condition, joint effort is essential for patient safety. Interdisciplinary communication allows health professionals to share vital information regarding patient medications, potential side effects, and substitutability. For instance, AlJassas et al. (2024) point out that intensive medication reviews by pharmacists can identify DDIs of high risk, facilitating a proactive approach in treatment management. Furthermore, CDS system implementation in EHRs enhances real-time detection of DDIs, but requires coordination between physicians, pharmacists, and nurses to ensure it is effectively implemented. By prioritizing collaboration, healthcare professionals can navigate the complexities of medication treatment, adapting patient schemes to eliminate symptomology and minimize adverse interactions, as noted by Praneetha et al. (2025).

7.4.5. Adjusting Dosages and Schedules

In the complex setting of pharmacotherapy, there is a need to adjust dosages and schedules due to the possibility of drug interactions that are capable of significantly altering drug metabolism as well as therapeutic action. Genetic variation, for instance, may result in different metabolic responses to drugs, necessitating adjustments in their administration. One study noted that over 80% of healthy volunteers demonstrated photoconversion following administration of CYP2C19 inhibitors, emphasizing the significant contribution of drug–drug interactions in metabolic profiles as well as in dosing regimens (Abouir et al., 2024). Furthermore, the application of physiologically-based pharmacokinetic (PBPK) modeling is a robust framework for predicting the pharmacokinetics of drugs under interacting agent conditions. Such modeling has illustrated the fact that certain combinations must have their dosing carefully optimized, particularly in the case of potent inhibitors or inducers, to avoid subtherapeutic responses or toxicity, demonstrating the necessity for tailoring treatment regimens within the context of possible interactions (Jia et al., 2024) (Figure 7 18).

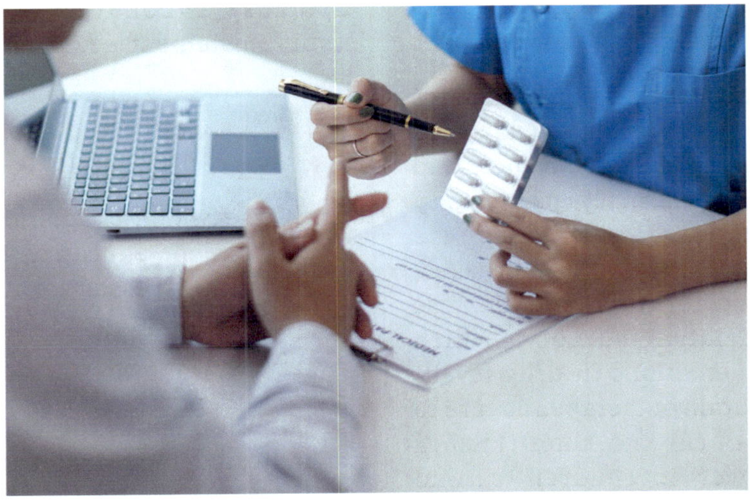

Figure 7.18. Adjusting dosages and schedules is paramount due to potential drug interactions that can significantly alter drug metabolism and therapeutic efficacy.

Source: https://staffingly.com/wp-content/uploads/2024/12/prior-authorization-dosage-adjustment.jpg.

7.4.6. Alternative Therapies and Options

Research on alternative interventions gives essential data on how to deal with drug interactions, especially in patients who require complementary treatment regimens alongside conventional drugs. For instance, the contemporary growth of antiretroviral treatments for HIV, as discussed in the EACS Guidelines, presents several first-line treatment guidelines that may be partnered with alternative interventions to enhance patient conditions and mitigate undesirable side effects of drug interactions (Ryom et al., 2022). Furthermore, the use of alternative treatments such as Veneto lax, a BCL-2 inhibitor, is indicative of the need to understand how other options may influence first-line therapies, particularly in oncological contexts where drug resistance is among the most significant challenges (Kapoor et al., 2020). Through emphasis on the safe combination of such alternative treatments, clinicians are better able to address the risk of drug interactions while practicing holistic care. This approach improves general knowledge about treatment efficacy and safety, ultimately leading to improved patient care and health outcomes.

7.4.7. Regular Monitoring of Drug Levels

The complexity of drug interaction necessitates regular monitoring of drug levels to guarantee optimal control of therapeutic effectiveness and safety. With rising polypharmacy, particularly among patients with chronic diseases, the danger of negative interactions is increased, as was shown in a study of chronic psychiatric treatment after bariatric surgery, which showed significant fluctuations in drug levels, necessitating re-evaluation of therapeutic care to avoid destabilization of chronic states (Pilková et al., 2024). Moreover, in children, careful monitoring of pharmacokinetic parameters has played a significant role in the prevention of concomitant medication-related adverse effects. A frequency of interaction between cyclosporine and rifampicin that was observed served to emphasize the vigilance required in keeping therapies at the highest drug levels and therapy outcomes (Kostyleva et al., 2022). Routine monitoring, therefore, not only serves as a safeguard against undesirable effects but is also part of achieving personalized patient care under circumstances of more than one treatment regimen (Figure 7.19).

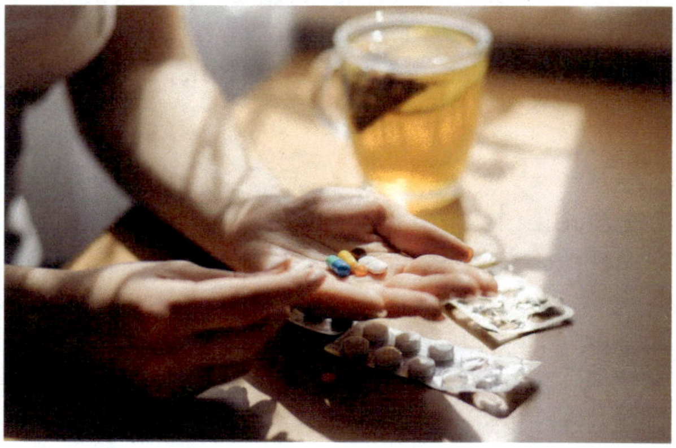

Figure 7.19. The complexity of drug interactions necessitates the regular monitoring of drug levels to manage therapeutic efficacy and safety effectively.

Source: https://www.accespharma.ca/uploads/_1920x9999_fit_center-center_99_none/ajustement-doses-medicaments.jpg.

7.4.8. Educating Patients on Potential Interactions

Part of the complex scenario of pharmacotherapy is that patient education on the risk of drug interactions is essential to safe and effective treatment. Patients who are prescribed lithium carbonate in the management of Bipolar Affective Disorder, for instance, must be educated about the risks of polypharmacy, as indicated by recent studies citing the fact that the patient would often be on different medications, risking higher likelihoods of adverse drug interactions (Jqão et al., 2025). Furthermore, self-medication by patients, particularly in those who have undergone kidney transplantation, contributes to the severity of this issue. High levels of self-medication can lead to the intake of OTC analgesics and other drugs that are themselves potentially harmful DDI with immunosuppressants, as is evident from study findings illustrating the prevalence of such risky behaviors (Demay et al., 2025). Hence, it is required of healthcare practitioners to implement robust education strategies that not only inform patients of the dangers of drug interactions but also encourage adherence to prescribed regimes and surveillance steps to mitigate the potential dangers.

7.4.9. Utilizing Technology in Managing Interactions

The integration of technology in health care has revolutionized the problem of drug interactions to enable specialists to provide more efficient and safer patient care. Advanced artificial intelligence (AI) systems, as stated by recent research, provide the capability to explore gigantic patient data, checking medication regimens for interactions with unmatched precision. For instance, AI programs can sift through a patient's drug histories and profiles and identify DDI that undermine patient safety in an instant (Chalasani et al., 2023). Furthermore, models like ChatGPT, through their natural language processing, are being explored as mediums to convey critical medication information to patients and enhance their education and adherence to treatment plans (Xue et al., 2023). This technology-driven approach not only minimizes the risks associated with polypharmacy but also fosters an interactive dialogue between healthcare practitioners and patients, ultimately leading to improved health outcomes and an informed patient group (Figure 7.20).

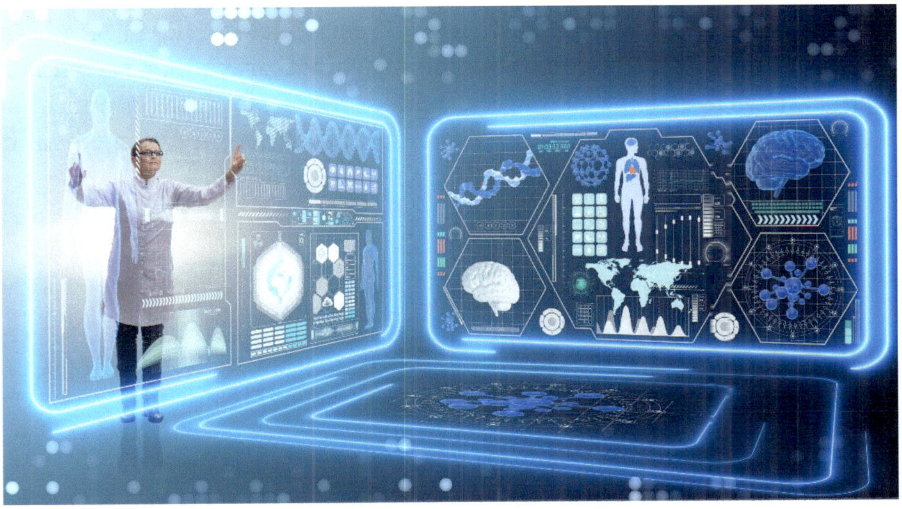

Figure 7.20. The integration of technology into healthcare has revolutionized the management of drug interactions, enabling professionals to provide safer and more effective patient care.

Source: https://esdst.eu/wp-content/uploads/2024/06/ai-in-health.jpg.

Test Your Knowledge

1. How can healthcare providers educate patients about the risks of drug interactions and ensure safe use of medications?
2. What are the best practices for managing drug interactions when prescribing drugs with known interaction potential (e.g., warfarin, antibiotics)?

Summary

Understanding drug interactions is crucial to the design of safe and efficacious pharmacological therapies. Complexity of interaction, particularly that of metabolic enzymes such as CYP3A4, emphasizes the value of rigorous research and strict adherence to current regulatory directives. New insights into the pregnane xenobiotic receptor (PXR) function indicate significant fields of drug exploration, revealing that its activation could be antagonized effectively by planned molecular-level design, as shown in Hall et al. (2021). Besides, the United States FDA's new 2020 guidelines, harmonized with closely aligned international standards from the EMA and the Japanese Pharmaceuticals and Medical Devices Agency, offer a model for robust and uniform drug interaction evaluations, as outlined in Sudsakorn et al. (2020). These developments combined facilitate a better understanding of drug interactions, with improved therapeutic efficacy and patient safety.

In evaluating the complexity of drug interactions, it is essential to incorporate pertinent findings that provide insight into their impact on patient care. Clarifying the type of interaction not only assists in minimizing adverse effects for healthcare professionals but also optimizes therapeutic effectiveness. Systematic reviews, according to the PRISMA 2020 guideline, have highlighted the importance of meticulous reporting standards to make the pharmacology assessment process more transparent (Page et al., 2021). Moreover, adherence to prescribed standards, such as those developed by the ESC and the European Atherosclerosis Society (EAS), emphasizes the need for medical practitioners to weigh clinical judgment against prevailing recommendations when prescribing medicines (Mach et al., 2019). As a whole, these support an omnidimensional drug interaction approach, with a call for constant research and adherence to medical best practices.

KEY TERMS FROM THIS CHAPTER

- Absorption rates
- Blood coagulability
- Enzyme inhibition
- Herb-drug interactions
- Over-sedation
- Pharmacodynamic parameters
- Analgesics
- Drug interaction
- GABAA receptors
- Jingyin granules
- Padsevonil
- Sedatives
- Antisense oligonucleotides (ASOs)
- Drug-protein interactions
- Genetic differences
- Non-alcoholic fatty liver disease
- Pathogens

Critical Thinking Questions

1. **What is a drug interaction?**
   a. A situation where a drug interacts with a disease
   b. A situation where one drug alters the activity of another drug
   c. A reaction between a drug and a patient's genetic makeup
   d. A condition where two drugs are given at the same time without affecting each other
2. **Which of the following is a potential consequence of a drug interaction?**
   a. Enhanced therapeutic effects
   b. Reduced drug absorption
   c. Increased toxicity
   d. All of the above
3. **Which type of drug interaction occurs when one drug affects the absorption of another drug?**
   a. Pharmacokinetic interaction
   b. Pharmacodynamic interaction
   c. Drug-food interaction
   d. Drug-drug interaction
4. **What is a pharmacodynamic drug interaction?**
   a. A drug interaction that alters the absorption rate of a drug
   b. A drug interaction that alters the effect of one drug on the other without changing their concentration
   c. A drug interaction that increases the metabolism of a drug
   d. A drug interaction involving a genetic predisposition to drug effects
5. **Which of the following mechanisms can cause a drug interaction involving cytochrome P450 enzymes?**
   a. Drug inhibition
   b. Drug metabolism
   c. Drug absorption
   d. Drug elimination

Answers to Critical Thinking Questions

1. (b); 2. (d); 3. (a); 4. (b); 5. (a).

Short Answer Questions

1. What is meant by a drug interaction, and how does it impact the efficacy and safety of drug therapy?
2. How can drug interactions influence the absorption, metabolism, and elimination of medications?
3. What are the different types of drug interactions, and how do they differ in terms of their mechanisms?
4. How can drug interactions result in therapeutic failure or adverse drug reactions (ADRs)?
5. What role do drug interactions play in polypharmacy, especially in elderly patients?

References

1. Abouir, K., Exquis, N., Gloor, Y., Daali, Y., & Samer, C. F. (2024). Phenoconversion due to Drug–Drug interactions in CYP2C19 genotyped healthy volunteers. *Clinical Pharmacology & Therapeutics, 116*(4), 1121–1129. https://doi.org/10.1002/cpt.3378Akkerman, O. W., Alffenaar, J. W. C., Bolhuis, M. S., et al. (2015). Role of therapeutic drug monitoring in pulmonary infections: Use and potential for expanded use of dried blood spot samples. https://core.ac.uk/download/55746955.pdf (accessed on 10th June 2025).
2. Aksoy, N., & Ozturk, N. (2023). A meta-analysis assessing the prevalence of drug–drug interactions among hospitalized patients. *Pharmacoepidemiology and Drug Safety, 32*, 1319–1330. https://www.semanticscholar.org/paper/865cf45e6ee29f4e49ee9ac2d295938562209555 (accessed on 10th June 2025).
3. AlJassas, S. M., Alzaidi, N. A., Algharqan, S. M., Aljawad, S. H., Alsofyani, B. M., & Hadadi, F. A. (2024). Evaluating the impact of drug–drug interactions in polypharmacy strategies for safe medication management. *Journal of Healthcare Sciences*. https://www.semanticscholar.org/paper/6ae6fe4db7636a1bc33058f907aaf6adc75781b8 (accessed on 10th June 2025).
4. Aydin, S., Karabacak, M., Vlachos, V., & Margetis, K. (2025). Navigating the potential and pitfalls of large language models in patient-centered medication guidance and self-decision support. *Frontiers in Medicine, 12*. https://www.semanticscholar.org/paper/fdbbb0f00891bd768904c6b15a96b4e45ad79905 (accessed on 10th June 2025).
5. Barzily-Rokni, M., Chapman, P. B., Cooper, Z. A., et al. (2012). Tumor micro-environment elicits innate resistance to RAF inhibitors through HGF secretion. https://core.ac.uk/download/323080472.pdf (accessed on 10th June 2025).
6. Bernardo, J., & Valentão, P. (2024). Herb-drug interactions: A short review on central and peripheral nervous system drugs. *Phytotherapy Research, 38*, 1903–1931. https://www.semanticscholar.org/paper/c4c3e53c2161bd19cd98e2be79ea2a021b63d341 (accessed on 10th June 2025).
7. Bharti, V., & Katiyar, D. (2025). Study on the adverse drug reactions and drug–drug interactions in elderly polypharmacy patients. *Journal of Neonatal Surgery*. https://www.semanticscholar.org/paper/effc897f0ed3b296cbaeea4b28cc8e51c80d1e7b (accessed on 10th June 2025).
8. Bleijs, M., van de Wetering, M., Clevers, H., & Drost, J. (2019). Xenograft and organoid model systems in cancer research. *The EMBO Journal, 38*. https://doi.org/10.15252/embj.2019101654.
9. Bogachev, V., Boldin, B., Komov, K. V., Abdoch, R., Kopnenkova, D. K., & Dzhenina, O. V. (2025). Fixed-dose ruscus extract combination and its place in current clinical guidelines for the treatment of chronic venous diseases. *Ambulatornaya Khirurgiya = Ambulatory Surgery (Russia)*. https://www.semanticscholar.org/paper/916464552754641a2ebf622e6c1f183a39005bbc (accessed on 10th June 2025).
10. Branch, C., Parson-Martinez, J., & Cory, T. (2024). Drug–drug interactions in HIV-infected patients receiving chemotherapy. *Expert Opinion on Drug Metabolism & Toxicology, 21*, 15–27. https://www.semanticscholar.org/paper/412a9250bda827a4e41bf17a0a1bbae3d8a40765 (accessed on 10th June 2025).
11. Bukić, J., Rušić, D., Turić, A., Leskur, D., Durdov, T., Božić, J., Kondža, M., et al. (2024). Evaluating pharmacists' knowledge of food–drug interactions in Croatia: Identifying gaps

and opportunities. *Pharmacy, 12*. https://www.semanticscholar.org/paper/98e51b9b4bedf818d23df0e0a7f6b596efe6a46d (accessed on 10th June 2025).

12. Capi, M., Curto, M., De Andrés, F., et al. (2016). Eletriptan in the management of acute migraine: An update on the evidence for efficacy, safety, and consistent response. https://core.ac.uk/download/74319151.pdf (accessed on 10th June 2025).
13. Casas, A. I., Nogales, C., Szepanowski, R. D., Elbatreek, M. H., Anastasi, E., Sadegh, S., Skelton, J., et al. (2025). Synergistic network pharmacology: Preclinical validation and clinical safety in acute ischemic stroke. *Journal of the American Heart Association*. https://www.semanticscholar.org/paper/41b6b49b9f6ca1d48ddcfc9c554f78ea38184d5c (accessed on 10th June 2025).
14. Chalasani, S. H., Syed, J., Ramesh, M., Patil, V., & Kumar, T. M. P. (2023). Artificial intelligence in the field of pharmacy practice: A literature review. *Exploratory Research in Clinical and Social Pharmacy, 12*, Article 100346. https://doi.org/10.1016/j.rcsop.2023.100346.
15. Chen, Y., Tripathi, L. P., Fujiwara, T., Kameyama, T., Itoh, M., & Mizuguchi, K. (2019). The TargetMine data warehouse: Enhancement and updates. *Frontiers in Genetics, 10*. https://www.semanticscholar.org/paper/12b85460797ae0919eda361457d5484845684f48 (accessed on 10th June 2025).
16. Coates, S. M., & Lazarus, P. (2023). Hydrocodone, oxycodone, and morphine metabolism and drug–drug interactions. *The Journal of Pharmacology and Experimental Therapeutics, 387*, 150–169. https://www.semanticscholar.org/paper/b2466bd98dee30aff9c536a3e90b73fad08ae495 (accessed on 10th June 2025).
17. Crooke, S. T., Vickers, T. A., & Liang, X. H. (2020). Phosphorothioate modified oligonucleotide–protein interactions. *Nucleic Acids Research, 48*, 5235–5253. https://doi.org/10.1093/nar/gkaa299.
18. Demay, E., Boissière, C., Laval, F., Vigneau, C., & Bacle, A. (2025). Prevalence of self-medication in kidney transplant patients: A single-center cross-sectional study. *Nephrology & Therapeutae, 21*(1), 5–11. https://www.semanticscholar.org/paper/87fad8cac5f495f4f8ed992035e8a71b40fb7934 (accessed on 10th June 2025).
19. Desai, N., Burns, L., Gong, Y., Zhi, K., Kumar, A., Summers, N., Kumar, S., et al. (2020). An update on drug–drug interactions between antiretroviral therapies and drugs of abuse in HIV systems. *Expert Opinion on Drug Metabolism & Toxicology, 16*, 1005–1018. https://www.semanticscholar.org/paper/2670923ef8cf2ffbd23887acea3ff41945c6d4b2 (accessed on 10th June 2025).
20. Diener, C., Keller, A., & Meese, E. (2022). Emerging concepts of miRNA therapeutics: From cells to clinic. *Trends in Genetics, 38*, 613–626. https://doi.org/10.1016/j.tig.2022.02.006.
21. Dunn, H. A., Orlandi, C., & Martemyanov, K. (2019). Beyond the ligand: Extracellular and transcellular G protein–coupled receptor complexes in physiology and pharmacology. *Pharmacological Reviews, 71*, 503–519. https://www.semanticscholar.org/paper/ccb7dfcd949428d210904b3c8e9861b78c5c192e (accessed on 10th June 2025).
22. Elvir-Lazo, O. L., White, P. F., Yumul, R., & Eng, H. C. (2020). Management strategies for the treatment and prevention of postoperative/post discharge nausea and vomiting: An updated review. *F1000Research, 9*, 983. https://doi.org/10.12688/f1000research.21832.1.
23. Fallon, M., Giusti, R., Aielli, F., Hoskin, P., Rolke, R., Sharma, M., & Ripamonti, C. (2018).

Management of cancer pain in adult patients: ESMO clinical practice guidelines. *Annals of Oncology, 29*(Suppl. 4), iv166–iv191. https://doi.org/10.1093/annonc/mdy152.

24. Fasinu, P. S., Bouic, P., & Rosenkranz, B. (2012). An overview of the evidence and mechanisms of herb–drug interactions. *Frontiers in Pharmacology, 3*, Article 69. https://doi.org/10.3389/fphar.2012.00069.

25. Fawzy, W. M. (2023). The interplay between experimental spectroscopy, theoretical, and computational quantum chemistry. *Journal of Chemistry and Interdisciplinary Research*. https://www.semanticscholar.org/paper/2036837b82f3c3573593ab53a2ee7836cbe75b05 (accessed on 10th June 2025).

26. Floerl, S., Kuehne, A., & Hagos, Y. (2020). Functional and pharmacological comparison of human, mouse, and rat organic cation transporter 1 toward drug and pesticide interaction. *International Journal of Molecular Sciences, 21*, 6871. https://doi.org/10.3390/ijms21186871.

27. Gordon, D. E., Jang, G. M., Bouhaddou, M., Xu, J., Obernier, K., White, K. M., O'Meara, M. J., et al. (2020). A SARS-CoV-2 protein interaction map reveals targets for drug repurposing. *Nature, 583*, 459–468. https://doi.org/10.1038/s41586-020-2286-9.

28. Hall, A., Chanteux, H., Ménochet, K., Ledecq, M., & Schulze, M. S. E. D. (2021). Designing out PXR activity on drug discovery projects: A review of structure-based methods, empirical and computational approaches. *Journal of Medicinal Chemistry*. https://www.semanticscholar.org/paper/c0265adcc80c8d662da0ad04b078acd80423af7f (accessed on 10th June 2025).

29. Jarrar, Y., Ghishan, M., Khirfan, F., & Hakooz, N. (2025). Genetic variants in *NUDT15* gene: Their clinical implications in cancer therapy. *Drug Metabolism and Personalized Therapy*. https://www.semanticscholar.org/paper/f9dec962af7d1ee05246dee3d378f9152a2d6c3e (accessed on 10th June 2025).

30. Jeong, E., Su, Y., Li, L., & Chen, Y. (2024). Discovering severe adverse reactions from pharmacokinetic drug–drug interactions through literature analysis and electronic health record verification. *Clinical Pharmacology & Therapeutics, 117*, 1078–1087. https://www.semanticscholar.org/paper/226ebe8dff0953f5a554d3285437a039147683f0 (accessed on 10th June 2025).

31. Jia, G., Ren, C., Wang, H., & Fan, C. (2024). Prediction of drug–drug interactions between roflumilast and CYP3A4/1A2 perpetrators using a physiologically-based pharmacokinetic (PBPK) approach. *BMC Pharmacology & Toxicology, 25*. https://www.semanticscholar.org/paper/c5a5eb67a256ce1ce1b26a5f0fd1f22c5aaaede1 (accessed on 10th June 2025).

32. Jia, X., Zhang, W., Du, S., Wen, L., Li, H., Yin, Z., Li, J., et al. (2021). What is the role of pharmacists in treating COVID-19 patients? The experiences and expectations of front-line medical staff. *Frontiers in Public Health, 9*, Article 778863. https://doi.org/10.3389/fpubh.2021.778863.

33. Juhi, A., Pipil, N., Santra, S., Mondal, S., Behera, J., & Mondal, H. (2023). The capability of ChatGPT in predicting and explaining common drug–drug interactions. *Cureus, 15*(3), e36272. https://www.semanticscholar.org/paper/95d7b47ddde5cbfb7e78caa41d73ad926795abd9 (accessed on 10th June 2025).

34. Kapoor, I., Bodo, J., Hill, B. T., Hsi, E. D., & Almasan, A. (2020). Targeting BCL-2 in B-cell malignancies and overcoming therapeutic resistance. *Cell Death and Disease, 11*. https://doi.org/10.1038/s41419-020-03144-y.

35. Khan, N., McGarry, K., Naqvi, A. A., Iqbal, M. S., & Haider, Z. (2020). Pharmacists' viewpoint towards their professional role in healthcare system: A survey of hospital settings of Pakistan. *BMC Health Services Research, 20*. https://doi.org/10.1186/s12913-020-05459-0.

36. Kharaba, Z., Farhat, J., Mahboub, B. S., Buabeid, M., Alfoteih, Y., Al-Worafi, Y. M., Jaber, A. A. S., et al. (2022). Current views of community and hospital pharmacists on pharmaceutical care services in the United Arab Emirates: A mixed methodological study. *F1000Research, 11*, 694. https://doi.org/10.12688/f1000research.110102.2.

37. Kleinpell, R., Grabenkort, W. R., Boyle, W. A., Vines, D., & Olsen, K. M. (2021). The Society of Critical Care Medicine at 50 years: Interprofessional practice in critical care: Looking back and forging ahead. *Critical Care Medicine, 49*, 2017–2032. https://doi.org/10.1097/ccm.0000000000005276.

38. Kolchinsky, A., Li, L., Lourenço, A., & Rocha, L. M. (2012). Evaluation of linear classifiers on articles containing pharmacokinetic evidence of drug-drug interactions. *arXiv*. http://arxiv.org/abs/1210.0734 (accessed on 10th June 2025).

39. Kostyleva, M., Strok, A., Postnikov, S., Gratsianskaya, A., & Ermilin, A. (2022). Pharmacotherapy in a multidisciplinary paediatric hospital: Polypharmacy and drug–drug interaction risk illustrated with a clinical case. *Safety and Risk of Pharmacotherapy*. https://www.semanticscholar.org/paper/02aa5c1a1eb617e731d3492664d5d705c35db6f2 (accessed on 10th June 2025).

40. Koziolek, M., Alcaro, S., Augustijns, P., Basit, A. W., Grimm, M., Hens, B., Hoad, C. L., et al. (2019). The mechanisms of pharmacokinetic food–drug interactions–A perspective from the UNGAP group. *European Journal of Pharmaceutical Sciences, 134*, 31–59. https://doi.org/10.1016/j.ejps.2019.04.003.

41. Kraus, B. J., Weir, M. R., Bakris, G. L., Mattheus, M., Cherney, D. Z. I., Sattar, N., Heerspink, H. J. L., et al. (2020). Characterization and implications of the initial estimated glomerular filtration rate 'dip' upon sodium-glucose cotransporter-2 inhibition with empagliflozin in the EMPA-REG OUTCOME trial. *Kidney International, 99*, 750–762. https://doi.org/10.1016/j.kint.2020.10.031.

42. La Via, L., Marino, A., Cuttone, G., Nunnari, G., Deana, C., Tesauro, M., Voza, A., et al. (2025). Critical care pharmacology of antiretroviral therapy in adults. *European Journal of Drug Metabolism and Pharmacokinetics, 50*, 105–118. https://www.semanticscholar.org/paper/d828e064fc5332d94060006b5c5112641503aa79 (accessed on 10th June 2025).

43. Lalagkas, P. N., Poulentzas, G., Kontogiorgis, C., & Douros, A. (2021). Potential drug–drug interaction between sodium-glucose co-transporter 2 inhibitors and statins: Pharmacological and clinical evidence. *Expert Opinion on Drug Metabolism & Toxicology, 17*, 697–705. https://doi.org/10.1080/17425255.2021.1921735.

44. Lee, J., Beers, J. L., Geffert, R. M., & Jackson, K. D. (2024). A review of CYP-mediated drug interactions: Mechanisms and *in vitro* drug–drug interaction assessment. *Biomolecules, 14*. https://www.semanticscholar.org/paper/a3cf21be52e2a1746f0b13140683236d2f4bca03 (accessed on 10th June 2025).

45. Levinstein, M. R., Budinich, R. C., Bonaventura, J., Schatzberg, A., Zarate, C. A., & Michaelides, M. (2025). Redefining ketamine pharmacology for antidepressant action: Synergistic NMDA and opioid receptor interactions? *The American Journal of Psychiatry*. https://www.semanticscholar.org/paper/6d16e70ffcc4a1f578db9dc7ebdec67704ea9f50 (accessed on 10th June 2025).

46. Lu, C., & Di, L. (2019). *In vitro* and *in vivo* methods to assess pharmacokinetic drug–drug interactions in drug discovery and development. *Biopharmaceutics & Drug Disposition, 41*, 3–31. https://doi.org/10.1002/bdd.2212.

47. Mach, F., Baigent, C., Catapano, A. L., Koskinas, K. C., Casula, M., Badimón, L., Chapman, M. J., et al. (2019). 2019 ESC/EAS guidelines for the management of dyslipidemias: Lipid modification to reduce cardiovascular risk. *European Heart Journal, 41*, 111–188. https://doi.org/10.1093/eurheartj/ehz455.

48. Maheta, D., Agrawal, S., Patel, J., Patel, M., Frishman, W. H., & Aronow, W. (2025). Curbside consult: Optimizing statin therapy in the elderly: A personalized approach to cardiovascular disease prevention. *Cardiology in Review*.

49. Manresa, A. P., Buendía López, S., Andión, M., Herrero, B., Lassaletta, Á., Ramírez, M., Ruano, D., et al. (2024). Safety and outcome of children, adolescents and young adults participating in phase I/II clinical oncology trials: A 9-year center experience. *Frontiers in Pediatrics, 12*. https://www.semanticscholar.org/paper/71d8c477fe00dd95da738877ed8d970ff667c645 (accessed on 10th June 2025).

50. Maseda, D., & Ricciotti, E. (2020). NSAID–gut microbiota interactions. *Frontiers in Pharmacology, 11*. https://doi.org/10.3389/fphar.2020.01153.

51. Mourão, J. Q., Castro, T. D., Vaz, J. B., da Silva, J. R., & do Nascimento, G. N. L. (2025). Mood stabilizers: Use, drug interactions, and lithium toxicity. *International Neuropsychiatric Disease Journal*. https://www.semanticscholar.org/paper/2638cd08a6c1d834c2dbc95f4e74dba83b8dd5c6 (accessed on 10th June 2025).

52. Murali, S., Damodaran, A., Jacob, N. M., Venugopal, A., Johnson, J., Vijayan, M., Pavithran, K., et al. (2024). Optimizing medication therapy in elderly patients: The impact of medication review using STOPP and START criteria version 2. *Journal of Oncology Pharmacy Practice*. https://www.semanticscholar.org/paper/a62d99fb03fbe8d4bdf6244ea0ee7713fd8471e5 (accessed on 10th June 2025).

53. Murray, C. J. L., Ikuta, K. S., Sharara, F., Swetschinski, L. R., Robles Aguilar, G., Gray, A. P., Han, C., et al. (2022). Global burden of bacterial antimicrobial resistance in 2019: A systematic analysis. *The Lancet, 399*, 629–655. https://doi.org/10.1016/s0140-6736(21)02724-0.

54. Najar, I., Pamu, S., Paul, A., Arora, P., Kaur, G., & Kumar, M. (2024). Pharmacokinetic drug interactions of piperine: A review of pre-clinical and clinical studies. *Current Drug Metabolism*. https://www.semanticscholar.org/paper/d9953c94b229ac8b018585e97ac34a301932ead2 (accessed on 10th June 2025).

55. Niu, J., Straubinger, R. M., & Mager, D. E. (2019). Pharmacodynamic drug–drug interactions. *Clinical Pharmacology & Therapeutics, 105*, 1395–1406. https://doi.org/10.1002/cpt.1434.

56. Page, M. J., Moher, D., Bossuyt, P. M., Boutron, I., Hoffmann, T., Mulrow, C. D., Shamseer, L., et al. (2021). PRISMA 2020 explanation and elaboration: Updated guidance and exemplars for reporting systematic reviews. *BMJ*. https://doi.org/10.1136/bmj.n160.

57. Peng, Y., Cheng, Z., & Xie, F. (2021). Evaluation of pharmacokinetic drug–drug interactions: A review of the mechanisms, *in vitro* and *in silico* approaches. *Metabolites, 11*. https://www.semanticscholar.org/paper/0642e3312fd3b7e7b750a9efd1a47b7fe4fda26b (accessed on 10th June 2025).

58. Pilková, A., Hartinger, J., Slanař, O., & Matoulek, M. (2024). Pharmacotherapy of carbamazepine-treated patient after bariatric surgery: A complex interplay between altered absorption and drug–drug interactions. *European Journal of Hospital Pharmacy*. https://www.semanticscholar.org/paper/4cffa31279869c9a65449c1ac14fce0c0a63070a (accessed on 10th June 2025).

59. Praneetha, A., Sathwika, M. H., Rahimunnisa, S., Lokeswari, P., Dikshitha, A., Ramya, S., & Krishna, K. (2025). Pharmacokinetics, disease, and equipment-related factors impacting intensive care unit patient outcomes: Comprehensive review. *Indian Journal of Pharmacy Practice*. https://www.semanticscholar.org/paper/00f7c1b30020f6f320c657f5a21c4fd203adcc0c (accessed on 10th June 2025).

60. Radu, A., Bungău, S., Corb Aron, R. A., Tarce, A. G., Bodog, R., Bodog, T. M., & Radu, A. (2024). Deciphering the intricate interplay in the framework of antibiotic-drug interactions: A narrative review. *Antibiotics, 13*. https://www.semanticscholar.org/paper/c2baddb406acd22527262b5d5f717477161ecc60 (accessed on 10th June 2025).

61. Rinella, M. E., Neuschwander-Tetri, B. A., Siddiqui, M. S., Abdelmalek, M. F., Caldwell, S. H., Barb, D., Kleiner, D. E., et al. (2023). AASLD practice guidance on the clinical assessment and management of nonalcoholic fatty liver disease. *Hepatology, 77*, 1797–1835. https://doi.org/10.1097/hep.0000000000000323.

62. Ryom, L., de Miguel Buckley, R., Cotter, A. G., Podlekareva, D., Béguelin, C., Waalewijn, H., Arribas, J. R., et al. (2022). Major revision version 11.0 of the European AIDS Clinical Society Guidelines 2021. *HIV Medicine, 23*, 849–858. https://doi.org/10.1111/hiv.13268.

63. Souto, E. B., Blanco-Llamero, C., Krambeck, K., Kiran, N. S., Yashaswini, C., Postwala, H., Severino, P., et al. (2024). Regulatory insights into nanomedicine and gene vaccine innovation: Safety assessment, challenges, and regulatory perspectives. *Acta Biomaterial, 180*, 1–17. https://doi.org/10.1016/j.actbio.2024.04.010.

64. Steffel, J., Collins, R., Antz, M., Cornu, P., Desteghe, L., Hæusler, K. G., Oldgren, J., et al. (2021). 2021 European Heart Rhythm Association practical guide on the use of non-vitamin K antagonist oral anticoagulants in patients with atrial fibrillation. *EP Europace, 23*, 1612–1676. https://doi.org/10.1093/europace/euab065.

65. Strilchuk, L. M., Fogacci, F., & Cicero, A. F. G. (2019). Safety and tolerability of available urate-lowering drugs: A critical review. *Expert Opinion on Drug Safety, 18*, 261–271. https://doi.org/10.1080/14740338.2019.1594771.

66. Sudsakorn, S., Bahadduri, P. M., Fretland, J., & Lu, C. (2020). 2020 FDA drug–drug interaction guidance—Comparison analysis and action plan by pharmaceutical industrial scientists. *Current Drug Metabolism*. https://www.semanticscholar.org/paper/bc2792e89d9d41dd366cc7e8422c8581ae4c11f6 (accessed on 10th June 2025).

67. Tarantino, G., Cataldi, M., & Citro, V. (2022). Could alcohol abuse and dependence on junk foods inducing obesity and/or illicit drug use represent danger to liver in young people with altered psychological/relational spheres or emotional problems? *International Journal of Molecular Sciences, 23*. https://www.semanticscholar.org/paper/315e5c1f62144d61e3131333caaf20ccff63a770 (accessed on 10th June 2025).

68. Thromboprophylaxis Working Group on Guidelines for, Covid Management of Anticoagulation in Hospitalized Pati, Embolism Pulmonary, Society Pulmonary Vascular Diseases Group of the Chinese T, Physicians Pulmonary Vascular Disease Working Committee of Ch, Prevention

National Cooperation Group on, Embolism Treatment of Pulmonary, et al. (2023). [Practice guidelines of thromboprophylaxis and management of anticoagulation in hospitalized patients with COVID-19]. *Zhonghua Yi Xue Za Zhi, 103*, 1–23. https://www.semanticscholar.org/paper/c8b4d7d12ee9930831851047b062a49d13bcba35 (accessed on 10th June 2025).

69. Tiwari, K., Kumar, B., Tiwari, A., Dhamija, P., Vardhan, G., Dehade, A., & Kumar, V. (2025). *In silico* analysis of Saroglitazar and ferulic acid binding to human ketohexokinase: Implications for metabolic dysfunction-associated steatosis liver disease (MASLD). *Cureus, 17*. https://www.semanticscholar.org/paper/5c8777b55aed80e0465bc0ebc78279be03f3f68c (accessed on 10th June 2025).

70. van Gerven, J., & Bonelli, M. (2018). Commentary on the EMA guideline on strategies to identify and mitigate risks for first-in-human and early clinical trials with investigational medicinal products. *British Journal of Clinical Pharmacology, 84*, 1401–1409. https://doi.org/10.1111/bcp.13550.

71. Verdegaal, A. A., & Goodman, A. L. (2024). Integrating the gut microbiome and pharmacology. *Science Translational Medicine, 16*. https://www.semanticscholar.org/paper/60d727fd5d8529e5e1e55f2cf60c27bfe3a86204 (accessed on 10th June 2025).

72. Visseren, F. L. J., Mach, F., Smulders, Y. M., Carballo, D., Koskinas, K. C., Bäck, M., Bénétos, A., et al. (2021). 2021 ESC guidelines on cardiovascular disease prevention in clinical practice. *European Heart Journal, 42*, 3227–3337. https://doi.org/10.1093/eurheartj/ehab484.

73. Volkow, N. D. (2020). Collision of the COVID-19 and addiction epidemics. *Annals of Internal Medicine, 173*, 61–62. https://doi.org/10.7326/m20-1212.

74. Wang, C., & Kurgan, L. (2018). Review and comparative assessment of similarity-based methods for prediction of drug–protein interactions in the druggable human proteome. *Briefings in Bioinformatics*. https://www.semanticscholar.org/paper/a848eae81c7b5ccaf3da67cd36bfe9d865701c7f (accessed on 10th June 2025).

75. Weinstein, Z. B., Kuru, N., Kiriakov, S., Palmer, A., Khalil, A. S., Clemons, P., Zaman, M., et al. (2018). Modeling the impact of drug interactions on therapeutic selectivity. *Nature Communications, 9*. https://www.semanticscholar.org/paper/56033e685144ec15451d81aa444506b6306e9f68 (accessed on 10th June 2025).

76. Wichmann, D. (2020). Autopsy findings and venous thromboembolism in patients with COVID-19. *Annals of Internal Medicine, 173*, 1030. https://doi.org/10.7326/L20-1206.

77. Wood, M., Daniels, V., Provins, L., Wolff, C., Kaminski, R., & Gillard, M. (2019). Pharmacological profile of the novel antiepileptic drug candidate Padsevonil: Interactions with synaptic vesicle 2 proteins and the GABAA receptor. *The Journal of Pharmacology and Experimental Therapeutics, 372*, 1–10. https://www.semanticscholar.org/paper/50c67a5308244ff5e65eb6d0de86ac3445ef9136 (accessed on 10th June 2025).

78. Xue, V. W., Lei, P., & Cho, W. C. (2023). The potential impact of ChatGPT in clinical and translational medicine. *Clinical and Translational Medicine, 13*, e1216. https://doi.org/10.1002/ctm2.1216.

79. Yildirim, E. S., Aydin, A., Ince, T., Varol, Z., Ünal, B., & Demir, A. (2024). Simethicone medication should be avoided in infants receiving oral lactase treatment. *Children, 11*. https://www.semanticscholar.org/paper/5e34202617b12aaea675c58fbf684d4b5aee9b1b (accessed on 10th June 2025).

80. Zhang, F., Liu, W., Huang, J., Chen, Q., Wang, D. D., Zou, L. W., Zhao, Y. F., et al. (2021). Inhibition of drug-metabolizing enzymes by Jingyin granules: Implications of herb–drug interactions in antiviral therapy. *Acta Pharmacological Sinica, 43*, 1072–1081. https://www.semanticscholar.org/paper/0466369d66c06a47d5855e20d9a0b7489771b079 (accessed on 10th June 2025).

81. Zhu, E., Gabriele, M., & Nguyen, M. (2021). The use of intravenous lidocaine in the setting of chronic dofetilide overdose: A case report. *Journal of Pharmacy Practice, 35*, 1054–1056. https://doi.org/10.1177/08971900211015053.

RATIONAL PRESCRIBING AND PRESCRIPTION WRITING

8

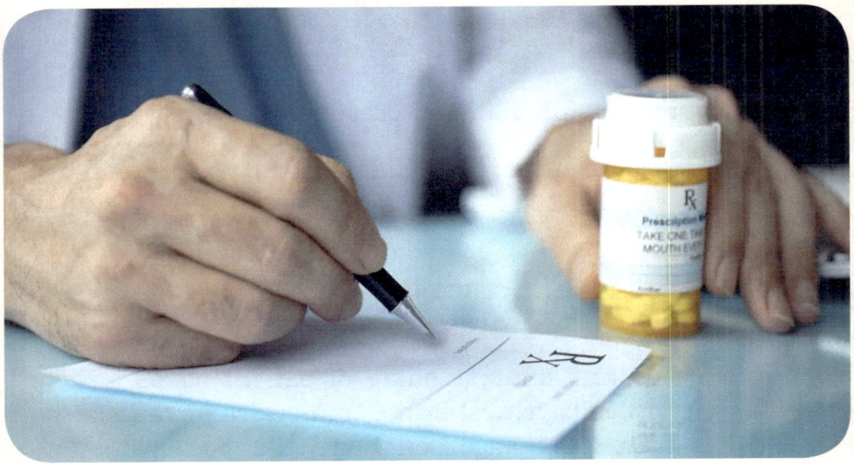

LEARNING OBJECTIVES

After studying this chapter, you will be able to:

1. Explain principles of rational prescribing
2. Identify components of effective prescription writing
3. Discuss challenges in rational prescribing
4. Focus on future directions in prescription practices

Introduction

In today's practice of medicine, rational prescribing and proper prescription writing have become the cornerstones of pharmacy and also of medical practice. When the patient care face is changing, a comprehension of drug management as an art becomes a necessity to safeguard patient outcomes. This chapter seeks to explain how rational prescribing goes beyond the selection of appropriate drug treatments but also patient factors, and thereby commences a whole regime of treatment. For instance, despite barriers in the delivery of pharmaceutical care services having been experienced by United Arab Emirates pharmacists, having complete prescribing practices integrated is crucial to maximal optimization of therapeutic effects (Kharaba et al., 2022). Moreover, increasing product complexity of such products as probiotics is utilized to highlight the need for evidence-based prescribing to minimize risks and maximize safety profiles, particularly among vulnerable populations (Piqué et al., 2019). Ultimately, rational prescribing's focus assists in improving the practice level of care.

8.1. Principles of Rational Prescribing

Learning Outcome

1. Understand patient needs and preferences
2. Explain evidence-based medicine and its role
3. Focus on pharmacological knowledge and drug interactions
4. Focus on consideration of patient demographics
5. Explain the cost-effectiveness of medications
6. Understand monitoring and follow-up strategies
7. Know the importance of clear communication with patients
8. Discuss adherence to clinical guidelines
9. Describe role of interdisciplinary collaboration

Rational prescribing is central to optimizing patient outcomes and drug-related complications. Central to this practice is the mandate that prescribing should be guided by guidelines and indicators that facilitate the effective use of drugs, as this approach highlights evidence that assesses prescribing trends for conditions, thereby enabling a comprehensive evaluation. For instance, based on a study of prescribing of antipsychotics, WHO core prescribing indicators were shown to be quite skewed towards atypical antipsychotics, with the need for ongoing monitoring of prescribing trends to ensure treatment safety and efficacy (Chandra et al., 2018). Similarly, drug prescribing practices of anti-glaucoma medications were an expression of best practice. Still, they emphasized the loophole of providing clear instructions on the usage of drugs—a characteristic that is most vital in optimizing therapeutic effects (Advani et al., 2018). Similarly, prescribing practices of anti-glaucoma medications exhibited good practice. Still, they insisted on the loophole to providing complex instructions on drug use—a characteristic that is most vital in optimizing therapeutic effects (Advani et al., 2018). These findings call for constant sensitization and education of healthcare professionals as a way to promote rational prescribing, consequently increasing patient care and resource utilization (Figure 8.1).

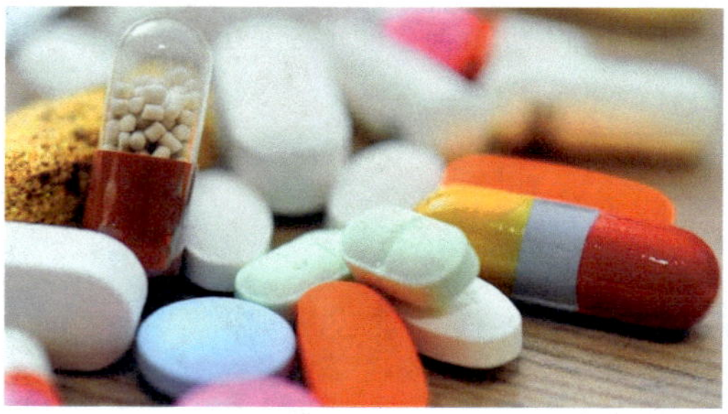

Figure 8.1. Rational prescribing.

Source: https://sp.kalantri.co.in/wp-content/uploads/2022/11/Drugs.jpg.

8.1.1. Understanding Patient Needs and Preferences

Accurate understanding of patient needs and wishes is critical in the framework of rational prescribing and prescription writing because they exert critical impacts on therapeutic outcomes. Engaging patients in the process of expressing their experience, expectations, and preferred treatment facilitates shared decision-making, which is essential for compliance with drugs. A study on E-prescription system integration indicates the sensitization of pharmacists regarding the benefits such systems can provide in tackling the problems of prescriptions, minimizing antibiotic consumption, and improving patient care (Majeed et al., 2023). In addition, adequate training of healthcare staff on the right usage of medicines must be delivered; some recent physicians demonstrate limited knowledge regarding drug selection and modes of prescribing (Kumar et al., 2019). By placing patient-centered strategies at the center of prescribing, healthcare professionals not only optimize medication adherence but also overall safety and effectiveness of treatment regimens as a whole, and thus health outcomes for patients.

8.1.2. Evidence-Based Medicine and Its Role

Integration of evidence-based medicine (EBM) into practice is necessary for ensuring logical prescribing and effective prescription writing. EBM encompasses the use of the best current science to make decisions regarding patient care to reduce polypharmacy risks. One of the severe problems with prescribing arises due to the increasing issue of polypharmacy, particularly among patients with psychiatric disorders, where complex drug treatment regimens lead to adverse drug interactions and inadequate management of adverse effects (Bhave et al., 2022). Besides, the formulation of treatment plans tends to wed official guidelines with customized adjustments, such as in exercise prescription, which combines scientific information and individual needs (Wackerhage et al., 2021). Compliance with EBM enables practitioners to support more efficient treatment while minimizing unwanted side effects, with a more structured approach to prescription practice that contributes to improved patient outcomes across diverse clinical settings (Figure 8.2).

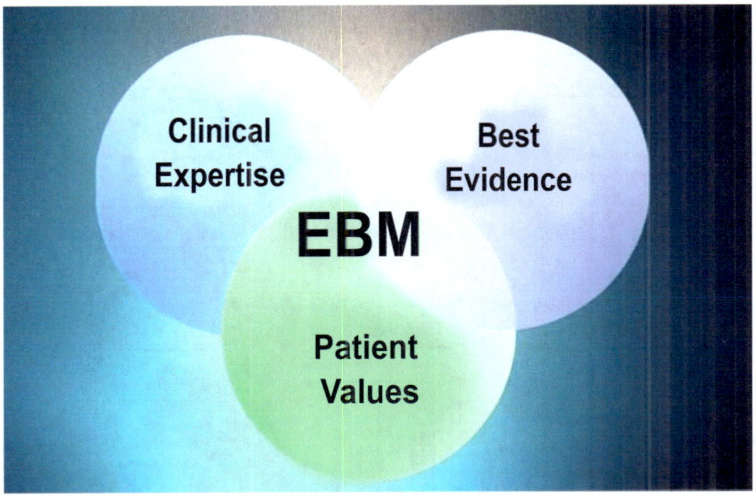

Figure 8.2. The integration of evidence-based medicine (EBM) into clinical practice is crucial for rational prescribing and effective prescription writing.

Source: https://www.cognibrain.com/wp-content/uploads/2023/01/Importance-of-Evidence-Based-Medicine-on-Research-and-Practice.jpg

8.1.3. Pharmacological Knowledge and Drug Interactions

In the context of rational prescribing and prescription, a good understanding of drug interactions and pharmacological knowledge is crucial in maximizing therapeutic benefits while promoting patient safety. Because most patients come in with a variety of comorbidities, particularly in elderly patients, polypharmacy and potentially inappropriate prescribing are risky. The development of instruments like the GheOP3S screening tool, which identifies potentially inappropriate medicines among older individuals, illustrates the utility of goal-directed pharmacovigilance in community pharmacy practice, thereby reducing adverse drug events (Boussery et al., 2015). In addition, the interaction between conventional medicine raises questions about the safety and effectiveness of various complementary and alternative therapies if not well regulated or comprehended. As highlighted in the One-World Medicine concept, combining traditional practice and EBM calls for strict standards for safe interactions of drugs so that patient well-being is ensured (Abdelfatah et al., 2019). Hence, a complete pharmacological framework is essential for effective prescribing (Figure 8.3).

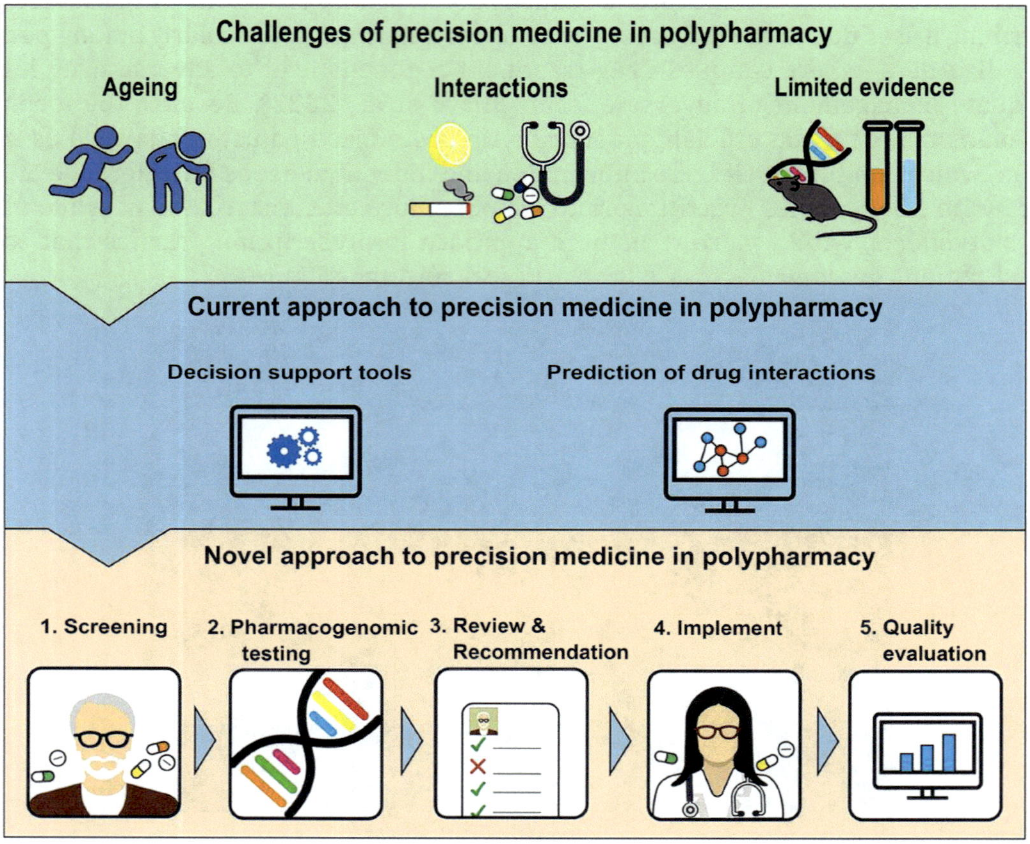

Figure 8.3. As patients often present with multiple comorbidities, particularly in older populations, the risk of polypharmacy and potentially inappropriate prescribing becomes significant.

Source: https://static.cambridge.org//content/id/urn%3Acambridge.org%3Aid%3Aarticle%3AS2752614323000108/resource/name/optimisedImage-S2752614323000108_figAb.jpg?pub-status=live.

8.1.4. Consideration of Patient Demographics

Patient demographics are a prime concern in the case of rational prescribing and prescription writing because they directly influence treatment outcomes and patient safety. Variances in age groups, socioeconomic status, and culture can influence how patients respond to drugs and adhere to treatment. For instance, a critique of steroid prescribing practice noted the fundamental significance of designing prescriptions, especially based on demographic information, to enhance patient safety and treatment outcomes (Ghutke et al., 2019). Second, demographic data also influence the identification of the demand and appropriateness of some medicines, as revealed in an analysis of Vitamins and Tonics prescriptive patterns across different populations, where intense disparities in prevalence were observed to arise based on patient demographics (Bhardwaj et al., 2018). With the integration of such data, healthcare professionals can reduce the probability of irrational prescribing and deliver more personalized treatment to patients, ultimately contributing to better health outcomes.

8.1.5. Cost-Effectiveness of Medications

In the backdrop of rational prescribing, the cost-effectiveness of medication serves as a pivotal point of deliberation that materially impacts patient care and healthcare systems in general. Effective drugs, particularly non-vitamin K antagonist oral anticoagulants (NOACs), have become increasingly well recognized to reduce the occurrence of stroke among patients with atrial fibrillation, which directly translates into reduced healthcare costs associated with stroke treatment and complications.

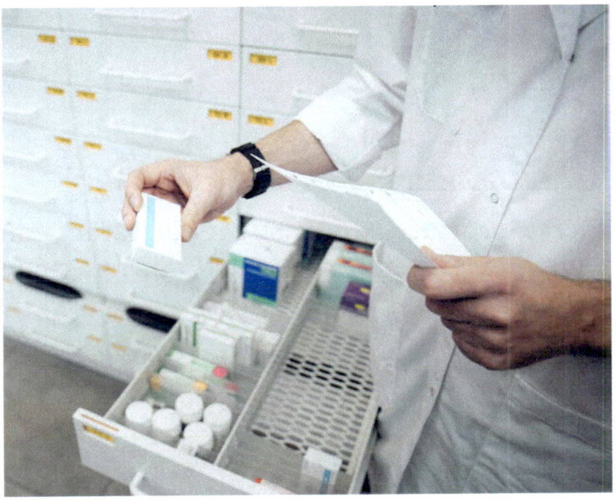

Figure 8.4. The cost-effectiveness of medications is a critical consideration that fundamentally impacts patient care and healthcare systems at large.

Source: https://web-assets.bcg.com/e7/41/299fd2d546e1be1d3fa2cb0ed231/navigating-the-inflation-reduction-act-impact-rectangle.jpg.

The European Heart Rhythm Association emphasizes the advantages of applying these agents because they have favorable safety profiles and greater patient compliance compared to traditional vitamin K antagonists, with potential for significant economic savings in the long run (Steffel et al., 2018). By considering both direct and indirect costs, health care providers can optimize their prescribing practice so that patients receive therapy that is not only clinically effective but cost-efficient as well (Steffel et al., 2021). The dual strategy optimizes the sustainability of health expenditure while guaranteeing quality patient care (Figure 8.4).

8.1.6. Monitoring and Follow-Up Strategies

Effective monitoring and follow-up actions are essential components of rational prescribing and prescription writing since they allow drugs to produce the intended clinical effects at the lowest adverse consequences. In the majority of healthcare settings, an organized mechanism for monitoring patient response can significantly improve prescribing patterns to result in better drug management. For instance, periodic auditing of prescription data can identify trends of drug use and determine areas for potential improvement. A study in Eswatini emphasized that even though an intervention that made use of prescription audit, feedback, and education was employed, it failed to significantly enhance rational prescribing practice, indicating more intricate interventions will be required to introduce change (Ncube et al., 2024). In addition, as highlighted under performance improvement rhetoric across disciplines, the integration of empathy within monitoring tools can enhance patient comprehension and challenge perception, thus facilitating more appropriately customized prescriptions according to specific needs (Buchheit et al., 2022). Through engagement in ongoing monitoring and individualized follow-up, healthcare professionals can maximize the safety and efficacy of therapeutic care.

8.1.7. Importance of Clear Communication with Patients

Good communication between healthcare providers and patients is essential in the construction of understanding, adherence, and safety in rational prescribing and prescription writing. Clear explanation of medication instructions, potential side effects, and the rationale for the treatment decision facilitates patients being actively engaged in their care. This is particularly crucial with the release of non-NOACs, which have also become the preferred treatment for atrial fibrillation and other conditions due to ease of handling and reduced monitoring needs (Steffel et al., 2018). Misconceptions are to blame for drug errors, which influence safety and efficacy of treatment. Clinical practitionersmust ensure that patients are aware not only of the technical aspects of their medicine but also of the underlying clinical reasons. This approach helps establish improved compliance and clinical results. This commitment to accurate communication forms the basis of the significance of rational prescribing in establishing cooperation in care (Figure 8.5).

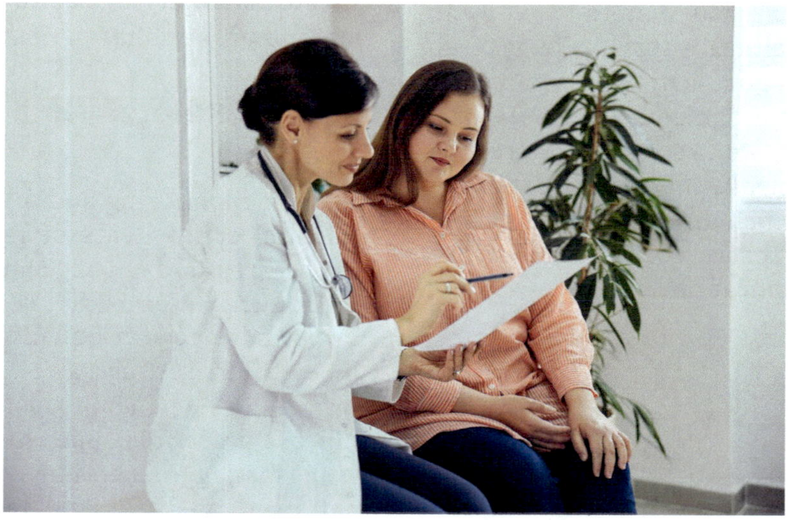

Figure 8.5. Effective communication between healthcare providers and patients is paramount in fostering understanding, compliance, and safety in the context of rational prescribing and prescription writing.

Source: https://publichealth.tulane.edu/wp-content/uploads/sites/3/2021/09/Strategies-for-Effective-Communication-in-Health-Care.jpg.

8.1.8. Adherence to Clinical Guidelines

Adherence to clinical guidelines is crucial for enabling rational prescribing and accurate prescription writing, as it directly impacts the success of therapy and patient safety. Sound evidence-based clinical guidelines provide clinicians with a framework to guide diagnosis and treatment in line with best practice. Irrational prescribing examples, as seen in studies where clinicians had large knowledge deficits regarding best drugs, show the total need to adhere to these standards (Kamuhabwa et al., 2013). Additionally, studies have shown that the prescriptions vary from national formularies, an indication of high degrees of variability in drug selection that could destabilize patient treatment (Iskandar et al., 2025). Hence, repeated training and continuous education of the health workers with a specific focus on current clinical guidelines are sine qua non. Such interventions may enhance compliance, eventually leading to better efficacy of treatment, reduced chances of issues with medication, and better utilization of healthcare resources.

8.1.9. Role of Interdisciplinary Collaboration

Interdisciplinary collaboration is at the heart of maximizing rational prescribing and prescribing through the integration of a diversity of professional perspectives and expertise. When medical professionals, such as exercise physiologists and general practitioners, combine drug and non-drug treatments, and they can develop comprehensive, worldwide treatment strategies. This is particularly important in the case of chronic disease management, where promotion of exercise can function as a low-cost measure supplementary to traditional medical practice (Albert et al., 2020). The opioid prescription epidemic currently also emphasizes the value of interprofessional teamwork between dental and medical educators, who are encouraged to revisit curricula that place emphasis on safe prescribing habits while being effective in managing patients' pain (Keith et al., 2017). These alliances improve patient treatment quality, foster a learning ethic from one another and ultimately lead to more evidence-based, rational prescribing practices in the health system (Figure 8.6).

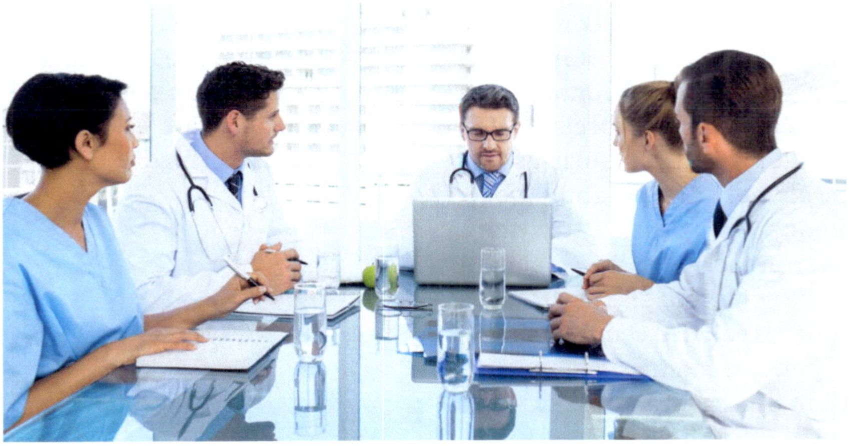

Figure 8.6. Interdisciplinary collaboration plays a pivotal role in enhancing rational prescribing and prescription writing by integrating diverse professional perspectives and expertise.

Source: https://www.sermo.com/wp-content/uploads/2023/02/effective-communication-img6-min-1050x555.jpg.

Test Your Knowledge

1. How can a prescriber ensure they are minimizing the risks of drug interactions when rationally prescribing medications?
2. What is the importance of considering the patient's age, medical history, and comorbid conditions when prescribing medicines?

8.2. Components of Effective Prescription Writing

Learning Outcome

1. Explain essential elements of a prescription
2. Know the importance of legibility and clarity
3. Discuss use of generic vs. brand names
4. Describe dosage forms and routes of administration
5. Understand duration of therapy and refills
6. Focus on patient education and counseling
7. Learn legal and regulatory requirements
8. Avoid common prescribing errors
9. Know the importance of electronic prescribing systems

Good prescribing handwriting is a component of rational prescribing, with important consequences for patient outcomes and compliance with drugs. An ideal prescription must have certain ideal features such as the patient's details, proper drug name, dose, route, and frequency. In addition to these crucial components, prescribers must ensure that prescriptions are complete and accurate to prevent the risk of error, as a WHO report revealed that almost 50% of patients fail to consume their drugs correctly due to prescription mistakes and misinterpretation (Das et al., 2017). Besides, the use of generic medicines and adherence to an essential drug list can enhance the quality of prescriptions, promoting both cost-effectiveness and accessibility. New research supporting comprehensive policy analysis highlights the need for a One Health approach to manage diverse prescribing patterns across industries and regions, thereby improving the effectiveness of drug use (Aarestrup et al., 2015).

8.2.1. Essential Elements of a Prescription

As far as rational prescribing and writing of prescriptions is concerned, familiarity with the key elements of a prescription assists in minimizing errors and maximizing patient safety. A good prescription would include the essentials of the prescribing physician's details, the patient's details, the accurate dosage of the drug, frequency, and the length of treatment. The present research is highlighting the importance of readability and legibility since the majority of the prescribing errors are a result of illegible or unreadable handwriting or omitted information, and therefore the need for standard forms of prescription (Bicknell et al., 2014). Moreover, the incorporation of behavior elements within the structure of prescription charts can significantly reduce errors, as noted in the IDEAS chart assessment, which found improved accuracy in prescribing through improved organization and readability (Bicknell et al., 2014). Similarly, it is vital to take into account the broader implications of prescribing practice, for example, their contribution to causing AMR, and thus the importance of safe prescribing in all healthcare environments (Figure 8. 7).

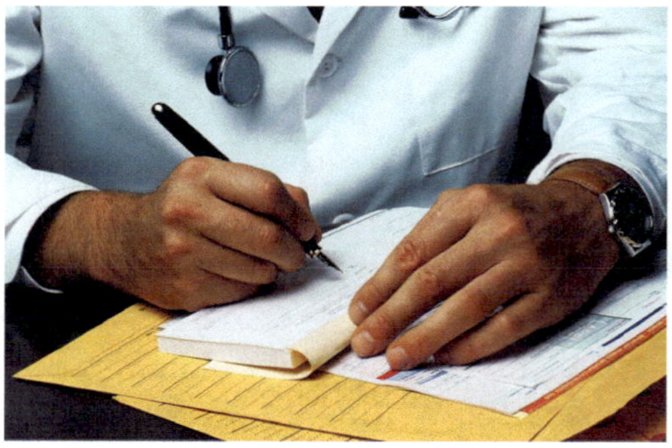

Figure 8.7. A well-structured prescription typically includes critical components such as the prescribing physicians details, patient information, specific drug dosage, frequency, and duration of therapy.

Source: https://www.verywellhealth.com/thmb/yDWxCo5Tojdxji6X6sn3B3NpeZg=/1500x0/filters:no_upscale():max_bytes(150000):strip_icc()/GettyImages-523437372-87574949a8d94a14ac8756588ce3288d.jpg.

8.2.2. Importance of Legibility and Clarity

In rational prescribing and prescription, clarity and legibility are most important. Legible prescriptions provide all of those people who are involved in the care of a patient with a crystal-clear understanding of the drug regimen without any ambiguity, thus reducing the risk of medication error. Aside from personal prescriptions, the impact of clarity extends to the broader environment of healthcare systems because good communication fosters patient-provider trust. This is particularly apparent in cases where patients must navigate complex health systems, typically molded by the social structures present within and around them. Successful prescription writing is a crucial juncture where medical science meets patient life, enhancing adherence and compliance. Identification of such dynamics offers the grounds for arguments on the evolving status of medical professionals to ensure that their practices comply with high levels of clarity and accountability (England, 2023; Lust, 2022).

8.2.3. Use of Generic vs. Brand Names

Discussion about the employment of generic versus brand-name drugs is at the core of sensible prescribing and prescribing practice. Generic drug, often supplied at reduced prices, promotes patient access and adherence to treatment courses, particularly in fiscally restricted health-care settings. The generic prescribing trend is capable of lowering healthcare spending significantly without compromising on effectiveness; for instance, one clinical audit highlighted that among a series of prescriptions, the frequency of both generic and brand names was noteworthy, pointing towards a combination of practices (Gawali et al., 2021). Nevertheless, even with such benefits, brand-name drugs generally have the advantage of having earned the trust already, along with perceived credibility both from the patients and practitioners. Thus, economic efficiency through generic substitution while prescribing has been achieved, and the same must be balanced against patient education, safety, and perception of similarity by generics. This cost and patient confidence balance is essential in achieving the best possible health outcomes (Rutto et al., 2024) (Figure 8.8).

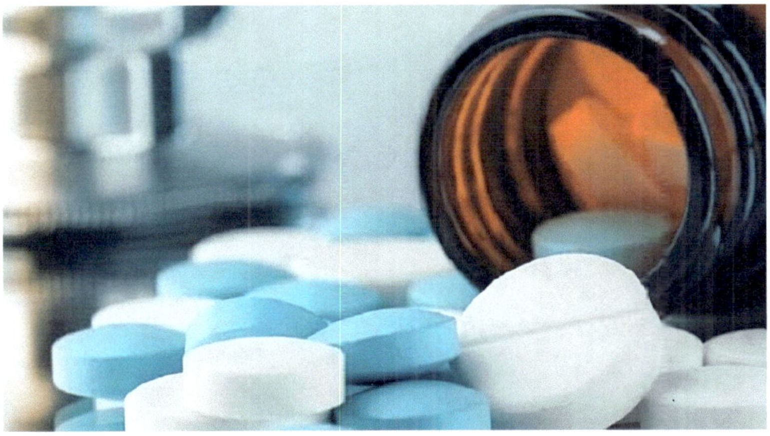

Figure 8.8. Generic drugs, often marketed at lower prices, enhance patient accessibility and adherence to therapeutic regimens, particularly in financially constrained healthcare settings.

Source: https://globelapharma.com/wp-content/uploads/2024/09/Generic-Medicines-scaled.jpeg.

8.2.4. Dosage Forms and Routes of Administration

In rational prescribing and writing out prescriptions, understanding dosage forms and routes of administration is fundamental to optimizing therapeutic efficacy. Tablets, injectables, and transdermal patches are formulated to maximize bioavailability and deliver drugs to sites of action in the body efficiently. Each of the four routes—oral, intravenous, intramuscular, and subcutaneous—has unique pharmacokinetic profiles, influencing the onset of action, peak effect, and duration of action of drugs. Additionally, route and dosage form can have a radical impact on patient outcome and compliance; for instance, injectables can be welcomed in cases of emergency for prompt action, while tablets orally can be more convenient in the case of chronic treatment. With the unprecedented surge in AMR, as pointed out in Salam et al. (2023a, b), the prescribing physicians should give these considerations serious thought to customize therapy that reduces exposure to unnecessary medication while also providing adequate treatment.

8.2.5. Duration of Therapy and Refills

The duration of treatment and refilling procedures is such a vital rational writing and prescribing issues that impose tremendous influence on patient compliance and therapeutic outcomes. Good medicine management is not just focused on the initial prescription, but also on how refill procedures are scheduled prudently to ensure continuity of care. Inadequate compliance, which affects nearly half of long-term medication patients, typically stems from various system-related problems, including complicated refill processes and patient-physician relationships (Khan et al., 2018). Moreover, the optimal dose and treatment duration, such as critical care fluid regimens, require tailoring treatment to the individual needs of patients without overloading the healthcare systems. This precision in prescription offers grounds for enhanced patient trust and participation, ultimately resulting in improved compliance and health outcomes (Malbrain et al., 2018). Rational prescribing should therefore choose both the duration of the therapy and refill conditions to maximize patient experience and efficiency (Figure 8.9).

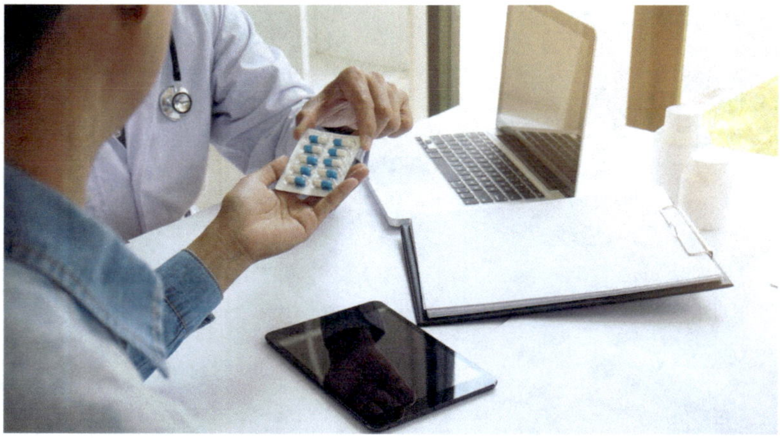

Figure 8.9. Effective medication management encompasses not only the initial prescription but also the careful consideration of refill protocols to ensure continuity of care.

Source: https://www.tigahealth.com/wp-content/uploads/2024/06/Preventing-Drug-Abuse-A-Joint-Effort-with-Government-Institutions2.jpg.

8.2.6. Patient Education and Counseling

Effective patient counseling and education are critical components of rational prescribing, as it equips patients with the knowledge needed to manage their medication and condition. Clinically, physicians have a direct role in influencing a patient's information concerning treatment regimens, potential side effects, and compliance with treatment. As in one study of community pharmacists, the pain management intervention shows the more general role of the pharmacist in patient education, proving not only their engagement with patients' needs but also indicating the need for continuous professional development and interprofessional practice in the healthcare system (Gazerani et al., 2024). Through the development of such a culture where patients are informed and empowered, problems related to medication mismanagement can be avoided, and therapeutic outcomes can be enhanced. The incorporation of comprehensive counseling strategies into routine practice thus supports rational prescribing, as well as patient safety and satisfaction with care overall (Devine et al., 2020).

8.2.7. Legal and Regulatory Requirements

Legal and regulatory compliance is of utmost significance in rational prescribing and prescription writing to ensure safety to the patient and effectiveness in treatment. The practitioners must work under a burdensome regulatory process prescribing drug administration, as these regulations are put in place to counteract the risks of drug abuse and side effects. For instance, management of non-NOACs necessitates careful consideration of patient factors such as age and renal function to align with the guidelines found in Steffel et al., (2021). Besides, a decentered approach to regulation, as illustrated in Black (2017), offers the compliance duty to extend beyond state structures to cover other stakeholders, thereby promoting a shared effort towards providing healthcare. This multifaceted regulatory model calls for complete training and sensitization of prescribers to ensure they remain informed about evolving standards and practices of pharmacotherapy (Figure 8.10).

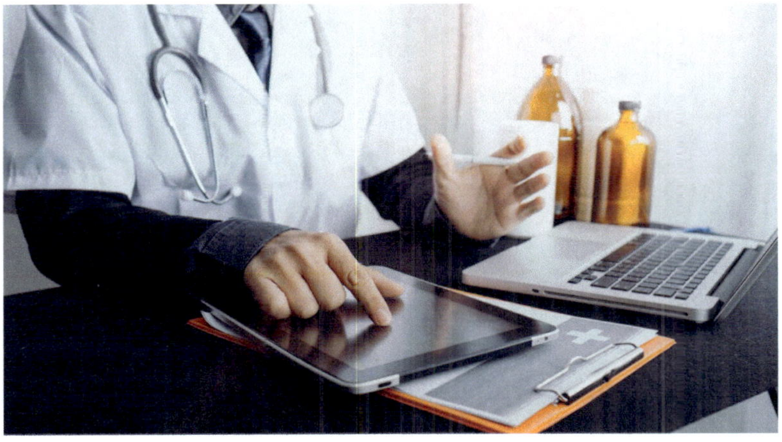

Figure 8.10. Healthcare providers must navigate a complex landscape of regulations that govern the prescribing of medications, as these requirements are designed to mitigate risks associated with drug misuse and adverse reactions.

Source: https://www.tigahealth.com/wp-content/uploads/2024/06/A-Compelling-Example-of-Institutional-Collaboration-Enhanced-Driving-Safety.jpg.

8.2.8. Avoiding Common Prescribing Errors

In rational prescribing, the avoidance of preventable prescribing errors is essential to preserve patient safety and ensure optimal therapeutic outcomes. Evidence shows that the majority of prescribing errors are system-related, including poor script, which was cited as being a significant issue in approximately 68% of prescriptions reviewed in a recent study (Bachewar et al., 2017). Moreover, the polypharmacy practice with 5.20 drugs per prescription is causing drug mismanagement and predisposing patients to adverse effects (Bachewar et al., 2017). To rectify these issues, ongoing education and training, like that imparted to medical interns, have proven helpful—demonstrating significant improvement in knowledge of prescriptions and compliance with rational prescribing guidelines after specific intervention. Thus, adopting routine prescription audits and enhancing prescriber education are significant steps towards the encouragement of responsible and effective prescription practices, reducing errors and optimizing clinical outcomes.

8.2.9. Importance of Electronic Prescribing Systems

Computerized prescribing systems have revolutionized the field of rational prescribing and prescription generation, and the management of drugs has been accurate and efficient. The systems significantly reduce the likelihood of handwriting or transcription errors resulting in adverse drug events, as evidenced by studies reporting their success in avoiding prescription errors (Davey et al., 2013).

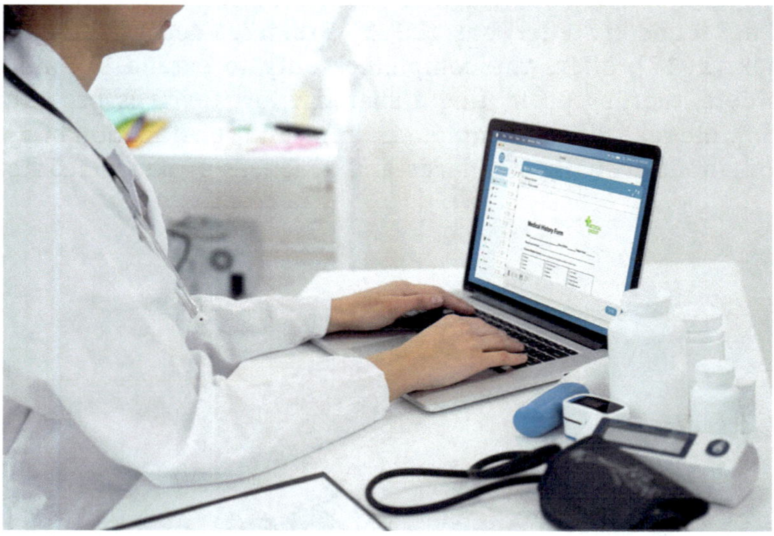

Figure 8.11. The integration of electronic prescribing systems has transformed the landscape of rational prescribing and prescription writing, enhancing the accuracy and efficiency of medication management.

Source: https://www.tigahealth.com/wp-content/uploads/2024/06/The-Evolution-of-Digital-Prescribing-with-Central-e-Prescription-885x615-1.jpg.

Moreover, automated patient medication histories and e-prescribing enhance access to detailed patient medication histories, reducing the risks of DDI and polypharmacy using delivering healthcare professionals information that supports evidence-based decision-making (McLellan, 2010). It is particularly beneficial in averting opioid crises, where improper prescribing has stringent consequences, as evidenced by the vast overdose fatality figures resulting from opioid prescription (McLellan, 2010) Ultimately, e-prescribing not only automates the prescribing process but also adheres to best practice for drug stewardship, promoting increased patient safety and improved outcomes (Figure 8.11).

Test Your Knowledge

1. What is the significance of specifying the route of administration in prescription writing?
2. How can prescribers ensure the use of the correct dosage form (e.g., tablet, liquid) in a prescription?

8.3. Challenges in Rational Prescribing

Learning Outcome

1. Understand polypharmacy and its implications
2. Explain the influence of pharmaceutical marketing
3. Discuss time constraints in clinical practice
4. Learn variability in patient responses to medications
5. Know access to drugs and healthcare disparities
6. Manage chronic diseases and complex cases
7. Describe resistance to change in prescribing habits
8. Discuss ethical dilemmas in prescribing
9. Learn strategies to overcome prescribing challenges

The complexities that underlie rational prescribing pose a significant challenge that can serve as a hindrance to effective pharmacotherapeutic care. A significant challenge includes the reframing of medical students' attitudes to prescription writing, which can be addressed through the application of tools such as threshold concepts. This is an educational approach that assists in nudging students to establish positive links to the core principles of rational prescribing, thereby enhancing their expertise in this area (Khurshid et al., 2020). In addition, the evolving world of drugs, particularly the use of non-NOACs, creates extra challenges. Practitioners must accommodate new-to-them therapeutic options, dosage alterations, and drug interactions in keeping with strict adherence to prescribed regimens (Steffel et al., 2018). Such challenges necessitate providing enduring education and thoughtful curriculum development to prepare future healthcare practitioners to tackle the challenges of rational prescribing in diverse clinical situations. As such, it is important to overcome such challenges to optimize patient outcomes and enable safe medication practices.

8.3.1. Polypharmacy and Its Implications

The practice of polypharmacy, where the patient is prescribed multiple drugs at one time, particularly among elderly patients, is a source of great concern regarding efficacy and safety in clinical practice. With the growing incidence of multimorbidity, there is a greater challenge to healthcare practitioners of rational prescribing that demands a critical appreciation for the consequences of polypharmacy. Central to the resolution of this issue is the concept of deprescribing, a purposeful reduction of drugs to reduce harm from polypharmacy. In a study included in the TAILOR drug synthesis, individualized approaches to deprescribing were highlighted as a necessity because both patients and clinicians are unclear on this (Reeve et al., 2022). Also, overuse of certain medicines, particularly antibiotics, is strongly linked with the overall public health issue of AMR to which holistic stewardship initiatives must be added to support prescribing (Godman et al., 2021). Thus, polypharmacy control is essential to enhance patient outcomes and minimize drug-related harm (Figure 8.12).

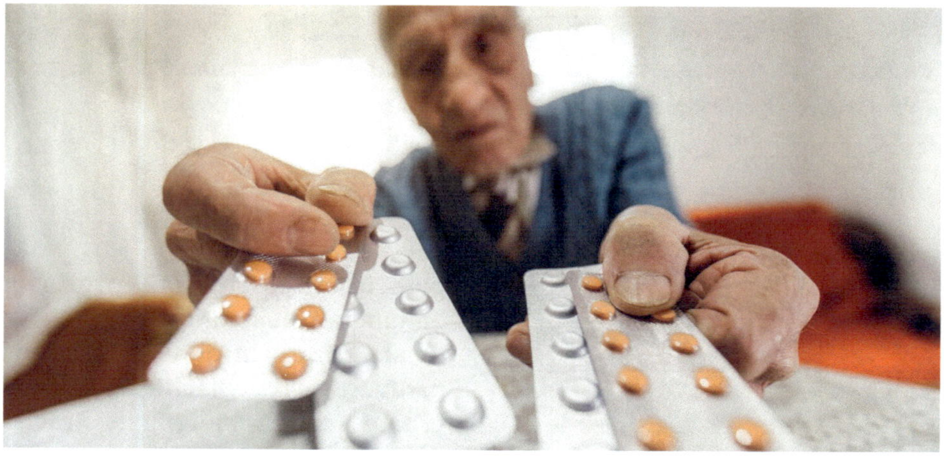

Figure 8.12. The phenomenon of polypharmacy, defined as the concurrent use of multiple medications by a patient, particularly among the elderly, raises significant concerns regarding both efficacy and safety in clinical practice.

Source: https://medizinonline.com/wp-content/uploads/2023/12/iStock-1149576100.jpg.

8.3.2. Influence of Pharmaceutical Marketing

The effect of drug promotion on physician prescribing practices is a significant factor in promoting rational prescribing. Drug company practices undertaken to promote drugs a tendency to influence the physicians' choices, as testified by several studies that document the dynamics of these influences across various groups. As an example, one study proved that marketing influences prescribing behavior among rural and urban doctors to a considerable extent, and certain media—like email—can be more effective in persuading urban doctors (Gupta et al., 2018). This highlights the importance of critically analyzing how such marketing can prioritize profits over patient care. Also, there is evidence that policy effectiveness in resistance against such influences has not been sufficiently studied because of advanced implementations under local rules and health infrastructure (Aarestrup et al., 2015). Overall, awareness regarding such marketing forces is required to make prescribing rational with a culture backing ethical practice and patients' requirements.

8.3.3. Time Constraints in Clinical Practice

In the clinical environment, stringent time constraints significantly hinder logical prescribing and best prescription writing. Physicians typically see large volumes of patients, leading to hurried consultations and compromised accuracy in drug regulation. The World Health Organization has indicated that almost 50% of patients fail to take their medication as prescribed because of mistakes caused by a lack of clear enough prescription, poor patient education, or lack of prescriber monitoring, all aggravated by time constraints (Das et al., 2017). Furthermore, the challenges of addressing care across various sectors—animal and human health, for example—make it challenging to establish integral prescribing strategies in resource-constrained settings (Aarestrup et al., 2015). These situations bring to the fore the imperative of coordinated interventions to maximize prescription behavior. By managing the multifaceted impact of time constraints, healthcare systems can construct a model that maximizes prescribing behavior and patient outcomes (Figure 8.13).

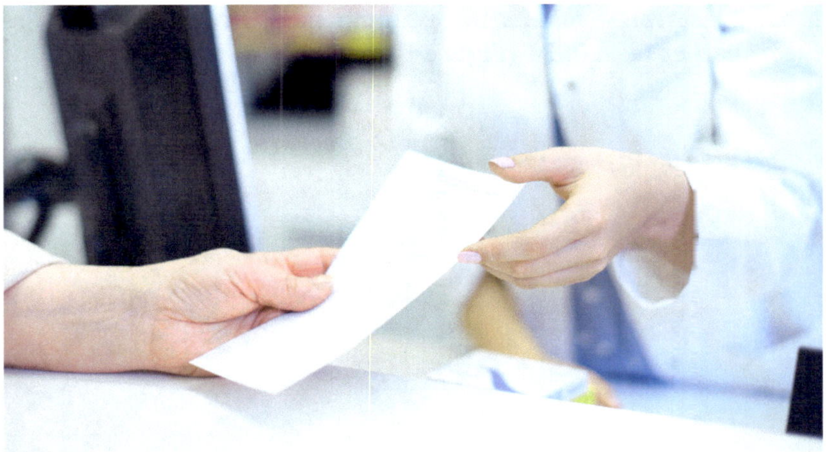

Figure 8.13. Time constraints significantly hinder the process of rational prescribing and effective prescription writing.

Source: https://www.tigahealth.com/wp-content/uploads/2024/06/The-Problem-Challenges-of-Traditional-Prescriptions-1.jpg.

8.3.4. Variability in Patient Responses to Medications

Variation in drug response in patients is a significant issue in the field of rational prescribing and writing prescriptions. Genetic variation, comorbid medical illnesses, and other drugs consumed at the same time are some of the factors that affect how individuals metabolize and respond to drugs. For instance, in elderly cancer patients, polypharmacy compiles treatment regimens unnecessarily due to interactions between the multiple medications for comorbid diseases and anticancer therapy (Khanal et al., 2019). Moreover, physicians sometimes apply off-the-shelf treatment strategies consistent with typical reactions rather than adapting them to the specific needs of individual patients. This tendency to conform to norms, while occasionally convenient, can fail to address the peculiarities of particular cases, causing suboptimal outcomes for those patients that require customized interventions (Frank et al.). Therefore, identifying and reacting to the natural variation in patient response is central to enhancing the effectiveness of therapies delivered and ensuring patient safety.

8.3.5. Access to Medications and Healthcare Disparities

Medication access remains an urgent issue that identifies health disparities throughout the globe, with significant effects on patient outcomes and prescribing practices. Socioeconomic conditions, proximity, and systemic discrimination often lead to unequal access, which may result in the marginalized group facing greater health risks and reduced medication adherence. This irregular landscape not only worsens health statuses but also highlights the limitations of rational prescribing, as practitioners may struggle to ensure their recommendations are compatible with the resources available in heterogeneous patient populations. Further, the evolution of antibiotic resistance is a witness to the need for equal access to effective interventions; without coordinated efforts to improve accessibility, the impacts of prescribed medications deteriorate. Addressing these matters of access in an innovative healthcare policy and consensual approach is crucial for building a society where rational prescribing results in optimum health returns for all, regardless of their situation or origin (Muteeb et al., 2023) (Figure 8.14).

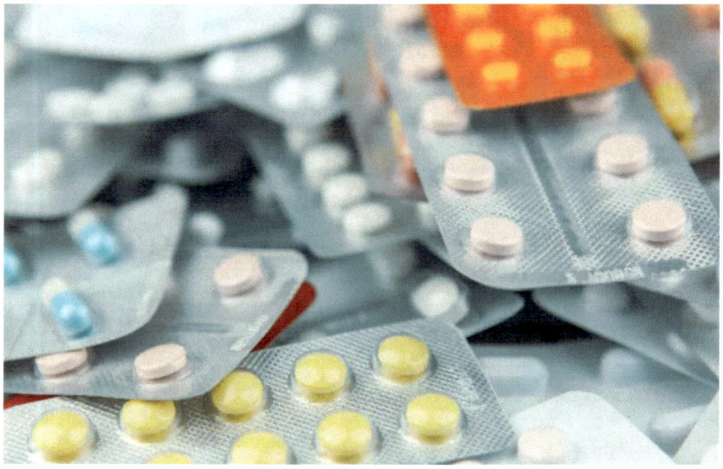

Figure 8.14. Access to medications remains a critical issue that underscores healthcare disparities globally, significantly affecting patient outcomes and prescribing practices.

Source: https://www.orfonline.org/public/uploads/posts/image/657dd90a2a20e.png.

8.3.6. Managing Chronic Diseases and Complex Cases

Ideal treatment of chronic diseases and complex cases demands that rational prescribing and prescription writing be treated delicately. As doctors handle complicated patients with intricate medical backgrounds, the merit of personalizing pharmacotherapy is self-evident. For instance, strict conformity to guidelines such as those presented by the WHO can significantly enhance therapy without diminishing the potential for adverse drug reactions (ADRs). Evidence indicates that the mean number of drugs prescribed per consultation can be over recommended levels, leading to potential polypharmacy and increased health spending (Iskandar et al., 2025). Additionally, it is essential to recognize the context of each condition; for instance, while acute conjunctivitis typically resolves without antibiotics, healthcare professionals tend to prescribe them, especially in vulnerable groups like children (Adomako et al., 2022). This highlights the need for continuous education and monitoring of prescribing practices in a bid to foster quality delivery of healthcare and avoid the risks of inappropriate use of drugs in the care of chronic ailments.

8.3.7. Resistance to Change in Prescribing Habits

Resistance to prescribing behavior change is a significant challenge in achieving rational prescribing and effective prescription writing. Practitioners are used to adhering to deep-rooted practices despite an excess of evidence for alternative approaches. Such resistance is frequently supported by systemic factors, including inadequate medical training and prescriber ignorance about the outcomes of their prescribing practice. For instance, the issue of misuse of antibiotics is compounded by myths among people about antibiotics. Therefore, there is a need for training programs to enhance knowledge and awareness, as stressed in Machowska et al. (2018). Furthermore, pharmaceutical marketing and organizational inertia can maintain rooted prescribing habits, thereby preventing clinicians from embracing updated guidelines. As seen in OECD's activities on AMR, these obstacles need to be solved to develop a more rational prescribing practice that is compatible with changing medical standards (Figure 8.15).

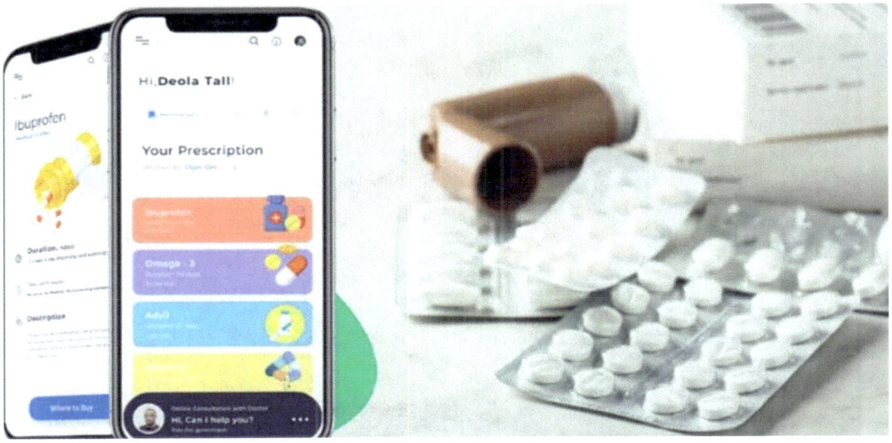

Figure 8.15. Resistance to change in prescribing habits presents a significant challenge in the pursuit of rational prescribing and effective prescription writing.

Source: https://www.jploft.com/posts/1718350562.webp.

8.3.8. Ethical Dilemmas in Prescribing

Ethical issues facing prescribers are multifaceted, interweaving clinical decision-making, patient autonomy, and systems. A principal concern is that some health professionals are minimizing the significance of consulting with patients, especially when they believe patients cannot make decisions on their behalf. Research has found that over 20% of doctors in specific contexts are not interested in involving patients in treatment planning, undermining the pillars of patient-centered care and autonomy (Howard et al., 2022). Non-involvement can lead to unfavorable health outcomes and increased doctor-patient conflict, particularly in contexts where trust in patients is prized. Secondly, ethical practice rises for professionals in low- and middle-income countries (LMICs), where the need to comply with regulatory needs is in a continuous strain against the urgent need for low-cost medicines (Amoako-Sakyi et al., 2022). The challenges leave prescribers with the compulsion to balance a delicate relationship between professional ethics and harsh realities, and therefore impacts the quality of care delivered to patients.

8.3.9. Strategies to Overcome Prescribing Challenges

The problems listed in the prescription of medicine, namely in the case of antibiotics, necessitate comprehensive steps towards encouraging logical prescription practices. One efficient method is the implementation of E-prescription systems, which can provide a cut in most of the issues associated with written prescriptions, including misuse and miscommunication, as attested by research on pharmacists attitudes towards such technology (Majeed et al., 2023). Besides, the fight against antibiotic resistance involves firm policy measures alongside educational campaigns that inform healthcare workers and patients on antimicrobial prudent use (Bloom et al., 2016). The presence of a proper working partnership among healthcare stakeholders can also create a convening framework that fosters optimal prescribing and ensures the quality of prescribed antibiotics. By integrating technological innovation with strategic governance frameworks, healthcare systems can enhance their capacity to promote rational prescribing and thereby reduce the aggregate burden of antibiotic resistance and improve patient outcomes (Figure 8.16).

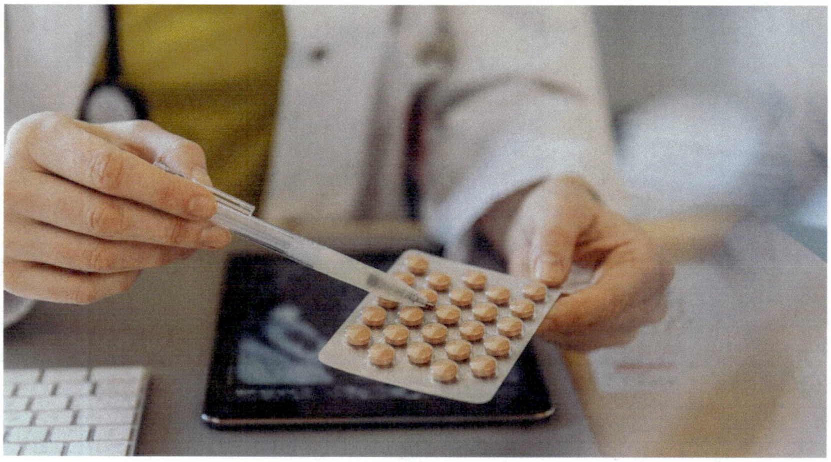

Figure 8.16. The challenges inherent in prescribing medications, particularly in the context of antibiotics, necessitate multifaceted strategies aimed at enhancing rational prescribing practices.

Source: https://web-assets.bcg.com/5d/34/55ad84ca4f0e84ed7f8f565341e8/wef-bcg-antimicrobial-resistance-rectangle-1.jpg.

Test Your Knowledge

1. What challenges do prescribers face when dealing with patients who have limited knowledge or understanding of their medications?
2. How do complex drug regimens or the unavailability of medications pose challenges in rational prescribing?

8.4. Future Directions in Prescription Practices

Learning Outcome

1. Know advances in pharmacogenomics
2. Explain the role of technology in improving prescribing
3. Understand the integration of artificial intelligence in decision-making
4. Discuss trends in personalized medicine
5. Know the importance of continuous education for prescribers
6. Enhance patient engagement in treatment decisions
7. Describe policy changes affecting prescription practices
8. Explain research and development in new medications
9. Learn global perspectives on rational prescribing

As the future of health care unravels, future prescription trends demand a paradigm shift towards more rationalized and innovative approaches. Greater emphasis on personalized medicine emphasizes the assumption that prescriptions are written to respond to the individualized genetic, environmental, and lifestyle traits of an individual patient, optimizing therapeutic response and minimizing side effects. Furthermore, the integration of new technologies—e.g., data analysis and artificial intelligence (AI)—into prescribing also holds the potential to improve decision-making by analyzing high amounts of patient data to ascertain the optimal treatment. Addressing the intellectual property-related ethical concerns and arrangements on costs for drugs is also crucial; shifts in intellectual property rights have a way of reconfiguring access to life-saving medication (Drahos, 2016). Lastly, having solid design principles for prescription writing will be essential in encouraging innovation and ensuring that future practice responds to the advanced challenges faced by healthcare systems (Fu et al., 2016).

8.4.1. Advances in Pharmacogenomics

The evolution of pharmacogenomics has significantly changed the practice of rational drug writing and prescribing, ushering in more personalized medical care. By integrating genetic information into prescribing practices, medical practitioners can better tailor drugs to the unique patient, ensuring maximum therapeutic gain with minimal risk of side effects. The innovation is particularly vital in addressing the complexity of heterogeneous populations, where genetic variations can influence drug metabolism and effectiveness.

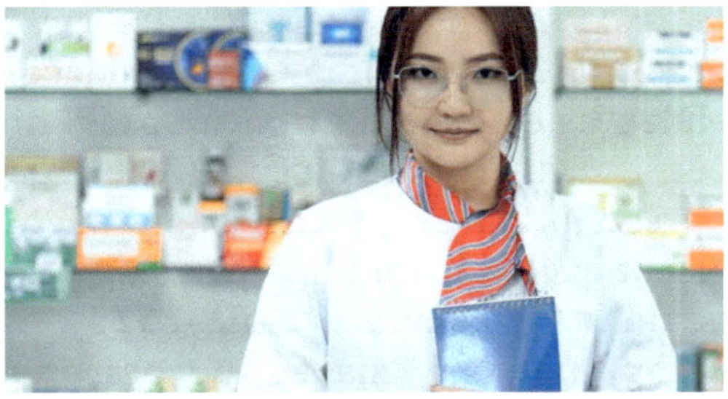

Figure 8.17. The evolution of pharmacogenomics has significantly transformed the landscape of rational prescribing and prescription writing, paving the way for more personalized medical approaches.

Source: https://aiin.healthcare/sites/default/files/styles/top_stories/public/2025-02/pharmacist.jpg.webp?itok=zALJzy0y.

With the growth of the field comes equally high ethical concerns, particularly how the field could be applied to discriminate against individuals based on genetics, as in research on the construct of race in medicine (Parver et al., 2008). Besides, to realize the potential of pharmacogenomics worldwide, practicing responsibly about traditional medicine while providing fair access to interventions, as in the case of the One-World Medicine program (Abdelfatah et al., 2019), will be necessary. Such steps will bridge gaps and enhance the overall efficacy of pharmacotherapy (Figure 8.17).

8.4.2. Role of Technology in Improving Prescribing

Technology application in prescribing processes has evolved as a primary source of enhancing patient care quality. E-prescription software, for instance, is employed to improve the rational use of drugs by avoiding issues associated with handwritten prescriptions, including compromising legibility and accuracy. A study highlights pharmacists' awareness of the potential of such systems in antibiotic stewardship improvement and facilitation of better patient outcomes, emphasizing their crucial role in today's healthcare practice (Majeed et al., 2023). Moreover, compliance with guidelines, as estimated through observational studies, exhibits that despite the generic drug prescription proportion being adequate, significant gaps remain in prescribing practice reasonability (Iskandar et al., 2025). Thus, technology not only makes the prescription process easier but also helps health providers deliver safer, more effective treatment, ultimately leading to improved outcomes and fewer drug side effects.

8.4.3. Integration of Artificial Intelligence in Decision-Making

The application of AI in decision-making represents a quantum leap towards evidence-based prescribing and prescription writing. Through the utilization of vast amounts of data, AI is capable of enhancing clinicians' ability to make informed decisions consistent with patient needs while lowering the potential risk of medication-related errors. For instance, machine learning algorithms can scan patient profiles and histories to provide tailored therapeutic options, thereby minimizing the risk of adverse drug interactions. Moreover, utilization of AI facilitates a closed-loop approach whereby treatment outcomes can be monitored to further improve prescribing practices. Data-driven decision making is critical in the contemporary healthcare setting where drug resistance makes treatment challenging (Muteeb et al., 2023). However, some challenges include ethical issues and the need for robust regulations to ensure confidence for the safe use of AI technologies within the healthcare setting. Addressing them is critical in achieving maximum patient care as well as maximum effectiveness of prescribed treatment (Figure 8.18).

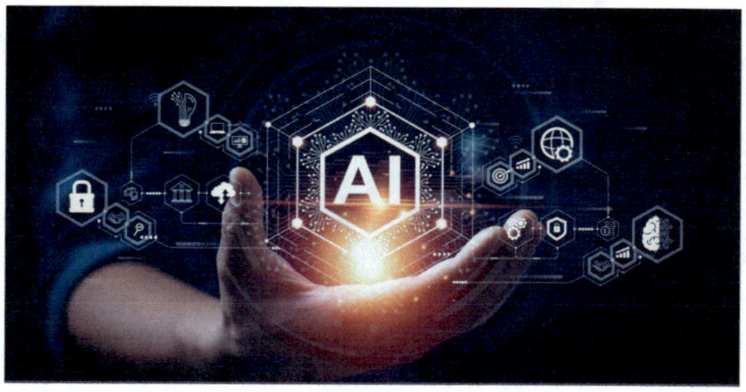

Figure 8.18. The integration of artificial intelligence (AI) in decision-making represents a transformative advancement in rational prescribing and prescription writing.

Source: https://healthcareitsm.com/wp-content/uploads/2023/06/Healthcare_AI-and-Healthcare_Systems.jpg.

8.4.4. Trends in Personalized Medicine

The advent of personalized medicine is a paradigm shift throughout the healthcare sector, with a focus on individualized treatment to cater to the particular genetic, environmental, and lifestyle determinants of individual patients. This approach is in concordance with rational prescribing paradigms that reinforce drug therapy following detailed assessment of patients rather than the "one size that fits all" approach. The integration of genetic and biomarker information into prescription practice allows doctors to maximize drug effectiveness while minimizing side effects, eventually leading to better patient outcomes. Furthermore, the vision of One-World Medicine seeks to unify conventional and traditional medicine practice, promoting integrative treatment modalities that respect cultural contexts and promote safety as well as effectiveness in therapeutic interventions (Abdelfatah et al., 2019). As healthcare systems worldwide grapple with rising costs, understanding co-occurrence in therapy response can unlock the door to innovative data-driven solutions that serve as the pillars of effective personalized medicine (Hsu et al., 2016).

8.4.5. Importance of Continuous Education for Prescribers

Within the ever-evolving healthcare setting, the importance of continuous education to prescribers cannot be overlooked. As there is increased medical knowledge and the development of new therapeutic options, prescribers must stay current in ensuring they deliver effective and safe patient care. Continuing education supports a greater awareness of newly arising issues. One of them is resistance to antibiotics, a problem which was prioritized by the unprecedented rise in microbial plasticity due to misuse of antibiotics (Muteeb et al., 2023). Continuing education also facilitates medical professionals in recognizing and coping with the complexity of pharmacology, including AMR mechanisms that counteract therapeutic efficacy (Salam et al., 2023). Through continual training, prescribers can make informed decisions, lower clinical errors, and support public health efforts against drug resistance. Putting a priority on ongoing education is thus essential for instilling rational prescribing practices that ultimately serve patient care and safeguard global health (Figure 8.19).

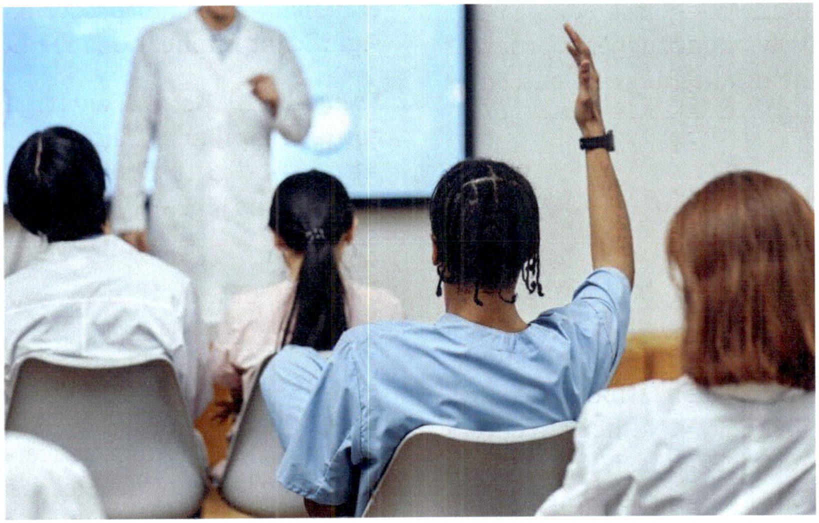

Figure 8.19. Continuous education facilitates a deeper understanding of emerging issues such as antibiotic resistance, a pressing concern highlighted by the alarming rise in microbial adaptability due to the misuse of antibiotics.

Source: https://careoptionsforkids.com/hubfs/Importance%20of%20Continuing%20Education%20for%20Nurses.jpg.

8.4.6. Enhancing Patient Engagement in Treatment Decisions

Patient involvement in treatment choice is central to the rational process of prescribing and writing prescriptions. Actively involving patients and health professionals not only establishes a partnership but also enhances compliance and satisfaction with treatment plans. Engaged patients are more likely to comply with medication regimens, as they become better informed about their medical conditions and the implications of their choices. This combined approach also addresses the rising problem of AMR, which has emerged primarily due to the misuse of drugs; thus, informed patients can make rational choices about the use of antibiotics, and this will help resist the silent pandemic of AMR (Salam et al., 2023). Moreover, the lack of well-defined guidance on treatment decision-making, particularly among older patients, jeopardizes health outcomes and emphasizes the need for effective communication and patient-centered strategies to mitigate falls and their complications (M-Odasso et al., 2022). Effective patient involvement suggests progress towards improved health literacy and outcomes in clinical practice.

8.4.7. Policy Changes Affecting Prescription Practices

Recent policy measures for enhancing rational prescribing practice have significant consequences for the provision of healthcare. For instance, the implementation of a PRF policy at Beijing's primary healthcare centers has been done to restrict excessive utilization of antibiotics and thus arrest the rising challenge of antibiotic resistance (Wushouer et al., 2023). Doctors and pharmacists were among the stakeholders who identified several challenges to the effective execution of PRF, including inadequate resources and varying review standards. Similarly, Thailand's RDU policy has led the focus towards quality improvement in healthcare through enhanced collaboration and training between healthcare providers (Intahphuak et al., 2022). Even with these interventions, enduring issues, including patient stress and management of drugs that have been obtained from external sources, render the attainment of desired objectives impossible. Lastly, these policies underscore the importance of systemic change that establishes a more informed and regulated prescribing environment, which is vital to safeguarding individual and public health (Figure 8.20).

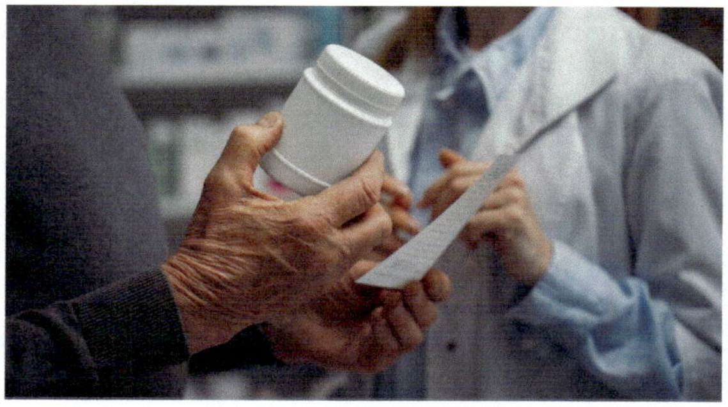

Figure 8.20. Recent policy changes aimed at enhancing rational prescribing practices have significant implications for healthcare delivery.

Source: https://www.tigahealth.com/wp-content/uploads/2024/06/Preventing-Drug-Abuse-A-Joint-Effort-with-Government-Institutions.jpg.

8.4.8. Research and Development in New Medications

The process of drug research and development is inherently linked with rational prescribing and prescription writing practice. As pharmaceutical companies seek to develop beneficial therapies, they typically face challenges that shape their approaches to the care of unique patients. For instance, while treatment must be individualized based on patients' specific needs, providers tend to resort to off-the-shelf treatments based on general population standards, a point posed by (Frank et al., 2025). This resort to pre-specified interventions adulterates the provision of customized care, especially in settings where infectious disease prevails, such as the situation in LMICs. In this, unethical prescribing practices, particularly with antibiotics, have serious consequences, including increased AMR, as noted by (Barker et al., 2015). Addressing these challenges through focused research can ensure maximum safety and efficacy of drugs and promote rational prescribing practices in the process.

8.4.9. Global Perspectives on Rational Prescribing

nternational rational prescribing is affected by differing regulatory environments and clinical behaviors, so the need to appreciate regional differences in strategy for coping with medication cannot be overestimated. Prescribing opioids has become a high-profile concern across most of the globe due to mounting diversion and addiction problems, particularly in the United States, where advice has emerged in the context of rising opioid-related death rates (Manchikanti, 2017). These suggestions aim to find an equilibrium between the valid interest in pain management and public safety and health needs. The concept of regulation, however, is questioned with a shift towards a decentred strategy recognizing various stakeholders like the community and the market as an integral aspect of good prescribing practice (Black J, 2017). This subtle appreciation develops an integrative strategy for rational prescribing, challenging medical professionals to look beyond clinical efficacy to the broader societal impacts of their prescribing practices.

Test Your Knowledge

1. What role could artificial intelligence and machine learning play in enhancing the decision-making process in rational prescribing?
2. How can the future of rational prescribing be shaped by personalized medicine and pharmacogenomics?

Summary

The importance of rational prescribing and sound prescription writing cannot be overstated, as these are the foundation blocks for therapeutic response and patient safety. The evidence is that patient-centered approaches to prescription based on preference and physiological variation significantly enhance outcomes and compliance. For instance (Sachs et al., 2013) recognizes the issue posed by the lack of age-suitable drug forms for children as patients as a clear need for drugs following children's and their guardians' preferences. Furthermore, the examination of policy structures shows that AMR should be managed by sophisticated and situation-specific interventions, as evidenced in Aarestrup et al., (2015). By advocating One Health policies, and for those that are responsive, healthcare practitioners can foster environments that promote safe prescribing habits and account for the diverse needs of their patient populations. In the end, continued focus and adaptability in these areas are necessary to ensure adequate healthcare provision.

The rational prescribing and prescription discussion emphasizes the need to address the increasing issue of AMR. The key strategy involves implementing C-reactive protein point-of-care testing (CRP POCT) to underpin clinical decision-making in primary care for respiratory tract infections (RTIs). This approach not only helps identify those patients who may potentially benefit from antibiotics but also improves effective practices of communication among patients and healthcare providers, thus reducing inappropriate prescriptions. In combination with delayed prescribing practices, CRP POCT has been proven to be a powerful driver in the prevention of unnecessary use of antibiotics, a powerful driver of AMR as established by current studies. The call for an interdisciplinary approach to these measures is urgent, requiring appropriate reimbursement, intensive training of doctors, and increased public education. Through cooperation at all levels of healthcare, the ultimate goal of antibiotic protection can be achieved, accentuating the importance of rational prescribing practice (Bjerrum et al., 2023, 2024).

KEY TERMS FROM THIS CHAPTER

- Antibiotic consumption
- Continuity of care
- Document
- Errors
- Exercise prescription
- Generic drug
- Healthcare professionals
- Legibility
- Pharmaceutical care services
- Probiotics
- Anti-glaucoma medications
- Demographic data
- E-prescription system
- Evidence-based medicine (EBM)
- General practitioners
- GheOP3S screening tool
- Healthcare systems
- Patient demographics
- Prescription
- Rational prescribing

CRITICAL THINKING QUESTIONS

1. **What is the primary goal of rational prescribing?**
   a. To prescribe the most expensive medication available
   b. To ensure the prescribed medication is appropriate, effective, and safe for the patient
   c. To prescribe the highest dosage of a drug
   d. To prescribe based on personal preferences
2. **Which of the following is an important principle of rational prescribing?**
   a. Prescribing the latest drug on the market
   b. Considering the patient's medical history and individual needs
   c. Prescribing medications with the shortest duration of action
   d. Prescribing the cheapest available medication
3. **What does the term "polypharmacy" refer to?**
   a. The use of a single drug for multiple conditions
   b. The use of multiple medications by a patient, particularly in elderly populations
   c. The prescription of medications with the same mechanism of action
   d. The practice of avoiding drug prescriptions altogether
4. **What should a healthcare provider consider when prescribing a medication?**
   a. The cost of the medication
   b. The patient's age, weight, and medical conditions
   c. The appearance of the medication
   d. Only the severity of the patient's symptoms
5. **What essential information must be included in a prescription?**
   a. The patient's favorite medication
   b. The drug's brand name only
   c. The patient's name, the drug name, dosage, route of administration, and frequency
   d. Only the drug's generic name

Answers to Critical Thinking Questions

1. (b); 2. (b); 3. (b); 4. (b); 5. (c).

Short Answer Questions

1. What is the primary goal of rational prescribing in clinical practice?
2. Which factors should be considered when making decisions about rational prescribing for a patient?
3. How does a healthcare provider determine the most appropriate drug for a patient?
4. What essential information should be included in a prescription to ensure it is clear and complete?
5. How does the inclusion of the correct dosage and frequency contribute to the effectiveness of a prescription?

References

1. Dar, O. A., Hasan, R., Schlundt, J., Harbarth, S., Caleo, G., Dar, F. K., Littmann, J., Rweyemamu, M., Buckley, E. J., Shahid, M., Kock, R., Li, H. L., Giha, H., Khan, M., So, A. D., Bindayna, K. M., Kessel, A., Pedersen, H. B., Permanand, G., . . . Heymann, D. L. (2015b). Exploring the evidence base for national and regional policy interventions to combat resistance. *The Lancet, 387*(10015), 285–295. https://doi.org/10.1016/s0140-6736(15)00520-6Abdelfatah, S., Abu-Darwish, M. S., Banerjee, M., Bhakta-Guha, D., et al. (2019). Biopiracy *versus* one-world medicine–from colonial relicts to global collaborative concepts. https://core.ac.uk/download/228178415.pdf (accessed on 10th June 2025).
2. Adomako, L. A. B., Alaverdyan, S., Appiah, F., Appiah-Thompson, P., et al. (2022). Appropriateness of antibiotic prescribing for acute conjunctivitis: A cross-sectional study at a specialist eye hospital in Ghana, *2021*. https://core.ac.uk/download/548487813.pdf (accessed on 10th June 2025).
3. Advani, M., & Jadhao, T. (2018). Study of prescription pattern of antiglaucoma drugs used in treatment of primary open angle glaucoma in ophthalmology outpatient department of a tertiary care hospital. https://core.ac.uk/download/543134216.pdf (accessed on 10th June 2025).
4. Albert, F. A., Crowe, M., Malau-Aduli, A. E. O., & Malau-Aduli, B. S. (2020). Physical activity promotion: A systematic review of the perceptions of healthcare professionals. *International Journal of Environmental Research and Public Health, 17*(12), 4358. https://doi.org/10.3390/ijerph17124358.
5. Amoako-Sakyi, D., Hamill, H., Hampshire, K., Mariwah, S., et al. (2022). "It is very difficult in this business if you want to have a good conscience": Pharmaceutical governance and on-the-ground ethical labour in Ghana. https://core.ac.uk/download/578087811.pdf (accessed on 10th June 2025).
6. Bachewar, N. P., Choudhari, S. R., & Dudhgaonkar, S. (2017). Assessment of prescription pattern using WHO drug prescribing indicators in medicine wards of a tertiary care teaching hospital: A retrospective observational study. https://core.ac.uk/download/539896789.pdf (accessed on 10th June 2025).
7. Balabalajee, J., Sakthibalan, M., Meher, B. R., Saravanan, S., et al. (2016). Effect of educational intervention on the knowledge and attitude on prescribing amongst interns of a tertiary care hospital: A questionnaire-based study. https://core.ac.uk/download/539896703.pdf (accessed on 10th June 2025).
8. Barker, C. I., Irwin, A., Le Doare, K., Sharland, M., et al. (2015). Improving antibiotic prescribing for children in the resource-poor setting. https://core.ac.uk/download/29469533.pdf (accessed on 10th June 2025).
9. Bharath Kumar, D. V., Lavanya, H. S., Kalpana, L. M., et al. (2019). Assessment on awareness of rational prescribing practices among medical interns in a tertiary care hospital: A questionnaire-based study. https://core.ac.uk/download/539895883.pdf (accessed on 10th June 2025).
10. Bhardwaj, V. K., Budania, N., Kumar, N., Kumar, R., et al. (2018). Evaluation of vitamins/tonics prescribing pattern in tertiary care teaching hospital and private sector. https://core.ac.uk/download/539896145.pdf (accessed on 10th June 2025).

11. Bhave, S., Kirpekar, V., & Gawande, S. (2022). Polypharmacy subtypes in psychiatry: The rational, the reasonable, the ridiculous & the hazardous. *Indian Journal of Psychiatry, 64*(Suppl. 1), S621. https://www.semanticscholar.org/paper/7a2e77d5624486b154fcb681c41a1cee96273ff8 (accessed on 10th June 2025).

12. Bicknell, C., Charani, E., Darzi, A., Franklin, B. D., et al. (2014). Redesigning the 'choice architecture' of hospital prescription charts: A mixed methods study incorporating *in situ* simulation testing. https://core.ac.uk/download/76995621.pdf (accessed on 10th June 2025).

13. Bjerrum, L., Gentile, I., Hopstaken, R., Llor, C., et al. (2023). Guidance on C-reactive protein point-of-care testing and complementary strategies to improve antibiotic prescribing for adults with lower respiratory tract infections in primary care. https://core.ac.uk/download/586370132.pdf (accessed on 10th June 2025).

14. Bjerrum, L., Gentile, I., Hopstaken, R., Llor, C., et al. (2024). C-reactive protein point-of-care testing in primary care—Broader implementation needed to combat antimicrobial resistance. https://core.ac.uk/download/614993936.pdf (accessed on 10th June 2025).

15. Black, J. (2017). *Critical Reflections on Regulation*. Routledge. https://doi.org/10.4324/9781351126816-2.

16. Bloom, G., Buckland Merrett, G., MacGregor, H., Wilkinson, A., et al. (2016). Towards the just and sustainable use of antibiotics. https://core.ac.uk/download/286048499.pdf (accessed on 10th June 2025).

17. Boussery, K., Mehuys, E., Petrovic, M., Somers, A., et al. (2015). Older patients' prescriptions screening in the community pharmacy: Development of the Ghent Older People's Prescriptions Community Pharmacy Screening (GheOP3S) tool. https://core.ac.uk/download/55843875.pdf (accessed on 10th June 2025).

18. Buchheit, M., & Allen, S. V. (2022). To optimize? First, empathize. *International Journal of Sports Physiology and Performance*. https://www.semanticscholar.org/paper/1a0ed96b94576cc9935b826e46015521cc686c48 (accessed on 10th June 2025).

19. Chandra, S., Karmakar, R., Kumar, S., Shaifali, S., et al. (2018). Drug utilization audit of antipsychotics using WHO methodology: Recommendations for rational prescribing. https://core.ac.uk/download/539896185.pdf (accessed on 10th June 2025).

20. Coleman, D. L., & Rosoff, P. M. (2011). The case for legal regulation of physicians' off-label prescribing. https://core.ac.uk/download/62564977.pdf (accessed on 10th June 2025).

21. Das, K., Routray, D., Sahoo, J., Singh, R., et al. (2017). Changing physician behavior: Interventions to improve prescription writing practices in a secondary level hospital in Delhi. https://core.ac.uk/download/551597320.pdf (accessed on 10th June 2025).

22. Davey, P., Brown, E., Charani, E., Fenelon, L., Gould, I. M., Holmes, A., Ramsay, C., et al. (2013). Interventions to improve antibiotic prescribing practices for hospital inpatients. *Cochrane Database of Systematic Reviews*. https://doi.org/10.1002/14651858.CD003543.pub3.

23. Devine, T., Jordan, J., Knoderer, C., McFarland, M., et al. (2020). *The Value-Driven Pharmacist: Basics of Access, Cost, And Quality* (2nd ed.). https://core.ac.uk/download/287886562.pdf (accessed on 10th June 2025).

24. Drahos, P. (2016). *A Philosophy of Intellectual Property*. https://doi.org/10.4324/9781315263786.

25. England, E. (2023). 'Show me you're trying, that's all...': Exploring the discursive impact of

punishments and incentives in the Welsh homelessness system as 'controlled conditionalities.' *Social Policy and Administration, 58*(1), 141–154. https://doi.org/10.1111/spol.12949.

26. Frank, R. G., & Zeckhauser, R. J. (2025). Custom made versus ready to wear treatments: Behavioral propensities in physician's choices. https://core.ac.uk/download/pdf/6586852.pdf (accessed on 10th June 2025).
27. Fu, K., Yang, M. C., & Wood, K. L. (2016). Design principles: Literature review, analysis, and future directions. *Journal of Mechanical Design, 138*. https://doi.org/10.1115/1.4034105.
28. Gawali, U., Gholve, P. B., Rizvi, S. H., & Mishra, P. (2021). Prescription pattern study of antiasthmatics drugs in tertiary care center. *International Journal of Basic and Clinical Pharmacology, 10*, 429. https://www.semanticscholar.org/paper/2ec4c4ed3f8a665e38023f1b6f68241e69b42156 (accessed on 10th June 2025).
29. Gazerani, P., & Mujtaba, S. H. (2024). Exploring the role of community pharmacists in pain management: Enablers and challenges. https://core.ac.uk/download/636678352.pdf (accessed on 10th June 2025).
30. Ghutke, B., Kachewar, A., Panekar, D., Shende, R., et al. (2019). Assessment of drug utilization pattern of steroids in a district general hospital in Amravati region. https://core.ac.uk/download/322817593.pdf (accessed on 10th June 2025).
31. Godman, B., Egwuenu, A., Haque, M., Malande, O. O., Schellack, N., Kumar, S., Saleem, Z., et al. (2021). Strategies to improve antimicrobial utilization with a special focus on developing countries. *Life, 11*(6), 528. https://doi.org/10.3390/life11060528.
32. Gupta, S., Khajuria, K., Khajuria, V., Kumar, R., et al. (2018). Comparative study of impact of marketing strategies of pharmaceutical houses on prescription practices of doctors: Rural vs urban. https://core.ac.uk/download/543133631.pdf (accessed on 10th June 2025).
33. Howard, P., Liang, Z., Liu, G., Xu, H., et al. (2022). Patient-centered care and patient autonomy: Doctors' views in Chinese hospitals. https://core.ac.uk/download/542340729.pdf (accessed on 10th June 2025).
34. Hsu, M. C. Y. (2016). A co-occurrence framework conceptualized for bridging the gap between basic science, clinical research and clinical practices. https://core.ac.uk/download/142068225.pdf (accessed on 10th June 2025).
35. Intahphuak, S., Lorga, T., & Tipwareerom, W. (2022). Community health nurses' perspective on the introduced rational drug use policy in primary care settings in Thailand: A descriptive qualitative study. *Tropical Medicine and Infectious Disease, 7*. https://www.semanticscholar.org/paper/d09776a530666bfb08c63cca89d1dd3c3929563c (accessed on 10th June 2025).
36. Iskandar, B., Febrina, M., Rahmadhani, R. O., & Agustini, T. T. (2025). Prescription patterns in the outpatient unit of XYZ Hospital, Pekanbaru: A study from 2022. https://core.ac.uk/download/653318982.pdf (accessed on 10th June 2025).
37. Kamuhabwa, A. A. R., & Silumbe, R. (2013). Knowledge among drug dispensers and antimalarial drug prescribing practices in public health facilities in Dar es Salaam. https://core.ac.uk/download/pdf/18174791.pdf (accessed on 10th June 2025).
38. Keith, D. A., Kulich, R. J., Bharel, M., Boose, R. E., Brownstein, J., Da Silva, J. D., D'Innocenzo, R., et al. (2017). Massachusetts dental schools respond to the prescription opioid crisis: A statewide collaboration. *Journal of Dental Education, 81*(12), 1388–1394. https://doi.org/10.21815/jde.017.098.

39. Khan, R., & Socha-Dietrich, K. (2018). Investing in medication adherence improves health outcomes and health system efficiency. *OECD Health Working Papers*. https://doi.org/10.1787/8178962c-en.

40. Khanal, S., Shrestha, S., & Shrestha, S. (2019). Polypharmacy in elderly cancer patients: Challenges and the way clinical pharmacists can contribute in resource-limited settings. https://core.ac.uk/download/287605655.pdf (accessed on 10th June 2025).

41. Kharaba, Z., Farhat, J., Mahboub, B. S., Buabeid, M., Alfoteih, Y., Al-Worafi, Y. M., Jaber, A. A. S., et al. (2022). Current views of community and hospital pharmacists on pharmaceutical care services in the United Arab Emirates: A mixed methodological study. *F1000Research, 11*, 694. https://doi.org/10.12688/f1000research.110102.1.

42. Khurshid, F., Bashir, S., & Noushad, B. (2020). Prescription writing through the lens of the threshold concept framework: A narrative review. *Research and Development in Medical Education, 9*, 11. https://doi.org/10.34172/rdme.2020.011.

43. Lust, E. (2022). *Everyday Choices*. https://doi.org/10.1017/9781009306164.

44. Machowska, A., & Stålsby Lundborg, C. (2018). Drivers of irrational use of antibiotics in Europe. *International Journal of Environmental Research and Public Health, 16*(1), 27. https://doi.org/10.3390/ijerph16010027.

45. Majeed, A. (2023). Perspectives and preferences of pharmacists about the role of e-prescription systems implementation in Pakistan to improve the rational use of antibiotics: A qualitative study and a quantitative survey. https://core.ac.uk/download/646179745.pdf (accessed on 10th June 2025).

46. Malbrain, M. L. N. G., Van Regenmortel, N., Saugel, B., De Tavernier, B., Van Gaal, P. J., Joannès-Boyau, O., Teboul, J. L., et al. (2018). Principles of fluid management and stewardship in septic shock: It is time to consider the four D's and the four phases of fluid therapy. *Annals of Intensive Care, 8*. https://doi.org/10.1186/s13613-018-0402-x.

47. Manchikanti, L. (2017). Responsible, safe, and effective prescription of opioids for chronic non-cancer pain: American Society of Interventional Pain Physicians (ASIPP) guidelines. *Pain Physician, 2*, S3–S92. https://doi.org/10.36076/ppj.2017.s92.

48. McLellan, A. T. (2010). Chronic noncancer pain management and opioid overdose: Time to change prescribing practices. *Annals of Internal Medicine, 152*(2), 123. https://doi.org/10.7326/0003-4819-152-2-201001190-00012.

49. Meena, V., Dubey, P., Kumar, D., & Meena, P. (2023). Survey of drugs prescribed in department of dermatology of a tertiary care center. *National Journal of Physiology, Pharmacy and Pharmacology.* https://www.semanticscholar.org/paper/5830aa7ac43e35240277c6a05b6ab7b6f383afdb (accessed on 10th June 2025).

50. Montero-Odasso, M., van der Velde, N., Martin, F. C., Petrović, M., Tan, M. P., Ryg, J., Aguilar-Navarro, S. G., et al. (2022). World guidelines for falls prevention and management for older adults: A global initiative. *Age and Ageing, 51*. https://doi.org/10.1093/ageing/afac205.

51. Muteeb, G., Rehman, M. T., Shahwan, M., & Aatif, M. (2023). Origin of antibiotics and antibiotic resistance, and their impacts on drug development: A narrative review. *Pharmaceuticals, 16*(11), 1615. https://doi.org/10.3390/ph16111615.

52. Ncube, N. B. Q., Chivese, T., Mukumbang, F. C., Bradley, H. A., Schneider, H., & Laing, R. (2024).

A combined strategies intervention on the World Health Organization prescribing indicators: A quasi-randomized trial. *African Journal of Primary Health Care & Family Medicine, 16*. https://www.semanticscholar.org/paper/96270b20af83d78478f83c734d39e50806216094 (accessed on 10th June 2025).

53. Parver, C. (2008). Patient-tailored medicine, part one: The impact of race and genetics on medicine. https://core.ac.uk/download/235399827.pdf (accessed on 10th June 2025).

54. Piqué, N., Berlanga, M., & Miñana-Galbis, D. (2019). Health benefits of heat-killed (tyndallized) probiotics: An overview. *International Journal of Molecular Sciences, 20*, 2534. https://doi.org/10.3390/ijms20102534.

55. Reeve, J., Maden, M., Hill, R., Turk, A., Mahtani, K. R., Wong, G., Lasserson, D., et al. (2022). Deprescribing medicines in older people living with multimorbidity and polypharmacy: The TAILOR evidence synthesis. *Health Technology Assessment, 26*, 1–148. https://doi.org/10.3310/aafo2475.

56. Rutoo, P., Mauli, S., & N. P. (2024). Clinical audit of drug prescription for skin disorders in dermatology OPD at a tertiary care centre. *Clinical Dermatology Open Access Journal*. https://www.semanticscholar.org/paper/82806c2a85c9cc4d85f7fe6628084035e6db1c73 (accessed on 10th June 2025).

57. Sachs, A. N., Nutt, C. T., Baguley, D., Notterman, D., Knoppert, D. C., Taylor, D. M., Ansah, E., et al. (2013). Children's medicines in Tanzania: A national survey of administration practices and preferences. https://core.ac.uk/download/pdf/11307828.pdf (accessed on 10th June 2025).

58. Salam, M. A., Al-Amin, M. Y., Salam, M. T., Pawar, J. S., Akhter, N., Rabaan, A. A., & Alqumber, M. A. A. (2023). Antimicrobial resistance: A growing serious threat for global public health. *Healthcare, 11*, 1946. https://doi.org/10.3390/healthcare11131946.

59. Saussure, F. de. (2017). *Course in General Linguistics*. Macat Library eBooks. https://doi.org/10.4324/9781912281732.

60. Smith, A. K. J. (2025). *The Sociology of Prescribing: A Narrative Review and Agenda*. https://unsworks.unsw.edu.au/bitstreams/3006e1a8-f109-4e18-999c-7bc5d5f99c0e/download (accessed on 10th June 2025).

61. Steffel, J., Collins, R., Antz, M., Cornu, P., Desteghe, L., Hæusler, K. G., Oldgren, J., et al. (2021). 2021 European Heart Rhythm Association practical guide on the use of non-vitamin K antagonist oral anticoagulants in patients with atrial fibrillation. *EP Europace, 23*, 1612–1676. https://doi.org/10.1093/europace/euab065.

62. Steffel, J., Verhamme, P., Potpara, T., Albaladejo, P., Antz, M., Desteghe, L., Hæusler, K. G., et al. (2018). The 2018 European Heart Rhythm Association Practical Guide on the use of non-vitamin K antagonist oral anticoagulants in patients with atrial fibrillation. *European Heart Journal, 39*(16), 1330–1393. https://doi.org/10.1093/eurheartj/ehy136 (accessed on 10th June 2025).

63. Subhashini, R., Bhuvaneswari, K., & Umamaheswari, A. (2020). Impact of a sensitization program on prescription order writing skills of second year MBBS students: A prospective study. *International Journal of Basic and Clinical Pharmacology, 9*, 906. https://www.semanticscholar.org/paper/471d35a3f7f66c3bc6711589f2ffe961682883fc (accessed on 10th June 2025).

64. Wackerhage, H., & Schoenfeld, B. (2021). Personalized, evidence-informed training plans and

exercise prescriptions for performance, fitness and health. *Sports Medicine, 51*, 1805–1813. https://www.semanticscholar.org/paper/1220476a749cae648362c2c794bec138aed5a824 (accessed on 10th June 2025).

65. Wushouer, H., Du, K., Chen, S., Li, H., Zhang, W., Yang, Y., Hu, L., et al. (2023). Evaluation of prescription review and feedback policy on rational antibiotic use in primary healthcare settings in Beijing, China: A qualitative study using the Theoretical Domains Framework and the Behavior Change Wheel. *JAC-Antimicrobial Resistance, 5*. https://www.semanticscholar.org/paper/1e7b6037b6831e6fa4e7fad28cfe35e4df22dd85 (accessed on 10th June 2025).

CLINICAL PHARMACOLOGY IN SPECIAL POPULATIONS

9

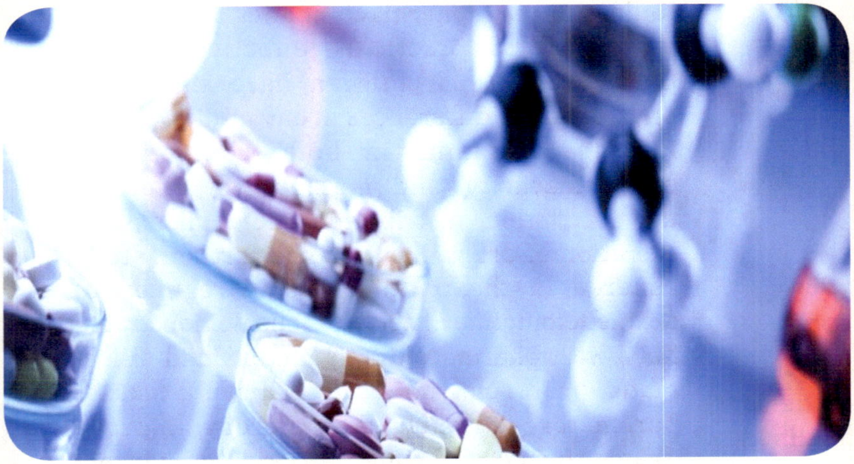

LEARNING OBJECTIVES

After studying this chapter, you will be able to:

1. Understand pediatric populations
2. Focus on geriatric populations
3. Discuss pregnant and lactating women
4. Explain patients with comorbidities

Introduction

Clinical pharmacology is an essential bridge between treatment and the management of special exceptional populations, who are generally children, the elderly, or patients with chronic disease. One should have an understanding of specific pharmacokinetic and pharmacodynamic characteristics in these patients to individualize the drug therapy for optimal benefit. For instance, factors such as weight, age, organ function, and comorbidities can significantly influence drug metabolism and effect. In addition, the arrival of new drugs has posed challenges of affordability and access, setting off an exploration of adaptive models of licensing. As mentioned above, MAPPs can bring forth new drugs with little data on effectiveness and safety, which may put patients at risk of using ineffective drugs (Schuurman et al., 2016). In addition, high-income countries are under mounting pressure to fund healthcare systems, and this necessitates strategic models to ensure equal access to these new therapeutics (Acurcio et al., 2014). These are strong aspects that indicate the imperative of individualized clinical pharmacological interventions in special populations.

9.1. Pediatric Populations

Learning Outcome

1. Understand pharmacokinetics in children
2. Know dosage considerations for pediatric patients
3. Focus on developmental pharmacology
4. Identify common medications used in pediatrics
5. Know adverse drug reactions in children
6. Explain ethical considerations in pediatric trials
7. Understand regulatory guidelines for pediatric pharmacology
8. Learn future directions in pediatric pharmacology research

Pharmacological therapy of pediatric patients presents unique challenges requiring modified approaches both to sustain efficacy and to preserve safety. Children, as opposed to adults, metabolize drugs differently due to variations in physiological development, particularly the ontogeny of drug-metabolizing enzymes. For instance, modeling research has demonstrated that although predictions of drug exposure in children aged two years and above can be pretty accurate, severe mispredictions are likely to occur in younger children because of the complexities of gut physiology and metabolic pathways in very young patients (Umehara et al., 2024). Additionally, the American Academy of Sleep Medicine offers evidence that disorders such as obstructive sleep apnea can be well treated in children with treatments like CPAP, given that professionals become experts in this area of advanced practice (Amos et al., 2022). These comments emphasize the need for individualized pharmacotherapy strategies based on both clinical experience and strong pharmacokinetic data to optimize outcomes in pediatric patients.

9.1.1. Pharmacokinetics in Children

Understanding pharmacokinetics in children is critical to practicing effective clinical pharmacology, as children have significant physiological differences from adults. These include variations in body composition, organ maturity, and metabolism, affecting the absorption, distribution, metabolism, and excretion of drugs. For instance, a recent study ushered in the optimal dosing regimen of dexmedetomidine in neonates and demonstrated how, with pharmacokinetic models and tailor-made protocols, one can achieve accurate parameter estimates and thereby improve drug efficacy and safety in the vulnerable population (Allegaert et al., 2019). Moreover, the heterogeneity of individual response necessitates scrupulous care with such variables as developmental status and genetic heterogeneity, particularly for high-stakes interventions such as antiretroviral therapy, where dosing variation is critical to avoid failure of treatment or resistance (Hentig et al., 2012). While clinical trials persist in improving dosing methods to greater precision, it becomes imperative to heed these individual pharmacokinetic profiles to maximize therapeutic benefit in pediatrics (Figure 9.1).

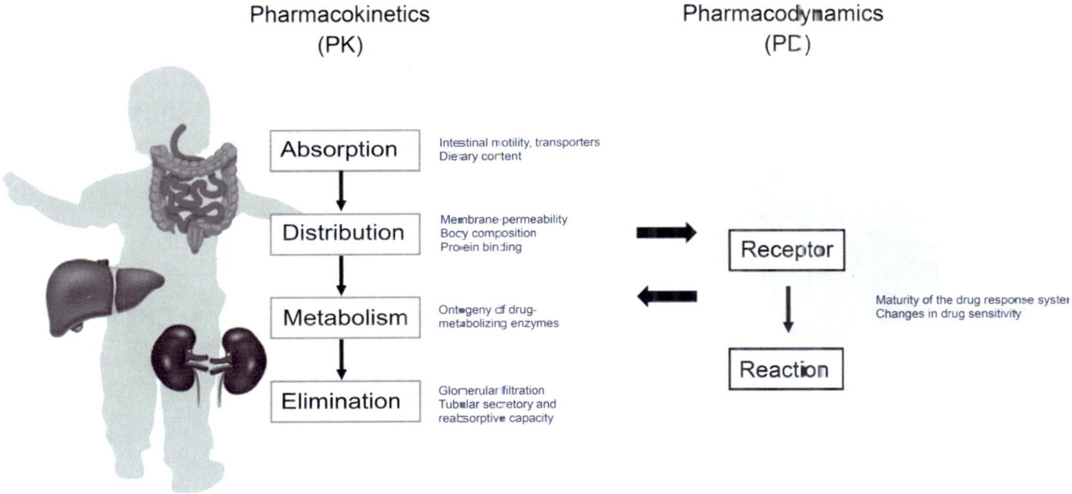

Figure 9.1. Understanding pharmacokinetics in children is crucial for effective clinical pharmacology, as pediatric patients exhibit significant physiological differences compared to adults.

Source: https://media.springernature.com/lw1200/springer-static/image/art%3A10.1007%2Fs00228-023-03598-x/MediaObjects/228_2023_3598_Fig1_HTML.png.

9.1.2. Dosage Considerations for Pediatric Patients

Optimum dose considerations in children are of highest concern in clinical pharmacology because they reflect the unique physiological characteristics and developmental orders that influence drug metabolism and action. Unlike adults, children have variable pharmacokinetics due to factors such as organ maturity, body composition, and processes of growth during childhood and adolescence. This diversity necessitates watchfulness in dosing, and therefore, there is a need for formulations designed for the aged and observation data to guide clinicians. Furthermore, as stated in the American Academy of Pediatrics and American Academy of Pediatric Dentistry guidelines for guaranteeing safety precautions and appropriate monitoring throughout procedures, the safety and effectiveness of pediatric sedation place a strong emphasis on careful planning, including a comprehensive pre-sedation evaluation and a solid grasp of pharmacokinetic principles (Coté et al., 2019). By integrating these, clinicians can maximize therapeutic benefits and minimize risks of pharmacotherapy in this susceptible population (Venkatakrishnan et al., 2021).

9.1.3. Developmental Pharmacology

Developmental pharmacology is a science that has a significant role in unraveling the intricate pharmacokinetics and pharmacodynamics, which vary considerably during different stages of human development, particularly in vulnerable populations such as neonates and children. As these groups have distinct physiological profiles, their response to drugs can be dissimilar from that in adults and hence calls for an adaptive approach to drug administration. For instance, recent studies of dexmedetomidine in mechanically ventilated neonates highlight the importance of developmental considerations in determining dosing regimens and pharmacokinetic profiles. Findings revealed that term neonates exhibited a 20% higher rate of clearance than predictions with the use of slightly older pediatric groups, pointing towards the requirement of age-defined clinical trial designs that consider developmental variability (Allegaert et al., 2019). Moreover, polymorphism detection in susceptibility genes is utilized to forecast drug response in a patient and is applied to maximize treatment regimen (Mueller et al., 2010). Developmental pharmacology is thus a foundation for maximizing the therapeutic gain in special groups through the utilization of knowledge-based and precise drug therapy (Figure 9.2).

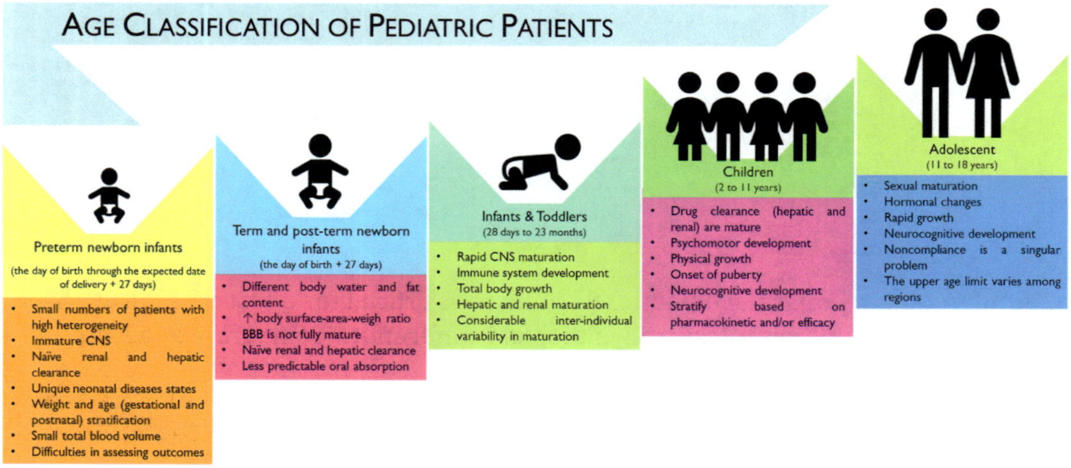

Figure 9.2. Developmental pharmacology.

Source: https://www.mdpi.com/pharmaceutics/pharmaceutics-15-02431/article_deploy/html/images/pharmaceutics-15-02431-g001.png.

9.1.4. Common Medications Used in Pediatrics

The landscape of child pharmacotherapy is dominated by a distinctive set of common drugs for everyday use tailored to the special anatomy and developmental variables of children. Among them, antibacterial drugs like amoxicillin are used to cure bacterial infections, whereas analgesics like acetaminophen are effective in curing pain and fever. Also, medications for the treatment of chronic diseases like inhalers for asthma and antihypertensives highlight the necessity of accurate dosing and surveillance in the younger age group. The moral implications of the use of such treatments are serious, especially considering the vulnerability of this population. The demand for safety and efficacy cannot be overstated, as seen in controversy around myopia control treatment, which calls for ethical consideration when prescribed to children (Drove et al., 2019). Furthermore, while probiotics are increasingly being applied to children for gastrointestinal disorders, the various outcomes necessitate familiarity with their risk-benefit profile about some pediatric conditions (Bennett et al., 2016).

9.1.5. Adverse Drug Reactions in Children

In pediatric populations, the occurrence of ADRs is usually a serious challenge, particularly in pediatric oncology, where drug administration off-label is common. Research has found that 44.44% of patients receiving chemotherapy developed ADRs, with the severity mostly categorized as moderate, highlighting the importance of vigilant observation under these conditions (Khajuria et al., 2024). Most frequent reactions were fever and vomiting, suggesting that clinicians should be alert enough to manage these reactions successfully. In addition, pharmacovigilance is essential in ensuring drug safety, particularly after marketing, for the identification of long-term and unexpected ADRs among children who are likely to have co-morbidities not typically accounted for in clinical trials (Manjhi et al., 2024). Therefore, an appreciation of the nature of ADRs in children demands a customized response to pharmacological management, with a focus on prevention and early intervention to maximize patient safety (Figure 9.3).

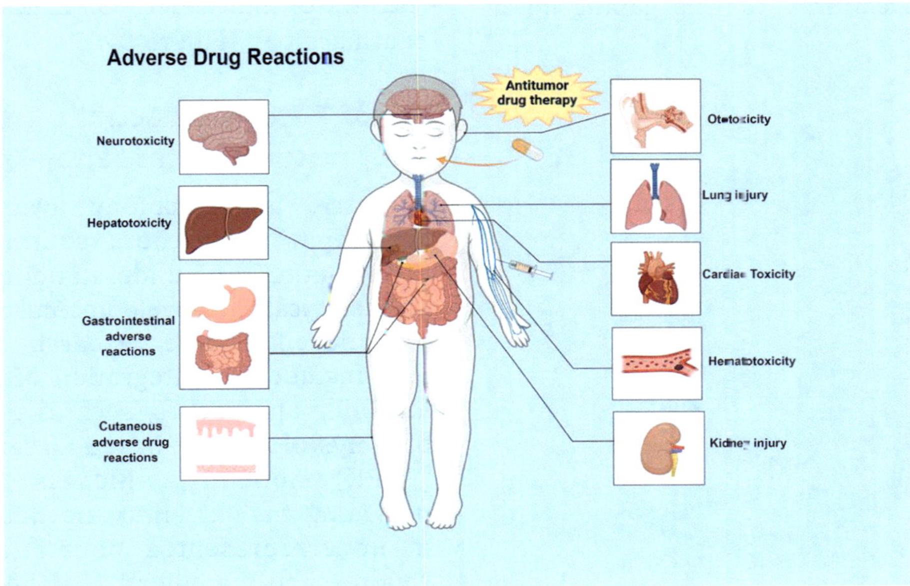

Figure 9.3. In pediatric populations, the occurrence of adverse drug reactions (ADRs) presents a significant challenge, particularly within oncology settings where the use of off-label medications is common.

Source: https://www.frontiersin.org/files/Articles/1329220/fphar-15-1329220-HTML/image_m/fphar-15-1329220-g001.jpg.

9.1.6. Ethical Considerations in Pediatric Trials

The ethical considerations within trials in children are a complex intersection of vulnerability, consent, and the demand for successful medical advancement. Children are often considered a vulnerable population due to their lack of ability to provide fully informed consent, and therefore, parents or guardians must provide this in their stead. This raises ethical issues of coercion and autonomy. Particularly in drug development for neonates, there remains an urgent unmet medical need for treatments, as determined by (Massaro et al., 2025). Moreover, new treatments such as cardiac xenotransplantation raise the ethical issue of child trials, where selection among child candidates would have to balance the potential benefit against significant risks, as argued in Hurst et al. (2024). Thus, researchers must work diligently through these ethical landscapes so that rigorous safeguards are in place to protect the welfare and rights of pediatric participants while advancing clinical pharmacology for this at-risk population.

9.1.7. Regulatory Guidelines for Pediatric Pharmacology

Regulatory guidance is essential in pediatric pharmacology to ensure the effectiveness and safety of drugs in this vulnerable population. Many drugs, including valuable oncology drugs, have long been underserved when it comes to dosing data and comprehensive safety information in children, leaving gaping holes in practice.

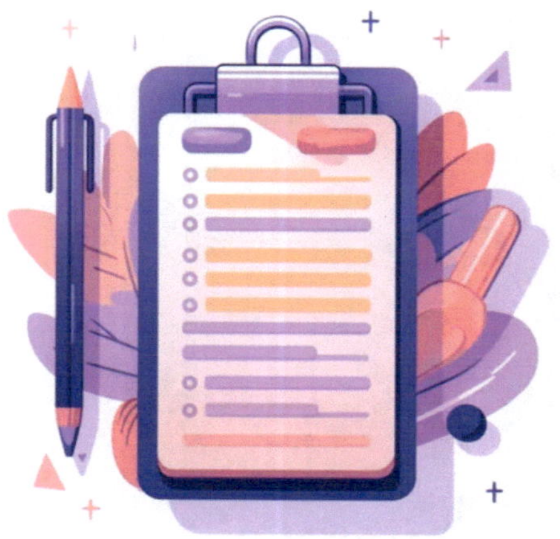

Figure 9.4. In the realm of pediatric pharmacology, regulatory guidelines play a crucial role in ensuring the safety and efficacy of medications for this vulnerable population.

Source: https://framerusercontent.com/images/mAd5yfzanPKOFYO6F59L1Qf9Y78.png.

This has prompted organizations like the FDA to put the process of updating prescribing guidelines in motion in response to evolving clinical experience and evidence (Balogh et al., 2019). Further, comparison of global guidelines reveals differences concerning the definition of monoclonal antibodies and their application in pediatrics, indicating the necessity for stringent regulatory mechanisms that are sensitive to these particular issues (Anvisa et al., 2018). Through the development of robust guidelines formulated in tune with children's growth and physiological peculiarities, pediatric patient protection can be maximized by regulatory authorities while encouraging therapy options and ease of clinical decision-making in pediatric pharmacology (Figure 9.4).

9.1.8. Future Directions in Pediatric Pharmacology Research

Pediatric pharmacology awaits extensive growth as researchers continue to refine their methods of understanding the unique physiological and developmental characteristics of children. Future research opportunities may include the integration of sophisticated modeling approaches, such as the application of physiologically-based pharmacokinetic (PBPK) modeling, which is promising in providing insights into the dosing of drugs in underrepresented populations, such as children and the elderly (Campo et al., 2021). Furthermore, use of quantitative systems pharmacology (QSP) can be of great help to understand pain treatment in pediatrics, to overcome inter-individual differences in response to treatment (Dijk et al., 2017). With these novel approaches in mind, researchers can predict pharmacokinetics and pharmacodynamics better in children, ultimately resulting in more effective and individualized therapeutic interventions. This shift not only indicates the requirement for individualized drug formulations but also the need to emphasize inclusivity in clinical trial models to best serve pediatric patients with the most appropriate pharmacological intervention.

Test Your Knowledge

1. What pharmacokinetic differences exist between neonates and older children?
2. How does gastric pH in infants affect oral drug absorption?

9.2. Geriatric Populations

Learning Outcome

1. Know age-related physiological changes
2. Explain polypharmacy and its implications
3. Discuss pharmacokinetics and pharmacodynamics in the elderly
4. Explain common health conditions in geriatric patients
5. Identify medication adherence challenges
6. Learn strategies for optimizing drug therapy
7. Describe the role of healthcare providers in geriatric pharmacology
8. Explain ethical issues in geriatric clinical trials
9. Focus on innovations in geriatric pharmacology

In the area of clinical pharmacology, older adults bring unique challenges that need a specialized strategy to manage drugs. This age group is prone to polypharmacy, the use of more than one drug, which is linked with significant side effects and treatment complications. As age progresses, physiological changes influence drug metabolism and drug action, which increases patients' vulnerability to drug errors as well as decreased quality of life. Health practitioners need to be vigilant to prevent such complications, particularly in care coordination and proper prescribing practices. (Anmolsingh et al., 2017) is eager to point out that awareness of the economic burden and health risks of polypharmacy, such as hospitalization because of drug-related complications, is essential. Implementing evidence-based practices to reduce polypharmacy rates will likely enhance therapeutic outcomes and protect the health of older adults. Thus, addressing the special needs of the geriatric population is necessary for improving clinical pharmacology in special populations.

9.2.1. Age-Related Physiological Changes

As age advances, a complex series of physiological changes occurs that significantly affects clinical pharmacology, particularly in special populations. Some of these changes with age include alterations in organ function, body composition, and drug metabolism.

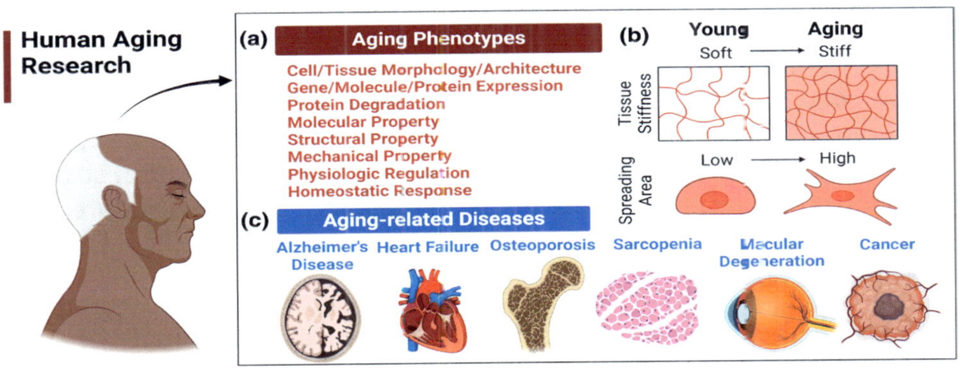

Figure 9.5. As individuals age, a multitude of physiological changes occurs that has significant implications for clinical pharmacology, particularly in special populations.

Source: https://onlinelibrary.wiley.com/cms/asset/b4e6a1c6-6a08-466b-bf5a-c945361abfec/acel14070-fig-0001-m.jpg.

For instance, decreased renal and hepatic function found among the elderly may lead to longer drug clearance and greater susceptibility to adverse drug effects. These physiological alterations demand modified dosing regimens in these individuals to achieve therapeutic effect with reduced risks. Further, the integration of multidisciplinary practices can optimize treatment outcomes, especially concerning complex situations like pregnancy, where physiological alteration is needed to modify pharmacotherapy to be administered safely.

Precisely, pregnancy-related physiological alterations, such as increased blood volume and altered drug metabolism, emphasize the need for individually tailored interventions (Net al., 2024). The dynamic interaction among the variations further supports an ongoing need for assessment and differential care strategies to optimize pharmacologic interventions across various age categories and conditions (Chavez et al., 2023) (Figure 9.5).

9.2.2. Polypharmacy and Its Implications

Polypharmacy, or the concurrent administration of two or more drugs, has significant consequences for patient safety, particularly among vulnerable groups such as the elderly. A growing incidence of polypharmacy has been linked to a myriad of side effects, such as drug errors, compromised quality of life, and hospitalization rates—all issues that require prudent healthcare interventions (Anmolsingh et al., 2017).

For older adults, the complexity of managing chronic illness necessarily results in long-acting medication, such as benzodiazepines, being prescribed, thereby exacerbating conditions. It has been found that physical health status and social isolation are predictors of higher benzodiazepine use among older adults, indicating how physical and mental conditions are connected with drug management (Chatterjee et al., 2017). Consequently, treatment of polypharmacy entails a broad range of interventions, including good prescribing practice along with extensive patient evaluation to minimize risk and promote an overall improved health status in special populations.

9.2.3. Pharmacokinetics and Pharmacodynamics in the Elderly

With the growing population of elderly patients, understanding the pharmacokinetic and pharmacodynamic complexity is more critical than ever. Physiological alterations with aging, i.e., body composition changes and organ function alterations, have a significant impact on the metabolism and excretion of drugs, leading to suboptimal therapeutic responses or even toxicity. For instance, the pharmacokinetics of neuromuscular agents such as sagamore show that aging alters their safety and efficacy profile, thereby making postoperative care in older patients complex (Bertoncello et al., 2017).

Moreover, elderly patients' underrepresentation in clinical trials often has dosing regimens that fail to address their unique pharmacological needs, hence posing higher risks of inefficacy or toxicity (Allegaert et al., 2017).

Therefore, the use of evidence-based methods for individualized dosing of drugs that counteract these pharmacodynamic differences in this vulnerable group is needed, eventually resulting in safer and more effective outcomes of pharmacotherapy (Figure 9.6).

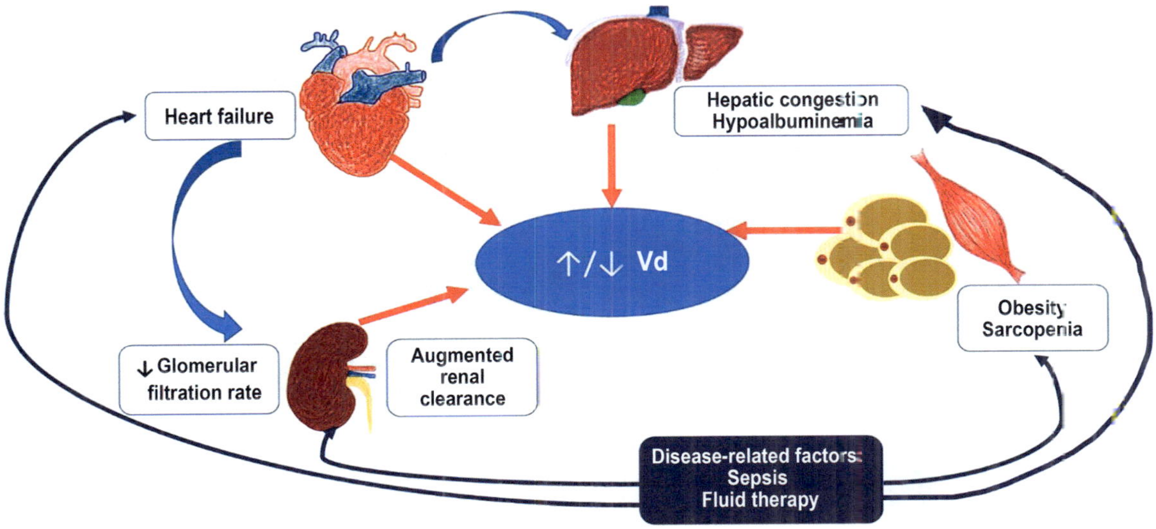

Figure 9.6. As the population of elderly patients continues to rise, understanding the intricacies of pharmacokinetics and pharmacodynamics becomes increasingly vital.

Source: https://www.mdpi.com/biomedicines/biomedicines-11-01633/article_deploy/html/images/biomedicines-11-01633-g001.png.

9.2.4. Common Health Conditions in Geriatric Patients

As the population of elderly people increases, it becomes increasingly important to know about the dominant health conditions among them, particularly given their multimorbid medical histories. Of these, asthma and mental diseases, including late-life depression, are prevalent and often intertwined. Many elderly patients have asthma as a part of comorbid conditions such as chronic obstructive pulmonary disease (COPD) and cardiovascular disease, which reflects the challenge of pharmacological treatment in the elderly population due to polypharmacy risks and pharmacokinetic alterations in older subjects (Khosa et al., 2023). Secondly, psychiatric disorders are surprisingly common, with estimates indicating that one in five older adults has a mental disorder, such as depression, which is often exacerbated by co-existing physical health conditions (Kazan et al., 2021). This multiple disorder interaction necessitates the incorporation of pharmacology practice into clinical care, specifically for older adults, in which treatments optimize physical as well as mental well-being.

9.2.5. Medication Adherence Challenges

Adherence to specific medications is an essential issue in special populations where the complexity of treatment therapies will complicate adherence. The reasons for non-adherence to medication include polypharmacy, which is prevalent in patients dealing with multiple chronic conditions, as it complicates dosing schedules and enhances the risk of side effects, thus discouraging future use (Anmolsingh et al., 2017). Moreover, the heterogeneity of healthcare experience and education across populations produces varied perceptions regarding the importance of adherence (Almarsdottir et al., 2024). The role of healthcare professionals in addressing these issues is paramount. Their role is to apply methods that enhance patient understanding and simplify treatment regimens to make the environment conducive to adherence. Eventually, medication adherence improves clinical outcomes and reduces the healthcare burden related to uncontrolled diseases, highlighting the importance of individualized interventions in clinical pharmacology (Figure 9.7).

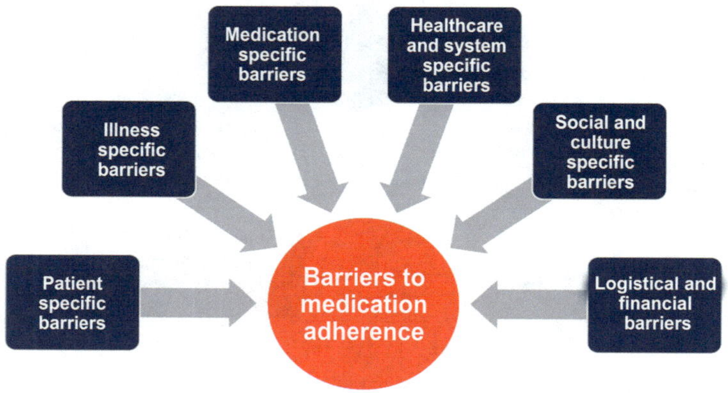

Figure 9.7. Medication adherence represents a critical challenge, particularly in special populations where the complexities of treatment regimens can hinder compliance.

Source: https://www.mdpi.com/pharmaceutics/pharmaceutics-13-01100/article_deploy/html/images/pharmaceutics-13-01100-g002.png.

9.2.6. Strategies for Optimizing Drug Therapy

Drug optimization plays a key role in optimizing treatment effectiveness, particularly in special groups, where pharmacokinetic and pharmacodynamic variability necessitates personalized intervention. Therapeutic drug monitoring (TDM) is one of the practical approaches by which clinicians can monitor drug levels and adjust doses accordingly to optimize therapeutic outcomes. For instance, in the therapeutic management of pulmonary infections, TDM has been crucial for antibiotics like gentamicin and voriconazole and demonstrated the role of dried blood spot methods in supporting such an approach (Akkerman et al., 2015). Additionally, adopting new strategies in disease treatment, as in the case of TB, is essential. The Global Tuberculosis Network emphasizes the use of a multidisciplinary strategy to investigate unmet therapeutic needs, particularly through the lens of pharmacokinetic observations from preclinical models. Such an approach not only promotes the identification of optimal drug regimens but also calls attention to the need to incorporate individual patient factors such as age and comorbidities into the optimization process (Alffenaar et al., 2020).

9.2.7. Role of Healthcare Providers in Geriatric Pharmacology

Healthcare professionals must manage geriatric pharmacology as the elderly population ages further and drug management complexity spreads. With patients experiencing polypharmacy, as in the concurrent use of multiple drugs, professionals are looking out for the complexity in prescribing and managing treatment, as well as the side effects. It is the duty of healthcare providers, particularly pharmacists and primary providers, to not only assess the appropriateness of prescribed medication but also coordinate care among various specialists to optimize therapeutic benefits. With communication and evidence-based intervention strategies, providers are in a position to minimize the hazards imposed by polypharmacy, typically resulting in medication errors, impaired quality of life, and hospitalizations (Anmolsingh et al., 2017). Ultimately, successful geriatric pharmacology depends on an interdisciplinary framework that emphasizes safety for the patient and personalized care (Figure 9.8).

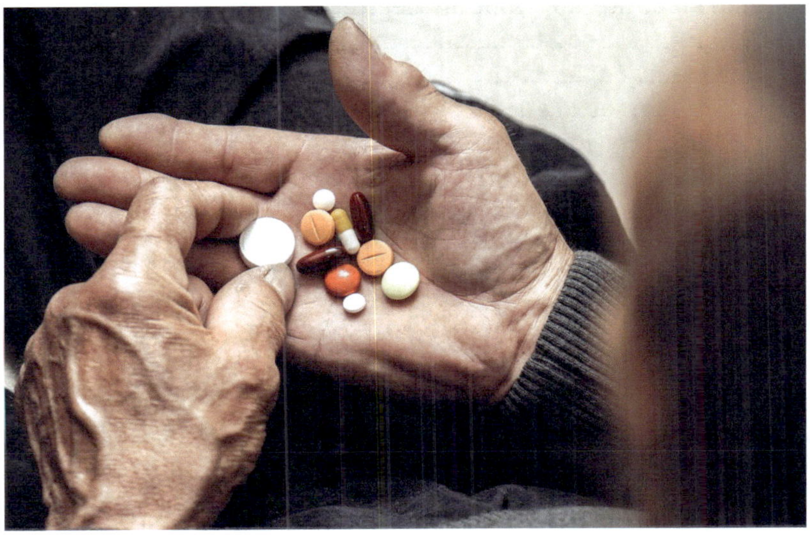

Figure 9.8. The role of healthcare providers in geriatric pharmacology is increasingly critical as the aging population continues to grow and complexity in medication management becomes more prevalent.

Source: https://d2jx2rerrg6sh3.cloudfront.net/images/Article_Images/ImageForArticle_24525_17065207532171781.jpg.

9.2.8. Ethical Issues in Geriatric Clinical Trials

The ethical landscape of geriatric clinical trials is complex with nuances that must be carefully considered, particularly in light of the unique frailties of older individuals. Given that this population of individuals typically has multiple health issues, it is necessary to ensure their inclusion in clinical trials without compromising their well-being and autonomy. Critical ethical issues, such as informed consent, are raised because compromised cognitive abilities may disable elderly persons from being well-informed regarding trial processes and hazards. Furthermore, there is widespread historical underrepresentation of elderly people in clinical trials, which compromises the generalizability of findings to them. Mitigating such ethical problems is a robust system that not only protects the rights and best interests of geriatric volunteers but also enforces strict ethical control. Lastly, involving older people in research can yield valuable information for optimizing pharmacological interventions, but it must be done with firm ethical integrity (Kolbin et al., 2023; Zur, 2023).

9.2.9. Innovations in Geriatric Pharmacology

The future of geriatric pharmacology is being reshaped with improved knowledge of the intricate pharmacokinetic and pharmacodynamic changes of the elderly. Recent innovations focus on the optimization of drug therapy to meet the unique health conditions of the elderly, balancing efficacy and safety. Elderly subjects have traditionally been underrepresented in clinical trials, perpetuating a paucity of evidence-based care for the elderly. As highlighted by current research, there has been a paradigm shift toward proactive prevention and individualized care being central to the improvement of health outcomes in aging communities (Terzic et al., 2019). However, the ambivalence toward pharmacotherapy among healthcare providers and society at large raises serious ethical issues. There is a need to balance the advantages and disadvantages of prescribed medication carefully, particularly against the background of enhanced susceptibility to side effects among elderly patients (Pepper et al., 1987). Such changes represent a landmark in promoting more advanced geriatric practice (Figure 9.9).

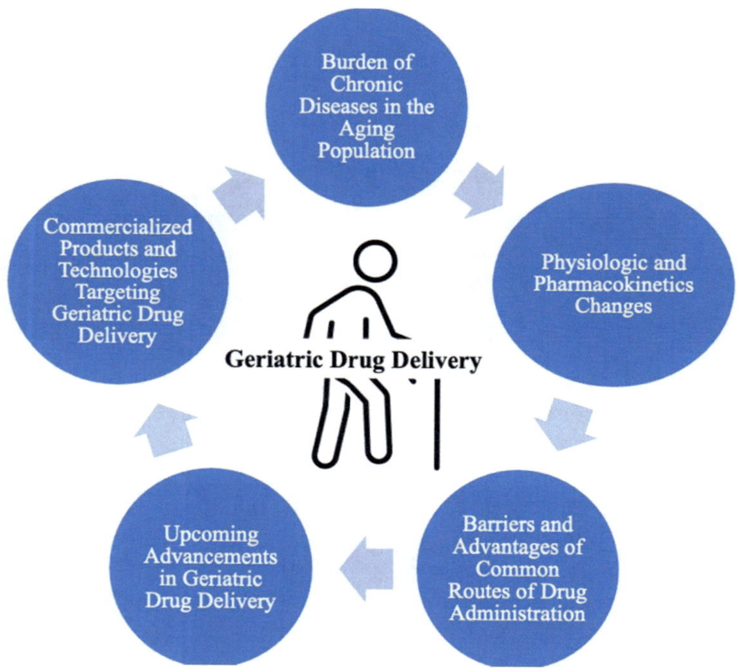

Figure 9.9. Recent innovations focus on tailoring drug therapies to meet the specific health challenges faced by older adults, balancing efficacy with safety.

Source: https://www.tandfonline.com/action/showGraphicalAbstractImage?doi=10.1080%2F1061186X.2024.2386626&id=idrt_a_2386626_uf0001_c.jpg.

Test Your Knowledge

1. Why are elderly patients more susceptible to adverse drug reactions (ADRs)?
2. How does polypharmacy contribute to drug interactions and complications in geriatric patients?

9.3. Pregnant and Lactating Women

Learning Outcome

1. Know physiological changes during pregnancy
2. Explain drug transfer to the fetus
3. Discuss the safety and efficacy of medications in pregnancy
4. Know common medications used during pregnancy
5. Understand lactation and drug excretion
6. Identify risks of untreated conditions in pregnant women
7. Focus on counseling for pregnant and lactating women
8. Learn regulatory considerations for drug approval
9. Focus on future research needs in this population

Pharmacotherapy in pregnant and lactating women presents unique challenges that require extensive consideration of maternal as well as fetal health. This category of women typically requires adjustment in the dosing of drugs due to physiological changes such as altered drug absorption and metabolism. Keeping in mind the risks of drug exposure during pregnancy, therapeutic requirements are to be weighed against potential undesirable effects on fetal growth by the physicians. For instance, the widely used psychoactive drug, caffeine, is a particular reason for concern; consumption of it leads to detrimental effects in vulnerable populations like pregnant and lactating women, as emphasized in a recent publication that sought to clarify safe levels of caffeine intake (Temple et al., 2017). Additionally, secondary conditions such as urticaria may complicate treatment as the effects of drugs chosen must be in terms of both efficacy and safety to both mother and child (Zuberbier et al., 2021). Therefore, an appreciable understanding of the effects of pharmacologic treatment in such a unique population is necessary to optimize clinical outcomes.

9.3.1. Physiological Changes During Pregnancy

Pregnancy brings about dramatic physiological changes that result in a remarkable impact on drug pharmacokinetics and pharmacodynamics, calling for due consideration in clinical pharmacology. Pregnancy brings about changes in plasma volume, organ function, and metabolism while the body adapts for fetal growth that can modify drug absorption, distribution, metabolism, and elimination. For instance, an increased plasma volume can lead to dilution of drug concentration, thereby necessitating appropriate dosage regimen adjustments to achieve therapeutic effect in pregnant patients. Moreover, application of pharmacometrics modeling, such as population pharmacokinetics (PopPK) and physiologically based pharmacokinetics (PBPK), is an advantageous method to predict drug behavior in this unique population, particularly keeping in mind the ethical considerations in carrying out clinical trials during pregnancy (Chaphekar et al., 2021). The lack of sound clinical evidence only serves to reinforce the need for novel strategies to optimize medication safety and efficacy in pregnancy, and to open the door to improved maternal and fetal outcomes for health (Teede et al., 2018) (Figure 9.10).

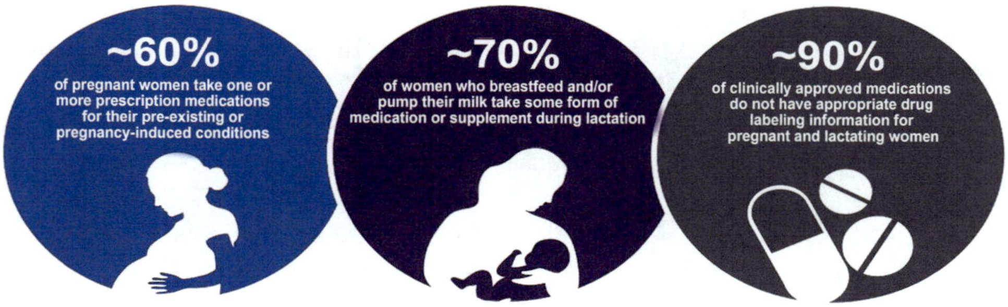
~60%
of pregnant women take one or more prescription medications for their pre-existing or pregnancy-induced conditions
~70%
of women who breastfeed and/or pump their milk take some form of medication or supplement during lactation
~90%
of clinically approved medications do not have appropriate drug labeling information for pregnant and lactating women

Figure 9.10. Pregnancy induces profound physiological changes that significantly impact the pharmacokinetics and pharmacodynamics of medications, necessitating careful consideration in clinical pharmacology.

Source: https://www.ajog.org/cms/10.1016/j.ajog.2021.04.227/asset/7332fc3c-7851-4c8b-95dc-c1f99feeac98/main.assets/gr1_lrg.jpg.

9.3.2. Drug Transfer to the Fetus

The transference of drugs to the fetus during pregnancy represents one of the main issues in clinical pharmacology because it impacts maternal and fetal health directly. The physiological changes present in pregnancy affect the pharmacokinetics as well as the pharmacodynamics of numerous medications, which require the judicious modification of dosing to avoid loss of therapeutic efficacy without creating risks for the developing fetus. Unfortunately, there is minimal data on fetal drug exposure since clinical trials in pregnant patients are morally objectionable. Thus, clinical clinicians have to resort to modeling and simulation methods, such as population pharmacokinetics and PBPK, to make predictions of drug transfer and optimize dosing regimens (Dowell et al., 2022). This emphasizes the urgent need for increased research in this area, particularly with the requirement for pharmacologic treatment of many conditions in pregnant patients with preservation of fetal safety (Dowell et al., 2022). Understanding of drug transfer dynamics is helpful in facilitating well-informed clinical decisions.

9.3.3. Safety and Efficacy of Medications in Pregnancy

The safety and efficacy of pregnancy drugs are critically important topics in clinical pharmacology since maternal well-being has a direct bearing on fetal growth and outcome. Physiological changes of pregnancy can affect the pharmacokinetics of drugs, and hence, tailored therapeutic approaches may need to be implemented to achieve optimal effectiveness with minimum risk. Pregnant females typically have specific problems, since the risk of teratogenic effects of some medications may jeopardize fetal health, caution naturally heightened due to a lack of robust clinical trials done on this population. Further, the treatment strategy for conditions like hidradenitis suppurativa (HS) is also more challenging in pregnant females, with HS possibly aggravating in pregnancy and necessitating an optimal therapeutic action versus maternal-fetal protection. Thus, further research and regulation measures are required to ensure that drugs administered to pregnant women for use are effective and safe and encompass these critical aspects of pharmacotherapy (Chung et al., 2024; Gupta et al., 2025) (Figure 9.11).

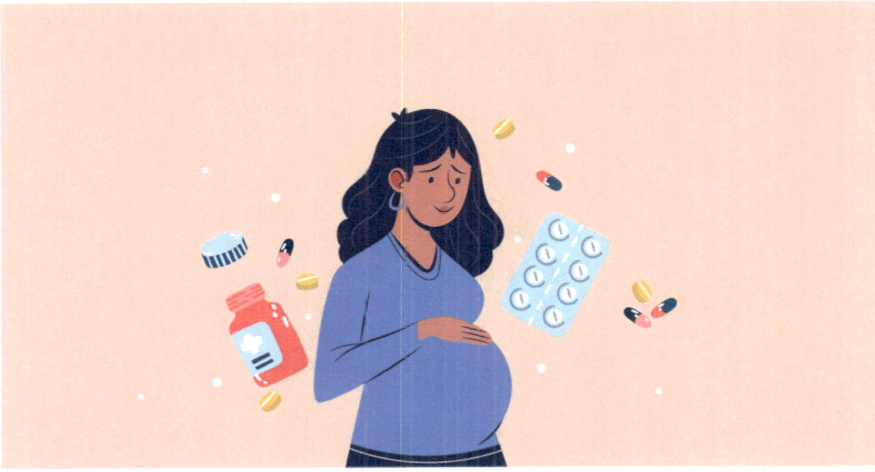

Figure 9.11. The safety and efficacy of medications during pregnancy are critically important considerations in clinical pharmacology, as maternal health directly impacts fetal development and outcomes.

Source: https://mpowerminds.com/assetOLD/images/What-Are-The-Impact-Of-Drug-Use-During-Pregnancy.jpg.

9.3.4. Common Medications used During Pregnancy

The employment of drugs during pregnancy presents unique challenges and complexities, and this makes careful pharmacological management of this exceptional group imperative. Among the usual drugs employed in pregnant patients are acetaminophen for pain and fever, which is overall safe if wisely employed. In contrast, non-steroidal anti-inflammatory agents such as ibuprofen are used with caution due to risks, particularly during the third trimester, whereby they affect fetal cardiovascular function. The problem is extended to medications such as burtons tyrosine kinase inhibitors (BTKis), whose safety profiles must be heavily tested to prevent adverse effects on both mother and fetus (Song et al., 2024). Further, growing insight into the impact of medication on the developing fetus underscores the importance of ongoing research to devise guidelines that ensure efficacy as well as safety at this critical period (Bukvi et al., 2024). This careful balance of benefit and risk is at the core of pharmacological practice in maternal health.

9.3.5. Lactation and Drug Excretion

The intricate interaction between drug excretion and lactation is significant in special population clinical pharmacology, particularly in the maintenance of medication safety in both breastfeeding women and infants. The majority of drugs during lactation are excreted through the breast milk, risking systemic exposure by the nursing infant. It is necessary to understand pharmacokinetic factors such as drug solubility, molecular weight, and protein binding to make an accurate prediction of drug transfer to breast milk. The FDA places a strong emphasis on evidence-based recommendations when prescribing medications to lactating women in addressing their therapeutic needs as well as ensuring the infants' safety (Clark et al., 2011). Furthermore, specific strategies, such as the timing of drug administration during breastfeeding, can reduce infant exposure to potentially toxic drugs.

Safe pharmacotherapy modifications are continually being investigated to balance the vulnerable equilibrium between maternal health and infant safety (Sears, 2013) (Figure 9.12).

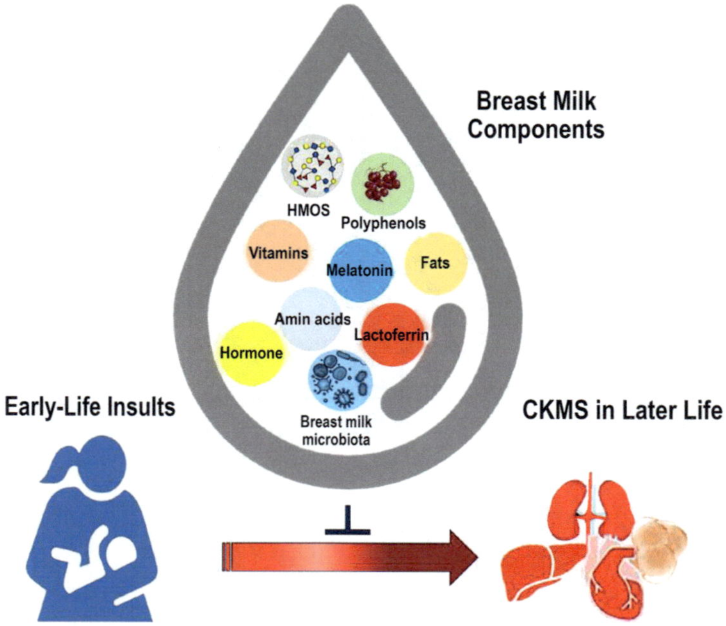

Figure 9.12. The intricate relationship between lactation and drug excretion plays a crucial role in the clinical pharmacology of special populations, particularly in guiding medication safety for breastfeeding mothers and their infants.

Source: https://pub.mdpi-res.com/nutrients/nutrients-17-00995/article_deploy/html/images/nutrients-17-00995-g001.png?1741773671.

9.3.6. Risks of Untreated Conditions in Pregnant Women

Pregnant women with unmanaged medical conditions are exposed to serious hazards compromising maternal and fetal health. Hypertension, gestational diabetes, and infection tend to progress unchecked, leading to severe complications like preeclampsia, preterm delivery, and fetal growth issues. More importantly, the complexities that come with successfully managing such conditions are worsened in the obstetric context, as evidenced in Clark et al., (2011). This accentuates the imperative need for evidence-based pharmacological treatment, specially tailored for pregnant patients. Furthermore, translational toxicology emphasizes the identification of such risks through assessing exposure at vulnerable windows of development, as per (Allen et al., 2013). Such interdisciplinary work strives to enhance further therapeutic strategies that not only treat conditions but also avert harmful health consequences. Lastly, treatment of untreated conditions during pregnancy is required to safeguard the mother's and the developing fetus's health in clinical pharmacology.

9.3.7. Counseling for Pregnant and Lactating Women

The counseling of pregnant and lactating women is an essential aspect of clinical pharmacology since it deals with the specific healthcare needs and potential hazards of drug exposure during this unique physiological status. Pregnant and lactating women require individualized advice regarding pharmacotherapy to avoid adverse effects on maternal health and fetal growth. Extensive counseling should address not only the most common drugs used in pregnancy and lactation but also the impact of environmental toxins, such as lead exposure. Proactive screening and treatment techniques are a crucial part of prenatal care since, according to recently proposed guidelines, lead exposure can have long-term negative consequences on the health of both mothers and infants. (Group CW on Pregnancy and Lead). In addition, evidence-based practice in lead exposure treatment and assessment is paramount in enabling desired health outcomes for such a vulnerable population. Therefore, effective counseling is a cornerstone in ensuring the health and safety of the mothers and their children (Figure 9.13).

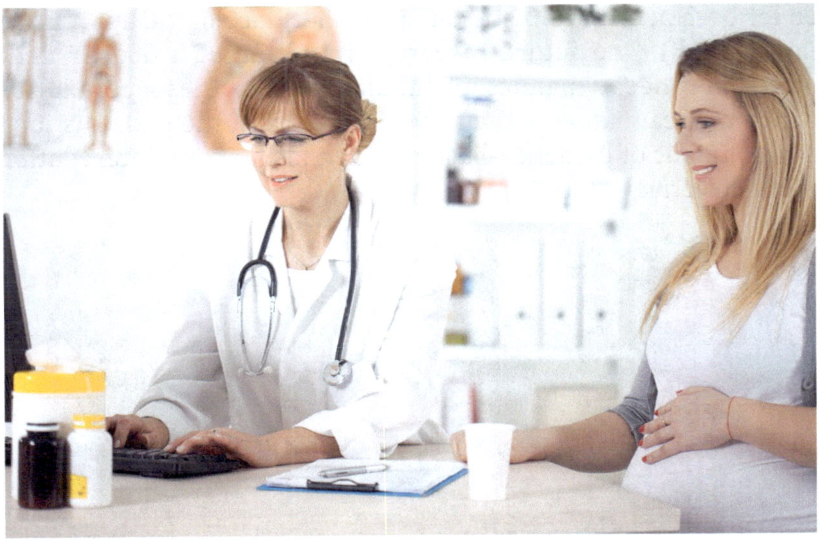

Figure 9.13. The counseling of pregnant and lactating women is a critical aspect of clinical pharmacology, as it encompasses the specific healthcare needs and potential risks associated with medication exposure during this unique physiological state.

Source: https://www.nwhjournal.org/cms/10.1016/j.nwh.2023.12.003/asset/587f56ef-943f-4dfe-90f3-23cfadd27bc5/main.assets/fx1_lrg.jpg.

9.3.8. Regulatory Considerations for Drug Approval

Governing the drug approval process is very difficult in the realm of clinical pharmacology among special populations. As the complexity of drug interactions and the range of physiological responses within such populations becomes more apparent, the methodologies of regulatory authorities will have to change to be able to embrace new information and knowledge. For instance, FDA initiatives to bring prescribing information for longstanding oncology drugs up-to-date are a growing recognition of the need for adaptive labeling processes aligned with current clinical practice, as outlined in Balogh et al., (2019). Similarly, the ethical considerations regarding myopia control therapies in kids highlight that the responsibility to provide safe and effective products rests with all concerned, including regulatory bodies. These evolving considerations are a reflection of the importance of a solid framework in regulatory processes, wherein effective therapy is delivered to all patients, particularly vulnerable ones, based on strong safety and efficacy evidence, as reported in Drove et al., (2019).

9.3.9. Future Research Needs in this Population

In considering future research priorities in special populations, such as neurocritical disease and osteoporosis, an interdisciplinary initiative is required to advance clinical pharmacology. Neuro-critically ill patients possess peculiar metabolic needs that call for discriminatory nutritional supply. Still, as noted earlier, there is an enormous deficit in systematic research into what those dietary requirements are and how they will respond pharmacologically (Kim et al., 2023). In addition to this, the old are also vulnerable to fractures and osteoporosis, and there is enough evidence that emphasizes the need for both pharmacological and non-pharmacological approaches for management and prevention (Fares, 2018). The future research would target a deeper understanding of the pharmacokinetics and pharmacodynamics of medications in these populations and the novel therapeutic approaches that can address their special needs. In the end, this focused research will contribute to the development of evidence-based guidelines, making interventions in these at-risk groups safer and more effective (Figure 9.14).

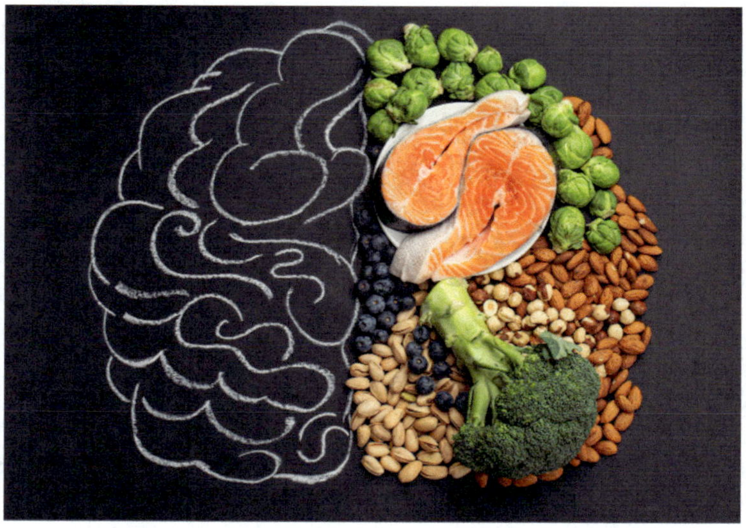

Figure 9.14. Neuro-critically ill patients face unique metabolic challenges that necessitate tailored nutritional interventions.

Source: https://www.elysiumhealthcare.co.uk/neurological/wp-content/uploads/sites/9/2024/05/Nutrition-In-Neurorehabilitation.1.png.

Test Your Knowledge

1. How should drugs be selected during pregnancy to minimize fetal risk?
2. What factors determine the extent of drug excretion into breast milk?

9.4. Patients with Comorbidities

Learning Outcome

1. Give a definition of comorbidities in clinical pharmacology
2. Know the impact of comorbidities on drug metabolism
3. Discuss drug interactions in patients with multiple conditions
4. Tailoring pharmacotherapy for comorbid patients
5. Learn case studies of comorbidity management
6. Discuss the role of interdisciplinary teams in treatment
7. Describe patient education and self-management strategies
8. Identify challenges in clinical trials for comorbid populations
9. Focus on future trends in managing pharmacotherapy for comorbidities

It is crucial in clinical pharmacology to appreciate the subtleties of managing patients with comorbidities since having more than one chronic disease would drastically alter the outcome of the treatment. Such patients might require differential therapeutic strategies to accommodate their unique physiological responses and drug interactions among the concomitant drugs. For instance, the therapeutic pattern of cancer treatment has been altered. Yet, ancient prescribing information remains available for the majority of oncology drugs, posing issues in their optimal application in patients with comorbidities (Balogh et al., 2019). Similarly, for autoimmune conditions like psoriatic arthritis, tumor necrosis factor inhibitors possess erratic pharmacokinetics and, therefore, a strict observation of the overall health of each individual as well as potential immunogenicity must be achieved (Kraft et al., 2017). Compliance with these nuances not only optimizes therapeutic efficacy and patient safety but also provides for a more personalized type of pharmacological treatment, with an emphasis on the importance of comorbidities to clinical judgment.

9.4.1. Definition of Comorbidities in Clinical Pharmacology

Knowing the definition of comorbidities in clinical pharmacology, particularly in observing special populations who usually have one or more diseases or disorders at the same time, is significant. Comorbidities refer to the presence of one or more additional diseases or disorders in addition to those patients with an initial disease that affect the results of pharmacological treatment. For instance, cardiovascular disease patients will also have diabetes, and thus drug interactions and side effects will have to be considered carefully because therapy can differ considerably across these comorbidities.

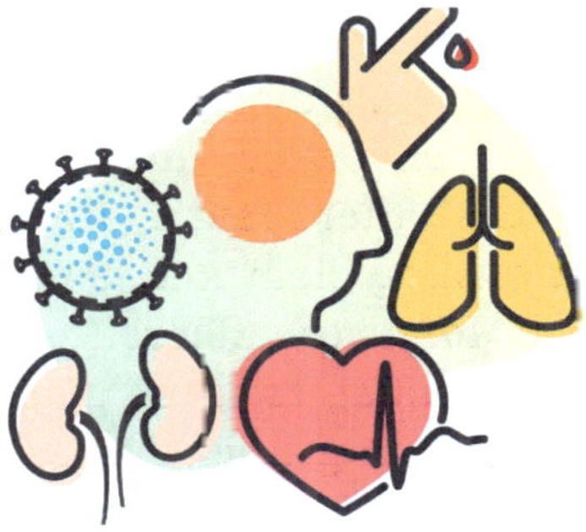

Figure 9.15. Comorbidities refer to the presence of one or more additional disorders or diseases in patients already diagnosed with a primary condition, affecting pharmacological treatment outcomes.

Source: https://www.cancertodaymag.org/wp-content/uploads/2022/06/12-Comorbidity-treating-whole-patient-1500.jpg.

The American College of Cardiology and American Heart Association emphasize that guidelines must assist clinicians in managing several complicated conditions simultaneously in a way that pharmacotherapy is safe and effective (Whelton et al., 2017; Mach et al., 2019). The impact on pharmacodynamics and pharmacokinetics of comorbidities is significant, requiring individualized approaches to drug selection and dosing. This is aimed at optimizing therapeutic response while minimizing adverse effects (Figure 9.15).

9.4.2. Impact of Comorbidities on Drug Metabolism

The interplay between comorbidities and drug metabolism is a significant issue in clinical pharmacology, particularly in special populations. Patients are often encountered with more than one chronic disease, such as diabetes and hypertension, that can significantly alter pharmacodynamics as well as pharmacokinetics. For instance, impairment of the kidney or liver that is usually found among such populations can lead to decreased clearance of drugs, which can cause potential toxicity or reduced therapeutic effect. As stressed by the ESC/EAS Guidelines, physicians must consider the specific health conditions of each patient upon prescribing and ensure that therapeutic strategies are designed concerning their unique needs (Mach et al., 2019). Moreover, adherence to clinical guidelines is essential, as these guidelines are founded on expanding scientific evidence for the complexity of drug interactions in comorbid patients (Cosentino et al., 2019). Therefore, healthcare professionals should be alert to monitoring and changing treatment courses to achieve optimum therapeutic results.

9.4.3. Drug Interactions in Patients with Multiple Conditions

The management of drug interactions in multibed patients is one of the biggest challenges in clinical pharmacology, particularly given the complexity of polypharmacy. As the patient might be on several drugs for various conditions, the risk of unwanted drug interactions rises, necessitating judicious and informed prescribing. Benefits of developments in data integration technology, including the heterogeneous biomedical data such as genomics and lifestyle factors, are significant in understanding these interactions. Clinicians apply integrative strategies for analyzing patients' profiles better, thus estimating the likely drug interactions and setting the optimal therapeutic regimens (Goldenberg et al., 2018). Moreover, organizations like the FDA are also being compelled to update prescribing labels for established oncology drugs with evolving knowledge about drug interactions based on large-scale clinical experience (Balogh et al., 2019). Hence, maximizing our practice of pharmacotherapy in complex patient populations is essential for ensuring safety and efficacy in treatment outcomes (Figure 9.16).

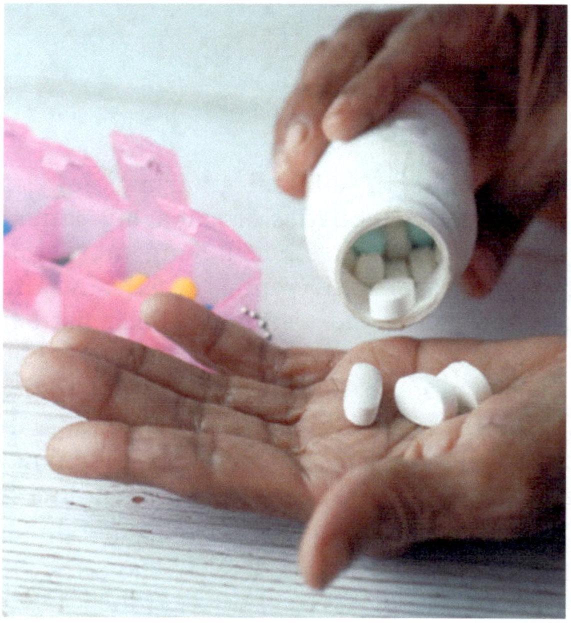

Figure 9.16. The management of drug interactions in patients with multiple conditions poses a significant challenge in clinical pharmacology, particularly when considering the complexity of polypharmacy.

Source: https://www.nia.nih.gov/sites/default/files/2021-08/older-adult-pills.jpg.

9.4.4. Tailoring Pharmacotherapy for Comorbid Patients

Comorbid treatment needs to be treated individually with a multimodal approach to pharmacotherapy that addresses the multifaceted nature of many concomitant diseases. Therapeutic regimens can be pretty complicated with comorbid disease and require close observation for drug interactions and response to drugs. In one study, it was discovered that combined treatment with individualized kinesiotherapy and regular pharmacological therapies resulted in significant clinical improvements in patients with chronic non-specific back pain and comorbid anxiety and depression, emphasizing the importance of individualized interventions (Golovacheva et al., 2024). Also, non-pharmacologic approaches like device therapies and lifestyle modifications are essential in disease management, including heart failure, particularly in special populations who may have unique challenges with a personalized treatment regimen (Dugal et al., 2024). Lastly, an approach involving both pharmacologic and non-pharmacologic factors may enhance patient outcomes and optimize therapeutic efficacy in comorbid patients (Figure 9.17).

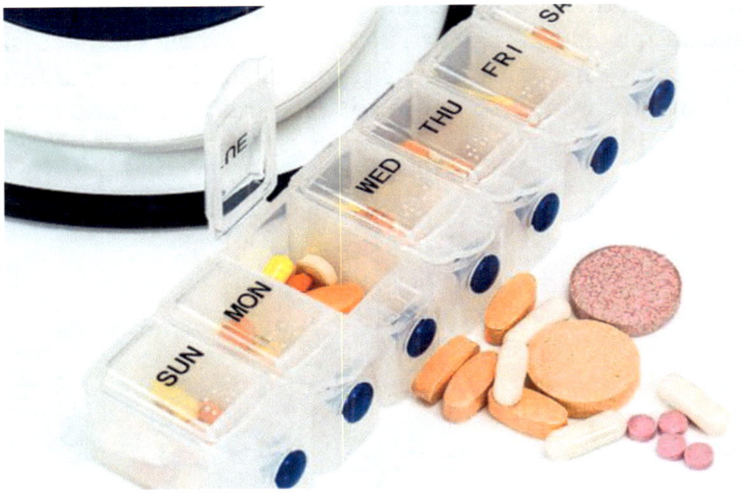

Figure 9.17. Comorbid conditions can significantly complicate treatment regimens, requiring careful consideration of drug interactions and individual patient responses.

Source: https://www.physio-pedia.com/images/thumb/6/64/Tablets_Polypharmacy.jpg/527px-Tablets_Polypharmacy.jpg.

9.4.5. Case Studies of Comorbidity Management

Education on comorbidity management via case studies provides insightful knowledge of clinical pharmacology in vulnerable populations. Case studies give a hint about the complexity of managing a patient with over one, sometimes interrelated, health condition needing a personalized pharmacological intervention to minimize drug interaction and maximize therapeutic effect. For example, managing a patient with both diabetes and hypertension requires judiciously selected antihypertensive medication that has no adverse effects on glucose regulation, and therefore, individually tailored drug therapy becomes a must. Additionally, assessing the use of off-label drugs becomes a necessity because drug control permits physicians to prescribe licensed drugs for off-labeled conditions and with inherent risks (Abbott et al., 2014). As the evidence for such interactions is accumulating, following precise reporting procedures is vital to track outcomes adequately, as emphasized in the study (Celli et al., 2015). Such case studies thus not only indicate practical uses but also highlight the value of evidence-based practice for clinical pharmacology.

9.4.6. Role of Interdisciplinary Teams in Treatment

Interdisciplinary collaboration enhances the efficacy of treatment approaches in clinical pharmacology, particularly in special populations. Multidisciplinary teams of professionals, which usually include doctors, nurses, pharmacists, and social workers, facilitate comprehensive care in managing the complex needs of patients. When managing chronic diseases such as Alzheimer's disease, for instance, collaboration among various healthcare professionals ensures personalized therapeutic intervention and effective monitoring of patient improvement. Alzheimer's prevalence is on the rise, with about 6.7 million Americans aged 65 years and older being affected, and the figure is likely to grow exponentially if innovations are not established. Moreover, interdisciplinary teams hold a key position in the treatment of the compounded issues presented by such diseases, such as management of medication and caregiver support, for which the necessity for the inclusion of a teamwork model in clinics becomes urgent (Lyon et al., 2022). This integrated strategy not only optimizes patient outcomes but also optimizes resource distribution across the spectrum of health (Figure 9.18).

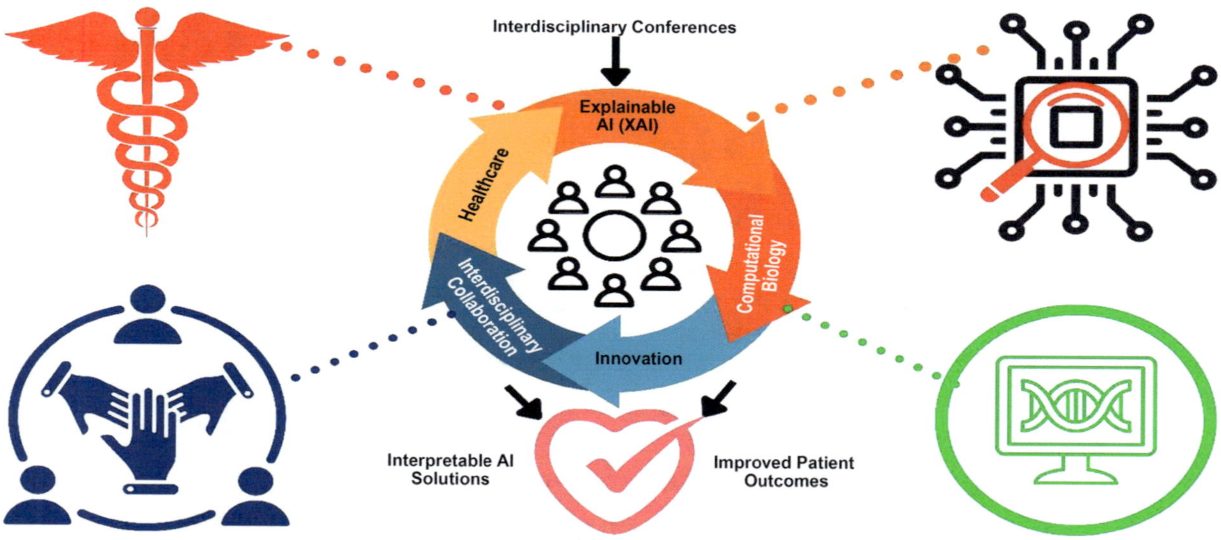

Figure 9.18. The efficacy of treatment approaches in clinical pharmacology, particularly in special populations, is significantly enhanced by the collaboration of interdisciplinary teams.

Source: https://pub.mdpi-res.com/biomedinformatics/biomedinformatics-04-00075/article_deploy/html/images/biomedinformatics-04-00075-ag.png?1716463367.

9.4.7. Patient Education and Self-Management Strategies

In clinical pharmacology, especially in special populations, patient education and self-management strategies are critical in achieving optimal health outcomes. Effective education empowers patients to make informed decisions about their therapy, with increased compliance with pharmacologic therapy and fostering self-care interventions. It is particularly relevant in this regard for vulnerable populations, such as children and the elderly, who may face special difficulties due to varying degrees of comprehension and ability. Strategies for both sharing information about treatment alternatives and the ethics involved in making such decisions are needed. For instance, health care practitioners are required to deal with the ethics of issuing treatments in children, for example, ensuring that parents and children are informed of the risks and benefits of interventions, as highlighted in Drove et al. (2019). Secondly, tailoring education efforts to the specific needs of different patient populations fosters a collaborative relationship between practitioners and patients, as recorded in the University (2018).

9.4.8. Challenges in Clinical Trials for Comorbid Populations

Clinical trials among comorbid populations are especially problematic, and they considerably complicate the measurement of efficacy and safety of drug therapies. One of the most significant difficulties is the heterogeneity of states and symptoms that can conceal drug effects, thereby making it difficult to obtain a clear insight into treatment effects. For example, while assessing ADHD treatment, interactions with numerous co-morbid conditions complicate prioritizing and treating symptoms, as described in Anderson et al. (2016).

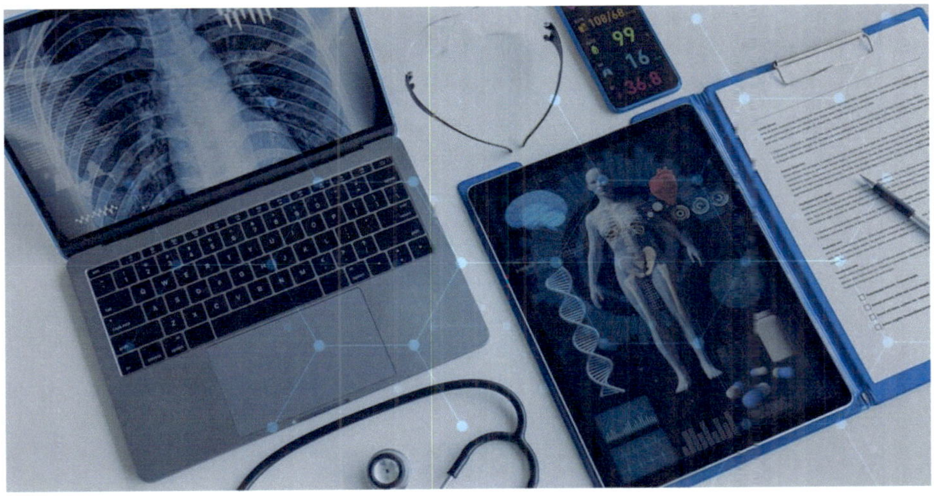

Figure 9.19. Conducting clinical trials within comorbid populations presents significant challenges that complicate the efficacy and safety assessment of pharmacological interventions.

Source: https://www.quanticate.com/hs-fs/hubfs/Therapeutic%20Areas.jpg?width=1042&height=549&name=Therapeutic%20Areas.jpg.

Furthermore, poor measurement tools for emotional and cognitive symptoms also contribute to such complications, hence the need for standard measures that capture the complexity of comorbidities. It has been proven by research that the lack of validated measures in determining cognitive impairment in mood disorders affects trial validity to a large degree, making it necessary to develop new assessment tools to optimize outcome monitoring and treatment effectiveness in these vulnerable populations, as testified by the outcome of Berent et al., (2007) (Figure 9.19).

9.4.9. Future Trends in Managing Pharmacotherapy for Comorbidities

As healthcare systems evolve to address the issue of treating patients with comorbidities, future pharmacotherapy will concentrate on patient-tailored medicine and combined care models. The trends will capitalize on the innovative science of pharmacogenomics to modify medication regimens based on the individual genetic profile of the patient, ultimately optimizing the effectiveness of treatment with minimal side effects. Furthermore, addressing the issues of polypharmacy, or the concomitant use of more than one drug, will become ever more fundamental to the future of health care as this diagnosis persists on an upward trajectory in different groups (Anmolsingh et al., 2017). Initiatives to improve medication adherence in patients, through the development of combination therapies and the application of digital health technologies, will also become increasingly fundamental to achieving favorable health outcomes. Notably, determinants of nonadherence, particularly in those with cardiovascular comorbidities, will assist clinicians in maximizing treatment adherence and healthcare spending management (Halava et al., 2016).

Test Your Knowledge

1. How can drug-drug and drug-disease interactions be minimized in these patients?
2. What role does clinical pharmacology play in designing individualized treatment plans for patients with comorbidities?

Summary

Clinical practice in pharmacology demands an adaptive approach that is sensitive to special needs of special groups, including children, the elderly, and patients with specific health conditions. An understanding of the principles of pharmacokinetics and pharmacodynamics influencing drug behavior in these groups is crucial for maximum therapeutic benefit. For instance, oncology drugs used extensively are often burdened with older labeling that motivates initiatives like the FDAs pilot program to enhance prescribing information in light of new clinical evidence (Balogh et al., 2019). Moreover, optimal control of diseases like peritoneal dialysis (PD)-associated peritonitis best demonstrates the evidence-based dosing practice imperative. The empiricism of vancomycin dosage with automated PD indicates the limitations of clinical understanding and the requirement for research to provide evidence-based pharmacologic decision-making (Kraft et al., 2020). By surmounting these issues, healthcare practitioners are able to deliver more efficient, safe, and personalized patient care in various clinical settings.

In studying clinical pharmacology in special populations, there are interesting findings that underscore the complexities of drug treatment in these populations. One such finding is the profound impact of physiological changes brought about by treatments such as ECMO on drug pharmacokinetics, resulting in differing drug efficacy or increased side effects, as documented for various medications (Aebi et al., 2017). In addition, cannabinoids represent another area of interest, i.e., cannabidiol (CBD), which is already reported to exhibit antiepileptic activity in children. CBD's low oral bioavailability and significant metabolism variations with or without food complicate its dosing and therapeutic effect (Albini et al., 2020). These findings highlight the need for customized pharmacotherapeutics and more clinical trials to ensure the safe and effective therapy of drugs in special populations to ultimately improve patient outcomes.

KEY TERMS FROM THIS CHAPTER

- Affordability
- Analgesics
- Clinical decision-making
- Composition
- Drug administration
- Drug errors
- Geriatric pharmacology
- Hidradenitis suppurativa (HS)
- Marketing
- Mounting pressure
- Age
- Children
- Comorbidities
- Dried blood spot methods
- Drug clearance
- Drug metabolism
- Guardians
- Lactating women
- Monoclonal antibodies
- Myopia

CRITICAL THINKING QUESTIONS

1. **Which of the following factors most affects drug dosing in neonates and infants?**
   a. Increased gastric acidity
   b. Decreased body water content
   c. Immature liver and kidney function
   d. Rapid gastric emptying
2. **Why do neonates often require different drug dosages compared to adults?**
   a. They metabolize drugs more quickly
   b. They have reduced protein binding and immature enzyme systems
   c. Their body fat is significantly higher than in adults
   d. Their blood-brain barrier is fully developed
3. **Which pharmacokinetic change is commonly seen in elderly patients?**
   a. Increased renal clearance
   b. Increased hepatic metabolism
   c. Decreased glomerular filtration rate (GFR)
   d. Increased total body water
4. **Why is polypharmacy a concern in geriatric pharmacology?**
   a. Older adults metabolize drugs faster
   b. It increases adherence to therapy
   c. It reduces the chances of drug-drug interactions
   d. It increases the risk of adverse drug reactions
5. **Which of the following is true regarding drug use in pregnancy?**
   a. All drugs are safe in the first trimester
   b. Drug metabolism is decreased during pregnancy
   c. The placenta acts as a complete barrier to drugs
   d. Certain drugs can cross the placenta and affect fetal development

Answers to Critical Thinking Questions

1. (c); 2. (b); 3. (c); 4. (d); 5. (d).

Short Answer Questions

1. How does the immaturity of liver and kidney function affect drug metabolism and elimination in neonates and infants?
2. What are the common pharmacokinetic changes seen in elderly patients?
3. How does pregnancy alter drug absorption, distribution, metabolism, and excretion?
4. How do multiple chronic conditions affect drug selection and dosing in patients with comorbidities?
5. What are the risks associated with polypharmacy in patients with complex medical histories?
6. Which population is most vulnerable to adverse drug reactions due to altered pharmacokinetics and pharmacodynamics?

References

1. Abbott, R., & Ayres, I. (2014). Evidence and extrapolation: Mechanisms for regulating off-label uses of drugs and devices. https://core.ac.uk/download/62566275.pdf (accessed on 10th June 2025).
2. Efferth, T., Banerjee, M., Abu-Darwish, M. S., Abdelfatah, S., Böckers, M., Bhakta-Guha, D., Bolzani, V., Daak, S., Demirezer, Ö. L., Dawood, M., Efferth, M., El-Seedi, H. R., Fischer, N., Greten, H. J., Hamdoun, S., Hong, C., Horneber, M., Kadioglu, O., Khalid, H. E., . . . Paul, N. W. (2018). Biopiracy versus One-World Medicine–From colonial relicts to global collaborative concepts. *Phytomedicine*, *53*, 319–331. https://doi.org/10.1016/j.phymed.2018.06.007Acurcio, F., Alkan, A., Brzezinska, A., Bucsics, A., et al. (2014). Are new models needed to optimize the utilization of new medicines to sustain healthcare systems? https://core.ac.uk/download/29181808.pdf (accessed on 10th June 2025).
3. Aebi, M., Shah, A. G., Anderson, M., Arlt, W., Barr, J., Barthelemy, R., Beiderlinden, M., et al. (2017). Medication complications in extracorporeal membrane oxygenation. https://core.ac.uk/download/129191716.pdf (accessed on 10th June 2025).
4. Akkerman, O. W., Alffenaar, J. W. C., Bolhuis, M. S., Hofman, T. J., et al. (2015). Role of therapeutic drug monitoring in pulmonary infections: Use and potential for expanded use of dried blood spot samples. https://core.ac.uk/download/55746955.pdf (accessed on 10th June 2025).
5. Albini, M., Cifelli, P., Di Bonaventura, C., Fanella, M., Giallonardo, A. T., Morano, A., & Palma, E. (2020). Cannabinoids in the treatment of epilepsy: Current status and future prospects. https://core.ac.uk/download/322821374.pdf (accessed on 10th June 2025).
6. Alffenaar, J. W., Cirillo, D. M., Dooley, K. E., Gumbo, T., et al. (2020). Integrating pharmacokinetics and pharmacodynamics in operational research to end tuberculosis. https://core.ac.uk/download/348665305.pdf (accessed on 10th June 2025).
7. Allegaert, K. M., van den Anker, J. N., van Hasselt, J. G. C., Knibbe, C. A. J., et al. (2017). Evidence-based drug treatment for special patient populations through model-based approaches. https://core.ac.uk/download/154412980.pdf (accessed on 10th June 2025).
8. Allen, D., Hughes, C., Obasanjo, I., et al. (2013). *Translational Toxicology: A Developmental Focus for Integrated Research Strategies*. https://core.ac.uk/download/235420438.pdf (accessed on 10th June 2025).
9. Almarsdottir, A. B., Benkő, R., Bennie, M., et al. (2024). *Introduction to Drug Utilization Research*. https://core.ac.uk/download/653281138.pdf (accessed on 10th June 2025).
10. Amos, L. B., Afolabi-Brown, O., Gault, D., Lloyd, R. M., Prero, M. Y., Rosen, C., Malhotra, R., et al. (2022). Age and weight considerations for the use of continuous positive airway pressure therapy in pediatric populations: An American Academy of Sleep Medicine position statement. *Journal of Clinical Sleep Medicine*. https://www.semanticscholar.org/paper/30e317b65e48fe26c4fbc4dea56f04a42e91ecd8 (accessed on 10th June 2025).
11. Anderson, R. H., & Mattingly, G. W. (2016). *Optimizing Outcomes in ADHD Treatment: From Clinical Targets to Novel Delivery Systems*. https://core.ac.uk/download/80495103.pdf (accessed on 10th June 2025).
12. Anmolsingh, R., Cornejo, K., Feldman, J., et al. (2017). *Dangers of Polypharmacy*. https://core.ac.uk/download/322431183.pdf (accessed on 10th June 2025).

13. Anvisa, Castaneda-Hernandez, et al. (2018). *Quality, Non-Clinical and Clinical Considerations for Biosimilar Monoclonal Antibody Development: EU, WHO, USA, Canada, and BRICS-TM Regulatory Guidelines*. https://core.ac.uk/download/287581236.pdf (accessed on 10th June 2025).

14. Balogh, E. P., Bindman, A. B., Eckhardt, S. G., Halabi, S., et al. (2019). *Challenges and Opportunities to Updating Prescribing Information for Longstanding Oncology Drugs*. https://core.ac.uk/download/286362252.pdf (accessed on 10th June 2025).

15. Bennett, W. E., Jr. (2016). *Quantitative Risk-Benefit Analysis of Probiotic Use for Irritable Bowel Syndrome and Inflammatory Bowel Disease*. https://core.ac.uk/download/46963153.pdf (accessed on 10th June 2025).

16. Berent, S., Bieliauskas, L. A., Caveney, A. F., Giordani, B., et al. (2007). *The Sensitivity and Psychometric Properties of a Brief Computer-Based Cognitive Screening Battery in A Depression Clinic*. https://core.ac.uk/download/213067709.pdf (accessed on 10th June 2025).

17. Bertoncello, F., Carron, M., & Ieppariello, G. (2017). Profile of sugammadex for reversal of neuromuscular blockade in the elderly: Current perspectives. *Core*. https://core.ac.uk/download/158825140.pdf (accessed on 10th June 2025).

18. Borbon Chavez, C. L., Becerra Macias, A. M., Armenta Bárcenas, C. del R., & Soqui Molina, A. I. (2023). Special considerations in pediatrics for rapid intubation sequence. *International Journal of Medical Science and Clinical Research Studies*. https://www.semanticscholar.org/paper/c481b918156c7c5fd69b0c7efdd5fd080f7aa476 (accessed on 10th June 2025).

19. Brown, J. D., Rivera Rivera, K. J., Crespo Hernandez, L. Y., Doenges, M. R., Auchey, I., Pham, T., & Goodin, A. (2021). Natural and synthetic cannabinoids: Pharmacology, uses, adverse drug events, and drug interactions. *The Journal of Clinical Pharmacology, 61*. https://doi.org/10.1002/jcph.1871.

20. Campo, C., García-Bea, A., Kim, C., Leal, S., et al. (2021). *Application of a Dual Mechanistic Approach to Support Bilastine Dose Selection for Older Adults*. https://core.ac.uk/download/547407070.pdf (accessed on 10th June 2025).

21. CDC Work Group on Lead and Pregnancy. (2025). *Guidelines for the Identification and Management of Lead Exposure in Pregnant and Lactating Women*. https://core.ac.uk/download/144198145.pdf (accessed on 10th June 2025).

22. Celli, B., Metzdorf, N., Miravitlles, M., Price, D., et al. (2015). Comorbidities of patients in tiotropium clinical trials: Comparison with observational studies of patients with chronic obstructive pulmonary disease. https://core.ac.uk/download/30435638.pdf (accessed on 10th June 2025).

23. Chaphekar, N., Dodeja, P., Shaik, I. H., Caritis, S. N., & Venkataramanan, R. (2021). Maternal-fetal pharmacology of drugs: A review of current status of the application of physiologically based pharmacokinetic models. *Frontiers in Pediatrics, 9*. https://doi.org/10.3389/fped.2021.733823.

24. Chatterjee, D., Gillman, G., Harari, D., Iliffe, S., et al. (2017). *Health Risk Appraisal in Older People 7: Long-Acting Benzodiazepine Use in Community-Dwelling Older Adults in London: Is It Related to Physical or Psychological Factors?* https://core.ac.uk/download/79558304.pdf (accessed on 10th June 2025).

25. Chung, C. S., Park, S. E., Hsiao, J. L., & Lee, K. H. (2024). A review of hidradenitis suppurativa in special populations: Considerations in children, pregnant and breastfeeding women, and the elderly. *Dermatology and Therapy, 14*, 2407–2425. https://www.semanticscholar.org/pa

per/57067b16b1bfc1dbfc7be4f62caf08387b1dca55 (accessed on 10th June 2025).

26. Clark, S. M., Denne, S. C., Easterling, T., Feibus, K., et al. (2011). *Pharmacotherapy and pregnancy: Highlights from the Third International Conference for Individualized Pharmacotherapy in Pregnancy*. https://core.ac.uk/download/62436354.pdf (accessed on 10th June 2025).

27. Cosentino, F., Grant, P. J., Aboyans, V., Bailey, C. J., Ceriello, A., Delgado, V., Federici, M., et al. (2019). 2019 ESC guidelines on diabetes, pre-diabetes, and cardiovascular diseases developed in collaboration with the EASD. *European Heart Journal, 41*, 255–323. https://doi.org/10.1093/eurheartj/ehz486.

28. Coté, C. J., & Wilson, S. (2019). Guidelines for monitoring and management of pediatric patients before, during, and after sedation for diagnostic and therapeutic procedures. *Pediatrics, 143*(6), e20191000. https://doi.org/10.1542/peds.2019-1000.

29. Dowell, D., Ragan, K., Jones, C. M., Baldwin, G., & Chou, R. (2022). CDC clinical practice guideline for prescribing opioids for pain—United States, 2022. *MMWR Recommendations and Reports, 71*, 1–95. https://doi.org/10.15585/mmwr.rr7103a1.

30. Drove, B., Gifford, K. L., Gonzalez-Meijome, J. M., Gray, S., et al. (2019). *IMI–Industry Guidelines and Ethical Considerations for Myopia Control Report*. https://core.ac.uk/download/293867276.pdf (accessed on 10th June 2025).

31. Dugal, J., Malhi, A., Ramazani, N., Yee, B., DiCaro, M. V., & Lei, K. (2024). Non-pharmacological therapy in heart failure and management of heart failure in special populations—A review. *Journal of Clinical Medicine, 13*. https://www.semanticscholar.org/paper/42b7c81b00125e01edb0c2f881eae13e89ed6af2 (accessed on 10th June 2025).

32. Fares, A. (2018). Pharmacological and non-pharmacological means for prevention of fractures among elderly. *International Journal of Preventive Medicine, 9*. https://www.semanticscholar.org/paper/8c30418f3e4657d524fac643acae0c45936afc32 (accessed on 10th June 2025).

33. Goldenberg, A., Hoffman, M. M., Leskovec, J., Nguyen, T., et al. (2018). Machine learning for integrating data in biology and medicine: Principles, practice, and opportunities. *arXiv*. http://arxiv.org/abs/1807.00123 (accessed on 10th June 2025).

34. Golovacheva, A. A., & Golovacheva, V. (2024). Complex treatment of patients with chronic non-specific back pain and comorbid disorders: A prospective clinical study. *Neurology, Neuropsychiatry, Psychosomatics*. https://www.semanticscholar.org/paper/85233582d67dca22da1cee9bd7c595994ca39a66 (accessed on 10th June 2025).

35. Gupta, K., & Sahu, K. K. (2025). Evaluating the safety and efficacy of pediatric medications: A comprehensive review of pharmacological interventions in children. *Journal of Neonatal Surgery*. https://www.semanticscholar.org/paper/02661d2c2ec7584949d887bbade28bae11739cae (accessed on 10th June 2025).

36. Halava, H. (2016). *Statin Adherence, Utilization, And Prescribing Patterns: Improving Effectiveness of Treatment* [Doctoral dissertation, University of Eastern Finland]. CORE. https://core.ac.uk/download/198003082.pdf (accessed on 10th June 2025).

37. Hurst, D., Padilla, L., Merlocco, A., Rodger, D., Bobier, C., Gray, W. H., Sorabella, R. A., et al. (2024). Pediatric cardiac xenotransplantation: Recommendations for the ethical design of clinical trials. *Transplantation, 108*, e292–e300. https://www.semanticscholar.org/paper/6eb967c97a231fffc2ec7d6d4ea671ee6dc8f0ad (accessed on 10th June 2025).

38. Kazan, J., & Gebara, M. A. (2021). Geriatric considerations for collaborative care for depression in rural populations. *Journal of the American Geriatrics Society, 70*. https://www.semanticscholar.org/paper/f335b7eb5fe71af1850157c95c6252d7d7a9ddea (accessed on 10th June 2025).

39. Khajuria, N., Menia, N., & Gupta, S. (2024). A prospective, observational study on adverse drug reactions in hospitalized pediatric cancer patients in a tertiary care teaching hospital. *Journal of Pharmacy & Bioallied Sciences, 16*, S3167–S3169. https://www.semanticscholar.org/paper/4b6f5dc242fa1ba96bed124cf1f0d790acdb66da (accessed on 10th June 2025).

40. Khosa, J. K., Louie, S., Lobo Moreno, P., Abramov, D., Rogstad, D. K., Alismail, A., Matus, M., et al. (2023). Asthma care in the elderly: Practical guidance and challenges for clinical management—A framework of 5 "Ps." *Journal of Asthma and Allergy, 16*, 33–43. https://www.semanticscholar.org/paper/4da61fc4788a7db3f26a1780f579f165411a216c (accessed on 10th June 2025).

41. Kim, J. H., Choo, Y. H., Kim, M., Jeon, H., Jung, H. W., Ha, E. J., Oh, J., et al. (2023). Neurocritical care nutrition: Unique considerations and strategies for optimizing energy supply and metabolic support in critically ill patients. *Journal of Neurointensive Care*. https://www.semanticscholar.org/paper/460c5b863fe4893171943d636b814064ef95f54e (accessed on 10th June 2025).

42. Kitsiou, A., Caforio, A. L. P., Porta-Sanchez, A., Vahanian, A., Iung, B., Carrera, C., Szymanski, C., et al. (2013). ESC core curriculum for the general cardiologist (2013). https://core.ac.uk/download/55756305.pdf (accessed on 10th June 2025).

43. Kljaic Bukvic, B., Kuzmanić Šamija, R., & Šegulja, S. (2024). Primjena ibuprofena u pedijatrijskoj populaciji. *Pediatric Croatica*. https://www.semanticscholar.org/paper/4448d36b64fd70576116cad97d0290e56d00a164 (accessed on 10th June 2025).

44. Kolbin, A., & Emelianova, L. (2023). Ethical issues in pediatric clinical trials. *Медицинская этика*. https://www.semanticscholar.org/paper/9d86b58fd4045dc6cd8ba64868fff7983d902ac9 (accessed on 10th June 2025).

45. Kraft, W. K., Lam, E., Lien, Y. T. K., Piraino, T., et al. (2020). Vancomycin in peritoneal dialysis: Clinical pharmacology considerations in therapy. CORE. https://core.ac.uk/download/322850154.pdf (accessed on 10th June 2025).

46. Kraft, W. K., Mantravadi, S., & Ogdie, A. (2017). Tumor necrosis factor inhibitors in psoriatic arthritis. CORE. https://core.ac.uk/download/83049994.pdf (accessed on 10th June 2025).

47. LeQuang, J., Bisney, J., Coluzzi, F., et al. (2018). *Gabapentin Use Disorder: Update for Clinicians*. https://core.ac.uk/download/188831513.pdf (accessed on 10th June 2025).

48. Lyon, A. R., López-Fernández, T., Couch, L. S., Asteggiano, R., Aznar, M. C., Bergler-Klein, J., Boriani, G., et al. (2022). 2022 ESC guidelines on cardio-oncology developed in collaboration with the European Hematology Association (EHA), the European Society for Therapeutic Radiology and Oncology (ESTRO) and the International Cardio-Oncology Society (IC-OS). *European Heart Journal, 43*, 4229–4361. https://doi.org/10.1093/eurheartj/ehac244.

49. Mach, F., Baigent, C., Catapano, A. L., Koskinas, K. C., Casula, M., Badimón, L., Chapman, M. J., et al. (2019). 2019 ESC/EAS guidelines for the management of dyslipidemias: Lipid modification to reduce cardiovascular risk. *European Heart Journal, 41*, 111–188. https://doi.org/10.1093/eurheartj/ehz455.

50. Madkhali, N. A. M., Alsomali, M. D. Y., Al-Dosari, Y. N. M., ALHarbi, S. T. A., ALRUWAILI, S. T. F., Alahdal, A. A. M., Almutiri, G. H. D., et al. (2024). A comprehensive multidisciplinary strategy for the management of musculoskeletal fractures throughout pregnancy: Evaluation, treatment, and maternal-fetal considerations. *Journal of Eco Humanism*. https://www.semanticscholar.org/paper/1fadbcf125a68de23b44a434dd67281b5ece527b (accessed on 10th June 2025).

51. Manjhi, P., Singh, M. P., & Kumar, M. (2024). Causality, severity, preventability and predictability assessments scales for adverse drug reactions: A review. *Cureus, 16*. https://www.semanticscholar.org/paper/528a7724f172a7e1a80325e972a60fac7d66d011 (accessed on 10th June 2025).

52. Massaro, A. N., Fletcher, E., Madabushi, R., Baer, G., & Green, D. (2025). A pediatric research imperative: Addressing neonates in drug development through understanding neonatal clinical pharmacology. *The Journal of Pediatric Pharmacology and Therapeutics, 30*(1), 8–16. https://www.semanticscholar.org/paper/13b4ddb89440e777ac68456eb7e4f86da2dc7b0c (accessed on 10th June 2025).

53. McCrory, P., Meeuwisse, W., Aubry, M., Cantu, R. C., Dvořák, J., Echemendía, R. J., Engebretsen, L., et al. (2013). Consensus statement on concussion in sport: The 4th International Conference on Concussion in Sport, Zurich, November 2012. *Journal of Athletic Training, 48*, 554–575. https://doi.org/10.4085/1062-6050-48.4.05.

54. Mueller, G. (2010). Personalized prognosis and diagnosis of type 2 diabetes—Vision or fiction? https://core.ac.uk/download/16432285.pdf (accessed on 10th June 2025).

55. Pepper, G. A., & Robbins, L. J. (1987). *Improving Geriatric Drug Therapy*. CORE. https://core.ac.uk/download/276285896.pdf (accessed on 10th June 2025).

56. Schuurman, A., Haycox, A., Bybau, A., Bucsics, A., Martin, A., Godman, B., et al. (2016). Payers' views of the changes arising through the possible adoption of adaptive pathways. https://core.ac.uk/download/77034413.pdf (accessed on 10th June 2025).

57. Sears, M. E. (2013). Chelation: Harnessing and enhancing heavy metal detoxification—A review. https://core.ac.uk/download/208557213.pdf (accessed on 10th June 2025).

58. Song, Z., Jiang, D., Yu, L., Chen, Y., Zhou, D., Li, Y., Wu, D., et al. (2024). Evidence-based expert consensus on clinical management of safety of Bruton's tyrosine kinase inhibitors (2024). *Chinese Journal of Cancer Research, 36*(3), 240–256. https://www.semanticscholar.org/paper/f8afc088b55284cf8d38fe9249925031dcd978c7 (accessed on 10th June 2025).

59. Teede, H., Misso, M., Costello, M., Dokras, A., Laven, J. S. E., Moran, L., Piltonen, T., et al. (2018). Recommendations from the international evidence-based guideline for the assessment and management of polycystic ovary syndrome. *Clinical Endocrinology, 89*, 251–268. https://doi.org/10.1111/cen.13795.

60. Temple, J. L., Bernard, C., Lipshultz, S. E., Czachor, J., Westphal, J., & Mestre, M. A. (2017). The safety of ingested caffeine: A comprehensive review. *Frontiers in Psychiatry, 8*, Article 80. https://doi.org/10.3389/fpsyt.2017.00080.

61. Terzic, A., & Waldman, S. A. (2019). *Health Care Evolves from Reactive to Proactive*. CORE. https://core.ac.uk/download/213444739.pdf (accessed on 10th June 2025).

62. Umehara, K., Parrott, N., Schindler, E., Legras, V., & Meneses-Lorente, G. (2024). PBPK modeling of entrectinib and its active metabolite to derive dose adjustments in pediatric

populations co-administered with CYP3A4 inhibitors. *Clinical Pharmacology & Therapeutics, 116*. https://www.semanticscholar.org/paper/9f16835436898f45be19eb9e826e9be05bf9b67b (accessed on 10th June 2025).

63. van Dijk, M., Goulooze, S. C., van der Graaf, P. H., Hankemeier, T., et al. (2017). *Towards Personalized Treatment of Pain Using a Quantitative Systems Pharmacology Approach*. https://core.ac.uk/download/154420864.pdf (accessed on 10th June 2025).
64. Venkatakrishnan, K., & Benincosa, L. J. (2021). Diversity and inclusion in drug development: Rethinking intrinsic and extrinsic factors with patient centricity. *Clinical Pharmacology & Therapeutics, 112*, 204–207. https://doi.org/10.1002/cpt.2416.
65. Virginia Commonwealth University. (2018). *Virginia Commonwealth University professional bulletin*. CORE. https://core.ac.uk/download/215485746.pdf (accessed on 10th June 2025).
66. von Hentig, N. (2012). *Personalizing HIV Therapy, Mission Impossible?* CORE. https://core.ac.uk/download/17028337.pdf (accessed on 10th June 2025).
67. Whelton, P. K., Carey, R. M., Aronow, W. S., Casey, D. E., Collins, K. J., Dennison Himmelfarb, C., DePalma, S. M., et al. (2017). 2017 ACC/AHA/AAPA/ABC/ACPM/AGS/APhA/ASH/ASPC/NMA/PCNA guideline for the prevention, detection, evaluation, and management of high blood pressure in adults: A report of the American College of Cardiology/American Heart Association Task Force on Clinical Practice Guidelines. *Hypertension, 71*. https://doi.org/10.1161/hyp.0000000000000065.
68. Zampieri, F. (2018). *Rise and fall of Achille De Giovanni's Clinical Anthropometry*. CORE. https://core.ac.uk/download/157767229.pdf (accessed on 10th June 2025).
69. Zuberbier, T., Abdul Latiff, A. H., Abuzakouk, M., Aquilina, S., Asero, R., Baker, D. R., Ballmer-Weber, B., et al. (2021). The international EAACI/GA^{2}LEN/EuroGuiDerm/APAAACI guideline for the definition, classification, diagnosis, and management of urticaria. *Allergy, 77*, 734–766. https://doi.org/10.1111/all.15090.
70. Zur, R. (2023). Protected from harm, harmed by protection: Ethical consequences of the exclusion of pregnant participants from clinical trials. *Research Ethics, 19*, 536–545. https://www.semanticscholar.org/paper/807180a8277a4c398b97fd696744cbc4d251088c (accessed on 10th June 2025).

PHARMACOGENETICS AND PHARMACOGENOMICS

10

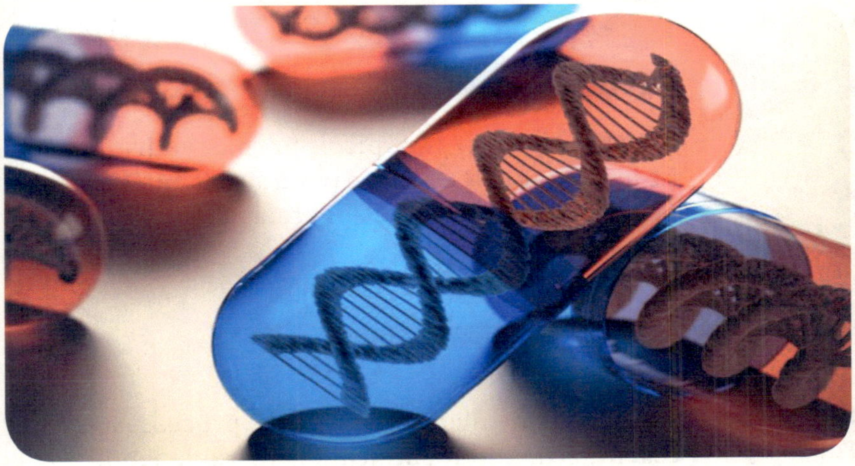

LEARNING OBJECTIVES

After studying this chapter, you will be able to:

1. Know the science of pharmacogenetics
2. Explain pharmacogenomics and drug development
3. Discuss clinical applications of pharmacogenetics and pharmacogenomics
4. Focus on ethical, legal, and social implications

Introduction

The advent of pharmacogenetics and pharmacogenomics is a milestone in the history of personalized medicine, founded on the understanding of individual genetic variations influencing drug efficacy and response. The discipline builds upon the foundation laid by the Human Genome Project, which established a genomic map for personalized treatment. As precision medicine advances, patients will be stratified into specific subgroups based on their genetic profiles to deliver more targeted clinical benefits (Wang et al., 2023). The integration of such genetic information into clinical practice has the potential to revolutionize treatment protocols, especially in oncology, where breakthroughs in pharmacogenomics have entered decision support systems that render prescribing more precise among healthcare professionals (Dodson et al., 2022). The chapter will explore further the implications of these fields, keeping in mind how they not only improve therapeutic outcomes but also minimize adverse drug effects.

10.1. The Science of Pharmacogenetics

Learning Outcome

1. Understand mechanisms of drug metabolism
2. Explain genetic polymorphisms and their effects
3. Discuss the role of enzymes in drug response
4. Learn case studies of pharmacogenetic variations
5. Know the impact of pharmacogenetics on drug efficacy
6. Explain pharmacogenetic testing methods
7. Discuss ethical considerations in pharmacogenetics
8. Know limitations of pharmacogenetic research
9. Understand future directions in pharmacogenetics

The science of pharmacogenetics moves to the forefront in creating tailored medication by identifying how genetic variation influences various individuals' reactions to drugs. By researching how an individual's genetic makeup is associated with his or her response to therapy, pharmacogenetics makes therapy more tailored, which will likely enhance the rate of efficacy while lowering side effects. Recent developments in pharmacogenomics have broadened this field, shifting from singular gene-drug interactions to the holistic perception that unites several -omics fields, including proteomics and metabolomics (Wée et al., 2023). The therapeutic implications for drug development are profound; as personalized medicine becomes more prevalent, regulatory bodies like the FDA increasingly license drugs by genetic biomarkers, showing more incorporation of pharmacogenomics into clinical practice (Senn, 2021). Widespread advances notwithstanding, it remains challenging to prove pharmacogenetic markers in diverse populations, necessitating ongoing research and collaboration in the healthcare community (Figure 10.1).

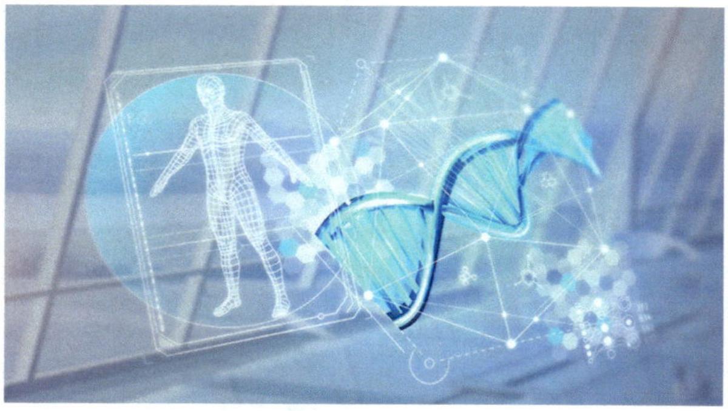

Figure 10.1. Pharmacogenetics.

Source: https://hospitalpharmacyeurope.com/wp-content/uploads/2024/02/Pharmacogenetics-What-pharmacists-need-to-know.jpg.

10.1.1. Mechanisms of Drug Metabolism

The study of drug metabolism processes is essential in the identification of explanations for differences in drug response among individuals, particularly in pharmacogenetics and pharmacogenomics. Drug metabolism refers to the process of biochemical transformations in drugs, primarily occurring within the liver. It can be classified into two main phases: phase I reactions, which include oxidation and reduction, and phase II conjugative reactions, which involve the excretion of metabolites. Genetic variation in enzymes that are implicated in such metabolic pathways can have a tremendous influence both on the efficacy and toxicity of drugs administered to patients. For instance, polymorphisms of cytochrome P450 enzymes can alter drug activation and clearance, leading to side effects or therapeutic failure, especially in chemotherapy drugs such as those for chemotherapy-induced nausea and vomiting (CINV) (Sugino et al., 2015). These genetic determinants are crucial for personalized medicine, enabling healthcare professionals to tailor drug therapies and achieve maximum therapeutic benefits with minimal side effects (Shivashankara, 2020).

10.1.2. Genetic Polymorphisms and Their Effects

Genetic polymorphisms play a critical role in pharmacogenomics and pharmacogenetics since these variations significantly affect drug responses at the individual level. Genetic polymorphisms, i.e., common variations in DNA sequences among individuals, can be a factor affecting drug metabolism, drug efficacy, and the risk of side effects. For instance, specific polymorphisms within the pharmacognosy may lead to variability of enzymatic function that directs drug metabolism, affecting the therapeutic action of some drugs, most significantly in cancer (Suarez-Kurtz et al., 2019). Furthermore, the ability to realize pharmacogenetic genotyping tests based on such an understanding makes personalized medicine possible through the capability to predict how a patient will respond to provided therapies. Thus, integration of these tests is emerging as central to optimizing drug therapies, enhancing effectiveness, and minimizing potential side effects, hence forming a cornerstone of modern pharmacological practices (Fenech et al., 2014). Lastly, discovery and integration of genetic polymorphisms into practice will revolutionize personalized treatment strategies (Figure 10.2).

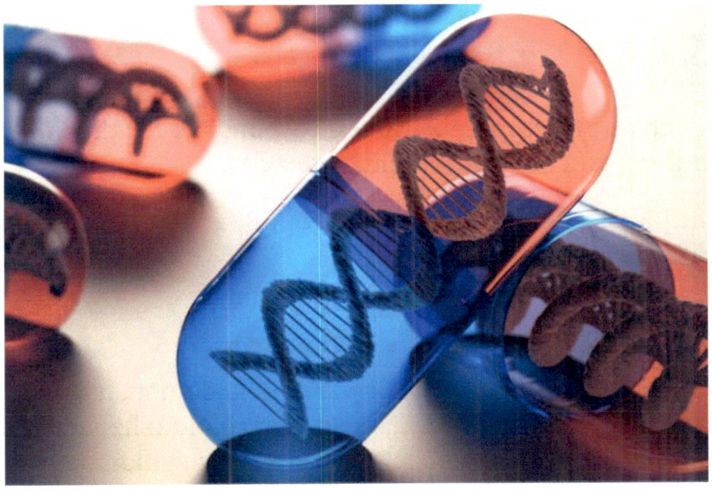

Figure 10.2. Genetic polymorphisms, which are common variations in DNA sequences among individuals, can affect drug metabolism, efficacy, and the risk of adverse effects.

Source: https://www.insideprecisionmedicine.com/wp-content/uploads/2019/09/Sep1_GettyImages_590279733_DNACapules-696x481.jpg.

10.1.3. Role of Enzymes in Drug Response

The role of enzymes in the action of drugs is at the heart of the science of pharmacogenetics and pharmacogenomics, as they enable the metabolism of the majority of pharmacologic medications. Enzymes such as cytochrome P450 are implicated in the biotransformation of many drugs, both their efficacy and possible toxicity. Genetic variation to code for the enzymes can lead to polymorphisms, and these lead to vast differences between individuals in drug metabolism and action. These genetic factors indicate the necessity of tailored therapeutic strategies; pharmacogenetic analysis can establish the risk of side effects or failure of treatment in patients and, hence, enable more effective treatment regimens. For instance, individualized medicine initiatives are now increasingly applying pharmacogenetic data to optimize the benefit/risk profile of medications in complex diseases like bipolar illness, where variability in response to treatment often leads to trial-and-error prescribing (Berghofer et al., 2014; Fenech et al., 2014). Through the alignment of drug treatment with a patient's genetic profile, healthcare providers can optimize patient safety and therapeutic outcomes (Figure 10.3).

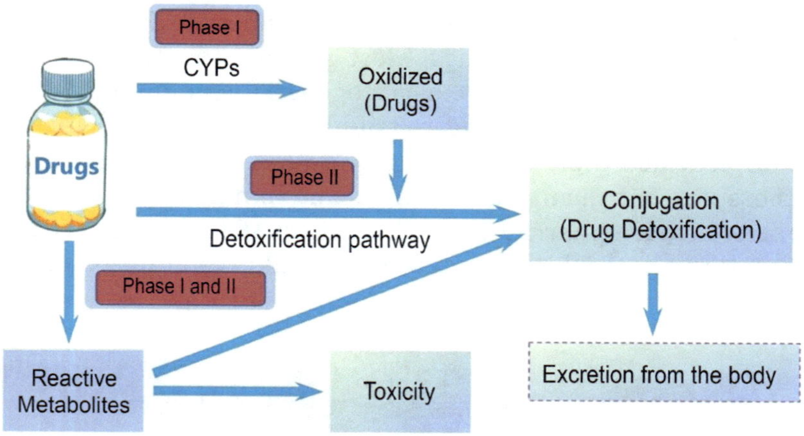

Figure 10.3. Enzymes such as cytochrome P450 are responsible for the biotransformation of many drugs, influencing both their efficacy and potential toxicity.

Source: https://pub.mdpi-res.com/ijms/ijms-22-12808/article_deploy/html/images/ijms-22-12808-g001.png?1638259059.

10.1.4. Case Studies of Pharmacogenetic Variations

The analysis of case studies in pharmacogenetic variations demonstrates the critical influence of genetic factors on drug efficacy and safety, emphasizing individualized treatment approaches. For instance, the identification of specific polymorphisms in key drug metabolizing genes can accurately forecast therapeutic efficacy as well as adverse reactions in different populations of patients. Expanding our understanding of such differences has made it possible to develop pharmacogenetic genotyping tests that yield patient-specific therapeutic strategies, hence enhancing patient outcomes and minimizing risks of standard therapies (Fenech et al., 2014). Also, next-generation sequencing (NGS) technology has revolutionized the field, allowing for larger-scale genotyping that can inform pharmacological treatment. However, practical implementation is constrained by heterogeneity and the lack of standard clinical protocols (Paepe et al., 2013). These case studies emphasize the increasing importance of pharmacogenetics and its role in the evolving face of personalized medicine.

10.1.5. Impact of Pharmacogenetics on Drug Efficacy

The impact of pharmacogenetics on drug efficacy is considerable, offering the potential for tailored therapeutic intervention, maximizing the response to therapy while minimizing adverse effects.

Pharmacogenetics can tailor drug therapy according to patients' genetic makeup, considerably maximizing drug efficacy by optimizing for addressing the delivery of the appropriate drug regarding each person's metabolic potential and susceptibility. This optimization is particularly pertinent in the instance of immunosuppressive therapy, where the therapeutic window is small and involves severe risks; under-treatment leads to organ rejection, while over-treatment risks exposing the patient to severe complications such as infections and nephrotoxicity. According to the Pharmacogenetics for Every Nation Initiative (PGENI), efforts to harmonize pharmacogenomic use have the potential to maximize drug treatment by developing population-specific markers and guidelines that offer targeted therapy as an acceptable alternative by way of various healthcare systems (Borg et al., 2012). Furthermore, the integration of pharmacogenetics and therapeutic drug monitoring (TDM) presents the possibility of improved clinical results, even when certain clinical benefits are not yet fully realized (Abboudi et al., 2012) (Figure 10.4).

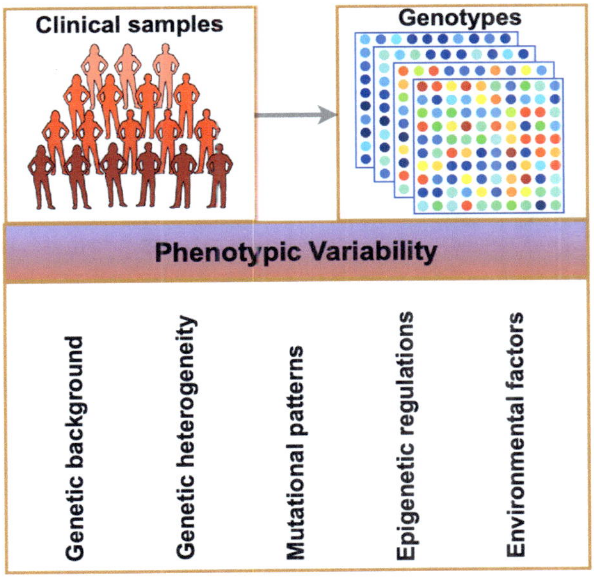

Figure 10.4. The impact of pharmacogenetics on drug efficacy is profound, offering the potential for tailored therapeutic strategies that maximize treatment outcomes while minimizing adverse effects.

Source: https://www.mdpi.com/pharmaceuticals/pharmaceuticals-17-00940/article_deploy/html/images/pharmaceuticals-17-00940-g002.png.

10.1.6. Pharmacogenetic Testing Methods

New technologies in the field of pharmacogenetic testing (PGT) have transformed personalized medicine, unveiling important information regarding how a person responds to various drugs. NGS has particularly transformed genotyping by making it possible to assess multiple genes at once, enhancing the precision of pharmacological treatment recommendations (Paepe et al., 2013). Despite such technical improvements, clinical use of PGT remains intermittent and is increasingly stimulated by inconsistent results between genetic variants and the absence of formalized guidelines for application. Furthermore, while several studies have delineated that pharmacogenetic tests are cost-effective, there is a significant gap in exploring their intrinsic value and clinical usefulness (Annemans et al., 2016). As scientists further develop these testing techniques and create sound evidence-based recommendations, the prospect for enhanced patient outcomes through individually adapted therapeutic approaches will more and more become an achievable goal, representing a significant advancement in pharmacogenetics and pharmacogenomics.

10.1.7. Ethical Considerations in Pharmacogenetics

As pharmacogenetics continues to drive the personalization of medicines, ethical concerns play a crucial role in determining its application in clinical care.

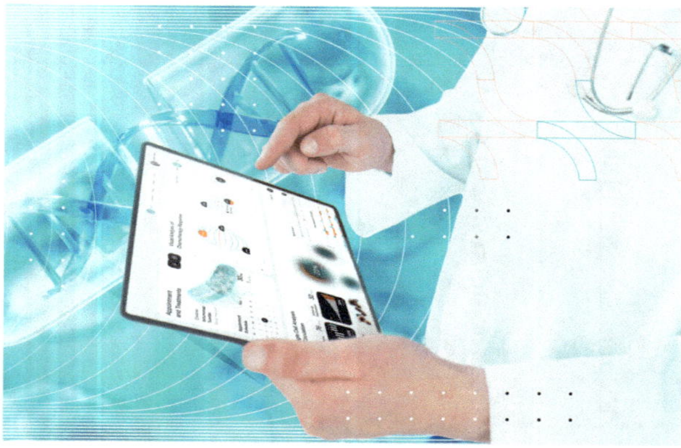

Figure 10.5. As pharmacogenetics continues to advance the personalization of medical treatments, ethical considerations play a crucial role in shaping its application in clinical practice.

Source: https://www.bgosoftware.com/blog/wp-content/uploads/2024/01/bgo-software-blog_post-size-%E2%80%93-Personalized-Medicine_no_title.png.

The addition of personalized genomic polygenic risk scores (PRS) opens new avenues to stratified treatment options. Still, it compromises patient privacy and informed consent, most notably how information is utilized and stored (Singh et al., 2024). In addition, the complexity of interpretation in pharmacogenomic data hinders the clinician's duty to inform patients about potential risks and benefits effectively. For instance, the variations in the efficacy of treating cardiovascular diseases highlight the importance of careful consideration of factors in individual patients along with genetic factors to facilitate equitable access to personalized therapy (Chatelin et al., 2017). These ethical issues must be resolved to protect public confidence and promote the ethical application of pharmacogenetics for improved patient outcomes along with minimizing any potential harm (Figure 10.5).

10.1.8. Limitations of Pharmacogenetic Research

Despite its promise, pharmacogenetic science is plagued by tremendous limitations that prevent it from being clinically useful. The most significant restriction comes from the overwhelming number of intricate genetic variations affecting drug response and metabolism. A multitude of mechanisms can account for a great deal of interindividual variation in treatment effect. Still, most studies have only focused on highly characterized genes, so functional effects of many rare variants remain unknown (Liu J-et al., 2022). In addition, while NGS technology has been able to identify thousands of genetic variations, accurate interpretation at the level of the individual remains elusive to us (Zhou et al., 2022). This is compounded by the limitations of current computational models, which themselves are not effective in forecasting the pharmacogenetic variant effects, thus necessitating more stable algorithms that are specifically tailored to this field. Hence, until such problems are addressed, the potential of pharmacogenetics as a mechanism for personalizing treatment regimens will remain mostly untapped.

10.1.9. Future Directions in Pharmacogenetics

As the field of pharmacogenetics develops, future directions must guarantee equal access and integrate testing into varied healthcare settings. Presently, PGT is confined to the big medical schools, causing unequal treatment, particularly for rural and underserved communities. A Montana-based study indicates the enthusiasm among healthcare stakeholders for implementing pharmacogenetics in community settings, with telehealth potentially being an access gap-filling solution (Killam et al., 2022). However, such challenges exist in the form of the complex nature of gene-drug interactions as it is presented through drugs like Thiopurine S-methyltransferase (TPMT) and Warfarin, where various genetic determinants and ethnic variations can yield conflicting results (Brazeau et al., 2009). Such complexities will be essential to overcome in developing the implementation schemes to ensure that pharmacogenetic advances reach all patients to ultimately create an increased and more effective healthcare environment (Figure 10.6).

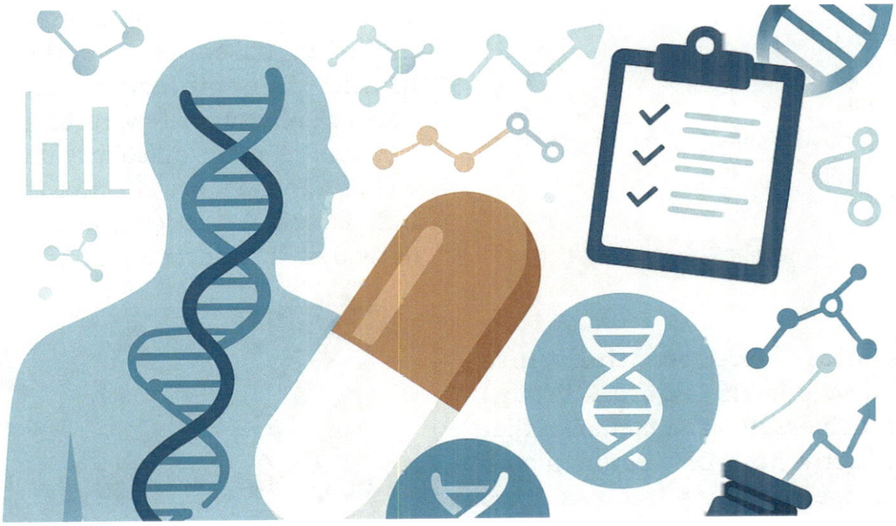

Figure 10.6. Currently, pharmacogenetic testing is primarily accessible in major academic medical centers, creating disparities in care, particularly for rural and underserved populations.

Source: https://media.licdn.com/dms/image/v2/D4D12AQF3CGXWNsy0Bw/article-cover_image-shrink_600_2000/B4DZZ2YSqkGgAQ-/0/1745742805363?e=2147483647&v=beta&t=IlYd7rN6hGzHYGFKrRZFgZlSWdNSpSViL5E6KCZiqhQ.

Test Your Knowledge

1. What role do cytochrome P450 enzymes (e.g., CYP2D6, CYP2C9) play in pharmacogenetics?
2. Why is it important to study genetic variability in drug targets and transporters?

10.2. Pharmacogenomics and Drug Development

Learning Outcome

1. Learn integration of genomics in drug discovery
2. Explain the role of biomarkers in pharmacogenomics
3. Discuss case studies of successful pharmacogenomic drugs
4. Identify challenges in implementing pharmacogenomics
5. Learn regulatory considerations for pharmacogenomic drugs
6. Discuss the economic implications of pharmacogenomics
7. Understand pharmacogenomics in clinical trials
8. Focus on personalized medicine and patient outcomes
9. Know future trends in drug development

Pharmacogenomics incorporation into pharmaceutical development is a breakthrough movement towards personalized medicine that enhances the effectiveness of treatment and minimizes the danger of side effects. As more is being investigated in the human genome, advances in genotyping technology enable the adjustment of drug dosing regulations based on genetic uniqueness, enhancing safety and clinical outcomes. For instance, the application of pharmacogenetics for immunosuppressive therapy shows a pressing need for tailored drug regimens to optimize patient outcomes in light of the narrow therapeutic index of such drugs (Abboudi et al., 2012). While significant progress has been made in the developed world, access to pharmacogenomic applications is lacking in most developing nations. Such initiatives like the PGENI are valuable toward mitigating these differences by promoting worldwide use and raising the level of awareness among practitioners (Borg et al., 2012). The future of pharmacogenomics holds the potential to revolutionize drug development, leading to more effective and safer treatments for diverse populations.

10.2.1. Integration of Genomics in Drug Discovery

The use of genomics in drug discovery represents a paradigm shift in pharmacogenetics and pharmacogenomics, fundamentally altering the paradigms of drug discovery and usage. This approach employs genetic data to identify biomarkers that direct drug responses, thereby enabling the development of personalized therapies based on the individual patient profile. By embracing the paradigms of network pharmacology, researchers can further streamline drug discovery methodologies to yield safer and more effective therapeutic agents that consider the complexities of biological networks (Marsh et al., 2010).

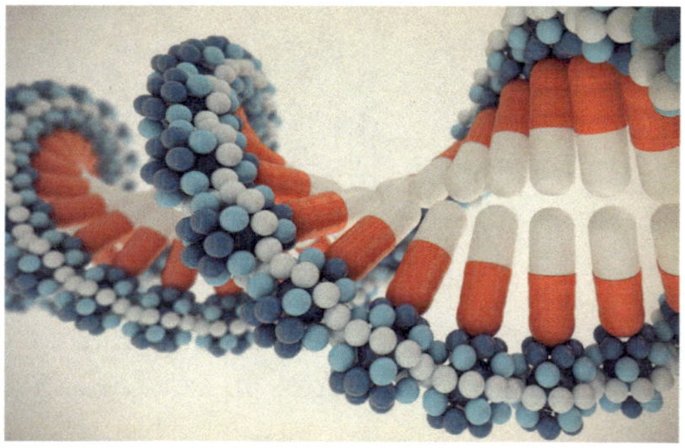

Figure 10.7. The integration of genomics into drug discovery represents a transformative advancement in pharmacogenetics and pharmacogenomics, fundamentally shifting the paradigms of how therapeutics are developed and applied.

Source: https://pharmaceutical-journal.com/wp-content/uploads/2021/01/pharmacogenomics-concept-ss-17.png.

Further advancement of pharmacogenomics has the possibility of improving novel modes of drug discovery and maximizing health outcomes through personalized medicine, essentially bridging the gap between genetic research and actual utilization in clinical practice (Bartlett et al., 2016). With genomics increasingly integrated into drug discovery paradigms, healthcare providers will need to modify practice to leverage this goldmine of genetic data (Figure 10.7).

10.2.2. Role of Biomarkers in Pharmacogenomics

In pharmacogenomics, biomarkers play a pivotal function to enhance the accuracy of drug therapy so that tailored treatment strategies are given to achieve optimum therapeutic gains at minimal cost of adverse effects. These biological indicators can alert clinicians about the genetic predisposition of a patient, which has a significant influence on drug metabolism, efficacy, and safety. For instance, immunosuppressive drugs, having a narrow therapeutic window, need careful monitoring so as not to trigger organ rejection or over-immunosuppression and consequent serious complications such as diabetes or nephrotoxicity. As mentioned, TDM presently guides treatment, but incorporation of pharmacogenomics can yet improve these approaches, enabling increasingly individualized management of patients (Abboudi et al., 2012). Also, with the NHS in the UK soon to make tremendous progress in genomic screening, there is a call to pharmacists to extend their understanding of drug response genes, which can revolutionize the prescribing and treating of drugs in clinical practice (Wright et al., 2020) (Figure 10.8).

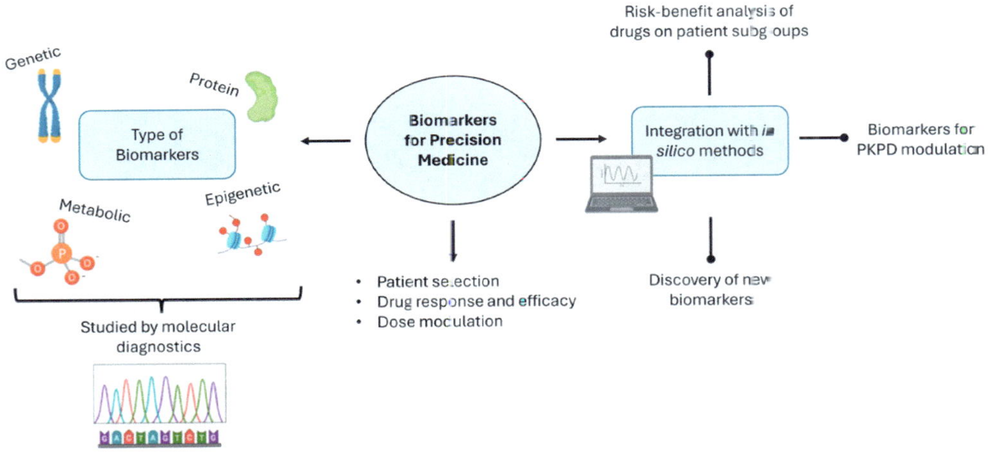

Figure 10.8. Biomarkers play a pivotal role in enhancing the precision of drug therapies, allowing for tailored treatment strategies that optimize therapeutic outcomes while minimizing adverse effects.

Source: https://www.mdpi.com/pharmaceutics/pharmaceutics-16-00332/article_deploy/html/images/pharmaceutics-16-00332-g002.png.

10.2.3. Case Studies of Successful Pharmacogenomic Drugs

The studies on pharmacogenomic drugs have offered numerous positive examples that show the application of tailored medicine for enhancing therapy. For instance, pharmacogenomic drug classification has highlighted the role of genes such as CYP2D6 in optimizing therapy for psychiatric illnesses and oncological treatment. A study highlighted the aspect that a majority of drug labels of FDA-approved medicines contain pharmacogenomic suggestions, and actionable guidance that supports clinicians in tailoring therapy based on genetic profiles, particularly for antidepressants and pain medications (Deb et al., 2024). Besides, enhanced understanding of genetic polymorphisms associated with fetal hemoglobin production in β-thalassemia and Sickle-cell disease has enabled clinicians to select the appropriate drug regimen and doses, with an evident correlation between the use of pharmacogenomics and improved patient outcomes (Gambari et al., 2024). All of this demonstrates the extent of genetic influence on achieving maximum effectiveness of drugs and minimizing side effects.

10.2.4. Challenges in Implementing Pharmacogenomics

Application of pharmacogenomics to clinical practice is plagued by several challenges that hinder its full potential in enabling personalized medicine. One of the main challenges is the low awareness and knowledge on the part of medical professionals, well-illustrated throughout the Middle East, including Lebanon, with only 67% of the participants reporting awareness of pharmacogenomics, in contrast to Qatar and Saudi Arabia (Shamieh et al., 2025). Also, cost barriers, such as genetic testing fees and reimbursement problems, pose additional barriers towards integration. Most notably, Lebanese clinicians expressed higher concerns about test costs, reflecting the highest-level barrier to access (Shamieh et al., 2025). Besides, the absence of standard operating procedures and scarcity of information on the clinical effectiveness of PGT add to resistance to adopting these practices. Addressing these issues entails customized educational programs and investments to create an environment that is hospitable to integrating pharmacogenomics into daily healthcare (Figure 10.9).

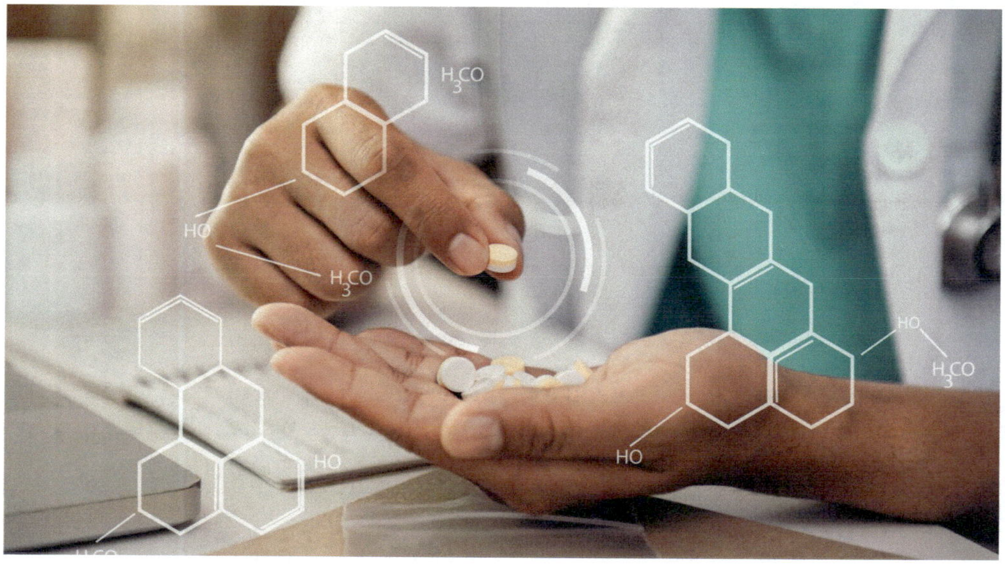

Figure 10.9. The implementation of pharmacogenomics in clinical settings faces numerous challenges that hinder its potential to enhance personalized medicine.

Source: https://media.licdn.com/dms/image/v2/D5612AQHpNl235a3Osg/article-cover_image-shrink_720_1280/B56ZUmI_QsHsAI-/0/1740101646432?e=2147483647&v=beta&t=nvkrixnt1TGqItkPdyPYltdVMVayp1aNgQjuQ-J9wrA.

10.2.5. Regulatory Considerations for Pharmacogenomic Drugs

The regulatory context of pharmacogenomic medicines is complex, in that it is the dynamic relationship between cutting-edge scientific advances and conventional healthcare systems. Addressing the institutional and ethical issues surrounding the use of pharmacogenomics is essential since it will increase medication efficacy and reduce adverse drug reactions (ADRs). While current literature mainly centers on regulatory obstacles, it fails to consider how clinicians perceive and integrate PGT in their practice. Interviews with healthcare professionals have found a divided acceptance of pharmacogenomics, expressing fears regarding patient exclusion from treatment based on genetic profiles and broader ethical issues surrounding genetic testing (Hedgecoe et al., 2006). Furthermore, the development of pharmacogenomic drugs is faced with a significant hindrance, in the form of costly research and legal liability issues, that can restrain innovation and postpone market access (Koch et al., 2012). Navigating these regulatory issues is crucial to take advantage of the complete potential of pharmacogenomics in clinical practice while ensuring patient rights.

10.2.6. Economic Implications of Pharmacogenomics

The economic impact of pharmacogenomics is significant, particularly as healthcare systems transition towards more personalized medicine practices. By tailoring drug treatments to one's genetic profile, pharmacogenomics has the potential likewise to have a drastic impact on reducing ADRs, which are said to cost enormous healthcare resources.

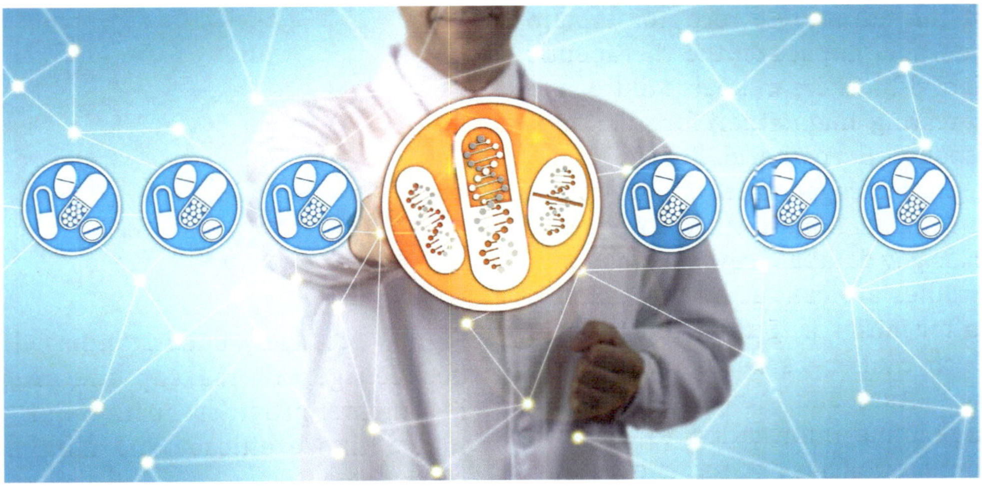

Figure 10.10. The economic implications of pharmacogenomics are profound, particularly as healthcare systems transition to more personalized medicine approaches.

Source: https://advancementsinoncology.com/wp-content/uploads/2024/05/Pharmacogenomics_dreamstime_xxl_118534269-scaled.jpg.

For instance, the NHS aims to apply genomic screening to increase patient outcomes and also minimize wasteful treatment costs—avoidance of medicines harm alone costs the NHS over £93.5 million annually. Further studies indicate that genetic factors can be responsible for 25-50% of drug response inappropriateness, which says a lot regarding the economic advantage of applying pharmacogenomic testing to customize drug selection (Hedgecoe et al., 2006). But successful implementation is contingent on the clinician uptake of pharmacogenomic technologies, whose attitudes may influence economic viability and ethical concerns in clinical practice (Hedgecoe et al., 2006). Therefore, integrating pharmacogenomics into medicine entails both economic benefits and potential issues of universal professional acceptance (Figure 10.10).

10.2.7. Pharmacogenomics in Clinical Trials

Pharmacogenomics integration in clinical trials is a paradigm shift approach of personalized medicine where drugs are tailored according to genetic patterns. By identifying genetic variations that affect drug efficacy and safety, pharmacogenomics enhances subject recruitment and optimizes clinical trial design. For example, research has shown that genetic variations of the adrenergic receptor system have a considerable impact on the therapeutic effectiveness of β-blockers in heart failure, and that genetic testing might therefore enhance treatment response (Barrese et al., 2014). Despite its potential, pharmacogenomics application in clinical trials remains limited since a review of the clinicaltrials.gov database revealed that 80% of relevant studies are conducted by academic institutions after initial drug approvals (Burt et al., 2013). Such challenges necessitate a shift in regulatory culture and greater recognition of pharmacogenomic information to improve drug development policies and patient therapy.

10.2.8. Personalized Medicine and Patient Outcomes

The evolution of personalized medicine, particularly by the sciences of pharmacogenetics and pharmacogenomics, has wide-ranging consequences for patient outcomes. Through a knowledge of how genetic variation affects response to medication, doctors can tailor medications that are optimized for maximum benefit and minimal side effects. As highlighted, pharmacogenetics focuses on particular genes, while pharmacogenomics deals with broader genetic interactions, both resulting in a more precise understanding of how individual variability shapes drug responses (Dash et al., 2024). Focused on its method, it not only enhances therapeutic usefulness but also results in improved safety profiles by obviating trial-and-error in drug and dosing choice. Particularly within anesthesia, pharmacogenomics plays a crucial role in tailoring anesthetic drugs to individual genetic profiles, thereby decreasing complications and shortening recoveries (Malviya et al., 2024). Thus, the trend for personalized medicine is an epoch-making development in medicine that aims to significantly enhance the quality of patient care and outcomes (Figure 10.11).

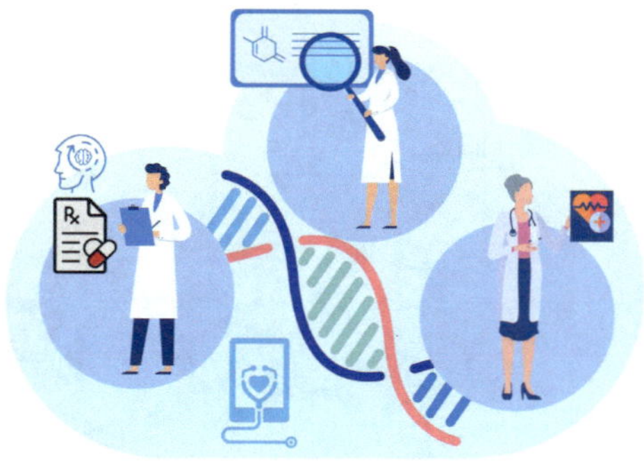

Figure 10.11. By understanding the interplay between genetic makeup and drug response, healthcare providers can tailor treatments that optimize efficacy and minimize adverse reactions.

Source: https://coreprescribingsolutions.co.uk/wp-content/uploads/2024/03/KEY-APPLICATIONS-OF-PHARMACOGENETICS-1024x679.jpg.

10.2.9. Future Trends in Drug Development

As the landscape of drug development continues to evolve, future trends increasingly center on the integration of pharmacogenetics and pharmacogenomics into individualized medicine. Both are based on the principle that genetic differences between individuals influence drug metabolism and therapeutic response. The emergence of personalized medicine is particularly pertinent in disciplines such as psychiatry, where polymorphic cytochromes, for example, CYP2D6 and CYP2C19, PGT has the potential to enhance treatment outcomes significantly and minimize adverse effects (Petek et al., 2009). Personalizing medication choice and dosing according to an individual's genetic profile enables clinicians to optimize therapeutic success, a development regarded as essential in today's clinical practice (Terzic et al., 2017). Furthermore, the ongoing development of nanotechnology enhances the potential for personalized treatment, leading to more precise and potent therapies that target not only specific diseases but also the unique genetic makeup of each patient.

Test Your Knowledge

1. How can stratifying clinical trial participants based on genetic profiles improve drug testing outcomes?
2. What challenges exist in integrating pharmacogenomic data into early-phase drug development?

10.3. Clinical Applications of Pharmacogenetics and Pharmacogenomics

Learning Outcome

1. Explain pharmacogenetic testing in clinical practice
2. Learn the impact on prescribing practices
3. Discuss case studies of clinical applications
4. Focus on pharmacogenomics in oncology, psychiatry, and cardiology
5. Understand patient education and engagement
6. Identify barriers to clinical implementation
7. Discuss the future of pharmacogenomic applications

The application of pharmacogenomics and pharmacogenetics in clinical settings is an innovative approach to personalized medicine that significantly influences treatment decisions. Pharmacogenomics and pharmacogenetics enable clinicians to tailor drug therapy based on an individual's genetic pattern, thereby enhancing the safety and efficacy of pharmacotherapy. As highlighted by recent studies, with the expanded capability for the detection of numerous genetic variants of drug response and metabolism, high-throughput molecular technologies are now able to be applied within the clinical setting (Schrijver et al., 2011). In addition to making the process more effective at identifying associated genetic markers, the movement also poses an interpretive challenge in the clinical environment. Moreover, as research continues to indicate that genetic variation is a driving force behind patient drug responses, pharmacogenetics becomes increasingly relevant to the design of targeted therapies, ultimately intending to improve patient outcomes and optimize treatment regimens (Fenech et al., 2007).

10.3.1. Pharmacogenetic Testing in Clinical Practice

PGT, as part of standard clinical practice, is a significant development in personalized medicine, facilitating individualized pharmacotherapy based on an individual's genetic profile. PGT enables identification of actionable variants potentially affecting drug metabolism, efficacy, and safety. For instance, studies have identified that over 95% of individuals have at least one pharmacogenetic variant that can impact drug treatment response, indicating the widespread influence of such testing (Mosch et al., 2024). Most notably in IBD, a concerted reverse phenotyping approach has revealed the prevalence of NUDT15 variants associated with thiopurine-induced toxicity, confirming the viability of tailored interventions minimizing adverse effects but achieving maximized therapeutic benefit (Roberts et al., 2024). As further evidence supporting pharmacogenetic panel testing is accrued, careful consideration of its utilization, including cost-effectiveness and the targeting of those at highest risk, will be essential for broad-scale clinical deployment (Figure 10.12).

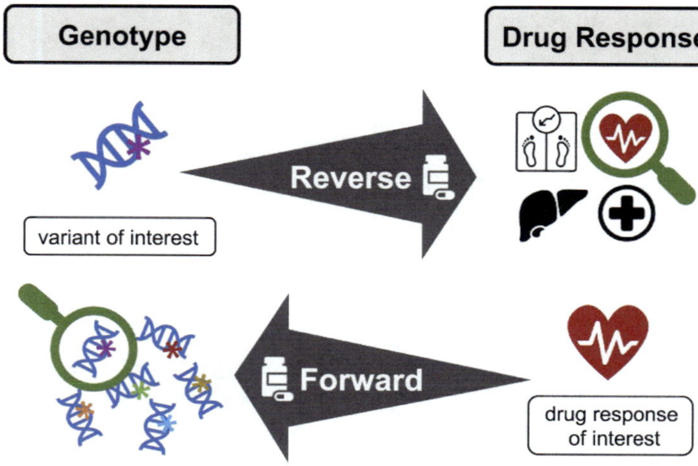

Figure 10.12. Pharmacogenetic testing facilitates the identification of actionable variants that can influence drug metabolism, efficacy, and safety.

Source: https://www.cell.com/cms/10.1016/j.xhgg.2022.100100/asset/ded767f5-ebb2-4230-826d-2aeba0baf11a/main.assets/gr4_lrg.jpg.

10.3.2. Impact on Prescribing Practices

The integration of pharmacogenomics and pharmacogenetics into clinical care is revolutionizing prescribing behavior toward a system of tailor-made medicine. The process eliminates the disparity in drug response in individuals, which can be initiated by genetic variability and contribute to up to 25-50% of drug-related adverse events (Wright et al., 2020). With the NHS preparing to add genomic screening as a standard aspect of care for patients, pharmacists are being increasingly requested to make suggestions based on the genetic makeup instead of simply on what can be observed (Wright et al., 2020). Also, the advent of EHR and clinical decision support (CDS) systems is facilitating the incorporation of pharmacogenomic data directly into the prescription. Yet, there are still barriers, such as clinician education and the usability of these systems, which must be overcome to optimally implement. Overcoming these barriers, pharmacogenomics has the potential to make a dramatic impact on medication safety and efficacy, thus improving patient outcomes overall (Figure 10.13).

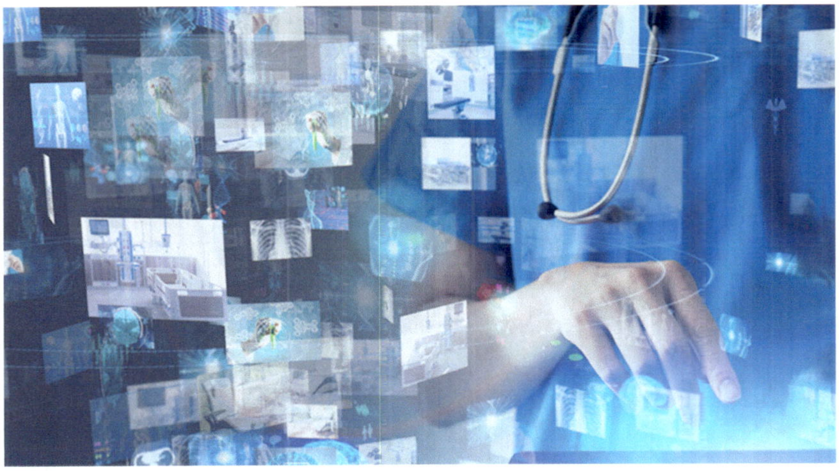

Figure 10.13. Development of electronic health records (EHR) and clinical decision support (CDS) systems is facilitating the incorporation of pharmacogenomic data directly into the prescribing process.

Source: https://www.facs.org/media/fawh2xyv/22sepbull-feat-clinical-decision-support-tools-hero.png?rnd=133069658382770000.

10.3.3. Case Studies of Clinical Applications

Pharmacogenetics' application in clinical practice has also yielded striking case reports demonstrating its possibilities and limitations. In oncology, for instance, the use of PGT to guide drug selection has illustrated both the promise and dangers of personalized medicine. Breast cancer and Alzheimer's clinicians have arrived with conflicting opinions about the ethical aspect of the application of genetic knowledge, i.e., excluding patients from receiving some medication based on genetic markers (Hedgecoe et al., 2006). The case studies reveal the complexities involved in using pharmacogenetics, especially amidst evolving evidence and variable results regarding the application of particular genetic variants. Even though next-generation sequencing (NGS) has significantly improved our capability for the affordable generation of pharmacogenetic profiles, challenges remain in translating genetic knowledge into clinical use daily, largely due to a lack of robust guidelines and delicate manipulation of genetic data (Paepe et al., 2013). Ultimately, these case studies advocate for ongoing debate and research in this area.

10.3.4. Pharmacogenomics in Oncology

The application of pharmacogenomics in oncology is a paradigm shift in the individualization of cancer treatment. Using genetic information, doctors can predict the patient's reaction to specific cancer treatments, thereby optimizing the treatment and lessening side effects. Despite its potential, the use of pharmacogenomics has not been maximally utilized, primarily due to drug development difficulties and the inability of routine genomic screening to become part of clinical practice. Emphasizing a delay in adoption, the majority of studies on pharmacogenomics are now carried out by academia as opposed to pharmaceutical companies (Burt et al., 2013). Furthermore, initiatives by organizations like the National Cancer Institute are targeted towards the necessity of the integration of pharmacogenomic markers within clinical trials, as well as coordinated biospecimen acquisition for investigative purposes (Allegra et al., 2010). Closing these gaps is critical to achieve the full potential of pharmacogenomics to enhance patient outcomes in oncology (Figure 10.14).

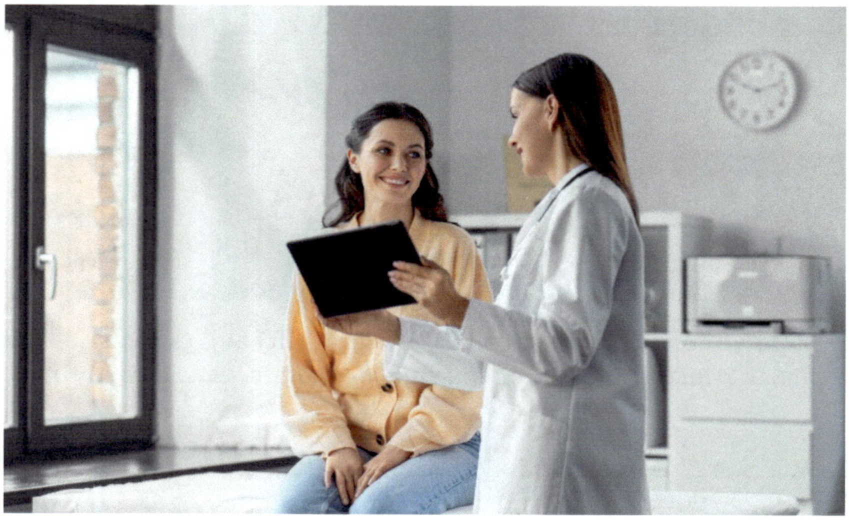

Figure 10.14. The integration of pharmacogenomics into oncology represents a transformative shift in how cancer treatments are personalized for patients.

Source: https://d1g9yur4m4naub.cloudfront.net/images/Article_Images/ImageForArticle_1351_17235438671248556.jpg.

10.3.5. Pharmacogenomics in Psychiatry

The application of pharmacogenomics in psychiatry introduces a revolutionary potential to optimize treatment regimens for mentally ill patients. As more evidence mounts on the utility of pharmacogenomic testing, there can be little doubt that personalized medicine will have a significant effect on drug prescription. For instance, the Clinical Pharmacogenetics Implementation Consortium (CPIC) has made recommendations for numerous psychiatric medications after identifying the urgent need for this approach among pediatric populations, particularly in light of the rising mental health crisis among young people (Miller et al., 2025). However, although pharmacogenomic use is promising, it is also problematic. A study of Slovak psychiatrists revealed that while they were familiar with the potential benefits of PGT, especially in the treatment-refractory patient, there are significant barriers such as the absence of unified guidelines and concerns over expense hindering widespread adoption (Krivosova et al., 2025). Overcoming such barriers is necessary in shaping the use of pharmacogenomics in psychiatry and improving patient care.

10.3.6. Pharmacogenomics in Cardiology

Pharmacogenomics in cardiology has been a paradigm shift towards personalized medicine, whereby treatment protocols are tailored to an individual's genes. With this technology, clinicians can predict the patients' response to cardiovascular drugs, thereby optimizing efficacy and minimizing side effects. For instance, genetic drug metabolism differences may significantly influence the effectiveness of anticoagulants such as warfarin, requiring dosage modifications using genetic tests. Furthermore, although evidence for the deployment of pharmacogenetics has grown at a rapid rate, deployment in the clinical setting remains shrouded in issues including economic factors and health care providers' lack of knowledge, as recent literature has shown (Jón-Espinosa et al., 2022). It's interesting to note that patient voice continues to be key because personal experience can provide valuable insights into the perceived value of PGT and its role in improving therapeutic results (Luzum et al., 2021). Ultimately, through cooperation among numerous stakeholders, the future will be one of realizing the full potential of pharmacogenomics in cardiology (Figure 10.15).

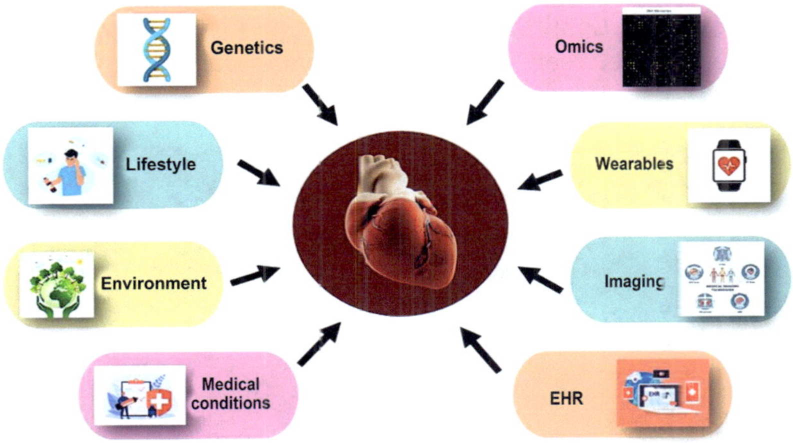

Figure 10.15. The integration of pharmacogenomics into cardiology represents a paradigm shift toward personalized medicine, wherein treatment strategies are tailored based on an individual's genetic makeup.

Source: https://www.thelancet.com/cms/10.1016/j.eclinm.2024.102660/asset/b5a89929-fe62-4705-b9a3-b345ef259057/main.assets/gr6_lrg.jpg.

10.3.7. Patient Education and Engagement

Patient education and participation are paramount within the practice of pharmacogenomics and pharmacogenetics to achieve optimal therapeutic outcomes. By effective communication of genetic information and how it influences customized drug regimens, health practitioners enhance patient understanding as well as treatment adherence. This is critical in the management of complex conditions such as autism spectrum disorder (ASD), where PGT may take a central role in finding the best psychotropic drugs for an individual based on a person's genetic profile (Genovese et al., 2023). In addition, precision psychiatry seeks to bridge the gap between practice and research through leveraging advances in genomics knowledge and neuroscience to guide day-to-day clinical decision-making, thereby allowing patients to be proactively involved in their treatment (Williams, 2022). Ultimately, gaining an informed set of patients not only improves health outcomes but also supports the larger endeavor of precision medicine in achieving effective and safe treatment models.

10.3.8. Barriers to Clinical Implementation

The application of pharmacogenetics and pharmacogenomics in clinical settings is hindered by several formidable barriers, which firmly inhibit their use despite the fact that they promise significant benefits to personalized medicine. Among the primary challenges identified is the need for standardized guidelines, processes, and protocols for the clinical application of pharmacogenetic information, something exceptionally experienced in Latin America and the Caribbean where studies are just beginning to roll out (Salas-Hernández et al., 2023). Furthermore, cost-effectiveness remains a paramount consideration, as the majority of healthcare systems are not ready to invest in pharmacogenomic testing unless there are apparent economic benefits. Despite increased awareness of pharmacogenomics among healthcare providers, resistance to clinical practice persists, indicating a need for more comprehensive medical school and residency training and education in genomic use (Padmanabhan et al., 2023). Combined, these challenges highlight the necessity of systematic approaches to close the gap between applied and theoretical research in pharmacogenomics (Figure 10.16).

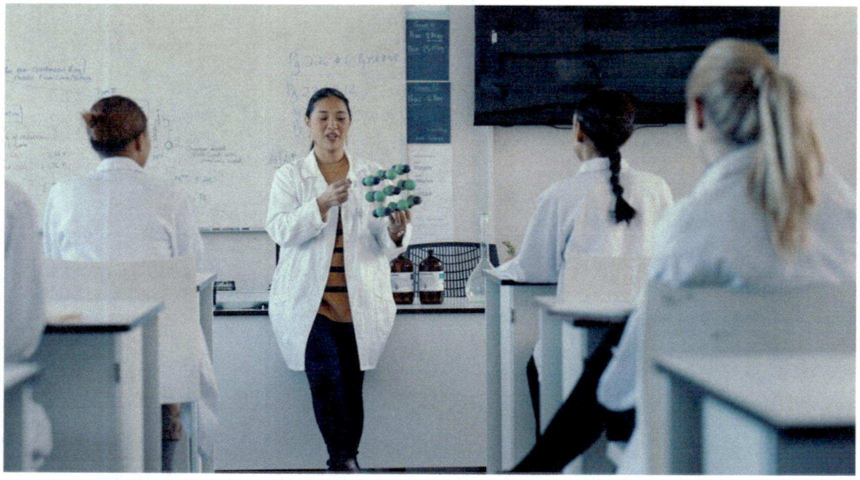

Figure 10.16. The integration of pharmacogenetics and pharmacogenomics into clinical practice faces several formidable barriers, significantly hindering their implementation despite their potential in personalized medicine.

Source: https://media.licdn.com/dms/image/v2/D5612AQH_XnidlwBWVA/article-cover_image-shrink_720_1280/article-cover_image-shrink_720_1280/0/1737393380739?e=2147483647&v=beta&t=NXVjDS2pkQ4kXLuUjvTHsRVX2EXlrA7QVsKhNBOsPIc.

10.3.9. Future of Pharmacogenomic Applications

The pharmacogenomic applications of the future have tremendous potential to revolutionize healthcare practice and improve patient outcomes by tailoring treatment regimens to individuals. By examining how genetic differences affect medication response, pharmacogenomics enables more individualized therapeutic approaches that enhance effectiveness with reduced adverse effects. Current research points to the potential for the incorporation of pharmacogenomic data into clinical practice, allowing the clinicians to make informed decisions from evidence derived from the unique genetic profile of a patient (Geetha et al., 2024). Despite existing barriers to its universal acceptance, including standardization and robust evidence for clinical utility, the future trajectory of pharmacogenomics is directed towards a role in revolutionizing medicine (Dash et al., 2024). With ongoing technological advancements and the increased availability of genetic testing, incorporating pharmacogenomic data into everyday clinical practice has the potential to transform patient treatment, ensuring that treatments are safe and effective across a broad range of populations.

Test Your Knowledge

1. How can pharmacogenomics improve treatment in cancer therapy?
2. In what clinical settings is pharmacogenetic testing routinely recommended?

10.4. Ethical, Legal, and Social Implications

Learning Outcome

1. Focus on privacy concerns in genetic testing
2. Understand discrimination based on genetic information
3. Describe informed consent in pharmacogenetic testing
4. Understand access to pharmacogenetic testing
5. Know public perception of pharmacogenomics
6. Explain regulatory frameworks governing pharmacogenomics
7. Focus on equity in healthcare and pharmacogenomics
8. Identify ethical dilemmas in genetic research
9. Explain future ethical considerations

The ethical, legal, and social impacts of pharmacogenomics and pharmacogenetics are increasing ever more significantly as these areas of research mature. Translating genetic screening into the clinical arena raises significant ethical concerns, particularly informed consent and patient autonomy. Unlike traditional genetic screening, the use of pharmacogenetic technologies directly impacts treatment regimens with the potential to generate exclusionary practices and penalties to particular groups of patients. Evidence indicates that there is a lack of understanding by clinicians concerning the ethical implications of PGT, more specifically their attitudes and the probability of biased treatment (Hedgecoe et al., 2006). In addition, the current pharmacogenomic policy framework remains underdeveloped, with it being challenging to navigate the complexities of informed consent and the ethical concerns that arise in this new area (Avard et al. 2007). Meeting these implications is necessary to uphold fair access and ethical utilization of pharmacogenetic progress in medicine.

10.4.1. Privacy Concerns in Genetic Testing

The development of pharmacogenetics and pharmacogenomics raises significant privacy concerns that need to be closely examined. With genetic screening increasingly becoming part of clinical practice, there is also the danger of unauthorized release of confidential genetic information. Discrimination can follow if the genetic information of people reveals them to be susceptible to certain diseases. This can have insurance and employment implications. Also, ethical informed consent considerations are central; the subjects must be made very clear about how they will use their genetic data will be used and shared. Existing literature presents that even though great attention is given to institutional barriers in the use of pharmacogenetic technology, ethical concerns, particularly privacy, are not yet addressed appropriately (Hedgecoe et al., 2006). The existing policy infrastructure for pharmacogenomics is still emerging and requires extension to capture these privacy challenges effectively (Avard et al., 2007). The stakeholders are therefore compelled to place importance on privacy to encourage trust in pharmacogenetic use (Figure 10.17).

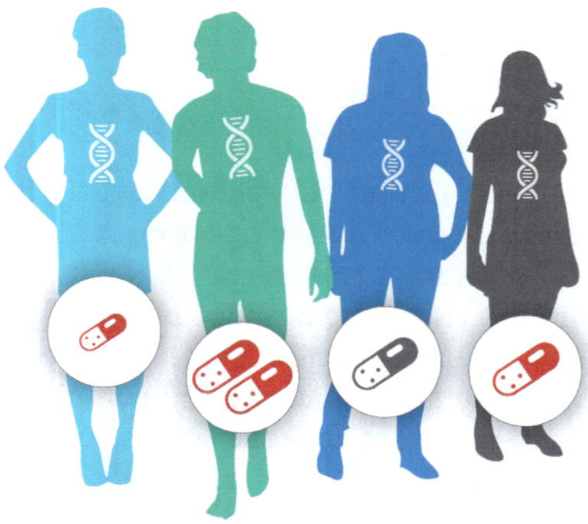

Figure 10.17. The advent of pharmacogenetics and pharmacogenomics presents significant privacy concerns that merit careful examination.

Source: https://images.squarespace-cdn.com/content/v1/611e9ed6b7bd816d2f8e42bb/258c2afe-ca5c-46a0-a624-80897869eeab/Rxight.png.

10.4.2. Discrimination Based on Genetic Information

Pharmacogenomics and pharmacogenetics can transform personalized medicine, but they also raise serious questions of genetic discrimination. As more genetic screening enters the clinical mainstream, there is an increasing risk that people will be discriminated against in the workplace, by insurers, or in access to healthcare because of their genes. According to (Matsuyama et al., 2023), proper population genetics frameworks must be established to prevent discrimination but allow for inclusive governance of pharmacogenomics. This is important not only for equity but also for optimizing the therapeutic effects of customized treatments. Yet, even with improvements in knowledge about how genetic variation influences drug response, as cited in Anghel et al. (2024), existing models of healthcare tend not to account for differences, enforcing a one-size-fits-all solution. Therefore, the application of genetic information to clinical practice needs to be supported by strong ethical frameworks to ensure protection from discriminatory actions.

10.4.3. Informed Consent in Pharmacogenetic Testing

Informed consent is a significant aspect of PGT, necessitating serious consideration of the ethical and legal aspects involved. Since pharmacogenetics can tailor medicine to the individual through adjustment of drug therapy based on the individual's genetic profile, it also raises significant challenges in terms of participant autonomy and knowledge of information. Because the pharmacogenomic policy landscape is still in its infancy, there is a critical need for clear guidance that ensures participants are adequately informed about the complexities of genetic testing and its potential implications for their health and treatment (Avard et al., 2007). Besides, as such treatment therapies advance from the development stage to clinical application, there is a requirement to overcome the many legal and regulatory barriers likely to burden informed consent processes. Ensuring that patients are not only well-informed but also engaged in decisions about their treatment is essential to the moral advancement of pharmacogenomics into practice (Evans et al., 2006) (Figure 10.18).

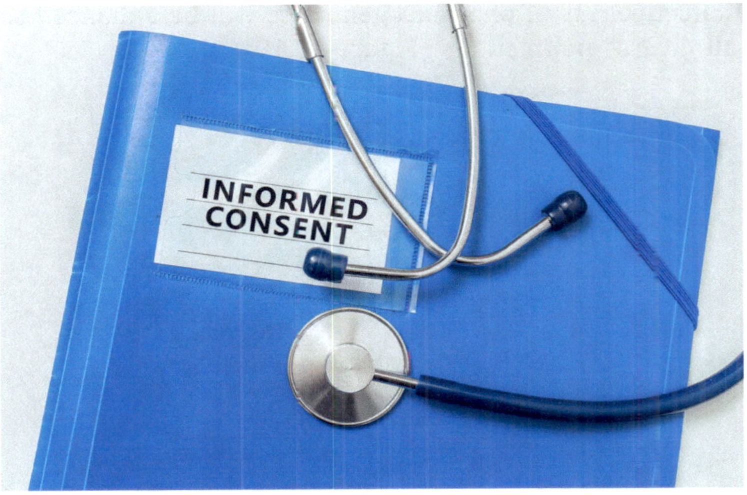

Figure 10.18. Informed consent is a pivotal aspect of pharmacogenetic testing, necessitating a nuanced understanding of its ethical and legal implications.

Source: https://aihcp.net/main/wp-content/uploads/2024/07/Depositphotos_102015738_S.jpg.

10.4.4. Access to Pharmacogenetic Testing

Accessibility of PGT remains the primary key to a successful implementation of personalized medicine. Differences in accessibility can make or break patient outcomes, as in the UK where the pharmacogenomic technology is yet to be adopted in routine practice. The latest drive for genomic screening in the NHS raises the imperative for doctors, and more so pharmacists, to be well informed about pharmacogenetics to reduce drug harm and increase the benefit of treatments (Wright et al., 2020). While literature tends to concentrate on institutional barriers to the use of PGT, it tends to neglect views of clinicians who are now beginning to integrate the tests into practice. Knowing what they believe regarding the moral implications of PGT, including how it disenfranchises patients from taking some medications, is imperative to further advancing this science (Hedgecoe et al., 2006). Hence, increasing access and acceptability of PGT is essential to optimizing patient care.

10.4.5. Public Perception of Pharmacogenomics

Public attitudes towards pharmacogenomics are crucial for shaping the future of personalized medicine, particularly given the increasing demand for individualized healthcare. Patient compliance with prescribed treatments, as well as public acceptance of pharmacogenomic procedures, can be impacted by awareness and knowledge about how genetic differences influence drug responses. Evidence suggests that despite the hopes of many patients for the advantages of gene testing, uncertainty about confidentiality and distress is present, which can successfully deter implementation at a whole level (Ashiq et al., 2023). Second, as pharmacogenomics has emerged, public health programs need to address ethical challenges regarding genetic information to foster confidence and cooperation in populations (Mak et al., 2024). Given the importance of pharmacogenomics' effects on treatment results, more educational outreach about the field is required in an effort to demystify the technology and make it easier to incorporate into everyday routines. Finally, through peer perceptions, the effectiveness of pharmacogenomics will be enhanced so that its advantages will be accessible to all diverse populations (Figure 10.19).

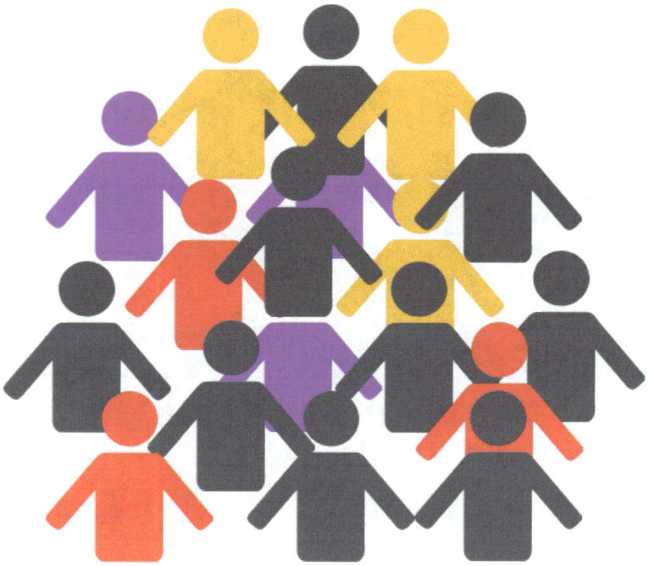

Figure 10.19. Awareness and understanding of how genetic variations affect drug responses can influence patient adherence to prescribed therapies and the overall acceptance of pharmacogenomic practices.

Source: https://www.labclinics.com/wp-content/uploads/2021/05/pharmacogeneticsAgena-3.png.

10.4.6. Regulatory Frameworks Governing Pharmacogenomics

Regulatory systems that cover pharmacogenomics are instrumental in facilitating genetic information to be effectively translated into the clinical setting, particularly as advances in sequencing technology like NGS continue to uncover complex genetic variations linked with drug response. Such frameworks must address the challenging issues posed by such new pharmacogenetic data, particularly regarding the proper interpretation of rare genetic variants that have been shown to have a considerable impact on drug metabolism and toxicity (Zhou et al., 2022). Given that ADRs rank among the leading causes of mortality in the developed world, precision pharmacovigilance emerges as an integral component of this regulatory landscape (Pretis et al., 2022). Regulatory bodies must simplify processes to integrate pharmacogenomic testing into clinical practice without compromising patient safety through efficient pharmacovigilance systems. A unifying regulatory strategy not only aids in personalized medicine but also averts risky drug therapy, substantially enhancing patient outcomes in the heterogeneity of clinical settings.

10.4.7. Equity in Healthcare and Pharmacogenomics

Incorporation of pharmacogenomics into health care presents a vital opportunity to bridge equity gaps, particularly for underserved populations. While the revolutionary potential of PGT is considerable, deployment has been virtually limited to academic urban medical centers, thereby excluding rural and community-based health systems. This absence of representation threatens to reverse much-needed health care parity, particularly for the subgroup populations with unique cultural and socioeconomic challenges, such as American Indians. A recent study discusses pharmacogenetics interest among stakeholders in these groups, with an emphasis on culturally competent implementation strategies that are access and equity-focused (Killam et al., 2022). Additionally, the research indicates a widespread ignorance of pharmacogenomics by these groups, reaffirming a critical need for education programs that foster awareness and acceptance (Davies et al., 2024). By community-based approaches and telemedicine choices, physicians can develop more inclusive pharmacogenomic approaches that address the varied needs of patients in an effective manner (Figure 10.20).

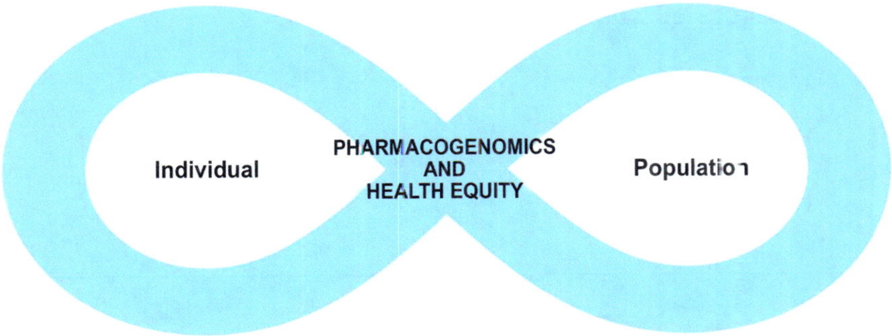

Figure 10.20. The integration of pharmacogenomics into healthcare presents a pivotal opportunity to address equity disparities, particularly among underserved populations.

Source: https://www.mdpi.com/pharmacy/pharmacy-11-00186/article_deploy/html/images/pharmacy-11-00186-g002.png.

10.4.8. Ethical Dilemmas in Genetic Research

The intersection of genetic investigation and ethical considerations is particularly relevant in the fields of pharmacogenetics and pharmacogenomics, where the implications of genetic individualization of drug therapy raise severe moral questions. As it advances to understand how genes affect drug responsiveness, the possibility of individualizing treatments based on an individual's genetic makeup is promising but problematic. Ethical problems are raised about access to these technologies; not every patient might be provided with equal care because of varying resources, potentially worsening current health inequalities. Additionally, discrimination based on genetic data adds another level of complexity to the issue. Literature shows that it is vital to address these ethical issues: The disease and its treatment must be dealt with in terms of genetic profiles to ensure efficiency and promote improved health outcomes (Dempton et al., 2011). Furthermore, the discovery of inter-patient variability in treatments for responses, particularly with chronic conditions like asthma, highlights the need for these ethics debates (Ellul-Micallef et al., 2016).

10.4.9. Future Ethical Considerations

With the development of pharmacogenomics and pharmacogenetics, the ethical aspects of their application become increasingly more complex. One such significant concern is the potential impact on patients' privacy, particularly about genetic data storage and retrieval procedures. Observance of individual confidentiality in personalized medicine is of most significant concern because failures may lead to discrimination or stigmatization. In addition, with such technologies enhancing the degree of customization in therapies, accessibility problems may arise; unequal access to genetic testing can exacerbate current health inequalities. Moreover, the implications of AI raised through various disciplines, such as education and archaeology, highlight the importance of rigorous ethical scrutiny; more reliance on algorithm-based decision-making in healthcare can contribute to bias or errors in interpreting genes (Rane, 2024; Tenzer et al., 2024). Next-generation ethical standards must not only shield against these risks but also create a culture that emphasizes well-informed consent and equitable treatment of all patients (Figure 10.21).

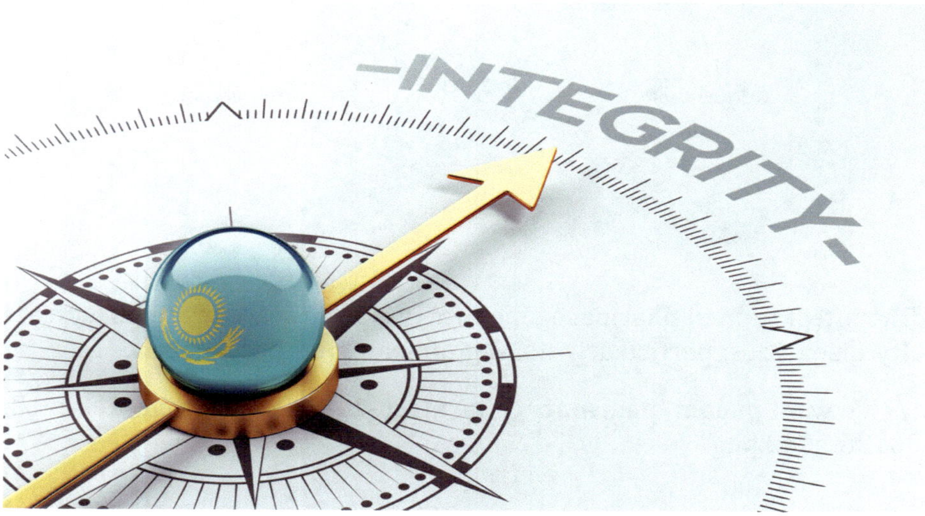

Figure 10.21. Ensuring that personalized medicine respects individual confidentiality is paramount, as breaches could lead to discrimination or stigmatization.

Source: https://aihcp.net/main/wp-content/uploads/2024/10/Ethic10-3.jpg.

Test Your Knowledge

1. What legal safeguards are in place to prevent genetic discrimination in healthcare or employment?
2. How might unequal access to pharmacogenomic testing worsen healthcare disparities?

Summary

The development of pharmacogenetics and pharmacogenomics holds much promise for the future of personalized medicine, particularly in enhancing drug performance and eliminating adverse effects. The use of genotyping is, nevertheless, limited in routine clinical practice due to conflicting results and a lack of standard guidelines for usage (Paepe et al., 2013). As the area of molecular genetics grows with technologies like NGS, the potential for more differentiated and personalized treatment options becomes an increasingly viable possibility. The translation into practice is hindered by issues like data quality, interpretation, and ethics, however. Besides, fields such as immunosuppressive therapy illustrate the intricacy of personalizing therapies using genetic profiles due to the importance of monitoring drug levels to maintain patient safety (Abboudi et al., 2012). To enhance the relevance of pharmacogenetic methods in clinical practice, long-term research and cooperation are needed.

Upon examining the key points of pharmacogenetics and pharmacogenomics, it becomes clear that these two fields represent a revolutionary approach to medicine, offering customized drug therapy choices based on genetic composition. The potential of PGT lies in its ability to customize pharmacologic treatments, more so for complex conditions such as BD, where responses to treatment can vary significantly across patients. Despite promising correlations between drug responses and gene markers, clinical adoption of PGT is presently limited due to a lack of certainty regarding validation and how to effectively implement this into decision-making (Berghofer et al., 2014). Furthermore, the inclusion of network pharmacology gives a robust framework for augmenting personalized medicine, emphasizing the necessity for new therapeutic methods based on genetics and world biochemical interactions (Marsh et al., 2010). Lastly, development in these areas of translational sciences has the potential to revolutionize drug discovery and improve therapeutic success for patients.

KEY TERMS FROM THIS CHAPTER

- DNA sequences
- Genetic variations
- Genotyping technology
- Immunosuppressive therapy
- Metabolomics
- Oncology
- Personalized genomic polygenic risk scores
- Pharmacogenetic testing (PGT)
- Phase II conjugative reactions
- Proteomics
- Genetic biomarkers
- Genomic map
- Human Genome Project
- Metabolites
- Next-generation sequencing (NGS) technology
- Patient privacy
- Personalized treatment
- Phase I reactions
- Precision medicine
- Thiopurine S-methyltransferase (TPMT)

Critical Thinking Questions

1. **What is the primary focus of pharmacogenetics?**
   a. How drugs alter organ function
   b. How genetic variations affect individual drug responses
   c. How to create synthetic drugs
   d. How food affects drug absorption
2. **Pharmacogenomics refers to:**
   a. Studying a single gene related to drug metabolism
   b. The interaction between a single drug and its target
   c. The study of the role of the entire genome in drug response
   d. The manufacturing of pharmaceuticals
3. **Which enzyme family is most commonly involved in pharmacogenetic variation?**
   a. Amylases
   b. Kinases
   c. Cytochrome P450 (CYP450)
   d. Proteases
4. **A patient with a CYP2D6 poor metabolizer phenotype is likely to experience:**
   a. Increased drug clearance
   b. Decreased drug effect
   c. Increased drug levels and risk of toxicity
   d. No change in drug response
5. **Which of the following drugs is commonly affected by pharmacogenetic variability in metabolism?**
   a. Paracetamol
   b. Codeine
   c. Ibuprofen
   d. Aspirin

Answers to Critical Thinking Questions

1. (b); 2. (c); 3. (c); 4. (c); 5. (b).

Short Answer Questions

1. What is pharmacogenetics, and how does it differ from pharmacogenomics?
2. How do genetic polymorphisms in drug-metabolizing enzymes affect drug response?
3. How is pharmacogenomic data used during the drug discovery and development process?
4. In what ways can pharmacogenomics reduce the failure rate of clinical trials?
5. How does pharmacogenetic testing guide the dosing of warfarin?
6. What are the potential ethical concerns related to the use of genetic information in prescribing drugs?

References

1. MacPhee, I., & Abboudi, N. (2012b). Individualized immunosuppression in transplant patients: potential role of pharmacogenetics. *Pharmacogenomics and Personalized Medicine*, 63. https://doi.org/10.2147/pgpm.s21743Anghel, S. A., Dinu-Pîrvu, C., Costache, M., Voiculescu, A. M., Ghica, M., Anuța, V., & Popa, L. (2024). Receptor pharmacogenomics: Deciphering genetic influence on drug response. *International Journal of Molecular Sciences, 25*. https://www.semanticscholar.org/paper/8a9ce86b5e6bc4a1f5bc1ea0694922363b05f50a (accessed on 10th June 2025).
2. Annemans, L., Berm, E. J. J., Boersma, C., de Looff, M., et al. (2016). Economic evaluations of pharmacogenetic and pharmacogenomic screening tests: A systematic review (second update of the literature). https://core.ac.uk/download/55807615.pdf (accessed on 10th June 2025).
3. Arnett, D., Avery, C. L., Bis, J. C., Boerwinkle, E., et al. (2015). Drug-gene interactions of antihypertensive medications and risk of incident cardiovascular disease: A pharmacogenomics study from the CHARGE consortium. https://core.ac.uk/download/42366925.pdf (accessed on 10th June 2025).
4. Ashiq, K., Ashiq, S., & Mustafa, N. (2023). Pharmacogenomics and the concept of personalized medicine for the management of hypertension. *Pakistan Heart Journal, 56*, 188–190. https://doi.org/10.47144/phj.v56i2.2553.
5. Ausi, Y., Barliana, M. I., Postma, M. J., & Suwantika, A. A. (2024). One step ahead in realizing pharmacogenetics in low-and middle-income countries: What should we do? https://core.ac.uk/download/653305168.pdf (accessed on 10th June 2025).
6. Avard, D., Joly, Y., Phillips, M. S., Silverstein, T., et al. (2007). Consent in pharmacogenomic research. https://core.ac.uk/download/46922901.pdf (accessed on 10th June 2025).
7. Barrese, V., Femminella, G. D., Ferrara, N., Rengo, G., et al. (2014). Tailoring therapy for heart failure: The pharmacogenomics of adrenergic receptor signaling. https://core.ac.uk/download/29469447.pdf (accessed on 10th June 2025).
8. Bartlett, M. J., & Shephard, E. A. (2016). The integration and interpretation of pharmacogenomics: A comparative study between the United States of America and Europe—Towards better health care. https://core.ac.uk/download/79517310.pdf (accessed on 10th June 2025).
9. Berghofer, A., Heils, A., Koski, A., Serretti, A., Szczepankiewicz, A., et al. (2014). *Towards the Clinical Implementation of Pharmacogenetics in Bipolar Disorder*. https://core.ac.uk/download/323064927.pdf (accessed on 10th June 2025).
10. Borg, J. J., Fenech, A. G., Grech, G., & Mitropoulos, K. (2012). Relevance of pharmacogenomics for developing countries in Europe: Implementation in the Maltese population. https://core.ac.uk/download/46602333.pdf (accessed on 10th June 2025).
11. Brazeau, D. A., & Brazeau, G. A. (2009). Role of the genomics revolution in pharmaceutics. https://core.ac.uk/download/146515647.pdf (accessed on 10th June 2025).
12. Burt, T., & Dhillon, S. (2013). Pharmacogenomics in early-phase clinical development. https://core.ac.uk/download/pdf/37750487.pdf (accessed on 10th June 2025).
13. Caputo, M., Corach, D., Flichman, D. M., et al. (2017). *Hepatitis C Virus Pharmacogenomics in Latin American Populations: Implications in The Era of Direct-Acting Antivirals*. https://core.ac.uk/download/159296291.pdf (accessed on 10th June 2025).

14. Cavallari, L. H., Hicks, J. K., Patel, J. N., Elchynski, A. L., Smith, D. M., Bargal, S. A., Fleck, A., et al. (2024). The Pharmacogenomics Global Research Network Implementation Working Group: Global collaboration to advance pharmacogenetic implementation. *Pharmacogenetics and Genomics*. https://www.semanticscholar.org/paper/de33a51c4fd7e2ec0808e93420c82ba2b59df0e2 (accessed on 10th June 2025).

15. Chatelin, J., Stathopoulou, M., Arguinano, A. A., Xie, T., & Visvikis-Siest, S. (2017). Pharmacogenomic challenges in cardiovascular diseases: Examples of drugs and considerations for future integration in clinical practice. *Current Pharmaceutical Biotechnology, 18*(3), 231–241. https://www.semanticscholar.org/paper/9a083090a38f2b18a244e2161b64b6fe170d318a (accessed on 10th June 2025).

16. Dash, B., Shireen, M., Pushpendra, M., Kumar, S., Goel, A., Semwal, P., & Rani, R. (2024). A comprehensive review: Pharmacogenomics and personalized medicine—Customizing drug therapy based on individual genetic profiles. *Chinese Journal of Applied Physiology, 40*, e20240011. https://www.semanticscholar.org/paper/247b582d7ab873598b3ec72eed5242c79ab0fd6b (accessed on 10th June 2025).

17. Davies, M. L. (2024). *Perspectives of Utilizing Pharmacogenomics to Inform Tobacco Cessation: Survey Results from An American Indian Community*. https://core.ac.uk/download/615798759.pdf (accessed on 10th June 2025).

18. De Paepe, A., & Vanakker, O. (2013). *Pharmacogenomics in Children: Advantages and Challenges of Next Generation Sequencing Applications*. https://core.ac.uk/download/55848729.pdf (accessed on 10th June 2025).

19. De Pretis, F., van Gils, M., & Forsberg, M. (2022). A smart hospital-driven approach to precision pharmacovigilance. *Trends in Pharmacological Sciences, 43*, 473–481. https://doi.org/10.1016/j.tips.2022.03.009.

20. Deb, S., Hopefl, R., Reeves, A., & Cvetkovic, D. (2024). ADME gene-related pharmacogenomic labeling of FDA-approved drugs: Comparison with Clinical Pharmacogenetics Implementation Consortium (CPIC) evidence levels. *Medicines, 11*. https://www.semanticscholar.org/paper/d1b5849ad6f8b6a645a782c7709a7eddefbb38f9 (accessed on 10th June 2025).

21. Dempton, J. L. (2011). *Genetic Intervention as A Lifestyle Approach: An Analysis of Disease and Treatment*. https://core.ac.uk/download/236291395.pdf (accessed on 10th June 2025).

22. Dhruv, F., & Farheen, F. (2023). A narrative review of advances in pharmacogenetics and personalized medicine in psychiatry. https://core.ac.uk/download/588466583.pdf (accessed on 10th June 2025).

23. Djeunang Dongho, G. B., Martinelli, A., Motshoge, T., et al. (2018). Human cytochrome P450 2B6 genetic variability in Botswana: A case of haplotype diversity and convergent phenotypes. https://core.ac.uk/download/154947683.pdf (accessed on 10th June 2025).

24. Dodson, C., & Layman, L. (2022). Refinement of a pharmacogenomics app for dosing guidelines for oncology: Findings from the usability evaluation. *Annals of Translational Medicine, 10*, 1261. https://doi.org/10.21037/atm-2022-68.

25. El Shamieh, S., Saleem, R., Halat, D. H., Fakhoury, H. M. A., Bastaki, K., Fawaz, M., Malki, A., et al. (2025). Integrating pharmacogenomics in three Middle Eastern countries' healthcare (Lebanon, Qatar, and Saudi Arabia): Current insights, challenges, and strategic directions. *PLOS One, 20*. https://www.semanticscholar.org/paper/0b0cbc35add8007dffb6678a4257e65e1a2247b8 (accessed on 10th June 2025).

26. Ellul-Micallef, R., & Fenech, A. G. (2016). *Pharmacogenetics of Asthma Therapeutics*. https://core.ac.uk/download/83019668.pdf (accessed on 10th June 2025).

27. Evans, B. J. (2006). What will it take to reap the clinical benefits of pharmacogenomics? https://core.ac.uk/download/46955240.pdf (accessed on 10th June 2025).

28. Fenech, A. G. (2007). *Pharmacogenetics: The Path to Personalized Prescribing*. https://core.ac.uk/download/83019753.pdf (accessed on 10th June 2025).

29. Freedman, A. N., Potosky, A. L., BIG Health Consortium, Cancer Centers Program, caBIG Community, et al. (2010). Cancer pharmacogenomics and pharmacoepidemiology: Setting a research agenda to accelerate translation. https://core.ac.uk/download/pdf/8484043.pdf (accessed on 10th June 2025).

30. Gambari, R., Waziri, A., Goonasekera, H., & Peprah, E. (2024). Pharmacogenomics of drugs used in β-thalassemia and sickle-cell disease: From basic research to clinical applications. *International Journal of Molecular Sciences, 25*. https://www.semanticscholar.org/paper/75a670923b46923bc57f7303ca49bef62029bb02 (accessed on 10th June 2025).

31. Geetha, K., Chandana, T., Sakshi, R., Chandu, C. S., & Ramarao, T. (2024). Pharmacogenomics in healthcare: Applications, challenges, and future directions with a focus on oncology. *International Journal of Health Sciences and Research*. https://www.semanticscholar.org/paper/2831472a14960f1801563eb3b3c25dc1ab5bad5e (accessed on 10th June 2025).

32. Genovese, A., & Butler, M. G. (2023). The autism spectrum: Behavioral, psychiatric and genetic associations. *Genes, 14*, 677. https://doi.org/10.3390/genes14030677.

33. Ginsburg, G. S., & Phillips, K. A. (2018). Precision medicine: From science to value. *Health Affairs, 37*, 694–701. https://doi.org/10.1377/hlthaff.2017.1624 (accessed on 10th June 2025).

34. Hedgecoe, A. M., Akhtar, A., Anderson, A., Anon, A., Bazell, C., Beauchamp, T., Beeson, D., et al. (2006). *Context, Ethics and Pharmacogenetics*. https://core.ac.uk/download/2708534.pdf (accessed on 10th June 2025).

35. Junaidi, A., Sazali, N., Gunawan, T., & Widiastuti, N. (2025). A mini review on advancements in membrane technologies for CO_2 separation: The role of polyphenylene sulfide fillers. *Journal of Applied Membrane Science & Technology*. https://www.semanticscholar.org/paper/ca7044be039b9ab7ed5d610fef25582b8bcc0d74 (accessed on 10th June 2025).

36. Killam, S. (2022). *Equitable Pharmacogenetic Testing Implementation for Rural and Underserved Populations*. https://core.ac.uk/download/534827834.pdf (accessed on 10th June 2025).

37. Koch, V. G. (2012). *Incentivizing the Utilization of Pharmacogenomics in Drug Development*. https://core.ac.uk/download/56355492.pdf (accessed on 10th June 2025).

38. Krivosova, M., Hutka, P., Hrtanek, I., Ondrejka, I., Maggioni, L., Marcatili, M., Clerici, M., et al. (2025). Slovak psychiatrists' perspective on the role of pharmacogenetic testing in mental health care. *International Journal of Neuropsychopharmacology, 28*, i281. https://www.semanticscholar.org/paper/a693e225a5005e602367584abf34393be1c4e1a8 (accessed on 10th June 2025).

39. Liu, J. S., Chen, Y., Shi, D., Zhang, B., & Pu, J. (2022). Pharmacogenomics—A new frontier for individualized treatment of Parkinson's disease. *Current Neuropharmacology, 21*, 536–546. https://doi.org/10.2174/1570159x21666221229154830.

40. Luzum, J. A., Petry, N., Taylor, A. K., Van Driest, S. L., Dunnenberger, H. M., & Cavallari,

L. H. (2021). Moving pharmacogenetics into practice: It's all about the evidence! *Clinical Pharmacology & Therapeutics, 110*, 649–661. https://doi.org/10.1002/cpt.2327.

41. Mak, S. S. S., & Chan, M. L. T. (2024). How nurses face a new era of genomics medicine and precision health: Oncology nurse clinicians' perspective. *Asia-Pacific Journal of Oncology Nursing, 11*, 100506. https://doi.org/10.1016/j.apjon.2024.100506.
42. Malviya, A. K., & Khanna, P. (2024). Precision medicine in anesthesia: Pharmacogenomics and personalized care. *National Board of Examinations Journal of Medical Sciences*. https://www.semanticscholar.org/paper/c23339ffda6b32e49ff331b27f7fa9cebe434e60 (accessed on 10th June 2025).
43. Mao, H. (2024). Advancements in filter technology: Evolution and applications. *Highlights in Science, Engineering and Technology*. https://www.semanticscholar.org/paper/fde450aca69ac70570abd3e224a3e7c39679839e (accessed on 10th June 2025).
44. Marsh, A., Singer, D. R. J., Taylor, P. C., & Watkins, P. B. (2010). Personalized medicine: The impact on chemistry. https://core.ac.uk/download/45676.pdf (accessed on 10th June 2025).
45. Matsuyama, K., Kurihara, C., Crawley, F., & Kerpel-Fronius, S. (2023). Utilization of genetic information for medicines development and equitable benefit sharing. *Frontiers in Genetics, 14*. https://www.semanticscholar.org/paper/492c0129d905b252fe50e32f1fbf3df552a7bb2f (accessed on 10th June 2025).
46. Miller, M. L., Seligson, N. D., Duong, B. Q., Elia, J., Hasan, S., Lacy, T., Blake, K. V., et al. (2025). Opportunities for pharmacogenomics in pediatrics: Prescribing trends of psychiatric medications with pharmacogenomic implications at a multistate pediatric health system. *The Journal of Pediatric Pharmacology and Therapeutics*. https://www.semanticscholar.org/paper/45abfc6285aca2cb98af86dc3c95584ede4b8b02 (accessed on 10th June 2025).
47. Mosch, R., van der Lee, M., Guchelaar, H., & Swen, J. (2024). Pharmacogenetic panel testing: A review of current practice and potential for clinical implementation. *Annual Review of Pharmacology and Toxicology*. https://www.semanticscholar.org/paper/e9ddbc40237099d5808e286ee6638138cccb10da (accessed on 10th June 2025).
48. Naik, D. (2019). Implementation of pharmacogenomics into electronic health record and clinical decision support. https://core.ac.uk/download/234018950.pdf (accessed on 10th June 2025).
49. Padmanabhan, S., du Toit, C., & Dominiczak, A. F. (2023). Cardiovascular precision medicine–A pharmacogenomic perspective. *Cambridge Prisms Precision Medicine, 1*. https://doi.org/10.1017/pcm.2023.17.
50. Petek, A., & Filaković, P. (2009). Personalized pharmacotherapy in psychiatry. https://core.ac.uk/download/14420495.pdf (accessed on 10th June 2025).
51. Pinzón-Espinosa, J., van der Horst, M. Z., Zinkstok, J., Austin, J., Aalfs, C. M., Batalla, A., Sullivan, P. F., et al. (2022). Barriers to genetic testing in clinical psychiatry and ways to overcome them: From clinicians' attitudes to sociocultural differences between patients across the globe. *Translational Psychiatry, 12*. https://doi.org/10.1038/s41398-022-02203-6.
52. Rane, N. (2024). Enhancing the quality of teaching and learning through ChatGPT and similar large language models: Challenges, future prospects, and ethical considerations in education. *TESOL and Technology Studies*. https://www.semanticscholar.org/paper/a73314f0c42eb5902e1ab5bb5b07455b5f9fb6e3 (accessed on 10th June 2025).

53. Roberts, C., Sazonovs, A., Smith, R., Bishara, M., Lin, S., Neil, C., Bewshea, C., et al. (2024). OP11: Exploring the potential clinical utility of NUDT15 pharmacogenetic testing in clinical practice: A 'focused reverse phenotyping' study in the UK IBD Bioresource. *Journal of Crohn's and Colitis*. https://www.semanticscholar.org/paper/ca8de5c63fb59b4a814528670a9105cab26c01b0 (accessed on 10th June 2025).

54. Sadée, W., Wang, D., Hartmann, K. E., & Toland, A. E. (2023). Pharmacogenomics: Driving personalized medicine. *Pharmacological Reviews, 75*(4), 789–814. https://doi.org/10.1124/pharmrev.122.000810.

55. Salas-Hernández, A., Galleguillos, M., Carrasco, M., López-Cortés, A., Redal, M. A., Fonseca, D. J., Esperón, P., et al. (2023). An updated examination of the perception of barriers for pharmacogenomics implementation and the usefulness of drug/gene pairs in Latin America and the Caribbean. *Frontiers in Pharmacology, 14*. https://doi.org/10.3389/fphar.2023.1175737.

56. Schrijver, I., & Wiita, A. P. (2011). Clinical application of high throughput molecular screening techniques for pharmacogenomics. https://core.ac.uk/download/323063319.pdf (accessed on 10th June 2025).

57. Senn, S. (2021). *Statistical Issues in Drug Development*. https://doi.org/10.1002/9781119238614.

58. Shivashankara, M. (2020). Pharmacogenomics. *Indian Journal of Medical and Paediatric Oncology, 41*, 550–551. https://www.semanticscholar.org/paper/6a8053a358b8a1b8a5158 4b866278e5911c7f8ca (accessed on 10th June 2025).

59. Singh, S., Stocco, G., Theken, K. N., Dickson, A. L., Feng, Q., Karnes, J. H., Mosley, J., et al. (2024). Pharmacogenomics polygenic risk score: Ready or not for prime time? *Clinical and Translational Science, 17*. https://www.semanticscholar.org/paper/85e27046715a4d95166 76fdfe48009a8327b2775 (accessed on 10th June 2025).

60. Suarez-Kurtz, G. (2019). Pharmacogenetic testing in oncology: A Brazilian perspective. https://core.ac.uk/download/268270134.pdf (accessed on 10th June 2025).

61. Sugino, S., & Janicki, P. (2015). Pharmacogenetics of chemotherapy-induced nausea and vomiting. *Pharmacogenomics, 16*(2), 149–160. https://www.semanticscholar.org/paper/db 325463b937208ce38630a7495a9cec8175229c (accessed on 10th June 2025).

62. Tenzer, M., Pistilli, G., Bransden, A., & Shenfield, A. (2024). Debating AI in archaeology: Applications, implications, and ethical considerations. *Internet Archaeology*. https://www.semanticscholar.org/paper/15e1d850ae113b1acf136f379c0eb1a22f4edbd8 (accessed on 10th June 2025).

63. Terzic, A., & Waldman, S. A. (2017). *Clinical Pharmacology & Therapeutics: Past, Present, and Future*. https://core.ac.uk/download/83049656.pdf (accessed on 10th June 2025).

64. Verbelen, M., Weale, M. E., & Lewis, C. M. (2017). Cost-effectiveness of pharmacogenetic-guided treatment: Are we there yet? *The Pharmacogenomics Journal, 17*, 395–402. https://doi.org/10.1038/tpj.2017.21.

65. Wang, R., & Wang, Z. (2023). Precision medicine: Disease subtyping and tailored treatment. *Cancers, 15*, 3837. https://doi.org/10.3390/cancers15153837.

66. Williams, L. M. (2022). Special report: Precision psychiatry—Are we getting closer? *Psychiatric News, 57*. https://doi.org/10.1176/appi.pn.2022.09.9.23.

67. Wright, D., & Youssef, E. (2020). *Pharmacogenomic Testing and Its Future in Community*

Pharmacy. https://core.ac.uk/download/288394496.pdf (accessed on 10th June 2025).

68. Zhou, Y., Tremmel, R., Schaeffeler, E., Schwab, M., & Lauschke, V. M. (2022). Challenges and opportunities associated with rare-variant pharmacogenomics. *Trends in Pharmacological Sciences, 43*(11), 852–865. https://doi.org/10.1016/j.tips.2022.07.002.

ANTIMICROBIAL PHARMACOLOGY AND STEWARDSHIP

11

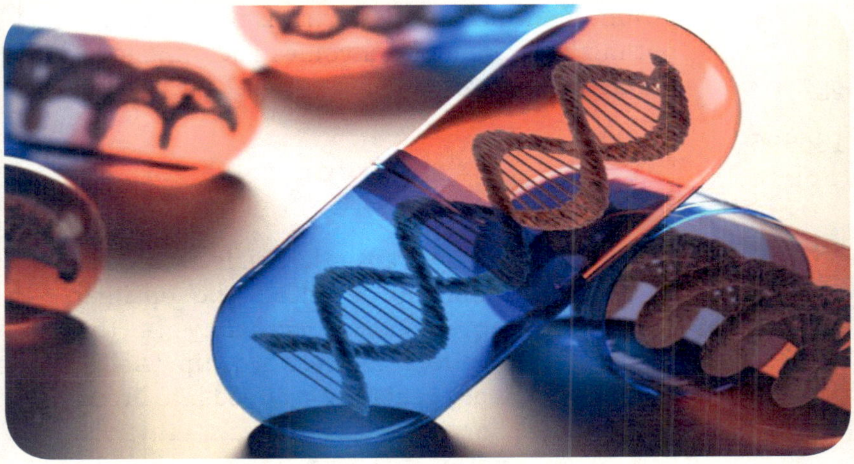

LEARNING OBJECTIVES

After studying this chapter, you will be able to:

1. Understand mechanisms of antimicrobial action
2. Focus on antimicrobial resistance
3. Learn principles of antimicrobial stewardship
4. Discuss future directions in antimicrobial pharmacology

Introduction

In recent years, the rising threat of antimicrobial resistance (AMR) has emerged as a priority public health issue, requiring re-evaluation of existing antimicrobial use strategies and stewardship. Inappropriate use of these lifesaving medications not only harms patient health but also compromises the efficacy of available treatments, leading to longer stays in the hospital and unnecessary deaths. Therefore, the integration of AMSP in healthcare organizations has also become imperative, with emphasis on a collaborative approach between healthcare professionals for optimized, appropriate selection and use of antimicrobials (Ahmad et al., 2018). The education regarding antimicrobial stewardship continues to be a persistent deficit in medical and pharmacy curricula, which systemically remain untreated despite its identification as a patient care determinant and interprofessional collaboration (Chin-Hong et al., 2017). Hence, these educational shortfalls have to be filled to equip future healthcare professionals with the necessary capabilities to tackle the pervasive issue of AMR and enhance patient outcomes (Figure 11.1).

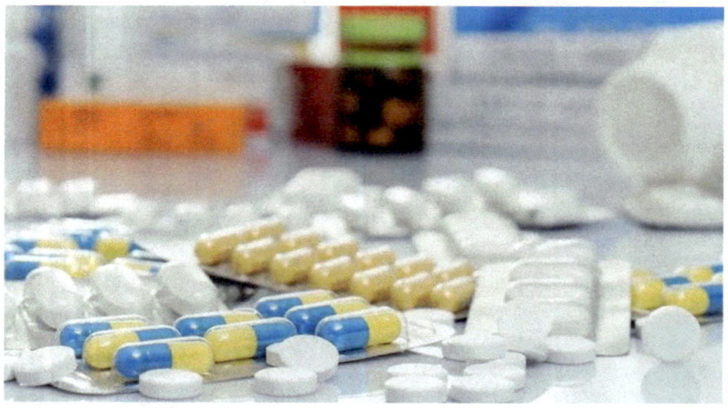

Figure 11.1. Antimicrobial pharmacology.

Source: https://cdn.britannica.com/95/186995-138-0E906776/antibiotics-overuse.jpg?w=800&h=450&c=crop.

11.1. Mechanisms of Antimicrobial Action

Learning Outcome

1. Understand the classification of antimicrobials
2. Explain mechanisms of action for antibiotics, antivirals, antifungals, and antiparasitic
3. Explain pharmacokinetics and pharmacodynamics
4. Discuss synergistic and antagonistic effects
5. Learn resistance mechanisms in pathogens
6. Know the role of biofilms in antimicrobial efficacy

Knowledge of antimicrobial mechanisms is critical to effective treatment design and resistance to the increasing menace of AMR. Antimicrobials work by disrupting particular structures or activities of bacteria, e.g., cell wall assembly inhibition, disruption of protein synthesis, or inhibition of nucleic acid replication. These targeted actions decrease microbial viability, leading ultimately to cell death or stasis. But bacteria can develop resistance mechanisms, such as altering target sites or employing efflux pumps that export the drug, making treatment difficult and conducive to the emergence of multidrug-resistant strains (McFall, 2021). In contexts like urinary tract infections, in which the prevalence of antibiotic prescription is considerably high, an understanding of these mechanisms aids stewardship interventions necessary for sustaining the efficacy of available antimicrobials and developing new therapeutic agents (Prieto et al., 2024). Hence, a clear vision of antimicrobial mechanisms is vital for optimizing treatment outcomes and enhancing public health programs.

11.1.1. Classification of Antimicrobials

The classification of antimicrobials is central to their mechanisms of action and optimal treatment approaches, specifically in the context of antimicrobial stewardship (AMS). Antimicrobials are generally grouped into broad categories, e.g., antibiotics, antifungals, antivirals, and antiparasitic, directed against specific pathogens. Antibiotics, further subclassified as beta-lactams and macrolides, demonstrate the nuance of antimicrobial therapy; they are used to treat a wide array of bacterial infections with a constantly changing spectrum of activity. The relevance of accurate antimicrobial classification is particularly keen when treating infections like intra-abdominal infections (IAI), where the timely selection of effective agents is essential in determining the outcome in patients (Strauss et al., 2016). Furthermore, the emergence of resistance is a significant challenge in antimicrobial pharmacology. As over 50% of antimicrobials are misused, the knowledge framed through accurate categorization goes a long way in informing prescribing behaviors and reducing the prevalence of resistant pathogens, which improves in AMS initiatives (Bodke et al., 2024) (Figure 11.2).

Category	Class (example)
Category I Very High Importance	• Carbapenems (Imipenem) • Cephalosporins (3rd & 4th gen) (Ceftiofur) • Fluoroquinolones (Enrofloxacin) • Glycopeptides (Vancomycin) • Glycylcyclines • Ketolides • Lipopeptides • Monobactams • Nitroimidazoles (Metronidazole) • Oxazolidinones • Penicillin-β-lactamase inhibitors (Amoxicillin/Clavulanic Acid) • Polymyxin (colistin, polymyxin B) • Therapeutic agents for TB
Category II High Importance	• Aminoglycosides (Gentamicin) • Cephalosporins (1st and 2nd gen - Cefapirin) • Fusidic acid • Lincosamides (Lincomycin) • Macrolides (Tulathromycin) • Penicillins • Quinolones (except fluoroquinolones) • Streptogramins (Virginiamycin) • Trimethoprim/sulfamethoxazole
Category III Medium Importance	• Aminocyclitols (Streptomycin) • Aminoglycosides • Bacitracins • Fosfomycin • Phenicols (Florfenicol) • Sulphonamides (Sulphathiazole) • Tetracyclines (Oxytetracycline) • Trimethoprim
Category IV Low Importance	• Flavophospholipols (Bambermycin) • Ionophores (Monensin)

Figure 11.2. The classification of antimicrobials.

Source: https://www.amstewardship.ca/wp-content/uploads/2018/07/ACER-Vets_V3_Table-2.png.

11.1.2. Mechanisms of Action for Antibiotics

The mechanisms of action for antibiotics are paramount in the recognition of their effectiveness in combating bacterial infections as well as in the advantages to antimicrobial stewardship. Antibiotics have numerous mechanisms of action, primarily inhibiting the synthesis of bacterial cell walls, proteins, nucleic acids, and biochemical processes. For instance, beta-lactams disrupt cell wall synthesis, leading to cell lysis. In contrast, aminoglycosides disrupt protein synthesis by inhibiting the binding of ribosomal subunits, with subsequent effects on bacterial growth and reproduction. The misuse of these agents can promote resistance, a risk noted in some studies that highlighted the importance of effective antimicrobial therapy in the control of infections like IAI (Strauss et al., 2016). Furthermore, there needs to be creative intervention programs to enhance public awareness about AMR and enlighten healthcare professionals since few studies have proved helpful in applying theoretical models to strengthen the understanding of behavior change in antibiotic prescribing (Davis et al., 2018).

11.1.3. Mechanisms of Action for Antivirals

Antiviral mechanisms of action are varied and a critical area of study in antimicrobial pharmacology, particularly in the face of rising resistance problems. Antivirals can target several steps in the virus life cycle, thereby inhibiting replication and reducing viral loads. Some antivirals, for instance, operate by inhibiting viral entry into host cells via mechanisms like receptor blockade or through altering host cell membranes. These others prevent viral enzymes that are used for replication from functioning, such as polymerases and proteases, which are essential for the creation of viral genetic material and proteins. Furthermore, understanding these mechanisms is indispensable for the development of stewardship programs for antivirals based on the rational use of the agents in order to prevent any resistance development. As indicated in previous research, the sensible use of antivirals is necessary to guarantee their efficacy in the context of increasing resistance pressures (Bradstreet et al., 2022; Laine et al., 2017) (Figure 11.3).

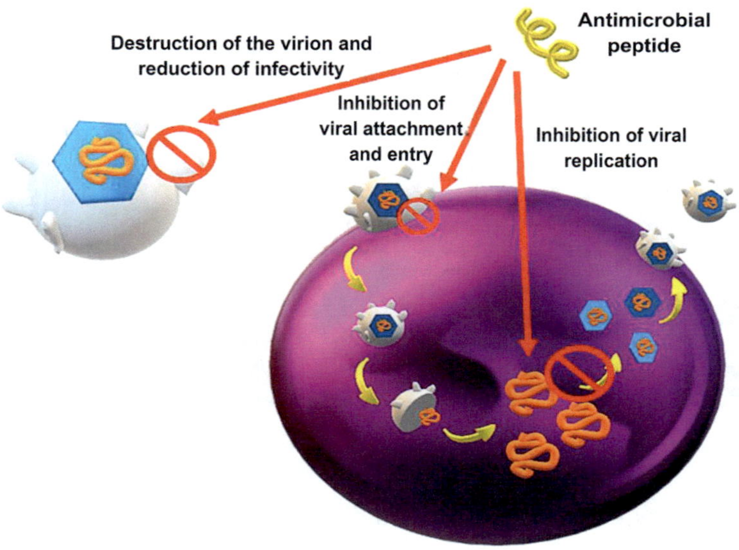

Figure 11.3. Antivirals can target various stages of the viral life cycle, thereby inhibiting replication and reducing viral load.

Source: https://onlinelibrary.wiley.com/cms/asset/2265bcdd-01d9-47f6-a4f3-9d5cb2d1b336/psc3534-fig-0001-m.jpg.

11.1.4. Mechanisms of Action for Antifungals

Understanding antifungal mechanisms of action is significant in the broader context of antimicrobial pharmacology and stewardship, particularly as the landscape of fungal infections continues to evolve. Antifungals primarily act against the unique cell structures and metabolic processes of fungi, which are significantly different from those of human cells. For instance, compounds like azoles inhibit the pathway of ergosterol synthesis, a critical component of the fungal cell membrane, thus compromising its integrity and leading to cell death. Other groups, including echinocandins, disrupt the cell wall's glucan synthesis pathway, thereby destabilizing the organism. This specificity is necessary to maintain collateral damage to the host microbiome at minimal levels, which is essential in the current scenario of rising AMR. The incorporation of data on antimicrobial activities, such as synergies between non-antibiotic drugs with antifungals (Barbosa et al., 2022), is also pivotal to the optimization of therapeutic approaches and better patient outcomes where there are issues of resistance (Strauss et al., 2016).

11.1.5. Mechanisms of Action for Antiparasitics

The therapeutic effectiveness of antiparasitic drugs depends on their different modes of action, which play a vital role in combating parasitic disease and checking the development of AMR. Among the well-documented classes of antiparasitics, the quinolines primarily inhibit heme polymerization, an essential process to the viability of Plasmodium species, and thus block vital metabolic processes in the parasites. Similarly, avermectins capitalize on glutamate-gated chloride channels, inducing paralysis and death in susceptible helminths and arthropods. Such understanding is essential not just to treat parasitic infections effectively but also for enhanced antimicrobial stewardship. Mismanagement of such treatments would result in resistance, as exemplified in ongoing studies demonstrating prevalent inappropriate prescribing behavior leading to AMR. Thus, the inclusion of complete educational frameworks tackling the mechanisms of antiparasitic action is crucial to bridge knowledge gaps in veterinary medicine and human medicine (Bradstreet et al., 2022; Bezuidenhout et al., 2023) (Figure 11.4).

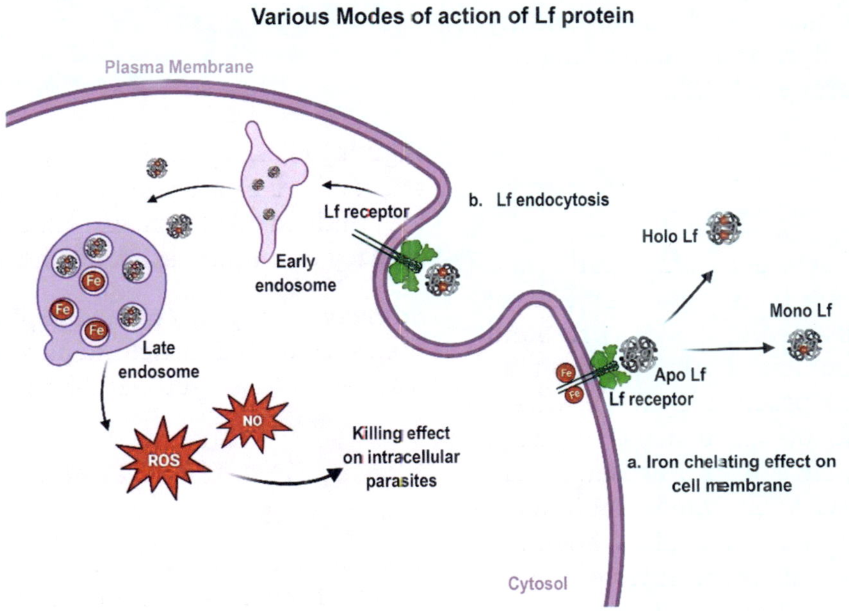

Figure 11.4. The efficacy of antiparasitic agents hinges on their distinct mechanisms of action, which are vital in combating parasitic infections and mitigating the risk of antimicrobial resistance.

Source: https://www.frontiersin.org/files/Articles/1330398/fpara-02-1330398-HTML-r2/image_m/fpara-02-1330398-g001.jpg.

11.1.6. Pharmacokinetics and Pharmacodynamics

In antimicrobial drug pharmacology, PK/PD is crucial to maximize therapeutic benefit while minimizing resistance. PK/PD analysis provides a rationale for understanding how drug concentration over time in the body correlates with its biological effect and thus with the dosage regimen to maximize benefit and minimize toxicity. For instance, the EMA emphasizes PK/PD studies to establish rational dosing regimens that involve *in vitro*, *ex vivo*, and *in vivo* models aimed at maximizing antibiotic usage and resistance prevention strategies (Ruiz et al., 2021). Furthermore, PK/PD-guided specialized dosing techniques are required in high-risk groups like neonates due to the interplay of pharmacological characteristics with physiological maturation. Using new technologies like model-informed precision dosing can enhance the exposure of antibiotics to maximize optimization with lower toxicity and improve collaboration among medical professionals (Berardi et al., 2023).

11.1.7. Synergistic and Antagonistic Effects

The relationship between synergistic and antagonistic effects is a key element of antimicrobial pharmacology with profound implications for outcomes of treatment as well as stewardship practice. Synergy, where the activity of two or more drugs is more than the sum of their separate activities, can optimize therapeutic effect while minimizing resistance development. Antagonism, however, may take place where drugs interfere with each other's activity, complicating treatment regimens and making therapeutic failure probable. Understanding these dynamics is crucial for maximizing drug combinations, particularly in light of the upcoming challenge posed by multidrug-resistant pathogens. For example, certain five-membered heterocycles form the cores of optimizing the design of good antimicrobial agents, wherein their structural features dictate the biological activity, including synergistic interactions that may maximize antibacterial activities while having an appreciable safety profile (Rusu et al., 2023). On the other hand, miscalibrated pairs may provide toxicities that negate the therapeutic purpose, reasserting the criticality of judicious pairing within AMSP (Kamel et al., 2024) (Figure 11.5).

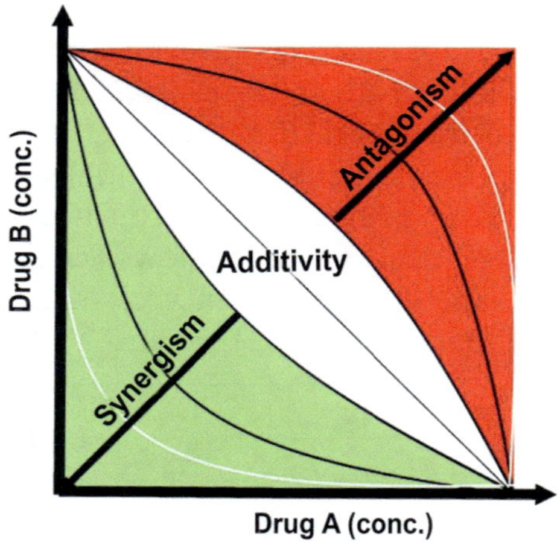

Figure 11.5. Synergy, where the combined effect of two or more agents exceeds the sum of their individual effects, can enhance therapeutic efficacy and limit resistance development.

Source: https://www.mdpi.com/toxics/toxics-03-00342/article_deploy/html/images/toxics-03-00342-g001-1024.png.

11.1.8. Resistance Mechanisms in Pathogens

The resistance to antimicrobials in pathogens is one of the most significant challenges facing public health and effective disease control. Pathogens employ mechanisms such as alteration of drug targets, enzymatic inactivation of the antimicrobials, and increased efflux of the drugs to be responsible for this resistance. The creation of multi-drug-resistant organisms, particularly among Gram-negative bacteria, has put healthcare professionals and researchers in a state of shock. These developments have been linked with excessive and inappropriate use of antibiotics, which favors the swift evolution of resistance. As mentioned by (Strauss et al., 2016), inappropriate initial antimicrobial therapy can lead to adverse results in patients, thereby stressing the necessity for broader awareness and rational use of these medicines. Similarly, Bradstreet et al. (2022) point to the imperative necessity of efficient AMSP to counter resistance and promote therapeutic success, emphasizing the interrelatedness of human, animal, and environmental health in addressing this crisis.

11.1.9. Role of Biofilms in Antimicrobial Efficacy

Biofilms, structured microbial communities implanted in a self-produced extracellular matrix, have a strong influence on antimicrobial efficacy and pose particular challenges to therapeutic strategies. Such complex systems enable bacteria to manifest enhanced resistance to antimicrobial compounds, primarily due to altered microenvironmental conditions and enhanced protective barriers to drug penetration. Biofilm formation has also been linked to mechanisms of quorum sensing and efflux pump usage, both of which have roles to play in resistance and persistence in hostile environments (Adu et al., 2019). Additionally, the unique structure of biofilms can disrupt effective delivery of therapeutic agents, complicating treatment protocols in clinical settings (Cooper et al., 2018). This resistance underscores the need for novel ideas in antimicrobial pharmacology, in particular aimed at biofilm-related infections and current research into naturally occurring compounds with anti-biofilm properties that may supplement existing treatment modalities under the auspices of stewardship programs (Figure 11.6).

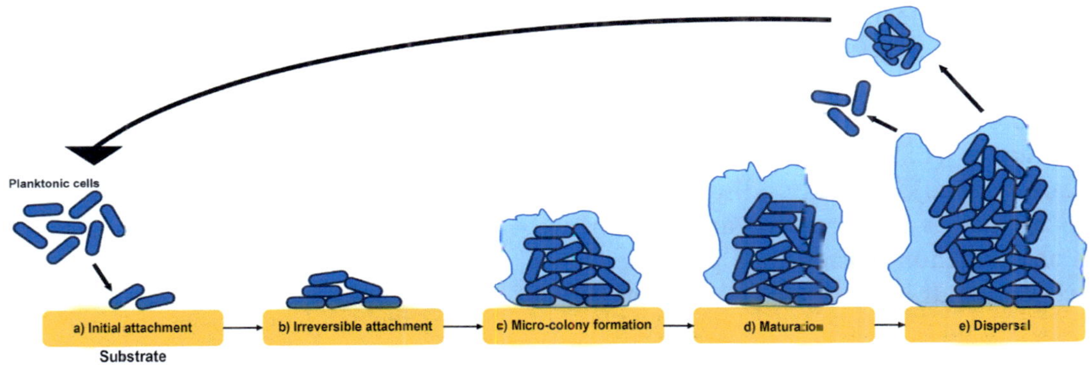

Figure 11.6. Biofilms, structured communities of microorganisms encased in a self-produced extracellular matrix, significantly influence antimicrobial efficacy and pose considerable challenges for treatment strategies.

Source: https://media.springernature.com/full/springer-static/image/art%3A10.1038%2Fs44259-024-00046-3/MediaObjects/44259_2024_46_Fig1_HTML.png.

Test Your Knowledge

1. What is the mechanism of action of aminoglycosides?
2. In what way does the mechanism of action of antifungal drugs differ from antibacterial agents?

11.2. Antimicrobial Resistance

Learning Outcome

1. Understand the definition and types of antimicrobial resistance
2. Know the causes of antimicrobial resistanceExplain the global impact of antimicrobial resistanceDiscuss surveillance and monitoring of resistance
3. Explain the role of healthcare settings in resistance
4. Focus on the economic implications of resistance
5. Learn strategies to combat resistance
6. Know the role of education in resistance prevention
7. Understand future directions in resistance research

The rise in the prevalence of AMR is a terrifying public health challenge, particularly in hospitals where the effectiveness of present-day antibiotics is compromised. Gram-negative bacteria, that is, Escherichia coli and Klebsiella pneumoniae, have emerged as the primary causative pathogens of severe infections through methods such as Extended-Spectrum Beta-Lactamases (ESBLs) and Metallo-Beta-Lactamases (MBLs) (Chattopadhyay et al., 2024). AMSP use is required in India, where the AMR phenomenon is especially prominent. AMSPs are being put in place for rational use of antimicrobials, improvement in patient outcomes, and reduction in unnecessary health care costs due to resistant infection (Shah et al., 2023). Implementation of effective AMSP, however, is foiled by numerous challenges, including scarce resources, poor laboratory infrastructure, and irrational prescribing. Overcoming these hurdles with integrative strategies is pivotal to avert the risk of AMR and preserve the efficacy of present antimicrobial agents.

11.2.1. Definition and Types of Antimicrobial Resistance

AMR is a world health issue, and this calls for cautious stewardship in the pharmacology discipline. AMR has been termed as when microbes such as bacteria, viruses, fungi, and parasites evolve to become resistant to drugs previously effective in targeting them, leading to treatment failure. AMR can be categorized into innate and acquired resistance, while the former can further be split into horizontal gene transfer and mutation processes. For instance, Helicobacter pylori exhibits acquired resistance through genetic alterations that complicate its treatment regimens and necessitate ongoing research and updated management strategies (Malfertheiner et al., 2022). Additionally, in children, inappropriate and overuse of antibiotics significantly complicate the issue, with a rise in multidrug-resistant organisms such as MRSA and carbapenem-resistant Enterobacteriaceae (Romandini et al., 2021). Fighting AMR calls for a multi-faceted approach that prioritizes judicious prescribing and new treatment methods to combat the threat of a post-antibiotic era (Figure 11.7).

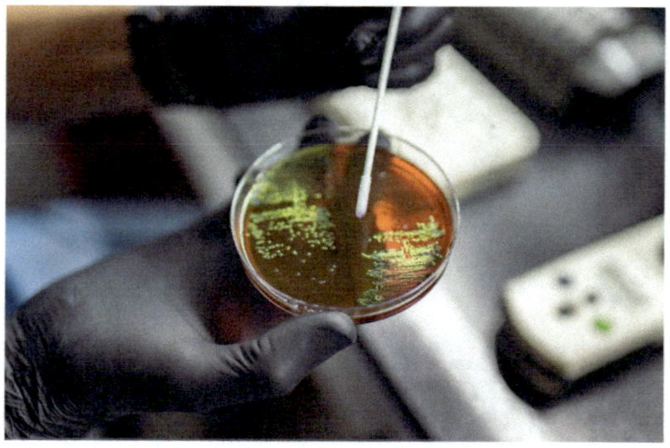

Figure 11.7. Antimicrobial resistance (AMR) represents a significant global health challenge, underscoring the need for vigilant stewardship in pharmacology.

Source: https://cdn.who.int/media/images/default-source/amr-lib/blink-shoot-malbran_sarah-pabst_00285.jpg?sfvrsn=dd75ea20_8.

11.2.2. Causes of Antimicrobial Resistance

AMR development is driven by a constellation of interrelated factors ranging from misuse of antibiotics in human and veterinary medicine to spread of resistant organisms in the environment. For instance, widespread misuse of colistin, which was once considered to be a last-line drug, has led to the emergence of colistin-resistant bacteria among multidrug-resistant Gram-negative Enterobacteriaceae. Such resistance results from gene changes blocking the drugs from being attached to bacterial membranes, emphasizing the subtle biological adaptations of pathogens under antimicrobial pressure (Gogry et al., 2021). Furthermore, veterinary care that encourages antimicrobial stewardship has shown that prudent antibiotic use can both assure improved patient outcomes and stop the emergence of resistance (Frey et al., 2022). Hence, it is critical to understand these causes and implement effective stewardship practices to promote the preservation of the effectiveness of existing antimicrobials and combat the impending increase of AMR worldwide.

11.2.3. Global Impact of Antimicrobial Resistance

The global burden of AMR is an increasing threat to public health that significantly undermines the efficacy of infection therapy in most healthcare settings. Aside from the added morbidity and mortality, it also has enormous economic consequences in the form of escalated costs and prolonged length of stay in the hospital. The intricate process of AMR, including enzymatic breakdown and biofilm development, aggravates it, rendering the common antibiotics ineffective (Sharma et al., 2024). Moreover, vulnerable populations such as cancer patients in low- and middle-income nations (LMICs) are at higher risk due to inadequate healthcare resources and ineffective infection control measures. It requires comprehensive strategies, including the strengthening of AMSP and greater international collaboration (Bulus et al., 2024). Without concerted global efforts to combat AMR, the full spectrum of its consequences will challenge the viability of modern medicine and compromise health security worldwide (Figure 11.8).

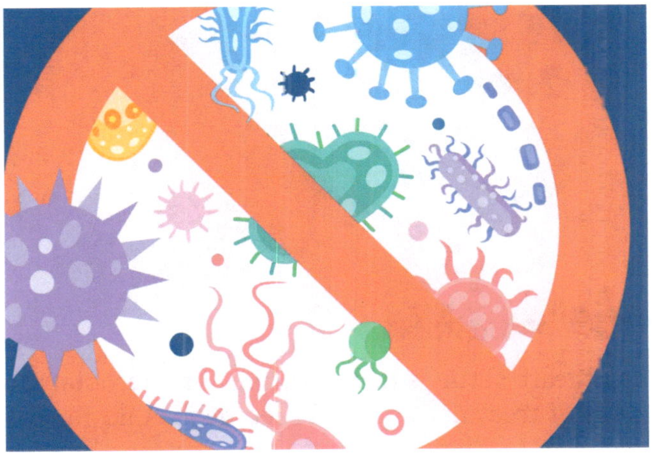

Figure 11.8. The global impact of antimicrobial resistance (AMR) is an escalating public health crisis that significantly undermines the efficacy of infection treatment across diverse healthcare settings.

Source: https://www.uicc.org/sites/default/files/styles/hero_extra_large/public/2023-10/Artboard%20981440.png.webp?itok=Qq0rTw-Y.

11.2.4. Surveillance and Monitoring of Resistance

Surveillance and monitoring for AMR are integral components in the overall framework of antimicrobial stewardship and pharmacology. A One Health approach, encompassing human, animal, and environmental health, needs to be applied to understand and act on the intricate reality of resistance (Häsler et al., 2016). The approach stresses the importance of applying combined surveillance systems that can identify resistant organisms in diverse ecosystems to finally inform policy and direct public health action. For example, South Africa's creation of a National Surveillance Centre and medicine supply early warning system reflects mounting recognition of the utility of such systems in the management of health outcomes (Godman et al., 2017). Beyond the facilitation of timely observation of trends in resistance, successful surveillance also facilitates broader societal gain, such as improved consumer confidence and enhanced animal welfare. Thus, organized surveillance is the foundation of combating resistance and sustaining the sustainability of healthcare systems internationally.

11.2.5. Role of Healthcare Settings in Resistance

The role of healthcare environments in the battle against AMR is critical, since they are both a treatment area and a petri dish for resistant microorganisms. Effective ASPs in such environments can significantly contribute to preventing the development of resistance by optimizing antibiotic use and promoting evidence-based prescribing.

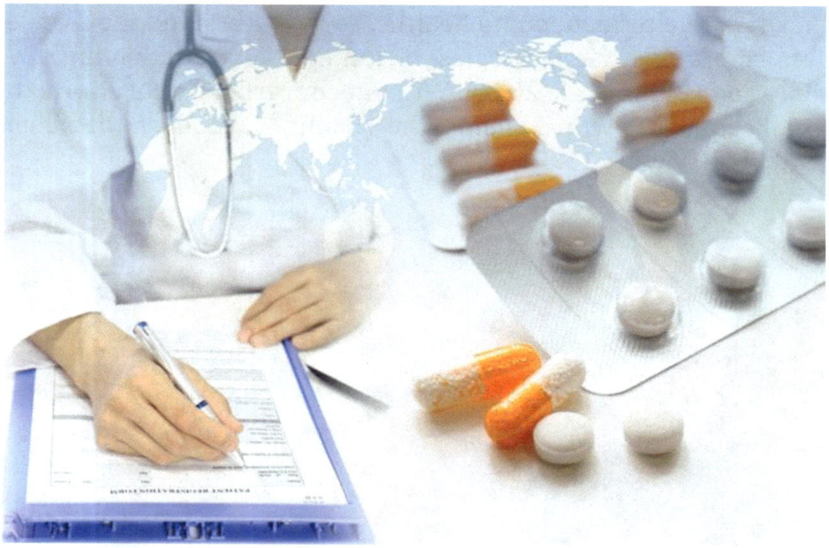

Figure 11.9. The role of healthcare settings in combating antimicrobial resistance (AMR) is critical, as they serve as both a locus of treatment and a breeding ground for resistant pathogens.

Source: https://www.cidrap.umn.edu/sites/default/files/styles/article_detail/public/images/news/global_abx_rx_0.jpg?itok=nM39ajeG.

For instance, studies show that EDs are open to cooperating in ASPs and acknowledge the need for having interventions with explicit use of clinical decision support (CDS) systems in EHRs (Dayan et al., 2017). Medical practitioners also consider AMR as an immediate issue and suggest improved antimicrobial prescribing and utilization of methods like prospective audits and continuous education (Chang et al., 2020). Thus, active involvement of healthcare organizations in the establishment of total ASPs is more crucial in the avoidance of resistance and public health protection (Figure 11.9).

11.2.6. Economic Implications of Resistance

The financial impacts of AMR extend well beyond healthcare expenses, penetrating deeply into society and the economy. As the prevalence of resistant infections grows, healthcare systems face escalating costs about more extended hospital stay, more expensive or more complex treatment, and lost workforce productivity. The treatment of infection is central to the activities of most clinicians (Lipman et al., 2019), and not treating or delayed treatment due to resistance can lead to high costs to patients and health workers. AMR also disrupts food production systems, leading to reduced consumer confidence and higher production costs of animal-source foods, as described within a One Health perspective. This model indicates that the costs of uncontrolled resistance dominate the investments required for effective surveillance and interventions, underlining the need for using integrated strategies that consider broader societal expenses (Häsler et al., 2016).

11.2.7. Strategies to Combat Resistance

The increasing prevalence of AMR necessitates embracing stringent measures to combat the extremely crucial challenge. A robust approach is the use of ASPs, which are aimed at optimizing antibiotic use across healthcare settings, including emergency departments. Evidence suggests that integrating CDS systems within EHRs will enhance antibiotic prescribing behavior, hence avoiding unnecessary use and making guideline following easier (Dayan et al., 2017).

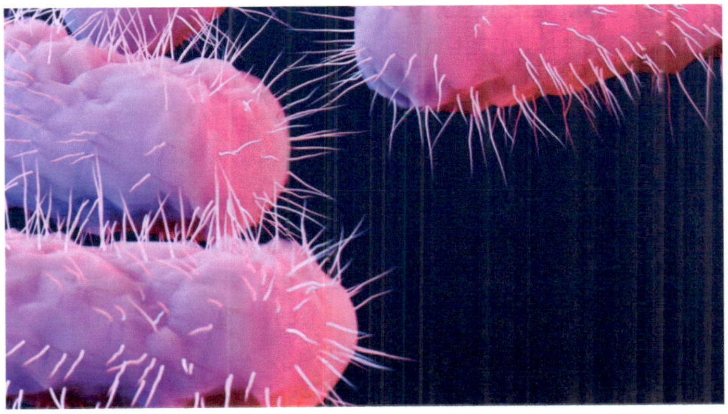

Figure 11.10. The increasing prevalence of antimicrobial resistance (AMR) necessitates the implementation of robust strategies to combat this formidable challenge.

Source: https://www.cdc.gov/antimicrobial-resistance/media/images/About-Antimicrobial-Resistance.jpg.

Interpreting and dispelling myths surrounding the safety and efficacy of antibiotics is also necessary since misinterpretation usually leads to overuse or misuse (Chakraverty et al., 2022). Optimizing proper antibiotic selection, duration, and indication through education can prevent the development of resistance by healthcare providers. These strategies together emphasize the importance of coordinated actions to ensure proper use of antibiotics, and, in the long run, improve patient outcomes without reducing the effectiveness of existing antimicrobial medicines (Figure 11.10).

11.2.8. Role of Education in Resistance Prevention

Prevention of AMR is provided by education, as it equips healthcare providers with the knowledge necessary to practice effective antimicrobial stewardship (AMS) measures. For instance, studies indicated that 69% of healthcare professionals questioned in India were trained and educated (E&T) regarding AMS during their medical professional training. Still, a clear imbalance was identified because most professionals were not provided with further training following basic education (Arora et al., 2019). Similarly, Russian information has revealed a disparity in AMS training, with over half of the respondents reporting a lack of postgraduate training, mirroring a pressing demand for programmatic education initiatives to enhance knowledge about the appropriate use of antibiotics (Bagin et al., 2021). These findings necessitate the emphasis on robust education systems that not only feature AMS training within undergraduate education but also emphasize opportunities for lifelong learning, ultimately building an educated workforce that can effectively handle AMR.

11.2.9. Future Directions in Resistance Research

With growing worldwide concern for AMR, future research goals in resistance must be directed towards new approaches to combat multidrug-resistant disease. Emerging technologies, such as whole genome sequencing and bioinformatics, play a crucial role in deciphering the genomic mutations that cause resistance and, consequently, in modulating the development of targeted therapies. For instance, the ongoing efforts towards surveillance programs globally, particularly that of Neisseria gonorrhoeae, highlight the need for programmatic data that informs both clinical practice and public health interventions (Bristow et al., 2019). Additionally, in low- and middle-income countries (LMIC), improved pediatric prescribing practices by evidence-based guidelines are essential because improper prescribing of antibiotics fuels resistance (Barker et al., 2015). These initiatives collectively emphasize the importance of concerted global response, drug development breakthroughs, and the utilization of sound policymaking to avert AMR and its implications for worldwide health (Figure 11.11).

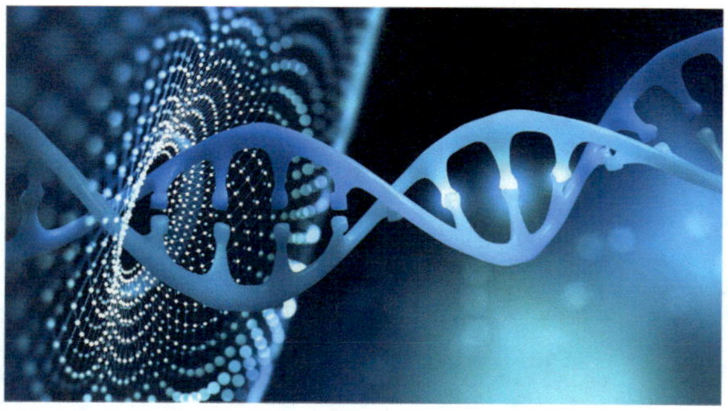

Figure 11.11. Emerging technologies such as whole genome sequencing and bioinformatics are pivotal in deciphering the genetic mutations associated with resistance, thereby guiding the development of targeted therapies.

Source: https://www.pharmaceutical-technology.com/wp-content/uploads/sites/24/2021/01/Genomics-Tech-Trends.jpg.

Test Your Knowledge

1. How can inappropriate use of antibiotics in agriculture contribute to resistance in humans?
2. What strategies can be employed to slow the emergence of antimicrobial resistance?

11.3. Principles of Antimicrobial Stewardship

Learning Outcome

1. Understand the definition of antimicrobial stewardship
2. Learn goals of antimicrobial stewardship programs
3. Identify key components of effective stewardship
4. Explain the role of healthcare professionals in stewardship
5. Discuss guidelines and protocols for prescribing
6. Perform monitoring and evaluation of stewardship efforts
7. Focus on patient education and engagement
8. Describe collaboration among healthcare teams
9. Learn case studies of successful stewardship programs

The antimicrobial stewardship principles are the foundation to minimizing the occurrence of AMR as a significant health risk globally due to the uncontrolled use of antimicrobial drugs in healthcare and veterinary medicine. Excellent stewardship is premised on an all-inclusive process that includes prescribing ethics, vigorous compliance with guidelines, and continuous education for healthcare professionals. By implementing policies such as limiting the spectrum of antibiotics, using culture and susceptibility testing, and promoting non-pharmaceutical alternatives, resistance development can be kept to a minimum. Also, by fostering coordination among farmers, public health representatives, and veterinarians through a platform such as the One Health approach, a holistic approach to AMR problems can be guaranteed. In Australia, several efforts have been made to incorporate these principles into veterinary practice, resulting in low AMR rates in food-producing animals, which highlights the importance of vigilant stewardship in guaranteeing animal and human health (Batey et al., 2024; House et al., 2024).

11.3.1. Definition of Antimicrobial Stewardship

Antimicrobial stewardship is a concerted set of actions for optimizing the use of antimicrobials in a manner that prevents the development of AMR while optimizing favorable treatment outcomes. The combined multifaceted strategy includes the exercise of good use, including proper diagnosis, suitable selection of agents, and strict conformity to guidelines that ensure the prudent use of these crucial drugs in the human, animal, and environmental health domains. There is pressure for such stewardship owing to the increasing incidence of AMR, which poses a significant threat to global public health and the efficacy of existing treatments. Australia has pioneered AMSP, understanding the importance of adopting a One Health approach that heeds the interconnectedness of human, animal, and environmental health (House et al., 2024). With new infections that present challenges in their treatment, antimicrobial stewardship is forever in the process of development, incorporating insights from ongoing research to optimize management and reduce risks of resistance (Malfertheiner et al., 2022) (Figure 11.12).

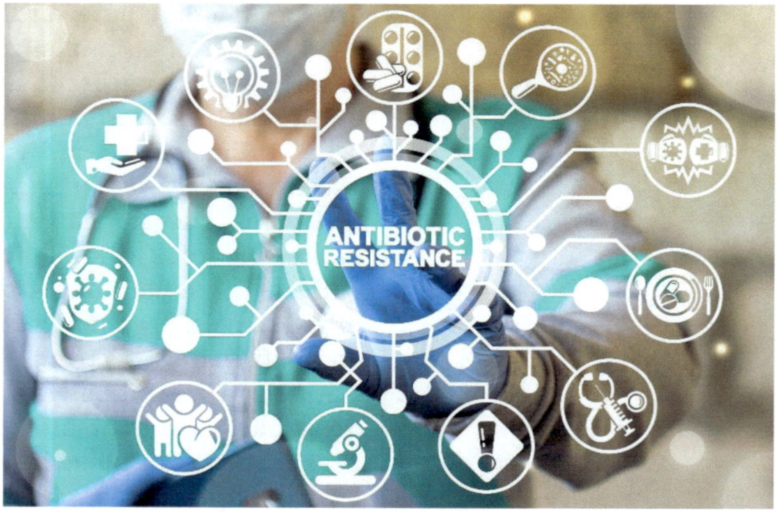

Figure 11.12. Antimicrobial stewardship refers to a coordinated set of strategies aimed at optimizing the use of antimicrobials to combat the development of antimicrobial resistance (AMR) while ensuring effective treatment outcomes.

Source: https://d2jx2rerrg6sh3.cloudfront.net/images/Article_Images/ImageForArticle_23902_16990099985066777.jpg.

11.3.2. Goals of Antimicrobial Stewardship Programs

ASPs are at the heart of addressing the mounting issue of AMR, with short-sighted goals aimed at optimizing the proper use of antibiotics in many healthcare settings. At the heart of the primary goals of these programs is the provision of rational antimicrobial selection, dosing, and course of antimicrobial therapy to optimize patient outcomes, minimizing toxicity and the likelihood of resistance emergence (Ahmad et al., 2018). Besides, ASPs also serve to improve the quality of diagnostics and facilitate appropriate prescribing, particularly in emergency departments, where the speed of interventions prompted by the urgency of instant action might lead to incorrect treatment (Dayan et al., 2017). Through multidisciplinary collaboration and application of resources such as CDS systems, ASPs contribute to improved implementation of guidelines and clinical pathways following best practices. Ultimately, these goals are all part of an integrated strategy that not only improves patient care but also protects public health by decreasing the spread of drug-resistant microorganisms.

11.3.3. Key Components of Effective Stewardship

Effective stewardship of antimicrobial drug use is essential to combat the growing threat of AMR. A primary component of stewardship is the integration into practice guidelines that encourage rational use of antimicrobials, such that treatment regimens are appropriate and effective against offending pathogens. For instance, in the management of intra-abdominal infection, it is essential to initiate empiric antimicrobial therapy broad enough to cover probable organisms since improper initial treatment may lead to poor outcomes and increase resistance (Strauss et al., 2016). Moreover, rigorous surveillance and education programs hold a pivotal position to promote correct prescribing by healthcare professionals. In countries like India, where rates of misuse of antibiotics are alarmingly high, the adoption of the WHO's AWaRe framework can guide national efforts towards prudent use of antibiotics and reduction in patterns of resistance (Gauthaman et al., 2022). Hence, stewardship measures in various dimensions must be utilized to combat the complexities in antimicrobial management effectively (Figure 11.13).

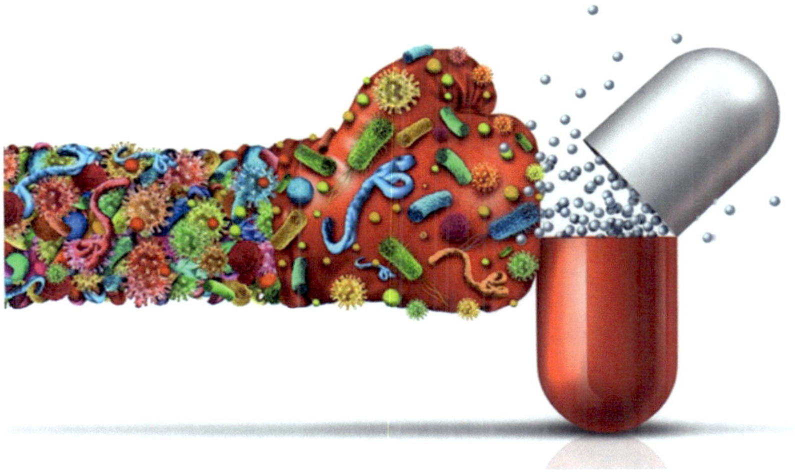

Figure 11.13. Effective stewardship in antimicrobial pharmacology is essential for combating the growing threat of antimicrobial resistance.

Source: https://d1g9yur4m4naub.cloudfront.net/image-handler/picture/2020/11/shutterstock_1061608160.jpg.

11.3.4. Role of Healthcare Professionals in Stewardship

The role of healthcare personnel towards antimicrobial stewardship lies at the core of the fight against the increasing threat of AMR. Effective stewardship initiatives rely on the concerted participation of different healthcare professionals, including physicians, pharmacists, and nurses, to enhance the utilization of antimicrobials. As indicated in research, many healthcare professionals recognize AMR as a critical problem and the importance of improving antimicrobial use by systematic audit and feedback processes and regular training programs (Chang et al., 2020). Furthermore, the implementation of interprofessional educational programs makes the future healthcare professionals' understanding of their respective roles in antimicrobial stewardship deeper, as it strongly enhances their confidence in the discussion of proper antimicrobial use (Chin-Hong et al., 2017). This collaborative approach not only generates improved patient outcomes but also induces a culture of accountability and responsibility in prescribing antibiotics, so vital in addressing the challenges posed by AMR in healthcare settings.

11.3.5. Guidelines and Protocols for Prescribing

In antimicrobial stewardship and pharmacy, adherence to set guidelines and policies for prescriptions is essential in order to optimize patient outcomes and minimize the possibility of resistance development. These policies serve as superior directives that assist in guiding healthcare providers in making decisions on whether or not to prescribe antibiotics. Evidence indicates that the implementation of institutional treatment guidelines significantly enhances prescriber knowledge and adherence to best practice, and this improves the overall quality of antibiotic prescribing (Onubogu et al., 2023). Moreover, it has been observed that healthcare institutions that have multidisciplinary antimicrobial stewardship teams and formal antimicrobial therapy guidelines have better compliance rates among healthcare professionals, as they recognize the importance of having these guidelines to combat AMR (Aboubreeg et al., 2022). With resistance still a significant global health issue, streamlining and enforcing such prescribing guidelines becomes imperative in safeguarding the effectiveness of existing antimicrobial products and supporting patient health outcomes (Figure 11.14).

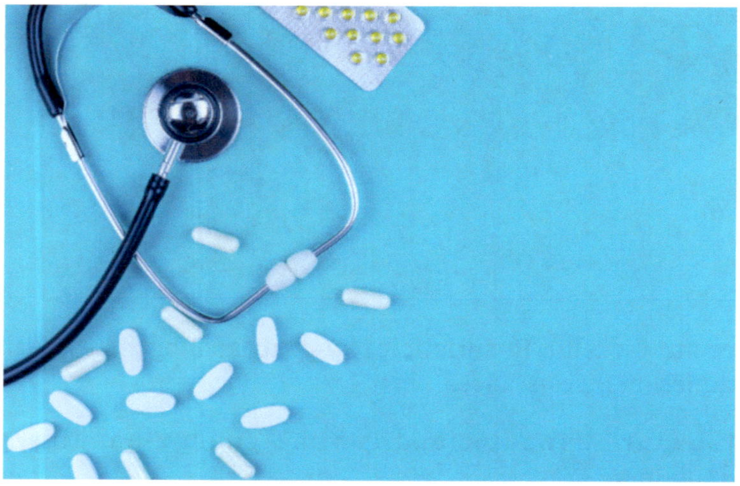

Figure 11.14. Adherence to established guidelines and protocols for prescribing is essential for optimizing patient outcomes and minimizing the risk of resistance development.

Source: https://assets.reflections.live/1699252243939-lomioqpd.png.

11.3.6. Monitoring and Evaluation of Stewardship Efforts

Observation and assessment of AMSP are essential in the fight against AMR, especially in high-risk individuals such as children. Systematic evaluation of the process involves monitoring of prescribing patterns and establishing the effect of interventions to maximize antibiotic use. For example, utilization of performance measures, such as the access percentage and the amoxicillin index, can uncover fundamental trends in antibiotic use between nations, offering insights into possible areas of quality improvement in stewardship practice (Bielicki et al., 2019). In addition, the application of guidelines, continuous training for healthcare personnel, and the integration of rapid diagnosis tests guarantee stewardship on an efficient level, as highlighted in pediatric population studies (Chine et al., 2020). Thus, robust monitoring structures are required to provide assurance that stewardship programs are effectively curtailing antibiotic misuse and enhancing patient safety in combating AMR.

11.3.7. Patient Education and Engagement

One of the most critical components of effective antimicrobial stewardship is robust patient education and engagement programs that empower patients to understand their role in managing AMR. Educating patients about the implications of unwanted antibiotic use enables physicians to promote awareness of medication compliance and adherence to prescribed regimens. This training is particularly useful for curbing the development of resistant bacterial strains, a significant public health challenge as outlined in current literature. As the ANA/CDC white paper reflects, enhancing nurses' involvement in stewardship programs is imperative because they can provide valuable information to patients and thereby improve education interventions and bridge knowledge gaps among healthcare professionals and patients. Second, patient participation through shared decision-making ensures that patients' input is considered in treatment decision-making. This practice has been shown to improve outcomes and reduce unnecessary antibiotic prescriptions (Ahmad et al., 2018) (Figure 11.15).

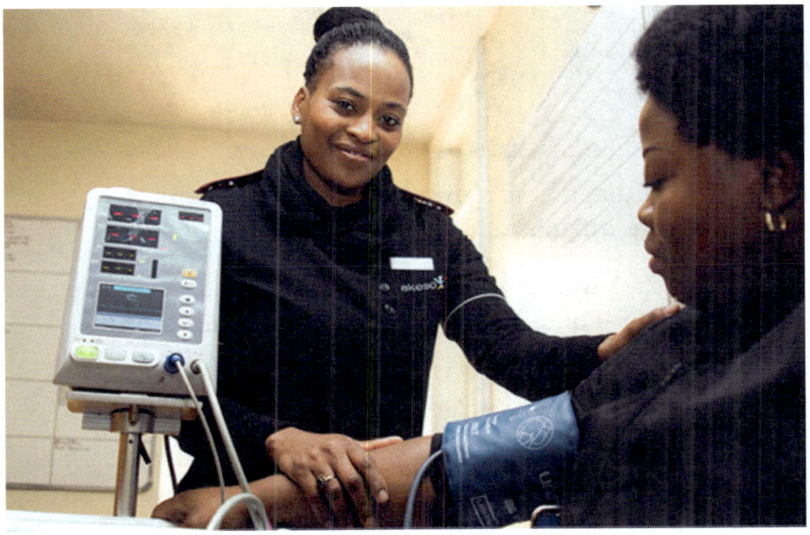

Figure 11.15. An essential component of effective antimicrobial stewardship involves robust patient education and engagement strategies that empower individuals to understand their role in combating antimicrobial resistance.

Source: https://www.reactgroup.org/wp-content/uploads/2020/05/patient-in-hospital-hush-naidoo-pa0uoltkwao-unsplash.jpg.

11.3.8. Collaboration Among Healthcare Teams

Excellent coordination between medical teams is central to the successful implementation of AMSP, especially in addressing the challenge of AMR. Coordination of different professionals like clinicians, pharmacists, and laboratorians develops an integrated approach to the care of patients, enhancing the quality of treatment as well as excellence in clinical decision-making. For instance, diagnostic stewardship collaboration helps teams rationalize testing processes that lead to timely and accurate diagnosis and, therefore, avoid unnecessary antimicrobial utilization. Clinical pharmacists' involvement has been most beneficial, such as in interventions that have led to improved carbapenem dosing protocol practices, emphasizing the importance of interprofessional collaboration in the inpatient setting (Tai et al., 2024). Besides, isolated episodes of cooperation, such as observing and reflecting, create a culture of continuous improvement and responsiveness to patient needs, culminating in better results in pediatric patients (sHoyt et al., 2025) (Figure 11.16).

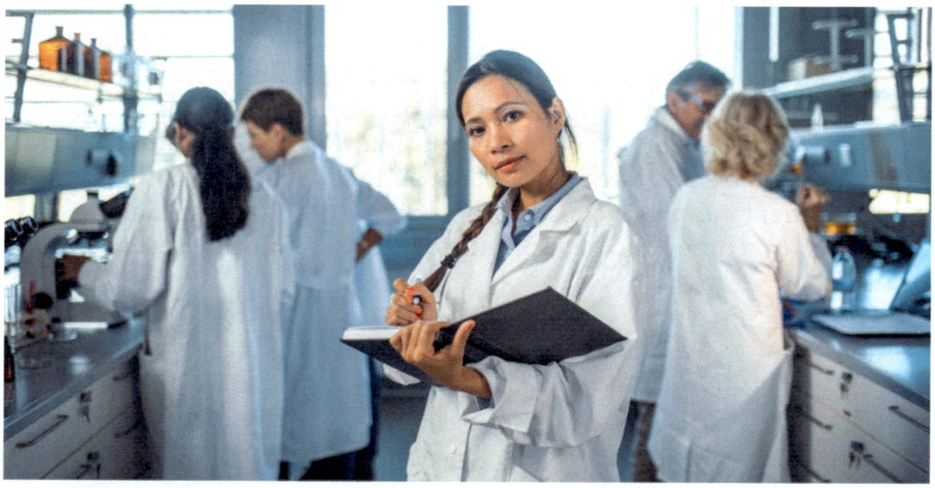

Figure 11.16. Collaboration in diagnostic stewardship allows teams to optimize testing practices that lead to timely and accurate diagnoses.

Source: https://s3.eu-north-1.amazonaws.com/cdn-site.mediaplanet.com/app/uploads/sites/44/2021/10/07155443/P9-Full-SC-bioMerieux-LifeStyle-Image.jpg.

11.3.9. Case Studies of Successful Stewardship Programs

The implementation of effective stewardship programs has signaled striking enhancements in antimicrobial utilization and patient outcomes, suggesting the use of educational efforts within programs. A practical example was the introduction of an interprofessional curriculum that combined medical and pharmacy students and enhanced participants' knowledge of the principles of antimicrobial stewardship. Following this curriculum, the capacity of students to describe the responsibilities of all professions involved in antimicrobial usage and to articulate interprofessional teamwork improved significantly, as indicated by survey results (Chin-Hong et al., 2017). Moreover, large reviews of AMSP in hospitals have revealed that these programs not only optimize antibiotic use but also yield considerable economic benefits. A study identified that hospitals where comprehensive stewardship programs were in use had mean cost savings of $732 per patient through reduced length of stay and lower spending on antibiotics, further underscoring the value of such programs (Apisarnthanarak et al., 2019). These types of scenarios highlight the significant contribution organized stewardship makes in preventing AMR while optimizing healthcare efficiency.

Test Your Knowledge

1. What roles do pharmacists and microbiologists play in antimicrobial stewardship?
2. How can diagnostic tools (e.g., rapid pathogen identification) enhance stewardship efforts?

11.4. Future Directions in Antimicrobial Pharmacology

Learning Outcome

1. Learn innovations in drug development
2. Explain the role of biotechnology in antimicrobial research
3. Understand personalized medicine and antimicrobial therapy
4. Focus on the development of rapid diagnostic tools
5. Discuss exploration of alternative therapies
6. Describe global initiatives for antimicrobial research
7. Know ethical considerations in drug development
8. Discuss the impact of policy on antimicrobial research
9. Identify future challenges in antimicrobial pharmacology

As AMR increases every day, the future of antimicrobial pharmacology must be strategically redirected so that therapeutic interventions become effective. The recent findings indicate an alarming pattern of excessive use of antibiotics, particularly in children, where empirical prescribing is common without guidelines (Gungam et al., 2018). This has been found to have a significant contribution towards the production of ADRs and increased rates of resistance, hence necessitating a more conservative approach in antibiotic stewardship. Furthermore, advancements in pharmacogenomics are pledged to bring about a personalized approach towards antibiotic therapy, thereby minimizing the risk of development of resistance but maximizing success in therapy (Gungam et al., 2018). These initiatives will necessitate strengthening cooperation between health professionals, establishing robust AMSP, and capitalizing on new technologies such as bioinformatics. This blended approach will not only enhance patient safety but also prolong the effective life of antibiotics currently in use in a more challenging therapeutic environment.

11.4.1. Innovations in Drug Development

The field of drug development has experienced breakthrough developments that are particularly significant in meeting the critical issue of AMR. New studies have focused on the discovery and optimization of novel compounds, particularly in antifungal therapy, to respond to the problem of resistant strains.

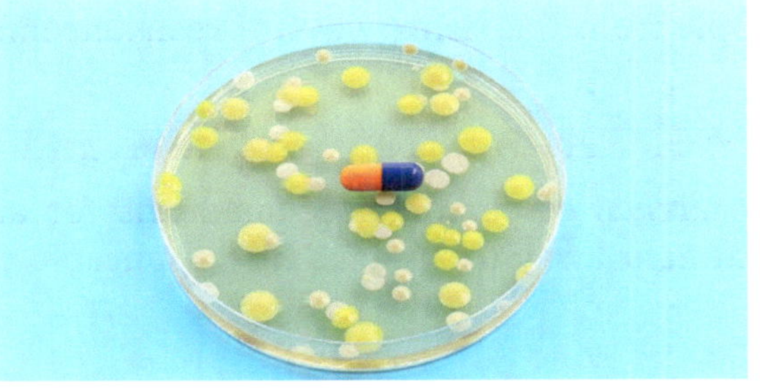

Figure 11.17. The landscape of drug development has witnessed transformative innovations that are particularly vital in combating the pressing issue of antimicrobial resistance.

Source: https://www.apexhospitals.com/_next/image?url=https%3A%2F%2Fbed.apexhospitals.com%2Fuploads%2FAntimicrobial_resistance2_3ff6e32da4.jpg&w=1920&q=75.

For instance, high-throughput screening technologies and synthetic biology are being applied to accelerate new antifungal compound discovery, as indicated by the alarming increase in severe fungal infections due to immunocompromised hosts as well as resistant pathogens such as Candida and Aspergillus spp. (Vitiello et al., 2023). Moreover, biotechnology techniques, such as the utilization of lignocellulosic biomass from agricultural waste, can develop sustainable drug formulation and manufacturing options, trending towards greener medicines (Mujtaba et al., 2023). Not only do these technologies enhance therapeutic options, but they also meet the principles of stewardship for antimicrobial pharmacology as they address the resistance problem and environmental impact (Figure 11.17).

11.4.2. Role of Biotechnology in Antimicrobial Research

The use of biotechnology in antimicrobial research has become increasingly important as the global menace of AMR continues to escalate. Breakthrough biotechnological methods, such as bacteriophage production, offer new remedies for conventional antibiotics by selectively combating and killing resistant bacteria (Todd et al., 2014). The reality is that bacteriophages, or phages, are a group of highly competent and adaptive viruses with the ability to infect and kill bacteria (Todd et al., 2014). This strategy not only provides a road map for new treatment modalities but also necessitates robust antimicrobial stewardship (AMS) systems to guide their effective utilization. AMS programs aim at preventing the misuse of antibiotics, as illustrated in ongoing global efforts to counter AMR challenges (Muhammad et al., 2023). By bringing together stewardship concepts and biotechnological advances, researchers can make therapy more effective while safeguarding people from the rising wave of resistant infections.

11.4.3. Personalized Medicine and Antimicrobial Therapy

The arrival of personalized medicine for antimicrobial therapy is a paradigm shift in infection treatment away from standards applicable to all towards more tailored approaches.

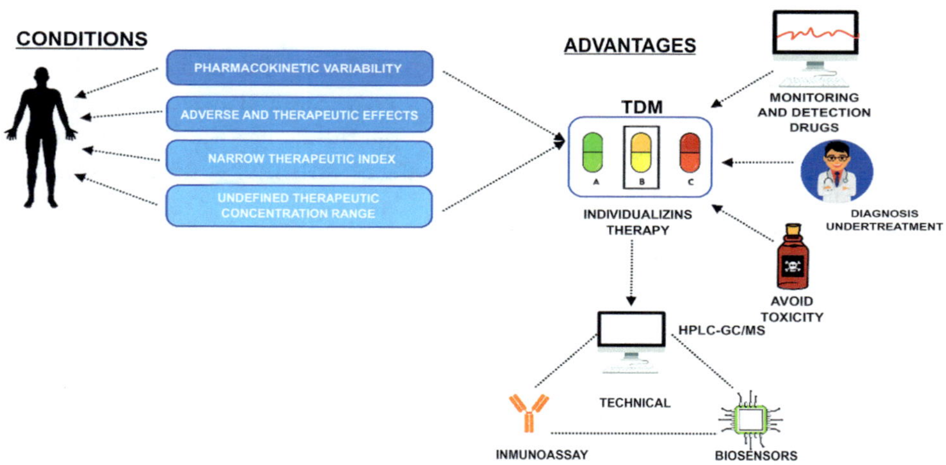

Figure 11.18. The emergence of personalized medicine in antimicrobial therapy represents a significant shift in how infections are managed, pivoting away from a one-size-fits-all approach toward more tailored interventions.

Source: https://pub.mdpi-res.com/jpm/jpm-10-00147/article_deploy/html/images/jpm-10-00147-ag.png?1601044227.

With the application of patient-related information like genetic, microbiological, and clinical variables, clinicians can optimally choose antibiotics and their doses to best treat infections at lower risks of side effects. This tailored approach is especially critical in the wake of rising dangers from AMR, which are driven primarily by unwarranted prescribing practices (Strauss et al., 2016). Through research, it has been proven that a systematic application of tailored strategies to infection management can effectively reduce the possibility of therapy failure and resistance (Afanasjeva et al., 2019).

Thus, integrating personalized medicine into antimicrobial stewardship not only promotes improved patient results but also allows for broader public health activities designed to safeguard the effectiveness of existing antimicrobial agents. As such, research studies and clinical models for this integration are essential to strengthening existing therapeutic measures (Figure 11.18).

11.4.4. Development of Rapid Diagnostic Tools

It is necessary to develop rapid diagnostic tests in the field of antimicrobial pharmacology and stewardship, particularly for maximizing the best use of antibiotics. With these emerging technologies, healthcare workers can rapidly diagnose pathogens and resistance patterns, enabling them to make rapid and specific treatment decisions.

As can be witnessed in the various studies, the integration of quick diagnostics into decision-making plans can significantly lower the risks caused by AMR, which is a prominent problem of concern in international health, particularly among vulnerable individuals such as neonates and children (Chine et al., 2020). Further, the implementation of such technology can help ensure the continuation of ASPs through improved antibiotic-prescribing habits in emergency departments where prompt action is vital (Dayan et al., 2017). Consequently, the strategic use of rapid tests not only encourages better patient outcomes but also plays a crucial role in avoiding overuse and misuse of antibiotics, thereby keeping them effective for generations to come.

11.4.5. Exploration of Alternative Therapies

Investigations into new treatments are now a central part of the fight against AMR, which is a basic challenge to modern medicine. With resistance bacteria and fungi ever more common as causes of infections, the need for new treatment modalities has never been more pressing. Other therapies, including the use of bacteriophages, antimicrobial peptides, and immunomodulators, offer practical alternatives for adjunct therapy together with traditional antibiotics. These alternatives not only address the instant medical issues but also prevent over-reliance on traditional antimicrobials and thus delay the development of AMR. Furthermore, raising public awareness of such treatments can result in a more informed approach to the use of antibiotics and ultimately improve overall health outcomes (Aminu et al., 2024). In parallel, research into these non-antibiotic therapeutic interventions is essential to maximize our intelligence and effectiveness in addressing AMR, as has been emphasized in recent reviews reporting the severity of this multifaceted threat (Aung et al., 2024) (Figure 11.19).

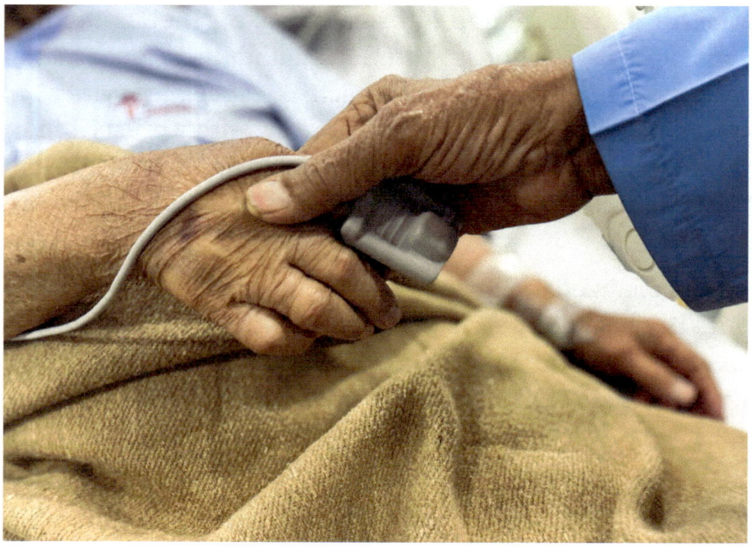

Figure 11.19. The exploration of alternative therapies has emerged as a pivotal component in the fight against antimicrobial resistance (AMR), which poses a critical challenge to modern medicine.

Source: https://360info.org/wp-content/uploads/2023/09/0fecbafbb21e1e09a6c1761ae6dd35d2ce4e2a8c8eb60e968cc70bff1c94393e-scaled.webp.

11.4.6. Global Initiatives for Antimicrobial Research

The increasing problem of AMR requires concerted international action to promote innovative research and development in antimicrobial pharmacology. Several programs, such as the Global Action Plan (GAP) and National Action Plans (NAPs), have been created to counteract the crisis of AMR by supporting antimicrobial stewardship (AMS) and enhancing surveillance of antibiotic use and resistance patterns. Recent reviews have further underscored the need for new treatment avenues, as the World Health Organization (WHO) has identified emerging pathogens that require attention, leading to the initiation of significant research initiatives focused on the threats. Even though there have been advances in antimicrobial agents, such as vaborbactam and cefiderocol, gaining approval, the overall pipeline is dismayingly weak and devoid of innovation (Mudenda et al., 2023). Accordingly, an integrated One Health approach is required for collaboration that synchronizes human, animal, and environmental health to break the barriers and achieve better world health outcomes (Mudenda et al., 2023).

11.4.7. Ethical Considerations in Drug Development

In the drug development context of antibiotics, ethics is of utmost concern because it spans the domains of public health, safety, and the new realm of precision medicine. The shift towards personalized paradigms of treatment necessitates a corresponding firm ethical framework that emphasizes the health of trial subjects as well as broad populations. As explained in recent publications, innovative in silico techniques have emerged as the key means of advancing drug development with reduced risks and facilitating more focused therapy aimed at the unique genetic signature of patients, in line with the aim of precision medicine (Marques et al., 2024). However, the ethical side of these innovations cannot be overlooked, particularly regarding data protection and consent. Additionally, with the industry embracing new ways of doing things, such as used in the production of cell-cultured foods, rigorous safety assessment plays an essential role in enabling the guarantee of new drugs and treatments before commercialization, justifying the assertion of the need for stringent ethical regulation for drug and food safety (Ong et al., 2021) (Figure 11.20).

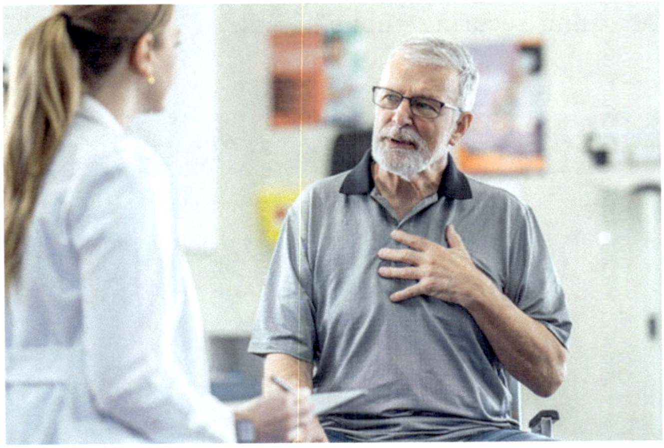

Figure 11.20. The shift towards individualized treatment paradigms necessitates a robust ethical framework that emphasizes the welfare of both trial participants and broader communities.

Source: https://health.ucdavis.edu/media-resources/contenthub/health-library/conditions/antibiotic-resistance-marquee.jpg.

11.4.8. Impact of Policy on Antimicrobial Research

Policy influence on antimicrobial research is invariably linked to the global phenomenon of AMR, and accordingly, it necessitates intersectoral frameworks and coordinated action. Effective policies are central to directing resources towards innovative research into resistance mechanisms and new antimicrobial agents. To support this, a One Health strategy is promoted, highlighting the interdependence of human, animal, and environmental health in research agendas. By prioritizing integrated surveillance systems across multiple health domains, policymakers are better positioned to comprehend and address the multidimensionality of AMR. Further, favorable policies for antimicrobial stewardship (AMSP) promote the sensible application of existing agents and prevent the transmission of resistant pathogens, significantly lowering healthcare costs and advancing patient outcomes (Ahmad et al., 2018). Lastly, well-structured policies not only support research advancement but also promote public health through long-term and dynamic antimicrobial use management, as highlighted in Häsler et al. (2016).

11.4.9. Future Challenges in Antimicrobial Pharmacology

As AMR is a growing challenge, the future of antimicrobial pharmacology teeters on the brink. The emergence of drug-resistant microbes bewilders treatment protocols, making effective infection control more difficult. Practitioners are faced with the daunting task of juggling the optimal application of antimicrobials with the need for resistance minimization, which necessitates innovative solutions in antimicrobial stewardship. These efforts are crucial because treatment of infection is a central aspect of the work of most clinicians (Lipman et al., 2019). Spread of resistant strains not only prolongs illnesses but also increases healthcare costs and hazards of medical intervention, further putting the spotlight on the necessity of efficient actions (Ahmad et al., 2018). The future of pharmacology will need to focus on optimizing existing agents as well as developing new therapeutic options and fostering interdisciplinary interaction to maximize solutions for the challenge of combating AMR and securing public health.

Test Your Knowledge

1. How is the study of the human microbiome influencing future antimicrobial strategies?
2. What innovations are being pursued to improve delivery systems for antimicrobial agents?

Summary

The need to combat AMR has prompted more focus on ASPs, which are the key frameworks for maximizing drug utilization in healthcare facilities. Though emergency department involvement in these efforts has been minimal, it is evident from recent studies that both ASP and emergency department leaders see the need for dedicated programs in these high-stakes care areas. Interestingly, the integration of CDS systems into EHRs seems to be a more preferable method for implementing ASPs in the emergency department environment, permitting more rational antibiotic prescribing practices (Dayan et al., 2017). Furthermore, the controlling AMR strategy revolves around a three-pillar approach comprising the judicious utilization of available antimicrobials, efficient infection control practices, and the advancement of environmental decontamination protocols (Ahmad et al., 2018). Therefore, reinforcing stewardship techniques in every healthcare setting is paramount to avoiding the threat from resistant organisms.

The antimicrobial pharmacology and stewardship landscape is inextricably linked with the combined energies of clinical pharmacists and medical physicians, as recent research on professional concordance regarding AMR and stewardship programs has indicated. Remarkably, an antibiotic practice study from the practitioners at Jinnah Sindh Medical University shows there is a moderate degree of agreement of 0.39 from these groups regarding antibiotic practices and thus a greatest possible need for improved communication and inter-group understanding in dealing with AMR (Zeeshan et al., 2024). Moreover, the development of targeted training materials for public health professionals in the UK illustrates a proactive approach to combating AMR through the encouragement of knowledge and self-reported intent to encourage antimicrobial stewardship (Taylor et al., 2024). These observations highlight the core intersection of education, collaboration, and education, all of which are crucial in promoting effective antimicrobial stewardship and addressing the global threat of AMR.

KEY TERMS FROM THIS CHAPTER

Antifungals
Antimicrobial stewardship
Antiparasitics
Avermectins
Bacteria
Biofilm formation
Clinical decision support (CDS) systems
Extended-Spectrum Beta-Lactamases
Gram-negative bacteria
Heterocycles
Antimicrobial resistance (AMR)
Antiparasitic
Antivirals
Azoles
Beta-lactams
Cell wall
Drug penetration
Extracellular matrix
Gram-negative Enterobacteriaceae
Intra-abdominal infections (IAI)

Critical Thinking Questions

1. Which of the following antibiotics inhibits bacterial cell wall synthesis?

a. Tetracycline

b. Ciprofloxacin

c. Amoxicillin

d. Erythromycin

2. Which class of antibiotics interferes with bacterial protein synthesis by binding to the 30S ribosomal subunit?

a. Macrolides

b. Fluoroquinolones

c. Aminoglycosides

d. Beta-lactams

3. Which of the following is a broad-spectrum antibiotic?

a. Penicillin G

b. Vancomycin

c. Chloramphenicol

d. Clindamycin

4. What is the mechanism of resistance for beta-lactamase producing bacteria?

a. Altered ribosomal binding sites

b. Decreased membrane permeability

c. Enzymatic degradation of antibiotics

d. Efflux pump activation

5. What is the primary goal of antimicrobial stewardship?

a. To promote the use of newer antibiotics

b. To reduce the cost of therapy

c. To ensure the appropriate use of antimicrobials to combat resistance

d. To replace all antimicrobials with herbal alternatives

Answers to Critical Thinking Questions

1. (c); 2. (c); 3. (c); 4. (c); 5. (c).

Short Answer Questions

1. What are the primary mechanisms by which antimicrobials inhibit or kill microorganisms?
2. How do beta-lactam antibiotics interfere with bacterial cell wall synthesis?
3. What are the major mechanisms by which bacteria develop resistance to antibiotics?
4. How do efflux pumps contribute to multidrug resistance in bacteria?
5. What are the key goals of antimicrobial stewardship programs (ASPs)?
6. How does appropriate antibiotic selection help reduce resistance and improve patient outcomes?
7. What are the current challenges in developing new antimicrobial agents?
8. How might bacteriophage therapy serve as an alternative to traditional antibiotics?

References

1. Sartelli, M., Labricciosa, F. M., Coccolini, F., Coimbra, R., Abu-Zidan, F. M., Ansaloni, L., Al-Hasan, M. N., Ansari, S., Barie, P. S., Caínzos, M. A., Ceresoli, M., Chiarugi, M., Claridge, J. A., Cicuttin, E., Dellinger, E. P., Fry, D. E., Guirao, X., Hardcastle, T. C., Hecker, A., . . . Catena, F. (2022). It is time to define an organizational model for the prevention and management of infections along the surgical pathway: a worldwide cross-sectional survey. *World Journal of Emergency Surgery*, *17*(1). https://doi.org/10.1186/s13017-022-00420-4Adu, F., Agyare, C., Boakye, Y. D., Danquah, R., et al. (2019). *Antimicrobial Agents: Antibacterial Agents, Anti-Biofilm Agents, Antibacterial Natural Compounds, And Antibacterial Chemicals*. https://core.ac.uk/download/322441236.pdf (accessed on 10th June 2025).

2. Afanasjeva, J., Anderson, K. C., Barreto, E. F., Beavers, K., et al. (2019). *PRN Opinion Paper: Application of Precision Medicine Across Pharmacy Specialty Areas*. http://deepblue.lib.umich.edu/bitstream/2027.42/149551/2/jac51107.pdf (accessed on 10th June 2025).

3. Ahmad, R., & Rehman, S. (2018). *Antimicrobial Stewardship: Need of the Hour*. https://core.ac.uk/download/539896609.pdf (accessed on 10th June 2025).

4. Aminu, R., Apollos, S. D., Enesi, K. O., Kwaga, J., et al. (2024). *Antimicrobial Resistance as A Global Public Health Threat: The Way Forward*. https://core.ac.uk/download/618203595.pdf (accessed on 10th June 2025).

5. Apisarnthanarak, A., Apisarnthanarak, A., Arco Del, A., Hohn, A., LaRocco Jr, A., Sick, A. C., Brink, A. J., et al. (2019). *Value of Hospital Antimicrobial Stewardship Programs (ASPs): A Systematic Review*. https://core.ac.uk/download/195292601.pdf (accessed on 10th June 2025).

6. Arora, A., Charani, E., Jenkins, A., Nathwani, D., et al. (2019). *The State of Education and Training for Antimicrobial Stewardship Programs in Indian Hospitals: A Qualitative and Quantitative Assessment*. https://core.ac.uk/download/195292330.pdf (accessed on 10th June 2025).

7. Aung, T. T., de la Fuente-Nunez, C., Hancock, R. E. W., Ho, C., et al. (2024). *Antimicrobial Resistance: A Concise Update*. https://core.ac.uk/download/622192219.pdf (accessed on 10th June 2025).

8. Bagin, V., Burasova, E., Domanskaya, O., Gordeeva, A., et al. (2021). *Current Antimicrobial Stewardship Practice and Education in Russian Hospitals: Results of A Multicenter Survey*. https://core.ac.uk/download/477968936.pdf (accessed on 10th June 2025).

9. Barbosa, L. B., Barroso, F. D. D., Cabral, V. P. F., Coutinho, A., et al. (2022). *Antimicrobial Activity of Selective Serotonin Reuptake Inhibitors in Bacteria and Fungi: A Systematic Review*. https://core.ac.uk/download/652318629.pdf (accessed on 10th June 2025).

10. Barker, C. I., Irwin, A., Le Doare, K., Sharland, M., et al. (2015). *Improving Antibiotic Prescribing for Children in The Resource-Poor Setting*. https://core.ac.uk/download/29469533.pdf (accessed on 10th June 2025).

11. Batey, R., Nilon, P., Page, S. W., Browning, G. F., & Norris, J. M. (2024). Antimicrobial prescribing guidelines for sheep. *Australian Veterinary Journal, 102*, 103–142. https://doi.org/10.1111/avj.13310.

12. Belay, W. Y., Getachew, M., Tegegne, B., Teffera, Z., Dagne, A., Zeleke, T. K., Abebe, R. B., et al. (2024). Mechanism of antibacterial resistance, strategies, and next-generation antimicrobials to contain antimicrobial resistance: A review. *Frontiers in Pharmacology, 15*. https://www.

semanticscholar.org/paper/d5a38deeb5968c243d99b6c446325c0aad44645a (accessed on 10th June 2025).

13. Berardi, A., Picone, S., Regazzi, M., & Tzialla, C. (2023). *Pharmacokinetic and Pharmacodynamic Considerations of Antibiotic Use in Neonates.* https://core.ac.uk/download/638792015.pdf (accessed on 10th June 2025).

14. Bezuidenhout, S., Engler, D., Godman, B., Meyer, J. C., et al. (2023). *Knowledge and Perceptions of Final Year Nursing Students Regarding Antimicrobials, Antimicrobial Resistance, And Antimicrobial Stewardship: Findings and Implications to Reduce Resistance.* https://core.ac.uk/download/593671834.pdf (accessed on 10th June 2025).

15. Bielicki, J. A., Hsia, Y., Jackson, C., Magrini, N., et al. (2019). *Consumption of Oral Antibiotic Formulations for Young Children According to the WHO Access, Watch, Reserve (AWaRe) Antibiotic Groups: An Analysis of Sales Data From 70 Middle-Income and High-Income Countries.* https://core.ac.uk/download/160810011.pdf (accessed on 10th June 2025).

16. Bodke, A. V., Dabhade, S. S., Gawari, N. C., Jadhav, R., et al. (2024). *Knowledge, Attitude, And Practice About Antimicrobial Stewardship Concepts Among Practitioners.* https://core.ac.uk/download/620835913.pdf (accessed on 10th June 2025).

17. Bradstreet, E. N. (2022). *The Impact of the COVID-19 Pandemic on Antimicrobial Stewardship Practices and Their Effect on Veterinary Medicine.* https://core.ac.uk/download/519803370.pdf (accessed on 10th June 2025).

18. Bristow, C. C., Cristillo, A. D., Dillon, J. A., Dong, F., et al. (2019). *Antimicrobial Resistance in Neisseria gonorrhoeae: Proceedings of the STAR Sexually Transmitted Infection-Clinical Trial Group Programmatic Meeting.* https://core.ac.uk/download/294625789.pdf (accessed on 10th June 2025).

19. Brown, C., Cars, O., Collignon, P., Dagan, R., DiNubile, M. J., et al. (2013). *Can We Prevent Antimicrobial Resistance by Using Antimicrobials Better?* https://core.ac.uk/download/29469446.pdf (accessed on 10th June 2025).

20. Bulus, A. D., Ezeh, E. C., Goldim, R. V., & Edache, A. E. (2024). Global impact of antimicrobial resistance on cancer care: Challenges and strategies in low- and middle-income countries. *World Journal of Advanced Research and Reviews.* https://www.semanticscholar.org/paper/68ff6db8658714b969f9ee384f755af4ea264630 (accessed on 10th June 2025).

21. Butler, M. S., Gigante, V., Sati, H., Paulin, S., Al-Sulaiman, L., Rex, J., Fernandes, P., et al. (2022). Analysis of the clinical pipeline of treatments for drug-resistant bacterial infections: Despite progress, more action is needed. *Antimicrobial Agents and Chemotherapy, 66.* https://doi.org/10.1128/aac.01991-21.

22. Chakraverty, R., Chauhan, J., & Pathan, S. (2022). *Antimicrobial Stewardship Program Activities in India: An Appraisal.* https://core.ac.uk/download/543133605.pdf (accessed on 10th June 2025).

23. Chang, J., Fang, Y., Gillani, A. H., Hayat, K., et al. (2020). *Perspective of Key Healthcare Professionals on Antimicrobial Resistance and Stewardship Programs: A Multicenter Cross-Sectional Study from Pakistan.* https://core.ac.uk/download/389312874.pdf (accessed on 10th June 2025).

24. Chattopadhyay, P., Das, S., Ghosh, R., & Saha, S. (2024). Exploring MBL detection along with ESBL co-expression of Gram-negative organism in clinical samples by phenotypic method in

a tertiary care hospital. *National Journal of Physiology, Pharmacy and Pharmacology*. https://www.semanticscholar.org/paper/90488f4f2efd4d4a7be18c2f658c2861273c6287 (accessed on 10th June 2025).

25. Chine, V., Esposito, S., Fanelli, U., Gismondi, P., & Pappalardo, M. (2020). *Improving the Quality of Hospital Antibiotic Use: Impact on Multidrug-Resistant Bacterial Infections in Children*. https://core.ac.uk/download/521222053.pdf (accessed on 10th June 2025).
26. Chin-Hong, P. V., Kim, L., MacDougall, C., Nanamori, M., et al. (2017). *An Interprofessional Curriculum on Antimicrobial Stewardship Improves Knowledge and Attitudes Toward Appropriate Antimicrobial Use and Collaboration*. https://core.ac.uk/download/323074459.pdf (accessed on 10th June 2025).
27. Cooper, C., Koonjan, S., & Nilsson, A. (2018). *Enhancing Whole Phage Therapy and Their Derived Antimicrobial Enzymes Through Complex Formulation*. https://core.ac.uk/download/160471288.pdf (accessed on 10th June 2025).
28. Davis, M., Flowers, P., Gozdzielewska, L., Langdridge, D., et al. (2018). *What Are The 'Active Ingredients' of Interventions Targeting the Public's Engagement with Antimicrobial Resistance and How Might They Work?* https://core.ac.uk/download/158172240.pdf (accessed on 10th June 2025).
29. Dayan, P. S., Gerber, J. S., Hersh, A. L., Kuppermann, N., et al. (2017). *Current State of Antimicrobial Stewardship in Children's Hospital Emergency Departments*. https://core.ac.uk/download/80495100.pdf (accessed on 10th June 2025).
30. Frey, E. C., Costin, M., Granick, J. L., Kornya, M., & Weese, J. S. (2022). 2022 AAFP/AAHA antimicrobial stewardship guidelines. *Journal of the American Animal Hospital Association, 58*(4), 1–5. https://doi.org/10.5326/1547-3317-58.4.1.
31. Gauthaman, G., Mathaiyan, J., & Meena, D. K. (2022). WHO AWaRe strategy and antimicrobial stewardship to combat antimicrobial resistance: An Indian perspective. https://core.ac.uk/download/539845693.pdf (accessed on 10th June 2025).
32. Godman, B., Defty, D., Steel, G., Zeeman, H., Stokes, J., et al. (2017). *Ongoing Initiatives to Improve the Quality and Efficiency of Medicine Use Within the Public Healthcare System In South Africa: A Preliminary Study*. https://core.ac.uk/download/132155450.pdf (accessed on 10th June 2025).
33. Gogry, F. A., Siddiqui, M. T., Sultan, I., & Haq, Q. M. R. (2021). Current update on intrinsic and acquired colistin resistance mechanisms in bacteria. *Frontiers in Medicine*, 8. https://doi.org/10.3389/fmed.2021.677720.
34. Gungam, P., Junapudi, S., & Yadav, Y. S. K. (2018). *Antibiotic Use in Pediatric Infections: A Study in Tertiary Care Hospital*. https://core.ac.uk/download/235920319.pdf (accessed on 10th June 2025).
35. Häsler, B., Queenan, K., & Rushton, J. (2016). A One Health approach to antimicrobial resistance surveillance: Is there a business case for it? https://core.ac.uk/download/45467944.pdf (accessed on 10th June 2025).
36. House, J. K., Izzo, M. M., Page, S. W., Browning, G. F., & Norris, J. M. (2024). Antimicrobial prescribing guidelines for dairy cattle. *Australian Veterinary Journal, 102*, 143–186. https://doi.org/10.1111/avj.13311.

37. Hoyt, B. M., Messacar, K., Sick-Samuels, A., Jaggi, P., Hamilton, S. L., Janelle, S., & Parker, S. K. (2025). Opportunities for collaboration: The synergy between antimicrobial and diagnostic stewardship in pediatrics. *Antimicrobial Stewardship & Healthcare Epidemiology*, 5. https://www.semanticscholar.org/paper/1296989261adc2d0d73407122007a5f08006c92c (accessed on 10th June 2025).

38. Kamel, M., Aleya, S., Alsubih, M., & Aleya, L. (2024). Microbiome dynamics: A paradigm shift in combatting infectious diseases. *Journal of Personalized Medicine, 14*, 217. https://doi.org/10.3390/jpm14020217.

39. Kinobe, R. T., Picard, J., & Sutcliffe, R. (2020). Utilization and evaluation of cooperative case-based teaching for integration of microbiology and pharmacology in veterinary education. https://core.ac.uk/download/303790668.pdf (accessed on 10th June 2025).

40. Laine, N. (2017). *Use of Antimicrobials in A Tertiary Children's Hospital*. https://core.ac.uk/download/132491357.pdf (accessed on 10th June 2025).

41. Lipman, J., & Lonsdale, D. O. (2019). Antimicrobial resistance: We must pursue a collaborative, global approach and use a "One Health" approach. https://core.ac.uk/download/287649693.pdf (accessed on 10th June 2025).

42. Malfertheiner, P., Mégraud, F., Rokkas, T., Gisbert, J. P., Liou, J. M., Schulz, C., Gasbarrini, A., et al. (2022). Management of *Helicobacter pylori* infection: The Maastricht VI/Florence consensus report. *Gut, 71*, 1724–1762. https://doi.org/10.1136/gutjnl-2022-327745.

43. Marques, L., Costa, B., Pereira, M., Silva, A., Santos, J., Saldanha, L., Silva, I., et al. (2024). Advancing precision medicine: A review of innovative *in silico* approaches for drug development, clinical pharmacology and personalized healthcare. *Pharmaceutics, 16*, 332. https://doi.org/10.3390/pharmaceutics16030332.

44. McFall, R. (2021). Antimicrobial resistance: Where are we now? *5*, 40. https://www.semanticscholar.org/paper/66b7e25485e960bb0253533c58af66ab0e7865e8 (accessed on 10th June 2025).

45. Mudenda, S., Chabalenge, B., Daka, V., Mfune, R. L., Salachi, K. I., Mohamed, S., Mufwambi, W., et al. (2023). Global strategies to combat antimicrobial resistance: A One Health perspective. *Pharmacology & Pharmacy, 14*, 271–328. https://doi.org/10.4236/pp.2023.148020.

46. Muhammad, K. M., & Shoge, M. O. (2023). Applications of antimicrobial stewardship and natural product chemistry in tackling antimicrobial resistance. https://core.ac.uk/download/595554889.pdf (accessed on 10th June 2025).

47. Mujtaba, M., Fraceto, L. F., Fazeli, M., Mukherjee, S., Savassa, S. M., de Medeiros, G. A., & Pereira, A. do E. S., et al. (2023). Lignocellulosic biomass from agricultural waste to the circular economy: A review with focus on biofuels, bio composites and bioplastics. *Journal of Cleaner Production, 402*, 136815. https://doi.org/10.1016/j.jclepro.2023.136815.

48. Ngoma, M. T., Sitali, D., Mudenda, S., Mukuma, M., Bumbangi, F., Bunuma, E., Skjerve, E., et al. (2024). Community antibiotic consumption and associated factors in Lusaka district of Zambia: Findings and implications for antimicrobial resistance and stewardship. *JAC-Antimicrobial Resistance, 6*. https://www.semanticscholar.org/paper/95fe6f846a22094184651893ab705bad2fd0e7a2 (accessed on 10th June 2025).

49. Ong, K. J., Johnston, J., Datar, I., Sewalt, V., Holmes, D., & Shatkin, J. A. (2021). Food safety considerations and research priorities for the cultured meat and seafood industry.

Comprehensive Reviews in Food Science and Food Safety, 20, 5421–5448. https://doi.org/10.1111/1541-4337.12853.

50. Onubogu, C. U., & Ugochukwu, E. F. (2023). Knowledge, practices, and influencers of antibiotic prescriptions of Nigerian doctors. https://core.ac.uk/download/639417407.pdf (accessed on 10th June 2025).
51. Prieto, J., Wilson, J., Tingle, A., Cooper, E., Handley, M., Rycroft-Malone, J., Bostock, J., et al. (2024). Strategies for older people living in care homes to prevent urinary tract infection: The StOP UTI realist synthesis (Vol. *28*(68), pp. 1–139). *Health Technology Assessment*. https://www.semanticscholar.org/paper/ed1dcd3d94f4b2305b8e7bfc582da643bd14da46 (accessed on 10th June 2025).
52. Ramesh, R., & Vadhwa, M. (2023). Prescription pattern of antibiotics in various clinical departments of a tertiary care health institution: A retrospective observational study. https://core.ac.uk/download/591404906.pdf (accessed on 10th June 2025).
53. Romandini, A., Pani, A., Schenardi, P., Pattarino, G., De Giacomo, C., & Scaglione, F. (2021). Antibiotic resistance in pediatric infections: Global emerging threats, predicting the near future. *Antibiotics, 10*(4), 393. https://doi.org/10.3390/antibiotics10040393.
54. Ruiz, A., Rodríguez Gascón, A., & Solinís Aspiazu, M. Á. (2021). The role of PK/PD analysis in the development and evaluation of antimicrobials. https://core.ac.uk/download/547406121.pdf (accessed on 10th June 2025).
55. Rusu, A., Moga, I., Uncu, L., & Hancu, G. (2023). The role of five-membered heterocycles in the molecular structure of antibacterial drugs used in therapy. *Pharmaceutics, 15*(11), 2554. https://doi.org/10.3390/pharmaceutics15112554.
56. Shah, A. M., & Shah, S. (2023). Antimicrobial stewardship program: Fighting antimicrobial resistance in India. *National Journal of Physiology, Pharmacy and Pharmacology*. https://www.semanticscholar.org/paper/c78984ef6ccaaa891d3138b70e4da8bebb0abda4 (accessed on 10th June 2025).
57. Sharma, D. (2024). Tackling antimicrobial resistance: Comprehensive review of mechanisms, trends, and strategies. *International Journal of Advanced Research*. https://www.semanticscholar.org/paper/523662f415617f6a61a5e3b8d082a891e4973167 (accessed on 10th June 2025).
58. Singh, S. (2016). Antimicrobial resistance and antibiotic stewardship: Knowledge, attitudes and perceptions amongst final-year undergraduate health professional students in a South African university. https://core.ac.uk/download/304374192.pdf (accessed on 10th June 2025).
59. Strauss, A., Teixeira Rodrigues, A., Holmes, A. H., Hernandez, B., Pope, C., Pulcini, C., et al. (2016). *Mapping the Decision Pathways of Acute Infection Management in Secondary Care Among Uk Medical Physicians: A Qualitative Study*. https://core.ac.uk/download/326247254.pdf (accessed on 10th June 2025).
60. Tai, T., Motoki, T., Yamaguchi, K., Watanabe, M., Ito, T., Yokota, K., Ishikawa, K., et al. (2024). Enhancing carbapenem antimicrobial dosing optimization: Synergy of antimicrobial stewardship teams and ward-based clinical pharmacists. *Antimicrobial Stewardship & Healthcare Epidemiology, 4*. https://www.semanticscholar.org/paper/5f871c7440b0381dae54b5276e78815e57bc17de (accessed on 10th June 2025).
61. Taylor, H., Mearkle, R. A., Huyton, R. A. M., & Ashiru-Oredope, D. (2024). Designing,

piloting and evaluating (through a matched pre- and post-implementation survey) a targeted e-learning resource on antimicrobial resistance for public health professionals. *European Journal of Public Health*. https://www.semanticscholar.org/paper/c35c9dd0b0c5013a5a4465727b0d2c31af23d043 (accessed on 10th June 2025).

62. Todd, K. (2014). The promising viral threat to bacterial resistance: The uncertain patentability of phage therapeutics and the necessity of alternative incentives. https://core.ac.uk/download/213020895.pdf (accessed on 10th June 2025).

63. Vitiello, A., Ferrara, F., Boccellino, M., Ponzo, A., Cimmino, C., Comberiati, E., Zovi, A., et al. (2023). Antifungal drug resistance: An emergent health threat. *Biomedicines, 11*(4), 1063. https://doi.org/10.3390/biomedicines11041063.

64. Zeeshan, F., Munawwar, R., Sultan, B., & Irshad, Z. (2024). The consonance between medical practitioners and pharmacists regarding antimicrobial stewardship practices: An observational study. *Journal of the College of Physicians and Surgeons–Pakistan, 34*(8), 897–903. https://www.semanticscholar.org/paper/6eb6dd63cda13e42cda527349e7ddf2a5a68ecba (accessed on 10th June 2025).

CARDIOVASCULAR DRUG THERAPY

12

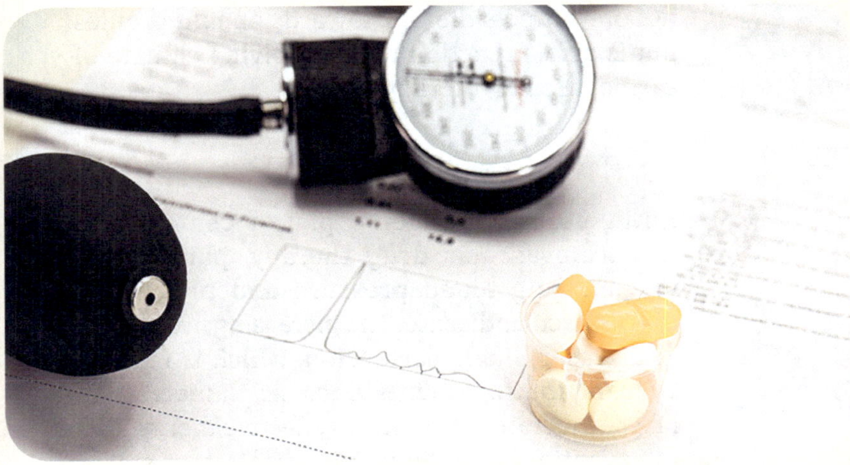

LEARNING OBJECTIVES

After studying this chapter, you will be able to:

1. Identify types of cardiovascular drugs.
2. Understand mechanisms of action.
3. Focus on clinical applications.
4. Know side effects and risks.

Introduction

The advent of cardiovascular drug therapy is a turning point in the management of cardiovascular disease, which remains a leading cause of morbidity and mortality across the globe. The overlap of various therapeutic drugs has revolutionized the face of management, allowing for improved prognosis and quality of life for the patient. The drugs target multiple mechanisms of cardiovascular pathology, including hypertension, hyperlipidemia, and thromboembolism, thereby addressing the multifaceted nature of heart disease. Significantly, the consequences of side effects, specifically metabolic complications linked to antiretroviral therapy, highlight the importance of a balanced approach to treatment. Specifically, cohorts like children and adolescents with diseases such as HIV are subject to special risks related to cardiovascular drug therapies due to metabolic complications, increasing cardiovascular diseases at a younger age (Muccini et al., 2024). Thus, an enlightened understanding of these processes is called for to optimize cardiovascular drug therapy (Montano et al., 2022) (Figure 12.1).

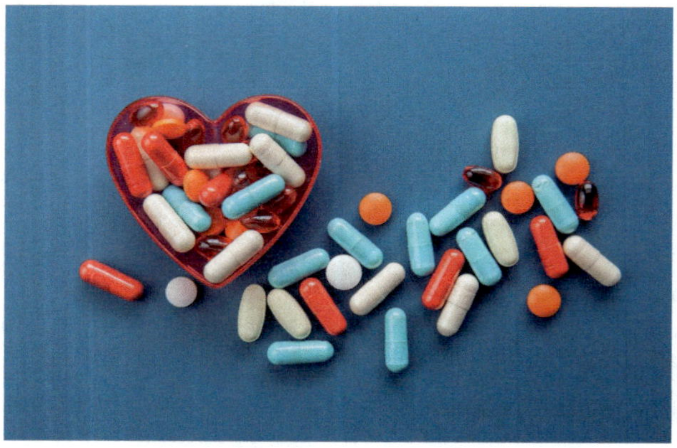

Figure 12.1. Cardiovascular drug therapy.

Source: https://www.practicenursing.com/media/wxgdg4y4/adobestock_132556299.jpeg.

12.1. Types of Cardiovascular Drugs

Learning Outcome

1. Understand antihypertensives, anticoagulants, antiplatelet agents, statins, and beta-blockers
2. Focus on ACE inhibitors
3. Discuss angiotensin II receptor blockers (ARBs)
4. Describe diuretics
5. Know calcium channel blockers

The diverse class of cardiovascular drugs is central to the treatment of cardiovascular diseases, curing many conditions with varying mechanisms of action. Among the leading classes are antihypertensives, which reduce blood pressure and protect against heart attack and stroke. Notable subgroups are ACE inhibitors and beta-blockers, each having distinct effects on cardiovascular function. Additionally, lipid-reducing medications, such statins, are essential for controlling cholesterol levels and minimizing the risk of atherosclerosis. Anticoagulants and antiplatelets, on the other hand, work by preventing thrombus, particularly among patients presenting with atrial fibrillation. Still further, current trends, as highlighted by recent literature, advocate for a shift towards the use of personalized medicine according to network pharmacology principles to enhance therapeutic safety as well as efficacy (Marsh et al., 2010; Whetstine et al., 2015). This tailored approach not only directs therapy towards patient profiles but is also a reaction to the evolving climate of cardiovascular therapy.

12.1.1. Antihypertensives

Antihypertensive agents play a central role in cardiovascular drug therapy, particularly in managing blood pressure and preventing cardiovascular disease. The increasing prevalence of diseases like hypertension, which is marked by contributing causes such as diabetes and lifestyle factors, necessitates effective therapeutic intervention. New findings indicate that statin, in addition to antihypertensive therapy, may enhance blood pressure control, demonstrating the synergistic effect, which may optimize the benefits of patients, especially in Type 2 Diabetes Mellitus comorbid patients (Besekar et al., 2025). In addition, the antihypertensive medication therapeutic response may be significantly influenced by genetic polymorphisms due to their effects on drug metabolism and therapeutic efficacy. Understanding such genetic determinants is essential so that treatments can be personalized, making therapy maximally optimal in individual patients (Rebrova et al., 2024). Ongoing advancements in the field will continue to illuminate the finesse of antihypertensive therapy and its integration into comprehensive cardiovascular care (Figure 12.2).

Antihypertensive Drug Classes

	Classes	Drug Names	Examples	Mechanism of Action	Main Effect on BP
A	ACE Inhibitors	"pril"	Lisinopril Enalapril	Inhibit ACE	↓ SVR, SV
A	ARBs	"sartan"	Losartan Valsartan	Block Angiotensin II Receptors	↓ SVR, SV
A	Alpha Blockers	"osin"	Doxazosin Terazosin	Block Alpha Receptors	↓ SVR
B	Beta Blockers	"lol"	Metoprolol Labetalol	Block Beta Receptors	↓ HR, SV
C	Calcium Channel Blockers (CCBs)	"dipine"	Amlodipine Nicardipine	Block Calcium Channels	↓ SVR
D	Diuretics	"ide"	Furosemide Hydrochlorothiazide	Facilitate Diuresis	↓ SV

**Alpha blockers refer to selective alpha-1 blockers, and calcium channel blockers refer to dihydropyridines

Figure 12.2. Antihypertensive medications.

Source: https://images.squarespace-cdn.com/content/v1/5e48489da899cd09424943db/1621867721364-KTYMJTN7B20MIWZYQVD1/austin+kosier+antihypertensive+medication+classes+drug+list+chart+examples+2.

12.1.2. Anticoagulants

The application of anticoagulants in cardiology cannot be overestimated, as they are pivotal in the prevention and treatment of thromboembolic disease, such as deep vein thrombosis (DVT) and pulmonary embolism. While older drugs like warfarin have been the standard, new anticoagulants such as rivaroxaban have gained favor since they are orally bioavailable and have predictable pharmacokinetics. However, as validated by challenging cases where the use of rivaroxaban was unsuccessful for the management of certain DVT patients, necessitating replacement with warfarin for a better prognosis, the choice of anticoagulant might significantly impact patient care (Adashek et al., 2017). In addition, the therapeutic setting is dynamic, with emerging evidence defining the overall health effects of vitamin K, which plays a crucial role in coagulation and cardiovascular disease, thereby connecting nutritional aspects with drug therapy (Araujo et al., 2020). Overall, the optimal use of anticoagulants relies on the possession of intricate knowledge on patient individualization, drug interactions, and up-to-date clinical evidence.

12.1.3. Antiplatelet Agents

Antiplatelet agents play a pivotal role in cardiovascular drug therapy, and their primary function is to inhibit the formation of thrombus under various cardiovascular disorders such as myocardial infarction and stroke. Antiplatelet agents not only block platelet aggregation but also manifest shear-dependent characteristics that enhance the fragility of thrombus and accelerate endogenous fibrinolysis, thus lending to their therapeutic effects. Both laboratory and clinical evidence suggest that the stability of thrombi in arteries, depending on the structural characteristics of the thrombus itself, plays a vital role in defining the level of infarction during coronary or cerebrovascular events

(Gast et al., 2018). By understanding the multi-dimensional actions of antiplatelet medications, clinicians can adjust treatment practices that decrease risks associated with cardiovascular diseases while maintaining consideration for the evolving drug regimens in comorbid patients with chronic conditions (Stuart, 2008). Thus, antiplatelet therapy remains a cornerstone in contemporary cardiovascular health management (Figure 12.3).

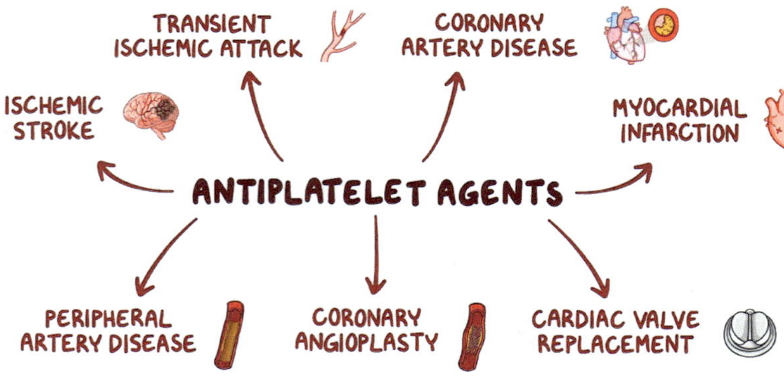

Figure 12.3. Antiplatelet agents.

Source: https://d16qt3wv6xm098.cloudfront.net/U1ni2OS8QKqV6KN_Dt6x7AZtT4OpY4zh/_.jpg.

12.1.4. Statins

Statins, chemically 3-hydroxy-3-methylglutaryl-coenzyme A reductase inhibitors, are an anchor medication for cardiovascular therapy, especially in patients with high levels of low-density lipoprotein cholesterol (LDL-c). Their ability to lower the concentration of serum LDL-c has made them first-line medications in the prevention of cardiovascular morbidity. While their advantages exist, statins have the potential to be linked with adverse effects, most prominently muscle pain and, in a small number of cases, rhabdomyolysis, highlighting the importance of careful monitoring during treatment. Studies have shown that although most patients comfortably tolerate statins, approximately 22.9% can present with some degree of adverse effect, for example, headache or insomnia, especially when drug interactions take place, as with simvastatin and nifedipine (Anni et al., 2009). Further, integrated metabolomic and lipidomic studies have the potential to describe factors that affect patient response to statins, enabling more effective and targeted cardiovascular treatments (Preiss et al., 2016).

12.1.5. Beta-Blockers

Beta-blockers have emerged as the cornerstone in the management of various cardiovascular illnesses, such as hypertension and heart failure. They achieve this by opposing the effects of epinephrine, thereby reducing heart rate and myocardial contractility, all contributing to achieving reduced blood pressure as well as decreased cardiac workload. They are essential in patients with illnesses like Cushing's syndrome, where there is increased risk of hypertension due to elevated levels of cortisol. In such cases, beta-blockers can help in reversing the hypertensive effect until the condition is treated correctly (Barbot et al., 2019). Furthermore, treatment of heart failure with beta-blockers has evolved, and evidence indicates their potential to improve survival and reduce hospitalization. However, a balance between efficiency and safety remains a target of ongoing research (Dans et al., 2014). Therefore, beta-blockers are a crucial therapeutic choice in the field of cardiovascular pharmacotherapy (Figure 12.4).

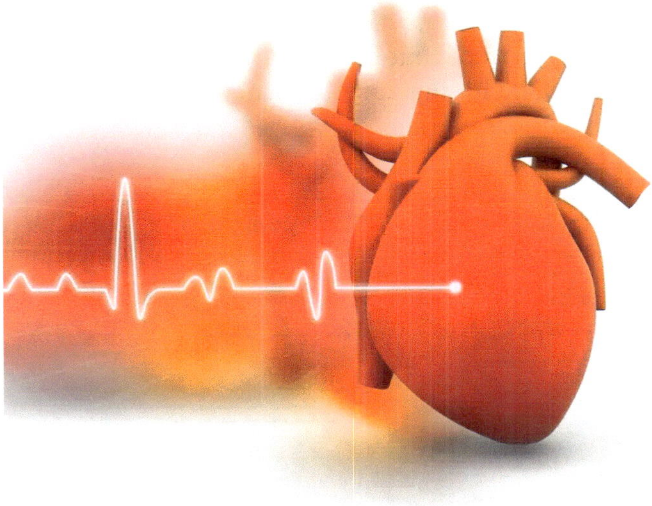

Figure 12.4. Beta-blockers have emerged as a cornerstone in the management of various cardiovascular conditions, notably hypertension and heart failure.

Source: https://m.economictimes.com/thumb/msid-100970095,width-1200,height-900,resizemode-4,imgsize-22688/beta-blockers-for-cardiovascular-diseases.jpg.

12.1.6. ACE Inhibitors

ACE inhibitors are pivotal in cardiovascular disease treatment, including hypertension and heart failure, by vasodilation and reduction of fluid retention. They act on the inhibition of the angiotensin-converting enzyme (ACE) involved in the conversion of angiotensin I to angiotensin II, a potent vasoconstrictor. Their clinical benefit is greater than lowering blood pressure; for instance, studies have confirmed that ACE inhibitors decrease oxidative stress and enhance vascular function, countering the deleterious actions of environmental pollutants like particulate matter (PM2.5) that cause cardiovascular disease in susceptible individuals. Specifically, captopril administration, an ACE inhibitor, exhibited significant improvements in mitigating PM2.5-induced hypertension and oxidative stress in model systems, indicating its positive cardiovascular implications (Kunti et al., 2024). Additionally, mounting evidence suggests that ACE inhibitors can counteract the undesirable effects of other cardiovascular drugs, such as those demonstrated by tyrosine kinase inhibitors, thereby further maximizing overall therapeutic potential in patients (Li et al., 2024).

12.1.7. Angiotensin II Receptor Blockers (ARBs)

Among cardiovascular drug treatments, Angiotensin II receptor blockers (ARBs) hold a significant position, particularly for the management of hypertension and heart failure. ARBs offer a targeted therapy through selective inhibition of the angiotensin II effect, leading to vasodilation and reduced blood pressure. Present studies indicate that while ARBs are generally well tolerated, they nonetheless possess unique safety profiles that influence prescribing. For instance, comparative evidence on the risks of cardiovascular events demonstrated that ACE inhibitors potentially yield improved outcomes among specific populations, undermining the relative advantage of ARBs in the prevention of cardiovascular events, especially for aged patients with type 2 diabetes mellitus (Zeng et al., 2025). Besides, profiles of adverse effects of other ARBs further confirm that individualized treatment approaches need to be embraced, that certain ARBs are associated with higher rates of risk for organ-specific complications, including cardiovascular complications (Ogura et al., 2025) (Figure 12.5).

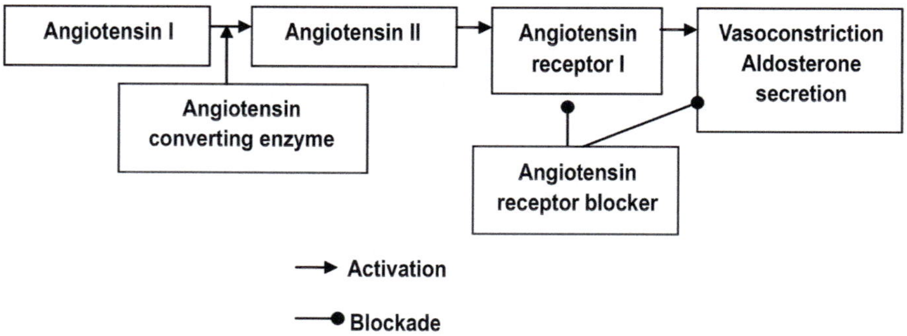

Figure 12.5. Angiotensin II receptor blockers (ARBs) play a significant role, particularly in the management of hypertension and heart failure.

Source: https://pub.mdpi-res.com/jpm/jpm-12-01253/article_deploy/html/images/jpm-12-01253-g001.png?1659167352.

12.1.8. Diuretics

Diuretics play a significant role in the treatment of cardiovascular diseases, and particularly in hypertension and heart failure. By facilitating sodium and water excretion, diuretics reduce the volume of blood, thereby reducing cardiac load and improving symptoms of the patient resulting from fluid overload. Studies have shown that successful diuretic therapy can affect overall patient prognosis in the presence of AHF since immediate and appropriate therapy when the patient is hospitalized is essential to optimize treatment interventions and improve long-term outcomes (Ambrosy et al., 2018). There is also growing curiosity about discovering possible interrelations between cardiovascular pharmacological therapies, e.g., diuretics, and psychological consequences. It has been described that while commonly prescribed antihypertensive drugs can influence mood disorders, the precise impact of diuretics like thiazides on psychological conditions requires more research (Boal et al., 2016). Thus, the multifaceted influence of diuretics is a strong area of study in cardiovascular pharmacotherapy.

12.1.9. Calcium Channel Blockers

Among cardiovascular drug treatments, calcium channel blockers (CCBs) are an important group of antihypertensive medications. They exert their effects by inhibiting calcium ion entry through L-type calcium channels with smooth muscle relaxation and consequent vasodilation. This mechanism significantly reduces peripheral vascular resistance and blood pressure. Therefore, CCBs are extremely valuable in the therapy of hypertension, which is increasingly becoming a problem among children, as evident from recent studies. Interestingly, secondary causes of hypertension, such as Cushing's syndrome, make its therapy even more difficult because elevated levels of cortisol result in vascular remodeling and chronic hypertension despite therapy (Barbot et al., 2019). Finally, heightened childhood and adolescent prevalence of hypertension highlights the need for evidence-based treatment regimens featuring CCBs as a component of other agents to tackle long-term cardiovascular morbidity (Agabiti-Rosei et al., 2016). As such, CCBs form a valuable weapon in the therapeutic arsenal against cardiovascular disease (Figure 12.6)

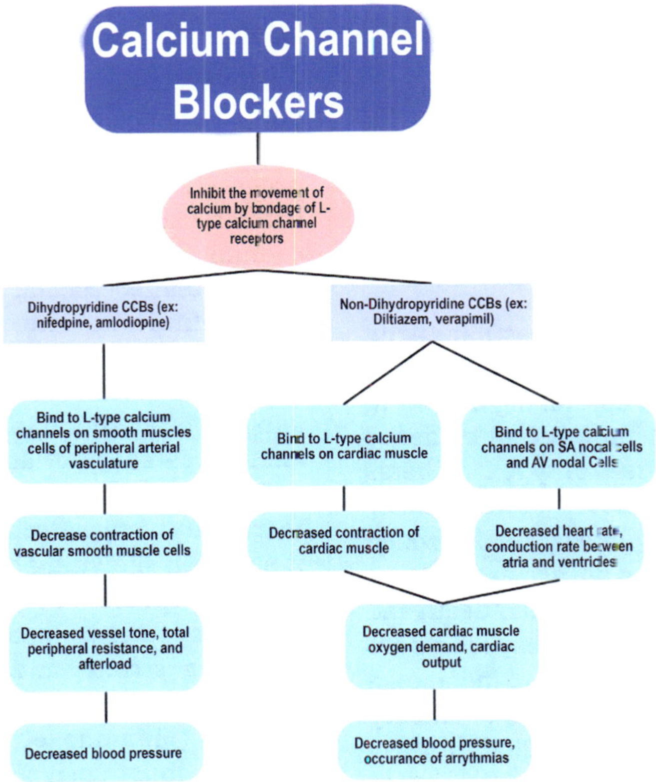

Figure 12.6. In the realm of cardiovascular drug therapy, calcium channel blockers (CCBs) serve as a pivotal class of antihypertensive agents.

Source: https://www.mdpi.com/cimb/cimb-46-00377/article_deploy/html/images/cimb-46-00377-g001.png.

Test Your Knowledge

1. What types of drugs are used in the management of heart failure?
2. Which lipid-lowering agents are most commonly prescribed in cardiovascular disease?

12.2. Mechanisms of Action

Learning Outcome

1. Understand how antihypertensives lower blood pressure
2. Explain the mechanism of action of anticoagulants
3. Discuss the role of antiplatelet agents in preventing clots
4. Describe statins and cholesterol reduction
5. Focus on beta-blockers and heart rate modulation
6. Know ACE inhibitors and vasodilation
7. Discuss ARBs and their impact on the renin-angiotensin system
8. Explain diuretics and fluid balance
9. Understand calcium channel blockers and vascular relaxation

Within the realm of cardiovascular drug treatment, familiarity with the mechanisms of action of therapy is key to optimizing benefit in the patient. For instance, more recent evidence has highlighted newer classes of type 2 diabetes drugs, such as sodium-glucose cotransporter 2 (SGLT2) inhibitors like empagliflozin, which have shown significant cardiovascular benefit, including reductions in cardiovascular death and hospitalization for heart failure. These effects are likely the result of hemodynamic and metabolic-driven pathways that enhance cardiac efficacy (Januzzi et al., 2017). Conversely, glucagon-like peptide–1 receptor agonists such as liraglutide and semaglutide have cardiovascular effects by other mechanisms, albeit slower, with variable effects on heart failure risk (Januzzi et al., 2017). In addition, administering metformin with statins in diabetics represents another form of drug interaction, considering that the combined action of both drugs on glucose and lipid metabolism can yield varied consequences when administered together or separately. Last but not least, knowledge of these mechanisms can help clinicians manage therapy in ways to reduce cardiovascular events in patients at risk.

12.2.1. How Antihypertensives Lower Blood Pressure

Antihypertensive medication plays a central part in managing high blood pressure through various mechanisms on diverse physiological processes. For instance, diuretics reduce blood volume via augmented excretion of water and sodium, subsequently reducing cardiac output and systemic vascular resistance. Conversely, ACE inhibitors and angiotensin receptor blockers (ARBs) inhibit the renin-angiotensin-aldosterone mechanism, leading to vasodilation and lowered blood pressure. Beta-blockers, another category of antihypertensives, reduce myocardial contractility and heart rate and therefore decrease cardiac work. Additionally, it has been shown that uncontrolled variability of blood pressure correlates with adverse outcomes, such as impaired functional recovery following stroke, and therefore emphasizes the importance of effective antihypertensive therapy (Manning et al., 2015). Also, some interventions, such as renal transplantation with concomitant nephrectomy, considerably reduce antihypertensive drug needs, endorsing the importance of targeted intervention in blood pressure control (Bahler et al., 2016) (Figure 12.7).

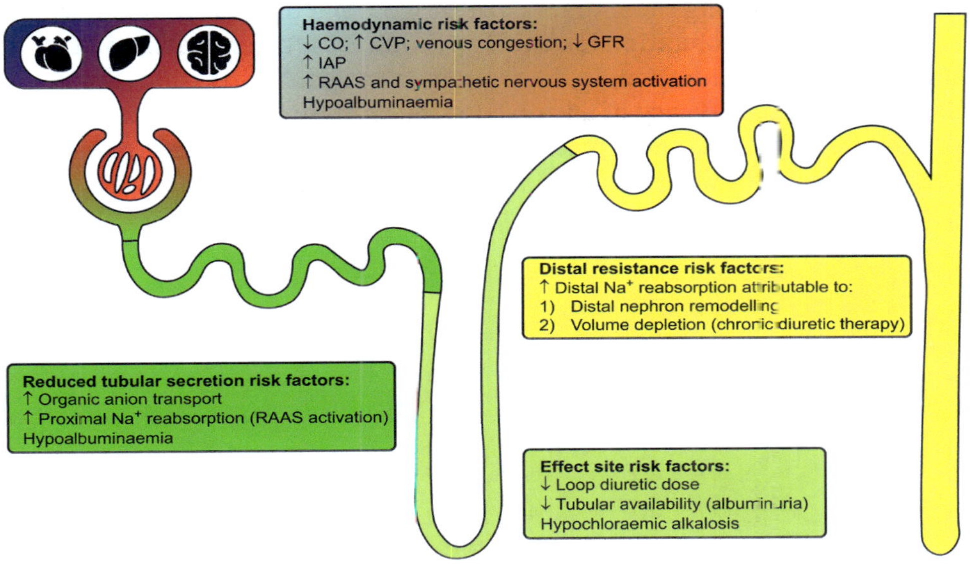

Figure 12.7. Diuretics reduce blood volume by promoting the excretion of sodium and water, which subsequently lowers cardiac output and systemic vascular resistance.

Source: https://www.bjanaesthesia.org.uk/cms/10.1016/j.bja.2025.02.032/asset/27a4a7d8-f7e9-48e6-8d50-7c1ba5ffc8b4/main.assets/gr1_lrg.jpg.

12.2.2. Mechanism of Action of Anticoagulants

Anticoagulants play a pivotal role in treating cardiovascular disorders by inhibiting several coagulation cascade steps with a reduced risk of thrombus formation. The traditional vitamin K antagonists, such as warfarin, primarily act by inhibiting the synthesis of vitamin K-dependent clotting factors, prolonging the prothrombin time, and reducing clot formation. But that was before direct oral anticoagulants (DOACs) came into the picture. Agents like dabigatran, which is a direct thrombin inhibitor, and factor Xa inhibitors rivaroxaban and apixaban offer more predictable pharmacokinetics, thus reducing the need for regular monitoring and dietary restrictions associated with warfarin therapy (Acharya et al., 2015). Besides, in acute coronary syndrome (ACS), novel combinations of antithrombotic agents, for example, DOACs, have promise for enhanced effectiveness in preventing major adverse cardiovascular events with the likelihood of inducing increased bleeding risk (Akhtar et al., 2020). Such a delicate balance of efficacy and safety renders anticoagulant therapy with cardiovascular drug regimens complex.

12.2.3. Role of Antiplatelet Agents in Preventing Clots

In the treatment of cardiovascular diseases, the application of antiplatelet drugs in preventing the formation of thrombus is most critical. The drugs are effective in inhibiting the aggregation of platelets, a primary mechanism towards the development of clots that precipitate disastrous vascular occurrences in the form of myocardial infarction and stroke. Moreover, recent findings highlight that antiplatelet therapy exhibits shear-dependent activity that enhances the fragility of developed thrombi, hence causing them to be more susceptible to endogenous fibrinolysis (Gast et al., 2018). The dynamic nature of antiplatelet therapy indicates its far-reaching benefits beyond its mere function in aggregation inhibition. In diseases such as atrial fibrillation, where clot formation is highly perilous, the relative efficacy of antiplatelet therapy about other forms of therapy, such as the Watchman's device, highlights their place in multidisciplinary treatment guidelines (Fladmo et al., 2019). Overall, antiplatelet drugs remain pivotal in cardiovascular morbidity prevention from thrombosis (Figure 12.8).

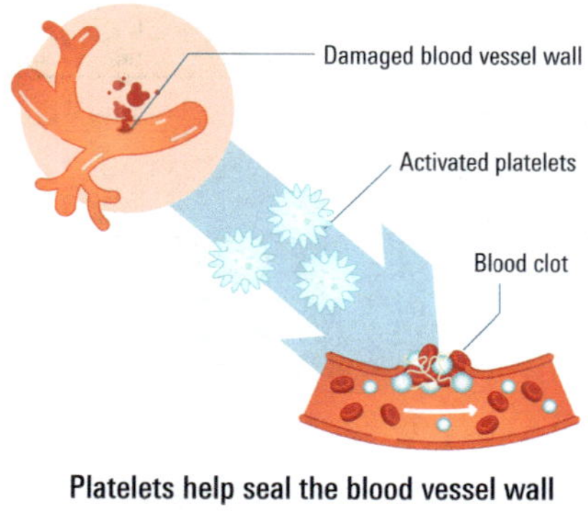

Figure 12.8. The role of antiplatelet agents in preventing thrombus formation is paramount.

Source: https://marley-storage.imgix.net/8fcb90ed-658c-43ee-92c2-bf285a0385b7/BL-platelets.png.

12.2.4. Statins and Cholesterol Reduction

Statins are now the cornerstone of cardiovascular risk reduction as a result of their high capacity for lowering cholesterol levels. Statins, in most instances, target LDL-C, which is typically compounded by an increased incidence of cardiovascular diseases (CVD). Statins' effectiveness is documented by their ability to profoundly reduce LDL levels, as well as cardiovascular event rates, particularly among those with established cardiovascular disease, as indicated by (Pichandi et al., 2011). But it is also understood that not all patients will attain optimal levels of LDL-C with statin monotherapy alone, so it becomes necessary for other or for adjunctive therapy in those who are intolerant or have a suboptimal response. Ezetimibe, for example, acts by inhibiting cholesterol absorption, providing a , proper therapeutic strategy for additional reduction of LDL-C and is regarded as safe and tolerable, adding to the therapeutic profile of cholesterol treatment in cardiovascular drugs, as highlighted in Dayspring et al. (2012).

12.2.5. Beta-Blockers and Heart Rate Modulation

The beta-blockers' action on heart rate modulation is a critical part of the treatment of heart failure and hypertension, as well as other cardiovascular diseases. By the mechanism of beta-adrenergic receptor antagonism, drugs produce this action by reducing myocardial contractility and heart rate, thereby lessening the workload of the heart and enhancing cardiac performance in general. In heart failure, this modulation is particularly beneficial, where beta-blocker therapy has been found to increase survival dramatically. The efficacy of beta-blockers, nonetheless, may vary among various people based on genetic differences, necessitating an individualized treatment strategy. Pharmacogenomics plays a significant role in explaining such variations since it studies genetic factors that affect drug response, which is very vital in the multisystem disease management of cardiovascular disease (Barrese et al., 2014). Also crucial is the control of factors contributing to hypertension since beta-blockers affect the vascular system too, influencing endothelial function and helping prevent the risks associated with elevated blood pressure (Cameron et al., 2016) (Figure 12.9).

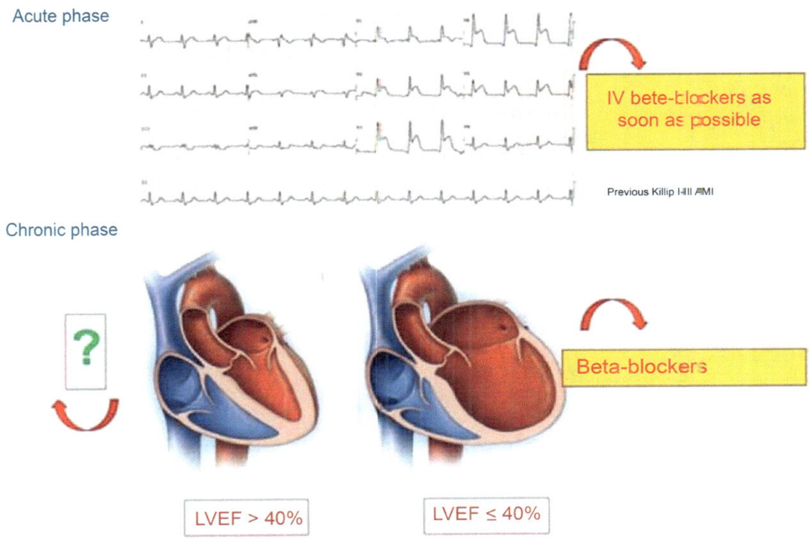

Figure 12.9. Current status of beta-blockers in the different phases of acute coronary syndrome. AMI, acute myocardial infarction; IV, intravenous; LVEF, left ventricular ejection fraction.

Source: https://www.revespcardiol.org/en-role-beta-blockers-in-cardiovascular-disease-articulo-S1885585719301860.

12.2.6. ACE Inhibitors and Vasodilation

ACE inhibitors are the key to managing cardiovascular disease due to their potent vasodilatory effects, which work to reduce blood pressure and improve cardiovascular health substantially. ACE inhibitors lead to the production of bradykinin, a peptide that promotes vasodilation, by inhibiting the ACE. This mechanism not only lowers systemic vascular resistance but also lowers the workload of the heart, thus making ACE inhibitors a cornerstone therapy in diseases such as hypertension and heart failure. Moreover, new data indicate that ACE inhibitors may lower oxidative stress and improve endothelial function, major determinants of cardiovascular pathology (Kunti et al., 2024). In addition, as regards the air pollution-induced cardiovascular effects, ACE inhibitors like captopril have been found effective in counteracting the adverse consequences of particulate matter exposure on vascular function, highlighting their therapeutic value in different formats (Mehrotra, 2025). Therefore, ACE inhibitors form an essential part of contemporary drug therapy for treating cardiovascular complications, highlighting their role in maximizing patient outcomes (Figure 12.10).

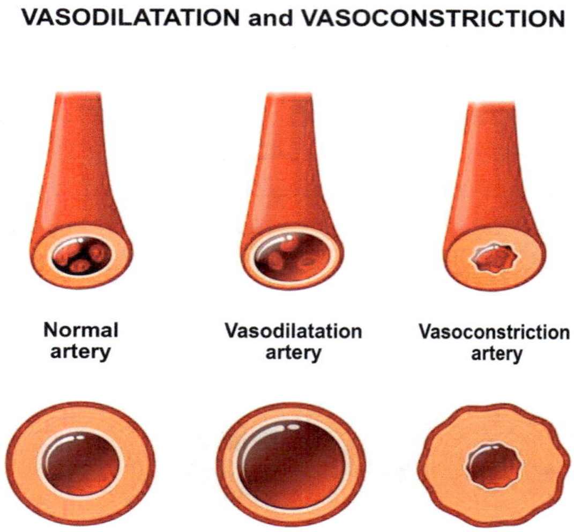

Figure 12.10. Vasodilation.

Source: https://facty.mblycdn.com/uploads/fh/2020/02/1163866175.jpg.

12.2.7. ARBs and Their Impact on the Renin-Angiotensin System

Angiotensin II receptor blockers (ARBs) are key to the modulation of the renin-angiotensin system (RAS), essential for cardiovascular homeostasis and blood pressure regulation. By selectively blocking the effects of angiotensin II, ARBs minimize vasoconstriction and facilitate vasodilation, thus lowering blood pressure and reducing cardiovascular strain. This mechanism is especially beneficial for heart failure and CKD, as the activation of RAS significantly contributes to the progression of disease and adverse cardiovascular outcomes. In patient populations suffering from hypertension and heart failure, ARBs have been proven to improve outcomes with reduced morbidity and mortality rates (Alzubi et al., 2024). Additionally, RAS blockade not only assists in blood pressure regulation but also serves a protective role in advancing kidney disease, particularly in diabetic patients, where the hypertensive condition is a crucial risk factor for complications (Banerjee et al., 2022).

12.2.8. Diuretics and Fluid Balance

Optimal fluid control, particularly in cardiovascular patients, often necessitates the use of diuretics. Such therapeutic modalities increase renal excretion of excess sodium and water and lead to a reduction of extracellular volume and blood pressure.

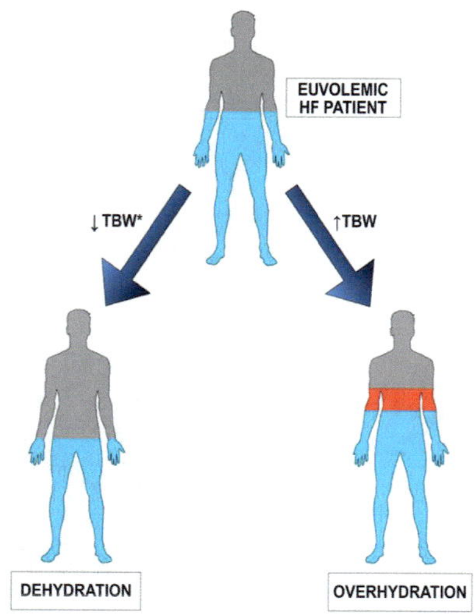

Figure 12.11. Effective management of fluid balance, particularly in patients with cardiovascular conditions, often necessitates the use of diuretics.

Source: https://pub.mdpi-res.com/biomedicines/biomedicines-11-02684/article_deploy/html/images/biomedicines-11-02684-g001.png?1696670549.

This is especially crucial in patients treated with therapies such as peritoneal dialysis (PD) where ideal fluid control can enhance overall outcome and therapy duration. Synergy between sodium restriction, diuretic therapy, and dietary therapy becomes essential in such cases, as volume control to the best possible level can directly impact morbidity and mortality (Agarwal et al., 2019). In children, hypertension treatment requires an orderly approach that includes both pharmacologic and non-pharmacologic intervention to maintain fluid balance along with management of related cardiovascular morbidity (Bruyne et al., 2014). Thus, diuretics are a fundamental component of the general approach to managing fluid imbalances and optimizing cardiovascular health for most categories of patients (Figure 12.11).

12.2.9. Calcium Channel Blockers and Vascular Relaxation

CCBs have an essential role to play in causing vascular relaxation and hence the management of hypertension and other cardiovascular disorders. The medication prevents the influx of calcium ions into the vascular smooth muscle cells, causing reduced contractility of the muscles and thus vasodilation. While CCBs are effective at lowering blood pressure, their effect on the vessels is not just relaxation; they also increase endothelial function, albeit less than Angiotensin converting enzyme inhibitors and Angiotensin II receptor blockers, which have a superior ability to inhibit the vascular remodeling and inflammation of hypertension (Cameron et al., 2016). Moreover, understanding the molecular mechanisms governing smooth muscle contractility enhances the therapeutic effects of CCBs in individualized therapy regimens for cardiovascular disease (Aggarwal et al., 2016). Overall, these features position CCBs at the forefront of cardiovascular drug therapy, both alleviating symptoms and addressing underlying vascular dysfunction.

Test Your Knowledge

1. How do calcium channel blockers like amlodipine help treat angina and high blood pressure?
2. Describe how statins work to lower cholesterol.

12.3. Clinical Applications

Learning Outcome

1. Focus on the treatment of hypertension
2. Management of heart failure
3. Prevention of myocardial infarction
4. Learn stroke prevention strategies
5. Discuss use in arrhythmias
6. Explain the role in coronary artery disease
7. Explain the management of peripheral artery disease
8. Describe post-operative cardiovascular care
9. Understand patient-specific considerations in therapy

The clinical applications of cardiovascular drug treatment are rapidly evolving due to advances in individualized medicine and emerging technologies. Through the use of human-induced pluripotent stem cells (iPSCs), researchers are creating patient-specific cardiovascular cells with the potential to revolutionize drug discovery and customized therapy. iPSCs provide a more natural model of cardiovascular diseases and, hence, overcome previous shortcomings in drug interaction and patient response (Chandy et al., 2020). Additionally, treatment strategies in the management of hypertension need to be individualized. The majority of antihypertensive treatments today are failing since they generalize complex disease mechanisms and unique patient responses. An accommodation of a more personalized approach that considers genetic histories and patient profiles is paramount to improving the management of hypertension as well as the cardiovascular system as a whole (Borghi et al., 2017) These converging strategies emphasize the promise that future drug therapy breakthroughs hold for making a significant impact on cardiovascular clinical outcomes.

12.3.1. Treatment of Hypertension

Treatment of hypertension is an essential component of cardiovascular drug therapy and mirrors the importance of effective treatment regimens in reducing cardiovascular risk. Current guidelines are for the administration of two-drug combinations as initial treatment because they are more effective compared to monotherapy. Specifically, the 2018 ESC/ESH Hypertension guidelines favor the use of combinations of angiotensin-converting enzyme (ACE) inhibitors, angiotensin-receptor blockers (ARBs), calcium channel blockers, and thiazide-type diuretics. There is empirical evidence to back up these recommendations, with the bonus that dual therapy not only enhances control of blood pressure but also lowers cardiovascular adverse events like heart failure and stroke (Cho et al., 2020).

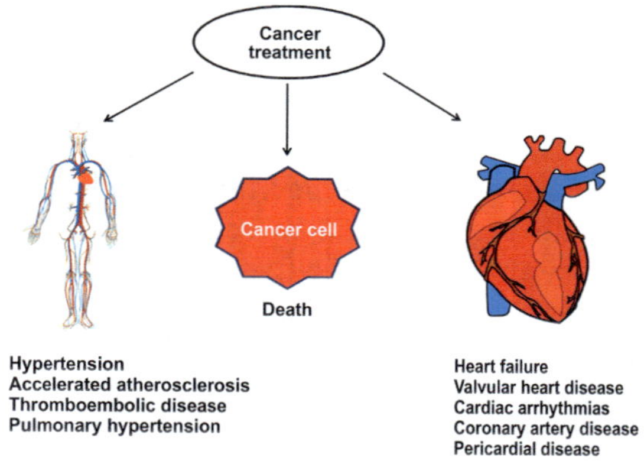

Figure 12.12. The treatment of hypertension is a critical aspect of cardiovascular drug therapy.

Source: https://media.springernature.com/m685/springer-static/image/art%3A10.1038%2Fs41371-020-0391-8/MediaObjects/41371_2020_391_Fig1_HTML.png.

However, it must be noted that the presence of cardiovascular risk factors together can reduce the response of patients to such therapies, as evidenced by studies showing decreased efficiency of treatment among hypertensive patients with other cardiovascular ailments (Charalampopoulos et al., 2014). Hypertension therapy on an individual basis is thus still a goal (Figure 12.12).

12.3.2. Management of Heart Failure

The management of heart failure has come a long way, particularly with pharmacological management, offering clinicians effective methods to improve the prognosis of their patients. Among the prospective treatment options, sodium-glucose co-transporter 2 (SGLT2) inhibitors have gained a lot of attention due to their positive effects on heart failure, particularly in patients who also have type 2 diabetes mellitus. These medications not only enhance glycemic control but also reduce hospitalization for heart failure by a considerable margin, leading the ESC to recommend their use as first-line therapy among drug-naïve patients (Gąsior et al., 2021). Also, inclusion of lifestyle interventions and AF monitoring plays an equally important role in the comprehensive management of heart failure. With ongoing study into long-term effectiveness of antiarrhythmic therapy and ablation interventions, the management landscape continually evolves, highlighting the requirement for tailored approaches to cope with the complex presentations of heart failure patients (Calkins et al., 2017).

12.3.3. Prevention of Myocardial Infarction

Prevention of myocardial infarction (MI) is a key focal point in cardiovascular drug treatment, particularly through the modulation of the renin–angiotensin–aldosterone system (RAAS). Prevention is rendered effective by the use of angiotensin-converting enzyme inhibitors (ACEis), which have been revealed to decrease the risk of MI considerably, particularly if started early in susceptible populations such as diabetes or hypertension (Sobhy et al., 2024). Moreover, the interaction between traditional risk factors and those for specific populations, such as HIV-infected patients, calls for an individualized approach to prevention. The high risk of MI in such patients cannot be attributed to traditional cardiovascular risk factors but also to the complexity of antiretroviral therapy and systemic inflammation (Protasov et al., 2024). Therefore, a comprehensive approach that incorporates pharmacological as well as lifestyle interventions is unavoidable for the prevention and management of myocardial infarction in multicultural patient populations (Figure 12.13).

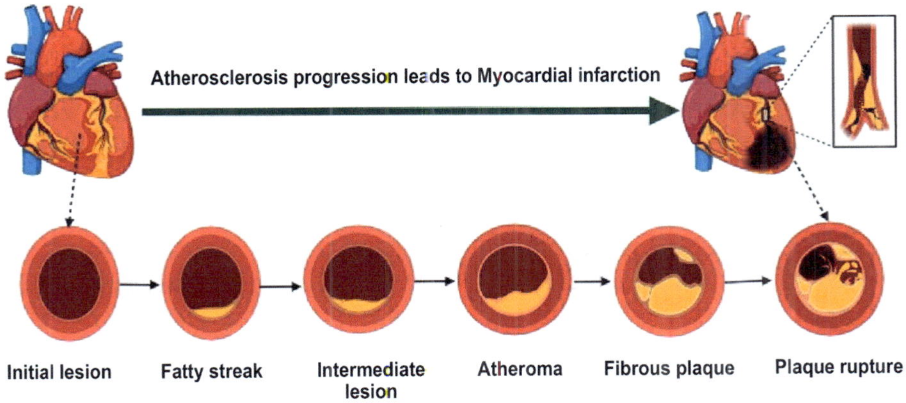

Figure 12.13. The prevention of myocardial infarction (MI) is a critical focus within cardiovascular drug therapy, particularly through the modulation of the renin–angiotensin–aldosterone system (RAAS).

Source: https://www.mdpi.com/cells/cells-13-01471/article_deploy/html/images/cells-13-01471-g001.png.

12.3.4. Stroke Prevention Strategies

Effective prevention of stroke is a key area in cardiovascular drug therapy since it prevents recurrent strokes and improves patient outcomes to a great extent. Antithrombotic drug compliance, such as aspirin and clopidogrel, is also essential in such measures; 96% of stroke patients adhered to at least one preventive drug after one year, where good compliance was particularly noted with aspirin and oral anticoagulation (Busse et al., 2003). Adherence to antihypertensive medication is also involved in stroke prevention since hypertension is a high-risk factor. Evidence suggests that early blood pressure control can result in less cardiovascular damage and events. While research in such a direction continues, it emphasizes the need to initiate antihypertensive therapy early to prevent the occurrence of stroke, pointing towards multi-dimensional prevention of stroke in cardiovascular drug treatment (Gallo et al., 2018).

12.3.5. Use in Arrhythmias

In cardiovascular pharmacotherapy, the management of arrhythmia is a significant part, particularly with the potential for severe complications, including sudden cardiac death. Drugs used to stabilize rhythm and heart rate are commonly employed in managing conditions such as atrial fibrillation and ventricular arrhythmias. This latter condition is specifically of concern in athletic groups, in whom there is a heightened risk of sudden cardiac death on exertion. Monomorphic ventricular arrhythmias, while often benign in athletes with no structural heart disease, need to be subjected to strict evaluation to rule out dangerous underlying pathology like hypertrophic cardiomyopathy. Successful treatment alternatives, such as radiofrequency catheter ablation, have promising outcomes, allowing many athletes to be returned safely to competitive sport once it is assured that there is no significant cardiac risk (Kitsiou et al., 2013; Aboulhosn et al., 2019). Thus, pharmacologic intervention knowledge is crucial in developing multidisciplinary treatment regimens for arrhythmia patients (Figure 12.14).

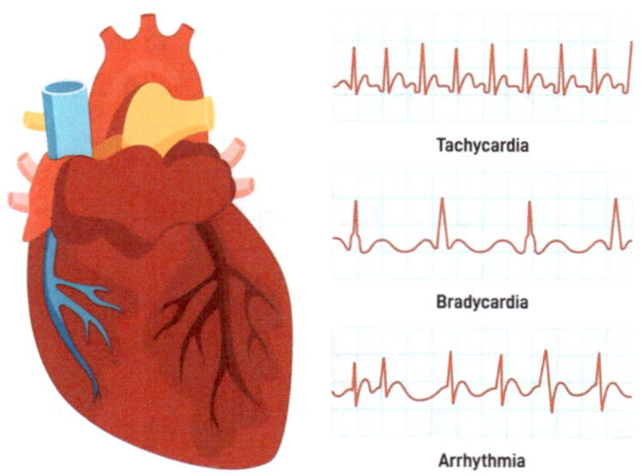

Figure 12.14. Antiarrhythmic medications are commonly employed to restore normal rhythm and heart rate, addressing conditions such as atrial fibrillation and ventricular arrhythmias.

Source: https://www.harleystreet.sg/img/pathological_arrhythmia.webp.

12.3.6. Role in Coronary Artery Disease

Coronary artery disease (CAD) is a pillar of cardiovascular disease, primarily because it is associated with arterial thrombus formation, and this can lead to ACS. CAD patients will require complex treatment strategies, including dual antiplatelet therapy (DAPT), with aspirin in combination with P2Y12 inhibitors, to avoid thrombotic event onset resulting in myocardial infarction (Farag et al., 2018). Additionally, background conditions such as hypertension, dyslipidemia, and even HIV infection play a significant role in CAD development and cardiovascular events. Studies indicated that the presence of coronary artery calcification (CAC) and mitral annular calcification (MAC) in the patient population can be employed as predictors of mortality and hence highlight the necessity for stringent screening and targeted treatment in susceptible groups (Bolger et al., 2015). Thus, effective cardiovascular drug therapy must mend the acute thrombotic risk as well as the underlying pathology of CAD.

12.3.7. Management of Peripheral Artery Disease

Management of peripheral artery disease (PAD) is essential not only for improving the quality of life of the patient but also in the prevention of cardiovascular complications of this disease. A multifaceted approach, including lifestyle modification and drug therapy, is necessary in management. Patients are initially motivated to engage in regular exercise regimes, which enhance walking ability and overall function. Additionally, antiplatelet medications such as aspirin and clopidogrel play a significant role in preventing thromboembolic complications, which are prevalent among PAD patients. Besides these medications, statins are generally employed to manage dyslipidemia and thereby prevent cardiovascular morbidity and mortality. The increased complexity of treatment also highlights the demand for personalized interventions, particularly since patients with PAD often have comorbid conditions such as diabetes and hypertension that require an integrated cardiovascular assessment and treatment regimen. Therefore, interdisciplinary coordination becomes imperative to optimize outcomes among this population of patients (Cameron et al., 2015) (Figure 12.15).

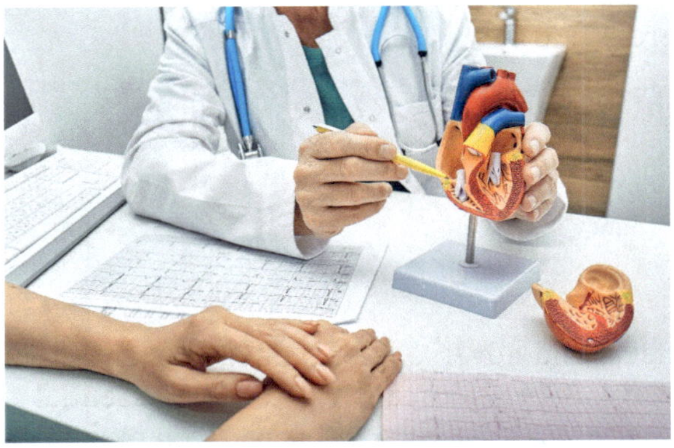

Figure 12.15. Managing peripheral artery disease (PAD) is crucial not only for improving patient quality of life but also for reducing cardiovascular risks associated with this condition.

Source: https://amscardiology.com/wp-content/uploads/2023/12/shutterstock_2167322485-scaled.jpg.

12.3.8. Post-Operative Cardiovascular Care

Postoperative management of the cardiovascular system is the most important consideration in the prevention of complications following surgery, particularly in patients with pre-existing cardiovascular disease. Careful vigilance strategies in the post-operative environment are key to ensuring early detection of potential cardiac insults, including myocardial infarction, which may arise as a consequence of perioperative stress. It has become realized that some cardiovascular care is needed, and the medical practitioners must conduct an adequate assessment of risk factors such as renal and pulmonary conditions, which are utilized to guide effective therapeutic interventions (Poldermans et al., 2009). Besides this, the role of cardiovascular drug therapy cannot be overestimated; beta-blockers and statins are examples of drugs that can not only be used for their chronic management ability but also their protective effects during the acute phase of the postoperative period (Kitsiou et al., 2013). Finally, a broad-based approach with an emphasis on careful monitoring and pharmacotherapy is essential in maximizing patient outcomes in post-operative cardiac care.

12.3.9. Patient-Specific Considerations in Therapy

Optimal cardiovascular drug therapy is a delicate application that is patient-specific and must be used to maximize the effectiveness of treatment. Comorbidities, age, and individual patient preference all contribute to determining the therapy.

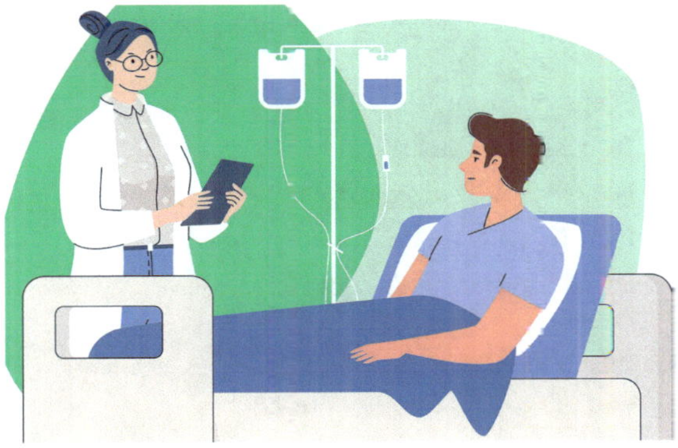

Figure 12.16. Effective cardiovascular drug therapy necessitates a nuanced approach that takes into account patient-specific considerations to optimize treatment outcomes.

Source: https://www.acc.org//-/media/Non-Clinical/Images/2025/01/CARDIOLOGY/02/Cardiotoxic-Cancer-Therapy-1200x800.jpg.

For instance, in patients with atrial fibrillation, the traditional method of vitamin K antagonists like warfarin can be made more challenging by diet interaction and monitoring, unlike newer agents like rivaroxaban that can provide easier and safer alternatives, particularly for patients with renal impairment or diabetes mellitus as demonstrated by real-world studies in terms of its safety profile (Dockrill et al., 2018). Besides, patient adherence to medication regimens is also a significant factor whereby therapies offering simpler dosing regimens, such as in the case of non-vitamin K OAC, enhance compliance and quality of life in general (Dockrill et al., 2018). Hence, individualization of therapy according to patient profiles facilitates a more patient-specific and effective method of cardiovascular therapy (Figure 12.16).

Test Your Knowledge

1. When is anticoagulant therapy indicated in cardiovascular care?
2. Which cardiovascular drugs are contraindicated during pregnancy and why?

12.4. Side Effects and Risks

Learning Outcome

1. Understand common side effects of antihypertensives
2. Identify risks associated with anticoagulants
3. Explain the adverse effects of antiplatelet therapy
4. Focus on statin-related muscle pain
5. Discuss beta-blocker side effects
6. Focus on ACE inhibitor cough and angioedema
7. Identify ARB-related renal complications
8. Focus on diuretic-induced electrolyte imbalances
9. Discuss calcium channel blocker side effects

The usage of cardiovascular drug therapy, while essential to address a variety of heart conditions, is not complication-free. One of the key things that should be remembered is the side effects and risks associated with these drugs since they can differ significantly based on the category of drug in question. For instance, patients with diabetes receiving antihyperglycemic treatment are at increased risk of cardiovascular complications, and this has been an issue raising confusion among clinicians on how to handle the therapy most appropriately. Current guidelines are to make an individualized consideration, which will encourage the treating physician to weigh each patient's unique health profile against the side effects and adverse effects of each agent (Agius et al., 2014). Moreover, it is also essential to observe that patients with severe mental illness possess prevalent co-occurring cardiovascular risk factors augmented by both drug side effects as well as comorbid diseases, such that management options become more complex and necessitate critical consideration of therapeutic interventions (Braga et al., 2018). It reiterates the importance of personalized risk assessments in cardiovascular drug therapy.

12.4.1. Common Side Effects of Antihypertensives

Antihypertensive medications, while effective in lowering blood pressure, are typically associated with other side effects that can affect patient compliance and overall treatment success. Dizziness, fatigue, and hypotension represent some of the more frequent undesirable effects, which can deter patients from taking these medications regularly. Specifically, diuretics induce electrolyte disturbances, manifesting as cramps or dehydration. Some patients also experience gastrointestinal disorders, which can significantly lower their quality of life. It is also noteworthy that antihypertensives are likewise linked with serious side effects of drugs, particularly when taken with other medications, like in cases where drug interactions lead to cardiovascular side effects (Adhikari et al., 2009).

As cardiovascular drug treatment continues to advance, and in the face of the increasing number of hypertension cases as well as their accompanying disorders (Freeman et al., 2013), there is a need to determine and even manage these side effects. Effective communication and observation are required for optimal therapeutic outcomes without risks (Figure 12.17).

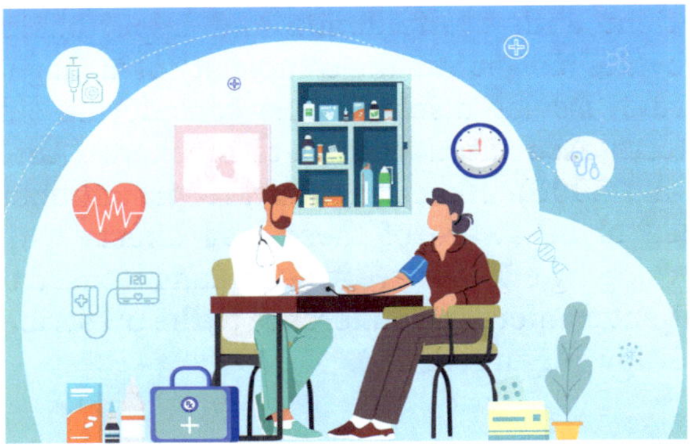

Figure 12.17. Antihypertensive medications, while effective in managing high blood pressure, are often associated with various side effects that can impact patient adherence and overall treatment outcomes.

Source: https://coreprescribingsolutions.co.uk/wp-content/uploads/2023/11/CLINICAL-PHARMACIST-INTERACTION.jpg.

12.4.2. Risks Associated with Anticoagulants

The use of anticoagulants, while imperative for thromboembolic events prevention in those with conditions such as atrial fibrillation, comes with immense risk that needs appropriate management. A significant limitation is the increased occurrence of bleeding events, which has been noted since the study comparison between OAC and antiplatelet (AP) therapy. Specifically, the patients who receive OAC and AP therapy have much higher rates of stroke and hemorrhagic events compared to their counterparts who receive only OAC, which necessitates follow-up and selection of the patient (Bassand et al., 2020). Furthermore, the interaction between hypertension and atrial fibrillation contributes to the risk factor, as uncontrolled blood pressure can predispose to disabling strokes and cardiovascular mortality in these patients (Sada et al., 2015). Thus, while anticoagulants are central to cardiovascular drug therapy, the risks associated therewith call for a balanced approach to treatment, with patient safety and adherence to therapeutic guidelines in mind

12.4.3. Adverse Effects of Antiplatelet Therapy

Antiplatelet therapy is a mainstay of the management of cardiovascular disease, particularly following ACS. Although useful in avoiding thrombotic complications, it is not without risk.

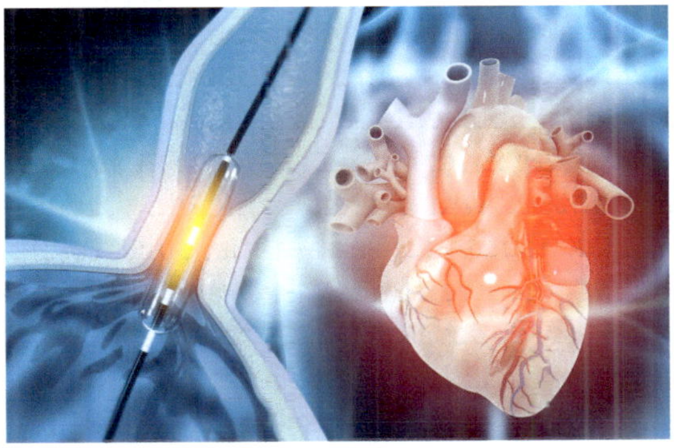

Figure 12.18. Antiplatelet therapy is a cornerstone in the management of cardiovascular conditions, particularly following acute coronary syndromes (ACS).

Source: https://medizinonline.com/wp-content/uploads/2023/11/iStock-1337210627-scaled.jpg.

Perhaps its most feared risk is an increased predisposition to bleed, which is a significant risk to patient safety. DAPT, especially following the use of drug-eluting stents, has been associated with variable bleeding complications. Evidence shows that despite shorter DAPT regimes (3–6 months) showing improved overall bleeding risk compared to more extended regimens (12–24 months), a risk for fatal bleeding complications still exists (Bulluck et al., 2014). Additionally, the use of adjunct therapies such as Very Low Dose Rivaroxaban also continues to augment bleeding risks, even though it has cardiovascular benefits in high-risk patients (Gorog et al., 2019). Hence, the adverse effects of antiplatelet therapy need proper selection and monitoring of the patient (Figure 12.18).

12.4.4. Statin-Related Muscle Pain

Being the first treatment of choice in hypercholesterolemia, statins form a foundation of cardiovascular drug therapy due to their capacity to lower cholesterol and prevent cardiovascular events. A key issue with the use of statins is statin-associated muscle soreness, which encompasses symptoms of myalgia, muscle weakness, and rhabdomyolysis in a minority of patients. These side effects will probably negatively influence patient adherence to treatment, with muscle pain being identified as a risk factor for non-adherence to lipid-lowering medication (Mitkova et al., 2024). Furthermore, research has revealed that the majority of patients experience different degrees of side effects in the muscles, highlighting the relevance of active follow-up of these symptoms by clinicians. Statin-induced muscle pain management is crucial for the optimization of patient results and ensuring that the benefits of these significant cardiovascular medications outweigh any possible threats to their use (Mahadevappa et al., 2024).

12.4.5. Beta-Blocker Side Effects

The use of beta-blockers within drug treatment for cardiovascular disease is not without issue, most notably with regard to their side effects, which can significantly impact patient compliance and effectiveness. Of treatment generally. Side effects such as fatigue, bradycardia, and worsening of asthma symptoms are particular issues for patients with pre-existing respiratory disease. Notably, although beta-blockers effectively decrease myocardial oxygen demand and heart rate, thereby alleviating symptoms such as angina, they also lead to dosing challenges due to patient intolerance (Silva et al., 2016). For example, a case report of a 58-year-old female patient with dyslipidemia and hypertension provides insight into the complexity of managing cardiovascular disease while considering side effects associated with beta-blockers (Abela et al., 2006). Hence, healthcare practitioners need to be aware of these side effects while developing effective treatment plans focused on patient comfort and adherence to the prescribed therapy (Figure 12.19).

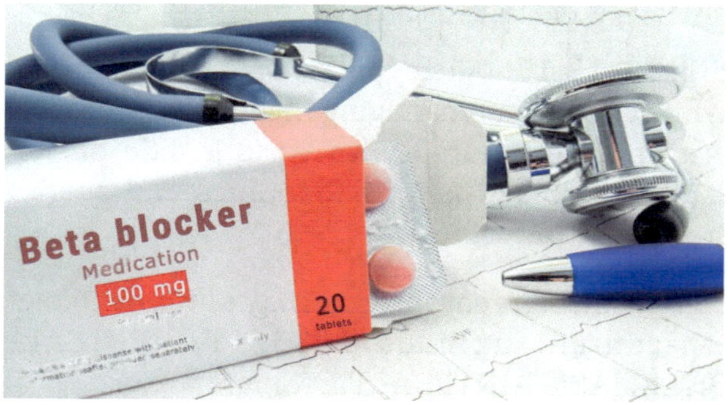

Figure 12.19. The use of beta-blockers in cardiovascular drug therapy is not without its challenges, particularly regarding their side effects, which can significantly impact patient adherence and overall treatment efficacy.

Source: https://bpincontrol.in/wp-content/uploads/2023/08/Beta-Blockers-Drugs-1200x675.jpg.

12.4.6. ACE Inhibitor Cough and Angioedema

Of the numerous side effects of angiotensin-converting enzyme (ACE) inhibitors, cough and angioedema stand out for their possible impact on compliance with treatment and therapeutic outcome. Dry, unproductive cough, which may last up to several weeks, is seen in approximately 5-20% of patients receiving ACE inhibitors via increased levels of bradykinin, which is irritating to the respiratory system. More concerning, however, is the potential for angioedema, a dangerous but uncommon disease that presents as swelling of inner skin layers, usually the throat and face. Both of these side effects require close observation and may lead healthcare providers to have to find other hypertension therapies. In comparative studies of different antihypertensive medications, the incidence of side effects such as angioedema was much lower in medications such as Clmesartan compared to enalapril, highlighting patient-specific drug planning in cardiovascular medication (Claggett et al., 2016; Kiranjit et al., 2018).

12.4.7. ARB-Related Renal Complications

Of cardiovascular medicine treatments, ARBs are particularly noted for the treatment of hypertension as well as the prevention of renal complications from cardiovascular conditions. ARBs have side effects, however, and are most concerning in their impact on renal function. Clinical practice teaches that while ARBs do enhance the prognosis of patients with chronic renal insufficiency, they will also cause acute renal failure in certain groups, most notably those with compromised renal perfusion or bilateral renal artery narrowing. Patients who initiate ARBs also often have to be closely monitored for renal function, particularly in the acute setting where temporary rises in serum creatinine are common. This underscores the necessity for international cardiovascular risk assessment before initiating therapy. With increasing public health interventions targeting hypertension among high-risk populations, it is necessary to understand such ARB-induced renal complications to optimize treatment regimens (Agabiti-Rosei et al., 2016; Cameron et al., 2018) (Figure 12.20).

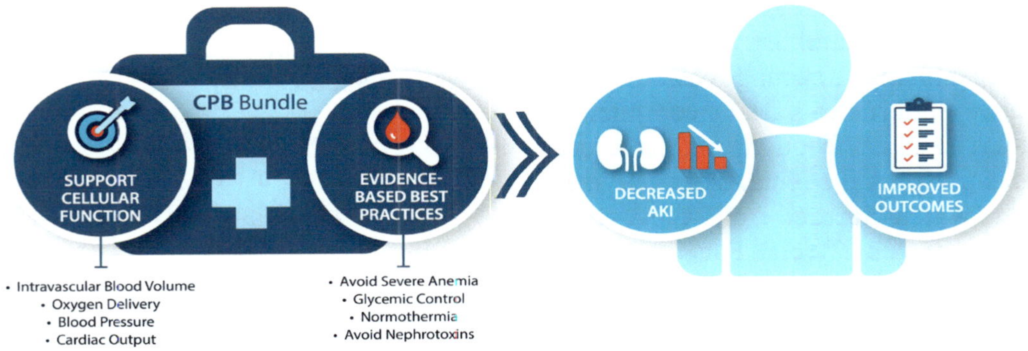

Figure 12.20. Patients initiating ARB therapy often require careful monitoring of renal function, particularly in the acute setting where transient elevations in serum creatinine are common.

Source: https://www.jcvaonline.com/cms/10.1053/j.jvca.2023.05.032/asset/0a11a550-7809-4f8f-90aa-ad6dd4788e41/main.assets/gr1_lrg.jpg.

12.4.8. Diuretic-Induced Electrolyte Imbalances

In cardiovascular drug therapy, diuretics are pivotal for managing hypertension and heart failure. Regrettably, their potency is usually earned at the expense of electrolyte homeostasis, one of the most significant of diuretic side effects with potentially far-reaching impacts for patient health. For instance, diuretics such as torsemide were revealed to induce hyponatremia and hypokalemia, as witnessed in a severe study that reported electrolyte serum changes upon administration (Agne et al., 2018). Furthermore, the use of diuretics in clinical settings, including intensive care units, usually led to extreme electrolyte disorders and necessitated vigilant monitoring by healthcare workers (Chitra et al., 2017). Diagnosing and treating diuretic-induced electrolyte imbalances is crucial because clinicians prescribe these life-saving medications, highlighting the necessity of a multidisciplinary care approach to both improve patient outcomes and prevent related complications in cardiovascular disease management strategies.

12.4.9. Calcium Channel Blocker Side Effects

CCBs are usually prescribed for hypertension and other cardiovascular conditions due to their capacity to dilate blood vessels and reduce the heart's workload. Their administration, however, is generally accompanied by a range of side effects that can easily undermine patient compliance and efficacy. The most frequent among these side effects is peripheral edema, dizziness, and constipation, which detract from the drugs' desirable therapeutic effects. For users, for example, edema can be a source of pain and dissatisfaction and potentially dissuade patients from adhering to their treatment plan. Clinically, as is the case with patients such as MB, with high blood pressure and elevated lipids, these side effects need specific consideration while planning treatment, as per clinical guidelines (Abela et al., 2006; Schembri et al., 2018). Surveillance and upkeep of such effects become essential in a bid to achieve maximum patient compliance and achieve desirable cardiovascular well-being, hence the need for personalized care in cardiovascular drug therapy (Figure 12.21).

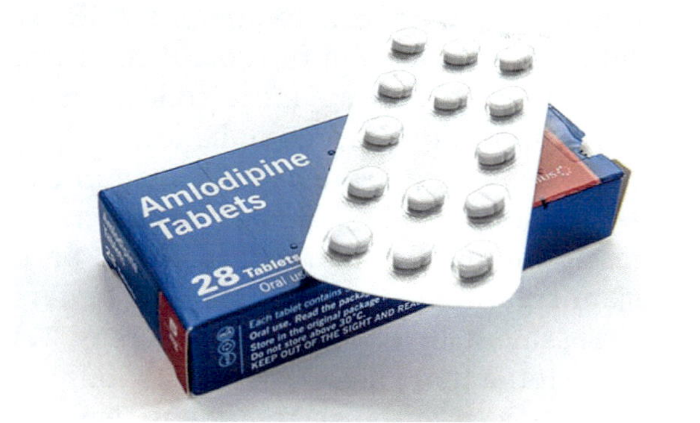

Figure 12.21. Calcium channel blockers (CCBs) are widely prescribed for managing hypertension and other cardiovascular conditions due to their efficacy in dilating blood vessels and reducing heart workload.

Source: https://www.bhf.org.uk/-/media/images/information-support/heart-matters/2018/august-2018/medical/calcium_channel_blockers_ssnoexp-620x400.jpg?rev=40de3fb0a5e04b48ac4840bc7c6f3064&la=en&h=400&w=620&hash=BE9DDCCF96E9A531C7381B4A34090B50.

Test Your Knowledge

1. What are the potential risks of long-term beta-blocker therapy?
2. Describe the bleeding risks associated with anticoagulant therapy.

Summary

Cardiovascular pharmacotherapy continues to evolve, emphasizing the need for research and clinical evaluation to ensure efficacy and safety. The analysis of dipeptidyl peptidase-4 inhibitors, such as vildagliptin, shows that, while they do not significantly impact left ventricular ejection fraction, they do result in left ventricular volume alteration, which poses questions regarding long-term clinical relevance (Bolli et al., 2017). Moreover, improvement in LDL-apheresis highlights the importance of multifaceted management and the establishment of updated guidelines based on current scientific evidence, reflecting changing patterns of cardiovascular treatment (Stefanutti et al., 2016). While clinicians grapple with the complexity of cardiovascular disease management, these findings highlight the necessity for tailored therapeutic interventions that consider patient-related factors and novel data to obtain maximal health outcomes in diverse groups. Therefore, ongoing innovation in cardiovascular drug therapy is still needed to improve patient care further.

When considering the changing environment of cardiovascular drug therapy, several noted points stand out that indicate the sophistication and imperatives of individualized treatment approaches. Advances of late underscore the transformative role of stem cells in treating heart pathology, with particular attention devoted to identifying viable sources and developing efficient mechanisms for myocardial regeneration. Some progenitor cells can restore damaged cardiomyocytes and enhance endothelium function, necessitating rigorous clinical trials to verify their efficacy (Kyryk, 2024). Moreover, pharmacogenetic factors play a vital role in individualization of treatment for ACS; the CYP2C19 gene polymorphisms have a determining effect on the reactions of patients to clopidogrel, leading to varied risks of hemorrhagic and thrombotic complications (Turaev et al., 2024). This identifies the necessity of tailoring cardiovascular drug regimens to individualized genetic profiles so as to ensure optimal therapeutic benefits and minimize adverse effects, and thus ensure optimal patient management in this critical field.

KEY TERMS FROM THIS CHAPTER

- Adolescents
- Antihypertensive agents
- Antihypertensive therapy
- Antiretroviral therapy
- Atherosclerosis
- Atrial fibrillation
- Beta-blockers
- Blood pressure
- Calcium channel blockers
- Cardiovascular pathology
- Cholesterol levels
- Cushing's syndrome
- Deep vein thrombosis (DVT)
- Diabetes
- Diuretics
- Hyperlipidemia
- Platelet aggregation
- Pulmonary embolism

Critical Thinking Questions

1. **Which of the following is a beta-blocker used in the treatment of hypertension and angina?**
   a. Enalapril
   b. Amlodipine
   c. Metoprolol
   d. Furosemide
2. **ACE inhibitors lower blood pressure primarily by:**
   a. Blocking calcium channels
   b. Promoting sodium reabsorption
   c. Inhibiting the conversion of angiotensin I to angiotensin II
   d. Increasing heart rate
3. **Which of the following drugs is a loop diuretic commonly used in heart failure?**
   a. Spironolactone
   b. Hydrochlorothiazide
   c. Furosemide
   d. Atenolol
4. **Nitrates relieve angina by:**
   a. Increasing myocardial oxygen demand
   b. Reducing heart rate
   c. Dilating coronary arteries and reducing preload
   d. Increasing blood volume
5. **Which of the following anticoagulants acts as a vitamin K antagonist?**
   a. Heparin
   b. Warfarin
   c. Dabigatran
   d. Rivaroxaban

Answers to Critical Thinking Questions

1. (c); 2. (c); 3. (c); 4. (c); 5. (b).

Short Answer Questions

1. What are the main classes of drugs used to treat hypertension?
2. How do antianginal drugs differ from antiarrhythmic medications?
3. How do beta-blockers reduce blood pressure and heart rate?
4. What is the mechanism of action of ACE inhibitors in managing hypertension and heart failure?
5. In which clinical conditions are nitrates most commonly used?
6. What is the role of diuretics in the treatment of heart failure?
7. What are the common side effects associated with ACE inhibitors?
8. Why must potassium levels be monitored when using loop or potassium-sparing diuretics?

References

1. Abela, J. C. (2006). *A Case of Hypertension*. https://core.ac.uk/download/46602086.pdf (accessed on 10th June 2025).
2. Hsu, J. J., Nsair, A., Aboulhosn, J. A., Horwich, T. B., Dave, R. H., Shannon, K. M., Boyle, N. G., Shivkumar, K., & Bradfield, J. S. (2019). Monomorphic ventricular arrhythmias in athletes. *Arrhythmia & Electrophysiology Review*, *8*(2), 83–89. https://doi.org/10.15420/aer.2019.19.3Acharya, T., & Deedwania, P. (2015). *An Evidence-Based Review of Edoxaban and Its Role in Stroke Prevention in Patients with Nonvalvular Atrial Fibrillation*. https://core.ac.uk/download/323310727.pdf (accessed on 10th June 2025).
3. Adashek, J., Ben-Zur, U. M., Nagar, M., Pietras, R., et al. (2017). *Incomplete Resolution of Deep Vein Thromboses During Rivaroxaban Therapy*. https://core.ac.uk/download/323077317.pdf (accessed on 10th June 2025).
4. Adhikari, P., Padmaja, U., & Pereira, P. (2009). *A Prospective Analysis of Adverse Drug Reactions in A South Indian Hospital*. https://core.ac.uk/download/pdf/87416.pdf (accessed on 10th June 2025).
5. Agabiti-Rosei, E., Cruickshank, J. K., Dominiczak, A., Erdine, S., et al. (2016). *2016 European Society of Hypertension Guidelines for The Management of High Blood Pressure in Children and Adolescents*. https://core.ac.uk/download/46165193.pdf (accessed on 10th June 2025).
6. Agarwal, R., Georgianos, P. I., Liakopoulos, V., Vaios, M., et al. (2019). *Assessment and Management of Hypertension Among Patients on Peritoneal Dialysis*. https://core.ac.uk/download/299809072.pdf (accessed on 10th June 2025).
7. Aggarwal, M., Brozovich, F. V., Degen, C. V., Gao, Y., et al. (2016). *Mechanisms of Vascular Smooth Muscle Contraction and The Basis for Pharmacologic Treatment of Smooth Muscle Disorders*. https://core.ac.uk/download/215937177.pdf (accessed on 10th June 2025).
8. Agius, R. (2014). *An Update on Pharmacotherapy for Type 2 Diabetes*. https://core.ac.uk/download/46602517.pdf (accessed on 10th June 2025).
9. Akhtar, Z., Farag, M., Gorog, D. A., Spinthakis, N., et al. (2020). *Is There a Role for Oral Triple Therapy in Patients with Acute Coronary Syndromes Without Atrial Fibrillation?* https://core.ac.uk/download/287582440.pdf (accessed on 10th June 2025).
10. Alacqua, M., Ambrosioni, E., Borghi, C., Brignoli, O., Caputi, A. P., Cricelli, C., Filippi, A., et al. (2009). *Adherence to Antihypertensive Medications and Cardiovascular Morbidity Among Newly Diagnosed Hypertensive Patients*. https://core.ac.uk/download/pdf/55068457.pdf (accessed on 10th June 2025).
11. Alzubi, A. S., Beshr, M. S., Abdelwahed, A., Abuajamieh, M., Elmesherghi, A. F., Ekreer, M., Alawi, Z. S. J., et al. (2024). Abstract 4144646: Assessing the impact of remote consultation strategies on optimizing guideline-directed medical therapy in heart failure patients: A meta-analysis. *Circulation*. https://www.semanticscholar.org/paper/f77ebe1e428fa3dd8c6603da943f74a14fafc763 (accessed on 10th June 2025).
12. Ambrosy, A. P., Antohi, E. L., Butler, J., Chioncel, O., et al. (2018). *Improving Post Discharge Outcomes in Acute Heart Failure*. https://core.ac.uk/download/228066233.pdf (accessed on 10th June 2025).
13. Ameer, B., & Weintraub, M. (2018). *Pediatric Obesity: Influence On Drug Dosing and Therapeutics*.

https://core.ac.uk/download/155271623.pdf (accessed on 10th June 2025).

14. Anni, A., Labado, R. O., Perwitasari, D. A., Udu, R. I., et al. (2009). *Safety Evaluation of Statin in Yogyakarta, Indonesia*. https://core.ac.uk/download/11820694.pdf (accessed on 10th June 2025).

15. Araujo, N. C. P., Marreiros, C., Simes, D., Viegas, I., et al. (2020). *Vitamin K as a Diet Supplement with Impact in Human Health: Current Evidence in Age-Related Diseases*. https://core.ac.uk/download/288958659.pdf (accessed on 10th June 2025).

16. Bahler, C. D., Goggins, W. C., Sharfuddin, A. A., Shumate, M. S., et al. (2016). *Native Nephrectomy with Renal Transplantation Decreases Hypertension Medication Requirements in Autosomal Dominant Polycystic Kidney Disease*. https://core.ac.uk/download/46964333.pdf (accessed on 10th June 2025).

17. Baker, A. H., Bradshaw, A. C., & Deng, L. (2016). *Role of Noncoding RNA in Vascular Remodeling*. https://core.ac.uk/download/46558277.pdf (accessed on 10th June 2025).

18. Banerjee, D., Winocour, P., Chowdhury, T., De, P., Wahba, M., Montero, R., Fogarty, D., et al. (2022). Management of hypertension and renin-angiotensin-aldosterone system blockade in adults with diabetic kidney disease: Association of British Clinical Diabetologists and the Renal Association UK guideline update 2021. *BMC Nephrology, 23*. https://www.semanticscholar.org/paper/6ae17910eef88141a71a3e6aaea42687dd418cc9 (accessed on 10th June 2025).

19. Barbot, M., Ceccato, F., & Scaroni, C. (2019). *The Pathophysiology and Treatment of Hypertension in Patients with Cushing's Syndrome*. https://core.ac.uk/download/211056096.pdf (accessed on 10th June 2025).

20. Barrese, V., Femminella, G. D., Ferrara, N., Rengo, G., et al. (2014). Tailoring therapy for heart failure: The pharmacogenomics of adrenergic receptor signaling. https://core.ac.uk/download/29469447.pdf (accessed on 10th June 2025).

21. Bassand, J. P., Camm, A. J., Dabrowski, E., Fitzmaurice, D. A., et al. (2020). Outcomes associated with oral anticoagulants plus antiplatelets in patients with newly diagnosed atrial fibrillation. https://core.ac.uk/download/287649753.pdf (accessed on 10th June 2025).

22. Beck, K. M., Liao, W., & Yang, E. J. (2018). Secukinumab in the treatment of psoriasis: Patient selection and perspectives. https://core.ac.uk/download/323063113.pdf (accessed on 10th June 2025).

23. Belch, J., Boc, V., et al. (2019). ESVM guideline on peripheral arterial disease. https://core.ac.uk/download/286715349.pdf (accessed on 10th June 2025).

24. Besekar, S., Jogdand, S., Patel, S. S., Shinde, R., & Kumar, S. (2025). Therapeutic evaluation of antidiabetic and antihypertensive therapy versus antidiabetic, antihypertensive and statins therapy in the management of type 2 diabetes mellitus patients with hypertension: A pragmatic clinical trial. *Journal of Clinical and Diagnostic Research*. https://www.semanticscholar.org/paper/325e70c5666cccc02bc0486c934ce63afa7e215a (accessed on 10th June 2025).

25. Bijlsma, M. J., Hak, E., Janssen, F., Vansteelandt, S., et al. (2016). The effect of adherence to statin therapy on cardiovascular mortality: Quantification of unmeasured bias using falsification endpoints. https://core.ac.uk/download/84046383.pdf (accessed on 10th June 2025).

26. Boal, A. H., Dominiczak, A. F., McCallum, L., Muir, S., et al. (2016). Monotherapy with major antihypertensive drug classes and risk of hospital admissions for mood disorders. https://core.ac.uk/download/46559113.pdf (accessed on 10th June 2025).

27. Bolger, A. F., Deeks, S. G., Glidden, D., Hsue, P., et al. (2015). Mitral annular and coronary artery calcification are associated with mortality in HIV-infected individuals. https://core.ac.uk/download/323074779.pdf (accessed on 10th June 2025).

28. Bolli, G. B., Kothny, W., Kozlovski, P., Krum, H., et al. (2017). Effects of vildagliptin on ventricular function in patients with type 2 diabetes mellitus and heart failure: A randomized placebo-controlled trial. https://core.ac.uk/download/96883576.pdf (accessed on 10th June 2025).

29. Borghi, C., Grassi, G., Agabiti-Rosei, E., Savoia, C., et al. (2017). Personalized medicine: A modern approach for the diagnosis and management of hypertension. https://core.ac.uk/download/96884785.pdf (accessed on 10th June 2025).

30. Borro, M., Di Sanzo, M., Fineschi, V., Frati, P., et al. (2017). Clinical applications of personalized medicine: A new paradigm and challenge. https://core.ac.uk/download/80315182.pdf (accessed on 10th June 2025).

31. Braga, O. G. (2018). Antipsychotic drug use: Managing cardiometabolic and cost effects. https://core.ac.uk/download/212899184.pdf (accessed on 10th June 2025).

32. Bulluck, H., Kwok, C. S., Loke, Y. K., Ryding, A. D., et al. (2014). Safety of short-term dual antiplatelet therapy after drug-eluting stents: An updated meta-analysis. https://core.ac.uk/download/41991335.pdf (accessed on 10th June 2025).

33. Busse, O., Diener, H. C., Glahn, J., Hamann, G. F., et al. (2003). Adherence to secondary stroke prevention strategies: Results from the German stroke data bank. https://core.ac.uk/download/16432868.pdf (accessed on 10th June 2025).

34. Calkins, H., Cleland, J. G. F., Heist, E. K., Kowey, P., et al. (2017). The burden of proof: The current state of atrial fibrillation prevention and treatment trials. https://core.ac.uk/download/80696856.pdf (accessed on 10th June 2025).

35. Cameron, A. C., Dobbin, S. J. H., Jones, R. J., Lang, N. N., et al. (2018). Toxicity of cancer therapy: What the cardiologist needs to know about angiogenesis inhibitors. https://core.ac.uk/download/161514882.pdf (accessed on 10th June 2025).

36. Cameron, A. C., Lang, N. N., & Touyz, R. M. (2016). Drug treatment of hypertension: Focus on vascular health. https://core.ac.uk/download/46559725.pdf (accessed on 10th June 2025).

37. Chandy, M., Paik, D. T., & Wu, J. C. (2020). Patient and disease-specific induced pluripotent stem cells for discovery of personalized cardiovascular drugs and therapeutics. https://core.ac.uk/download/323062894.pdf (accessed on 10th June 2025).

38. Charalampopoulos, A., Connolly, S. B., Davies, R. J., Gibbs, S., et al. (2014). Response to pulmonary arterial hypertension drug therapies in patients with PAH and cardiovascular risk factors. https://core.ac.uk/download/76996385.pdf (accessed on 10th June 2025).

39. Chitra, B. (2017). Study on drug utilization pattern of diuretics at a tertiary care teaching hospital. https://core.ac.uk/download/235666163.pdf (accessed on 10th June 2025).

40. Cho, J., Hripcsak, G., Jung, S., Lee, D., et al. (2020). Comparison of first-line dual combination treatments in hypertension: Real-world evidence from multinational heterogeneous cohorts. https://core.ac.uk/download/323077278.pdf (accessed on 10th June 2025).

41. Claggett, B., Desai, A. S., Lefkowitz, M., McMurray, J. J. V., et al. (2016). Efficacy of sacubitril/valsartan vs. enalapril at lower than target doses in heart failure with reduced ejection fraction: The PARADIGM-HF trial. https://core.ac.uk/download/323073560.pdf (accessed on 10th June 2025).

42. Dans, A. L., Guyatt, G. H., Hood, W. B., et al. (2014). Digitalis for treatment of heart failure in patients in sinus rhythm. https://core.ac.uk/download/20480211.pdf (accessed on 10th June 2025).

43. Dayspring, T. D., Phan, B. A. P., & Toth, P. P. (2012). *Ezetimibe Therapy: Mechanism of Action and Clinical Update*. https://core.ac.uk/download/323069011.pdf (accessed on 10th June 2025).

44. De Bruyne, P., & Vande Walle, J. (2014). *Management of Hypertension in Children and Adolescents*. https://core.ac.uk/download/55853879.pdf (accessed on 10th June 2025).

45. de Graaf, A. A., Groen, A. K., & van Stee, M. F. (2018). *Actions of Metformin and Statins on Lipid and Glucose Metabolism and Possible Benefit of Combination Therapy*. https://core.ac.uk/download/519006314.pdf (accessed on 10th June 2025).

46. De Silva, R., & Giavarini, A. (2016). *The Role of Ivabradine in The Management of Angina Pectoris*. https://core.ac.uk/download/77017505.pdf (accessed on 10th June 2025).

47. Dockrill, S. J., Gorog, D., & Vimalesvaran, K. (2018). *Role of Rivaroxaban in The Management of Atrial Fibrillation: Insights from Clinical Practice*. https://core.ac.uk/download/287581671.pdf (accessed on 10th June 2025).

48. Einsle, F., Klotsche, J., Labeit, A. M., & Lehnert, H. et al. (2012). *Changes in the Prevalence, Treatment and Control of Hypertension in Germany: A Clinical-Epidemiological Study of 50,000 Primary Care Patients*. https://core.ac.uk/download/14528086.pdf (accessed on 10th June 2025).

49. Farag, M., Hirsh, J., Ibanez, B., Mega, J. L., Park, K. W., Suh, J. W., & Valgimigli, M. (2018). *More, More, more: Reducing Thrombosis in Acute Coronary Syndromes Beyond Dual Antiplatelet Therapy—Current Data and Future Directions*. https://core.ac.uk/download/287581674.pdf (accessed on 10th June 2025).

50. Farrugia, C. (1999). *The Antiplatelet Activity of Aspirin*. https://core.ac.uk/download/46604499.pdf (accessed on 10th June 2025).

51. Ferlini Agne, G. (2018). *Orally Administered Torsemide in Horses: Pharmacokinetic and Pharmacodynamic Studies*. https://core.ac.uk/download/650416154.pdf (accessed on 10th June 2025).

52. Fladmo, E. (2019). *Embolus Prevention: Anticoagulant Therapy in Comparison to Watchman's Procedure in Patients with Atrial Fibrillation*. https://core.ac.uk/download/524633922.pdf (accessed on 10th June 2025).

53. Freeman, D., Huda, S., Jarvie, E., & McKenna, S., et al. (2013). *How to Assess and Manage Hypertension During and After Pregnancy*. https://core.ac.uk/download/19888252.pdf (accessed on 10th June 2025).

54. Gallo, G., Tocci, G., & Volpe, M. (2018). *Is Early and Fast Blood Pressure Control Important in Hypertension Management?* https://core.ac.uk/download/153366055.pdf (accessed on 10th June 2025).

55. Gąsior, M., Kułaczkowska, Z. M., Rokicka, D., & Strojek, K. et al. (2021). *Metformin in Patients with Type 2 Diabetes Mellitus and Heart Failure: A Review*. https://core.ac.uk/download/427160022.pdf (accessed on 10th June 2025).

56. Gast, A., Michelson, A. D., Labarthe, B., Shen, B., Patrono, C., Ammollo, C. T., Capodanno, D., et al. (2018). *Potentiation of Thrombus Instability: A Contributory Mechanism to The Effectiveness*

of Antithrombotic Medications. https://core.ac.uk/download/287581673.pdf (accessed on 10th June 2025).

57. Gorog, D. A., Gue, Y. X., Kanji, R., & Srinivasan, M., et al. (2019). *Rationale and Design of "Can Very Low Dose Rivaroxaban (VLDR) in Addition to Dual Antiplatelet Therapy Improve Thrombotic Status in Acute Coronary Syndrome (VaLiDate-R)" Study*. https://core.ac.uk/download/287582404.pdf (accessed on 10th June 2025).

58. Januzzi, J. L., Petrie, M. C., Sattar, N., Zinman, B., et al. (2017). *Novel Diabetes Drugs and The Cardiovascular Specialist*. https://core.ac.uk/download/82893969.pdf (accessed on 10th June 2025).

59. Joshi, J., Rubart, M., & Zhu, W. (2020). *Optogenetics: Background, Methodological Advances and Potential Applications for Cardiovascular Research and Medicine*. https://core.ac.uk/download/299809076.pdf (accessed on 10th June 2025).

60. Kiranjit, & Singh, P. (2018). *A Prospective Study to Analyze the Side Effects of Olmesartan Medoxomil and Enalapril in Hypertensive Subjects*. https://core.ac.uk/download/477854280.pdf (accessed on 10th June 2025).

61. Kitsiou, A., Caforio, A. L. P., Porta-Sanchez, A., Vahanian, A., Iung, B., Carrera, C., Szymanski, C., et al. (2013). *ESC Core Curriculum for The General Cardiologist (2013)*. https://core.ac.uk/download/55756305.pdf (accessed on 10th June 2025).

62. Kuntić, M., Junglas, T., Kuntić, I., Oelze, M., Strohm, L., Ubbens, H., Zheng, J., et al. (2024). Mitigation of PM2.5-induced cardiovascular damage by statins and ACE inhibitors. *RedoXplore*. https://www.semanticscholar.org/paper/98edd374c52026adb21a301dd3bb7ae4397956c4 (accessed on 10th June 2025).

63. Kyryk, V. (2024). Stem cell therapy for cardiac regeneration: Key points. *Cell and Organ Transplantology*. https://www.semanticscholar.org/paper/6a1b536f3691ad0d162e4187a4a2e2ffd1507b5f (accessed on 10th June 2025).

64. Li, J., Zhang, L., Ge, T., Liu, J., Wang, C., & Yu, Q. (2024). Understanding sorafenib-induced cardiovascular toxicity: Mechanisms and treatment implications. *Drug Design, Development and Therapy, 18*, 829–843. https://www.semanticscholar.org/paper/2bf33ebd969e9461b5e71d74b1aede8eeb5debee (accessed on 10th June 2025).

65. Manjappa Mahadevappa, Hussain, S., Dharwadkhar, S., & Madapat, K. J. (2024). Lipid-lowering therapy–associated erectile dysfunction and testicular pain: A rare case report. *Hospital Pharmacy, 60*, 215–220. https://www.semanticscholar.org/paper/50b68cf885048cf60d634f8398e588c03d5bcd75 (accessed on 10th June 2025).

66. Manning, L. S., Potter, J. F., Robinson, T. G., Rothwell, P. M., et al. (2015). Prognostic significance of short-term blood pressure variability in acute stroke. https://core.ac.uk/download/41990664.pdf (accessed on 10th June 2025).

67. Marsh, A., Singer, D. R. J., Taylor, P. C., Watkins, P. B., et al. (2010). Personalized medicine: The impact on chemistry. https://core.ac.uk/download/45676.pdf (accessed on 10th June 2025).

68. Mehrotra, K. (2025). Nanoparticles in renal hypertension therapy: Advances, mechanisms, and future perspectives. *International Journal for Research in Applied Science and Engineering Technology*. https://www.semanticscholar.org/paper/91e2717dc9956066a029d3d2829738c2b1a0f549 (accessed on 10th June 2025).

69. Mitkova, Z., Dimova, A., Petrova, G., & Dimitrova, M. (2024). Adverse drug reactions of cardiovascular classes of medicines—Data for Bulgarian population. *Biomedicines, 12*. https://www.semanticscholar.org/paper/14b195b690d1a233f7985d4211ff83307700e515 (accessed on 10th June 2025).

70. Montano, M., Landay, A., Perkins, M., Holstad, M., Pallikkuth, S., & Pahwa, S. (2022). HIV and aging in the era of ART and COVID-19: Symposium overview. *Journal of Acquired Immune Deficiency Syndromes (1999), 89*(Suppl 1), S3–S9. https://www.semanticscholar.org/paper/fe892dc8c1f6190a9dbcabd6f44e8e2a0aeacf57 (accessed on 10th June 2025).

71. Muccini, C., Bottanelli, M., Castagna, A., & Spagnuolo, V. (2024). Cardiometabolic complications in children and adolescents with HIV on antiretroviral therapy. *Expert Opinion on Drug Metabolism & Toxicology, 20*, 893–905. https://www.semanticscholar.org/paper/4b1b7577c815056caa25f4aa2ebd6b8c0a089483 (accessed on 10th June 2025).

72. Ogura, T., & Shiraishi, C. (2025). Comparison of adverse events among angiotensin receptor blockers in hypertension using the United States Food and Drug Administration Adverse Event Reporting System. *Cureus, 17*. https://www.semanticscholar.org/paper/62d65abdf6954cf1695b324e6e5558d8cfd8f256 (accessed on 10th June 2025).

73. Pichandi, S., Pasupathi, P., Rao, Y. Y., Farook, J., Ambika, A., Ponnusha, B. S., Subramaniyam, S., et al. (2011). The role of statin drugs in combating cardiovascular diseases: A review. https://core.ac.uk/download/pdf/14696.pdf (accessed on 10th June 2025).

74. Poldermans, D., Bax, J. J., Boersma, E., De Hert, S., Eeckhout, E., Fowkes, G., Gorenek, B., et al. (2009). *Guidelines for Pre-Operative Cardiac Risk Assessment and Perioperative Cardiac Management in Non-Cardiac Surgery: The Task Force of the ESC and ESA*. https://core.ac.uk/download/55798032.pdf (accessed on 10th June 2025).

75. Preiss, D., Rankin, N. J., Sattar, N., Welsh, P., et al. (2016). Applying metabolomics to cardiometabolic intervention studies and trials: Past experiences and a roadmap for the future. https://core.ac.uk/download/46567783.pdf (accessed on 10th June 2025).

76. Protasov, K. V., Eniseeva, E. S., & Plotnikova, Y. K. (2024). Myocardial infarction in patients with HIV infection: Incidence, risk factors, pathogenesis, clinical performance and treatment. *Russian Journal of Cardiology*. https://www.semanticscholar.org/paper/664dec4a34b9788d945d3c62f3ed05c0ad6d5e56 (accessed on 10th June 2025).

77. Rebrova, E., & Shikh, E. V. (2024). *The Effect of Genetic Polymorphism of Genes Encoding the Target of Action on The Variability of The Response to Antihypertensive Therapy*. Clinical Pharmacology and Therapy. https://www.semanticscholar.org/paper/ad8d07920be3a9941963ed32c680592cdeb3e81c (accessed on 10th June 2025).

78. Sada, L., Savoia, C., & Volpe, M. (2015). Blood pressure control versus atrial fibrillation management in stroke prevention. https://core.ac.uk/download/54519414.pdf (accessed on 10th June 2025).

79. Schembri, K. (2018). Management of hypertension in primary care. https://core.ac.uk/download/286457814.pdf (accessed on 10th June 2025).

80. Sobhy, M., Eletriby, A., Ragy, H., Kandil, H., Saleh, M., Farag, N., Guindy, R., et al. (2024). ACE inhibitors and angiotensin receptor blockers for the primary and secondary prevention of cardiovascular outcomes: Recommendations from the 2024 Egyptian Cardiology Expert Consensus in collaboration with the CVREP Foundation. *Cardiology and Therapy, 13*, 707–

736. https://www.semanticscholar.org/paper/30b3dbbdb4da5b6fd4fcdecb4c00ed4d186d0ffc (accessed on 10th June 2025).

81. Stefanutti, C. (2016). The 1st and 2nd Italian Consensus Conferences on low-density lipoprotein apheresis: A practical synopsis and update. https://core.ac.uk/download/98341266.pdf (accessed on 10th June 2025).

82. Stuart, B. C. (2008). How disease burden influences medication patterns for Medicare beneficiaries: Implications for policy. https://core.ac.uk/download/71352038.pdf (accessed on 10th June 2025).

83. Turaev, F. K., Abdullaev, S. P., Gafurov, F. S., Gonturyev, N. N., Tuchkova, S., Mirzaev, K., & Sychev, D. A. (2024). *Patients' Pharmacogenetic Characteristics and The Risk of Cardiovascular Events to Antiplatelet Therapy with Clopidogrel: Case reports. Therapist's Bulletin*. https://www.semanticscholar.org/paper/341e1d85808fea3c7442d83491b2c8349571b9cf (accessed on 10th June 2025).

84. Whetstine, L. M. (2015). Cognitive enhancement: Treating or cheating? https://core.ac.uk/download/231877482.pdf (accessed on 10th June 2025).

85. Zeng, W., Wang, T., Stürmer, T., He, N., Shen, P., Lin, H., Guan, X., et al. (2025). Comparative effectiveness of angiotensin-converting enzyme inhibitors and angiotensin II receptor blockers on cardiovascular outcomes in older adults with type 2 diabetes mellitus: A target trial emulation study. *Cardiovascular Diabetology, 24*. https://www.semanticscholar.org/paper/3c45c52ce145bcd8be371955dddf4f6a970ce0e0 (accessed on 10th June 2025).

CNS DRUG THERAPY

13

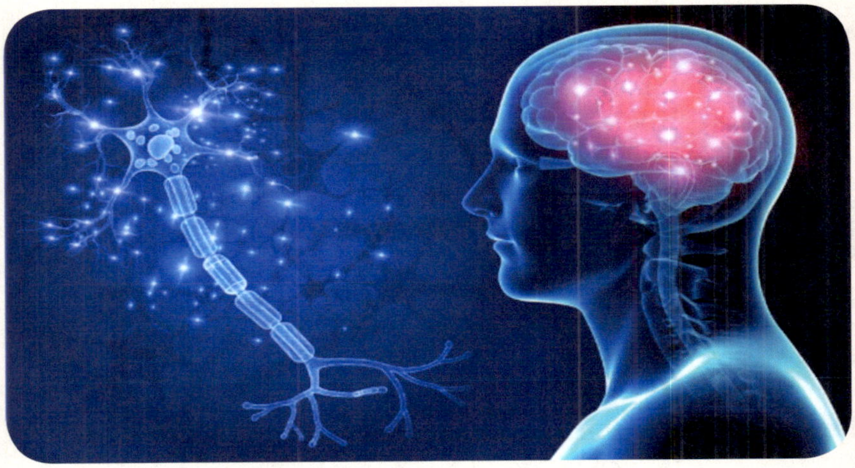

LEARNING OBJECTIVES

After studying this chapter, you will be able to:

1. Explain types of CNS drugs
2. Understand mechanisms of action
3. Discuss clinical applications

Introduction

An introduction to the subtleties of Central Nervous System (CNS) drug therapy is crucial to grasp the ongoing challenges of neuro disorder therapy. The complex structure of the blood-brain barrier (BBB) highly restricts drug passage, necessitating novel strategies to deliver therapeutic action. As highlighted in recent reviews, invasive and non-invasive strategies have emerged to breach such barriers. Notably, research into the properties of nasal mucosa for drug delivery is promising, but it is still in experimental stages (Carafa et al., 2017). Recent symposia such as the HIV Cure and Reservoir Symposium also indicate the intersection between pharmacology and immunology, with emphasis on advances in therapy that not only aim for viral eradication but also consider the unique CNS compartments where reservoirs exist (Cole et al., 2018). Thus, an overview provides the foundation for a detailed discussion of CNS drug therapy, illuminating both technological advances and enduring clinical issues in this critical field (Figure 13.1).

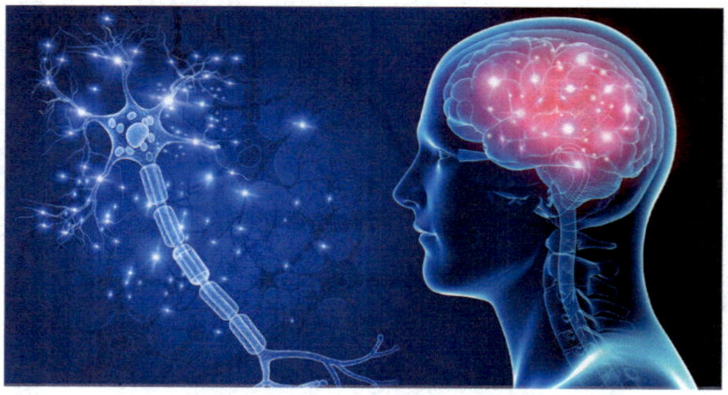

Figure 13.1. Central nervous system (CNS) drug therapy.

Source: https://www.mdanderson.org/images/publications/cancerwise/Graphics/CNS%20lymphoma.png.

13.1. Types of CNS Drugs

Learning Outcome

1. Understand antidepressants and their mechanisms
2. Explain antipsychotics and their classifications
3. Learn anxiolytics and their therapeutic uses
4. Focus on mood stabilizers and their role in treatment
5. Discuss stimulants for attention disorders
6. Know antiepileptic drugs and seizure management
7. Discuss neuroprotective agents and their significance
8. Describe opioids and their impact on CNS pain management
9. Identify emerging CNS drug classes

Medications in the CNS are mainly involved in the treatment of many neurological and psychiatric illnesses. They can be grouped into many broad categories based on their mechanisms and therapeutic applications. Most prominent among these are the anticonvulsants, which are mainly employed to treat seizure disorders, and the antidepressants, which are designed to treat the symptoms of depression and anxiety. In addition, antipsychotics form the basis of the management of conditions such as schizophrenia by targeting neurotransmitter mechanisms to restore equilibrium in brain processes. It is crucial to note that the effects of the drugs will vary significantly depending on genetic, biological, and environmental factors that affect the drug's metabolism and efficacy. Recent evidence emphasizes the role of individualized medicine approaches in CNS drug treatment, as exemplified by research on genetic markers in acute lymphoblastic leukemia (ALL) that may influence treatment decisions (Shertzer et al., 2020). Further, research into HIV latency has also suggested the significance of CNS reservoir knowledge and the potential for site-specific therapeutic targeting that might enhance CNS drug efficacy (Alvarez-Carbonell et al., 2017).

13.1.1. Antidepressants and Their Mechanisms

The mechanisms through which antidepressants influence the CNS are multifaceted and most vital in explaining their role in therapeutic therapy. Mainly, the drugs are aimed at altering neurotransmitter levels, predominantly serotonin, norepinephrine, and dopamine, improving mood and relieving depressive symptoms. Selective serotonin reuptake inhibitors (SSRIs), for instance, enhance serotonergic activity through inhibition of its reuptake, thereby increasing synaptic content. Furthermore, the neurogenic hypothesis suggests that antidepressants can induce neurogenesis in the hippocampus, thereby resulting in long-term mood stabilization. This mechanism is particularly relevant in the case of such conditions with chronic pain where antidepressants can be employed for modulating pain circuits and achieving optimal overall pain control regimens (Cruccu et al., 2018). Along with the improvement of the understanding of these mechanisms, additional research is required to establish the optimal combinations of treatments and dosages to be applied to the individual patient, especially as some antidepressants have side effects (Coluzzi et al., 2015) (Figure 13.2).

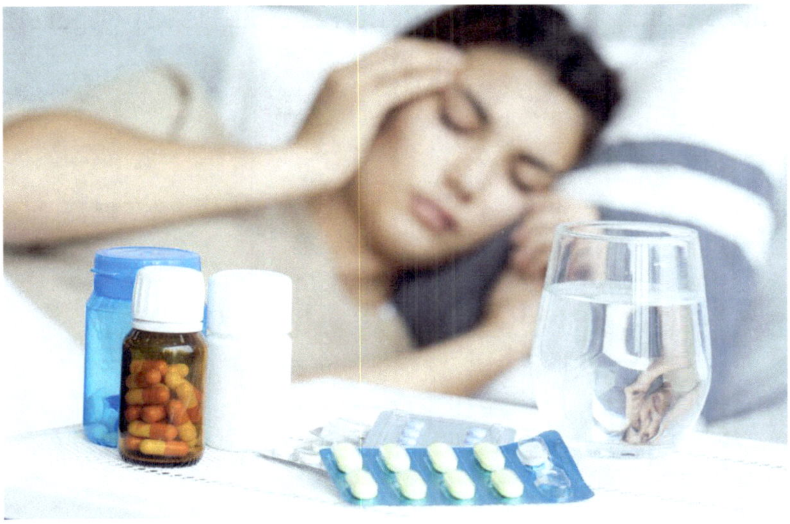

Figure 13.2. Antidepressants.

Source: https://cdn-prod.medicalnewstoday.com/content/images/articles/314/314790/sleeping-pills.jpg.

13.1.2. Antipsychotics and Their Classifications

The antipsychotic typology is crucial in the treatment of a variety of mental illnesses, such as schizophrenia and bipolar disorder (BD). Antipsychotics can be divided mainly into two groups: typical and atypical drugs. Typical antipsychotics, predominantly phenothiazines, have been employed since the 1950s and are widely known for their capability to control positive symptoms of schizophrenia, such as delusions and hallucinations, through blockade of the D2 receptor (Anderson et al., 2022). On the contrary, atypical antipsychotics possess a broader therapeutic effect by both targeting the positive and negative symptoms and also influencing serotonergic activity. New advances in immune psychiatry suggest that the immune system involvement in psychotic disorders will provide new pathways to more targeted treatment approaches, hinting towards the detection of biosignatures for early intervention (Pandarakalam et al., 2022). This two-pronged approach of purifying classifications and incorporating immunological knowledge serves to promote an enhanced understanding of psychotic disorders and, ultimately, CNS drug therapy.

13.1.3. Anxiolytics and Their Therapeutic Uses

Anxiolytics are a class of CNS drugs that are central to treating anxiety disorders, which are becoming increasingly prevalent in current society. The drugs are directed at increasing the action of gamma-aminobutyric acid (GABA), the major inhibitory neurotransmitter, hence bringing about relaxation and alleviation of anxiety. For instance, research cites the action of vigabatrin, a GABA-transaminase irreversible inhibitor that significantly elevates brain concentrations of GABA and possesses anxiolytic properties in model systems (El-Hwuegi et al., 1996). Pioneering drugs, novel anxiolytics, are emerging with advantages over traditional therapies, including reduced side effects and better-dosing regimens. Pharmacists need to remain up-to-date with these advances to properly suggest newer drugs, making sure they take into consideration potential side effects and drug interactions while enabling patient care (Gutierrez et al., 1992) (Figure 13.3).

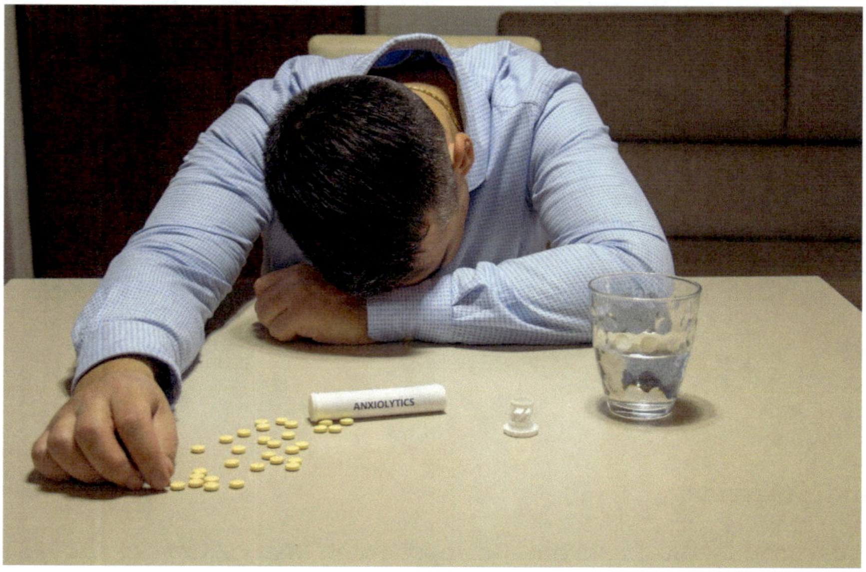

Figure 13.3. Anxiolytics.

Source: https://cdn.apollohospitals.com/health-library-prod/2022/07/shutterstock_2110621637-scaled.jpg.

13.1.4. Mood Stabilizers and Their Role in Treatment

Mood stabilizers play an role in mood disorder management, particularly in disorders such as BD, where patients fluctuate between mania and depression. Mood stabilizers allow for equilibrium of mood and minimize the occurrence of severe manic episodes and depressive states. As mood stabilizers can affect the neurobiological processes for mood regulation, efficacy is significant with certain drugs like lamotrigine. This agent has come to not only be an effective mood-stabilizing agent in the bipolar spectrum but also because of its minimal ability to induce depression relief without triggering mania, thus filling an essential gap in treatment (Prabhavalkar et al., 2015). Moreover, the interconnection between mood disorders and circadian rhythm has resulted in research on using light-based therapies and neurotrophins as adjunct treatment options, enhancing our understanding of mood regulation and developing therapeutic strategies (Iannitelli et al., 2015). All these advances demonstrate the prominence of mood stabilizers in multimodal CNS drug therapy.

13.1.5. Stimulants for Attention Disorders

The treatment of ADHD relies mainly on CNS stimulants that enhance the neurotransmission of norepinephrine and dopamine to improve attention, impulse regulation, and hyperactivity in the patient. Though commonly used are the drugs methylphenidate and amphetamines, which are stimulant drugs, their potential for abuse and dependence is still a matter of concern. In response to them, other medicines like viloxazine have been brought in. As a selective norepinephrine reuptake inhibitor, viloxazine presents a non-stimulant option with a well-documented safety profile and FDA indication for the treatment of ADHD in pediatric patients, suggesting efficacy on par with stimulant therapy (Haddad et al., 2022). Furthermore, findings indicate that pharmacologic intervention, including stimulants, reduces the likelihood of developing Alzheimer's disease in older age, offering a key, multifaceted consideration in ADHD therapy management (H-Flores et al., 2024). Hence, the search for stimulant options continues to be critical in optimizing the treatment of attention disorders (Figure 13.4).

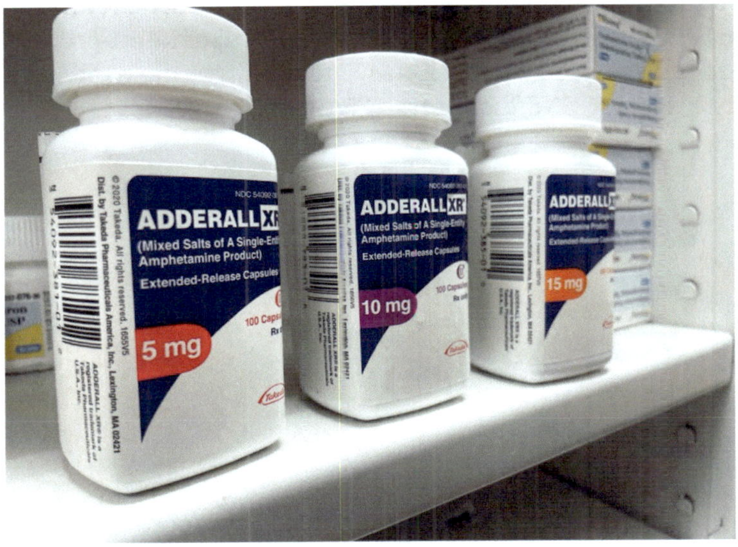

Figure 13.4. Stimulants for attention disorders.

Source: https://www.mentalhealth.com/wp-content/uploads/2025/03/Attention-Deficit-Hyperactivity-Disorder-ADHD-Stimulants.jpeg.

13.1.6. Antiepileptic Drugs and Seizure Management

Antiepileptic drugs (AEDs) form the core of seizure control, particularly in light of the complex, multifactorial nature of epilepsy as a chronic neurological disorder with spontaneous recurring seizures and frequently related to loss of consciousness (Kumari et al., 2023). Treatment has become exponentially complicated with the application of a host of both traditional and novel AEDs that exhibit distinctive mechanisms of action with distinct side effect profiles. Conventional medications, i.e., valproate and phenytoin, have opened doors to seizure therapy, but more recent therapies such as levetiracetam are more effective, particularly in drug-resistant cases (Anand et al., 2024). Besides drug therapy, complementary therapies such as herbal preparations are gaining more attention since, while needing better scientific evidence, they are becoming more accepted due to their potentially lesser side effects. This three-stranded approach emphasizes the importance of individualized treatment planning to optimize outcomes for epilepsy patients.

13.1.7. Neuroprotective Agents and Their Significance

The role of neuroprotective agents in the treatment of CNS diseases cannot be overstressed, particularly when neurodegenerative ailments such as Alzheimer's are concerned. With the zeal for effective therapies that can reverse disease progression coming at such a critical time, identification of novel compounds has gained momentum. Latest research points to the promise of natural flavonoids, which have been recognized as neuroprotective agents capable of rescuing neurons from cell damage. For instance, p-morpholinyl flavone screening proved their effectiveness in the preservation of human neuroblastoma cells from oxidative stress and amyloid beta cytotoxicity, suggesting their therapeutic use in Alzheimer's (Evans et al., 2019). Moreover, strategies in drug design enabled the production of new indole derivatives with dual cholinesterase and monoamine oxidase inhibiting properties, broadening the therapeutic path of neuroprotective pharmacotherapy (Agbaba et al., 2014). Together, these advances serve to highlight the need for novel neuroprotective approaches in the battle against CNS disorders (Figure 13.5).

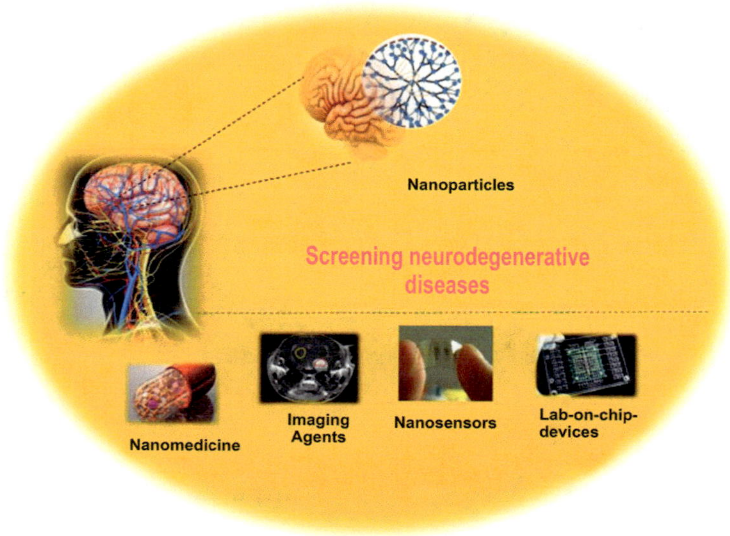

Figure 13.5. The significance of neuroprotective agents in CNS drug therapy cannot be overstated, particularly in the context of neurodegenerative diseases such as Alzheimer's.

Source: https://advance.sagepub.com/users/847771/articles/1235501/master/file/figures/image1/image1.png.

13.1.8. Opioids and Their Impact on CNS Pain Management

Opioid use for treating CNS pain is complex, reflecting their efficacy and consequent hazards. Even though morphine and other opioids are efficient in pain relief for severe pain, they are also accompanied by severe issues like their potential adverse impact on bone mineralization and increased risk of falls due to CNS-related side effects like dizziness and somnolence. According to the recent literature, prolonged intake of analgesics has been reported to lead to the occurrence of symptoms such as opioid-induced hypogonadism that has a link with osteoporosis, making monitoring among prolonged users vital (Coluzzi et al., 2015). Moreover, standard opioid therapy may not always be the best approach in postoperative pain control since the disadvantages of morphine could be better enhanced by other opioids like sufentanil. This opioid presents a good therapeutic profile with the promise of new strategies in analgesia that could lead to better patient outcomes with reduced risk (Coluzzi et al., 2016).

13.1.9. Emerging CNS Drug Classes

The advent of novel CNS drug classes is a turning point in the history of CNS drug therapy, particularly in the management of conditions such as neurodegenerative diseases and pain. New approaches employ new mechanisms of action, including neuroprotection and modulation of neuroinflammation, to target more specifically pathophysiological mechanisms. It has recently been established that retinal ganglion cells, and hence glaucoma and other CNS disorders, are of paramount importance to preserve, with pressure-independent pharmacotherapeutic interventions being an imperative (Cordeiro et al., 2021). Nanomedicine has also emerged as an innovative strategy, with plastic, targeted therapeutics that are capable of surmounting serious medical challenges while maximizing therapy performance and safety profiles (Aslund et al., 2020). With each new class of novel drugs moving to the clinic, they also have the potential to revolutionize the treatment paradigm and ultimately improve patient quality of life and outcome for CNS disorders (Figure 13.6).

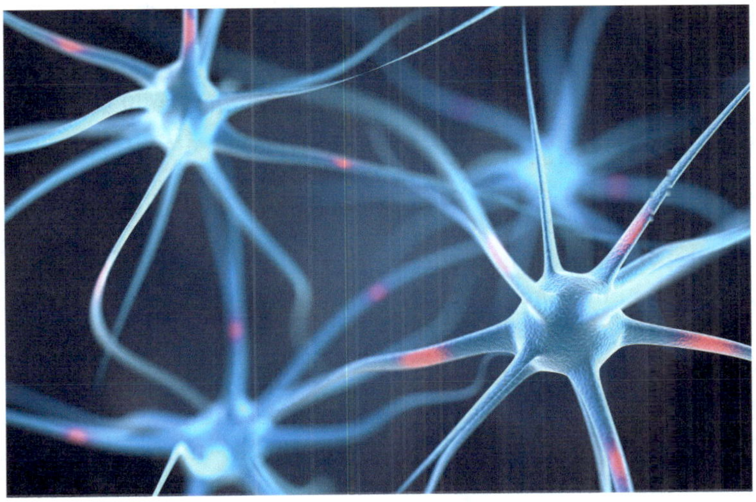

Figure 13.6. The development of emerging Central Nervous System (CNS) drug classes marks a pivotal advancement in the field of CNS drug therapy, particularly in addressing conditions such as neurodegenerative diseases and chronic pain.

Source: https://admin.americanaddictioncenters.org/wp-content/uploads/2017/03/Neurons-in-the-brain-71524651.jpg.

Test Your Knowledge

1. Which CNS drugs are commonly used for seizure management?
2. What are the key differences between SSRIs and tricyclic antidepressants?

13.2. Mechanisms of Action

Learning Outcome

1. Understand neurotransmitter systems involved in CNS therapy
2. Know receptor interactions and drug efficacy
3. Explain the pharmacokinetics of CNS drugs
4. Discuss pharmacodynamics and therapeutic outcomes
5. Define the blood-brain barrier and drug delivery
6. Identify genetic factors influencing drug response
7. Know side effects and adverse reactions
8. Describe drug interactions in CNS therapy
9. Understand innovations in drug design and delivery

The pharmacological actions of CNS medication therapies are multifaceted and often include interacting with the neurotransmitter systems, neuroinflammation pathways, and cellular responses in the brain. Examples include probiotics and their inactivated derivatives, paraprobiotics, which have been recognized as a potential therapeutic intervention, influencing gut microbiota composition, hence modulating the gut-brain axis. This interaction is believed to decrease neuropsychiatric symptoms by altering neurotransmitter levels, cytokine release, and neuronal signaling pathways, ultimately leading to improved emotional stability and mental function (Mudaliar et al., 2024). In addition, recent studies of SGLT2 inhibitors show other ways in which these agents are neuroprotective through the reduction of oxidative stress and inhibition of inflammatory processes in the CNS. By acting directly on SGLT receptors found in the brain, these drugs can effectively manage several neurological disorders such as Alzheimer's disease and ischemic stroke, thereby enhancing CNS therapy outcome (Sobczyk et al., 2024).

13.2.1. Neurotransmitter Systems involved in CNS Therapy

The interaction between multiple neurotransmitter systems is vital to the pathogenesis and efficacy of CNS drug therapies. Neurotransmitters such as dopamine, serotonin, and acetylcholine are not only integral to mood and cognition control but also to the regulation of neuroinflammatory processes occurring in numerous CNS diseases. Experimental data, for instance, suggest that these neurotransmitters have the capability of modulating immunological responses, which are progressively implicated in the pathogenesis of such diseases as Alzheimer's disease. Recent studies have shown that pharmacologically active molecules for dementia may raise the levels of neurotransmitters, possibly having a modulatory effect on inflammation and neurodegeneration (Giubilei et al., 2016). Additionally, the therapeutic action of cannabinoids in CNS pharmacotherapy is evidence of the dynamics of neurotransmitter interactions, particularly the way in which non-Δ9-tetrahydrocannabinol Phyto cannabinoids can use the endocannabinoid systems' therapeutic potential, marking a significant change in treatment paradigms (Adams et al., 2011). Such developments emphasize the paramount importance of neurotransmitter systems for fostering effective CNS treatments (Figure 13.7).

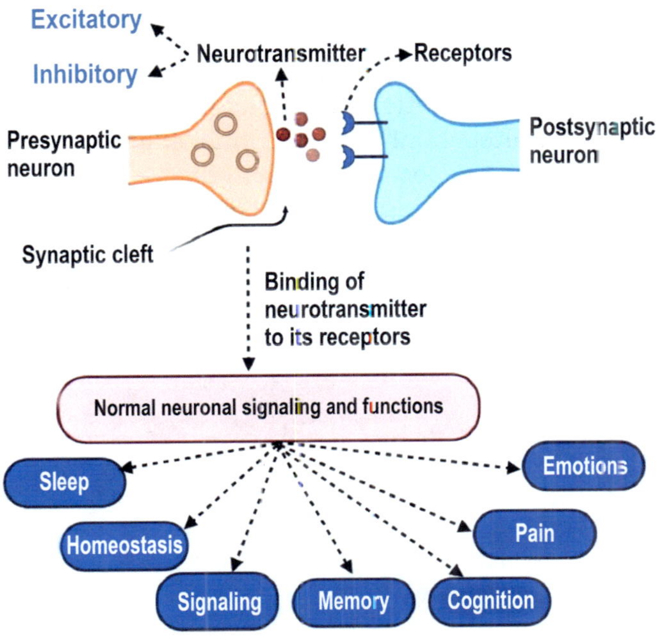

Figure 13.7. Neurotransmitters such as dopamine, serotonin, and acetylcholine are not only fundamental in regulating mood and cognition but also in modulating neuroinflammatory responses associated with various CNS disorders.

Source: https://www.mdpi.com/molecules/molecules-28-00210/article_deploy/html/images/molecules-28-00210-g001.png.

13.2.2. Receptor Interactions and Drug Efficacy

Action of drugs within the CNS is dependent to a large extent on receptor interactions that have a determining influence on the mediation of physiological action to pharmacological agents. Understanding these interactions is essential, particularly regarding tailoring treatment to specific neurological disorders. For instance, the advancement of targeted therapies, such as the use of Osimertinib to treat non-small-cell lung cancer, demonstrates how receptor selectivity can enhance the efficacy of treatment; the drug selectively inhibits both EGFR-TKI–sensitizing and EGFR T790M resistance mutations, hence showing the importance of specificity of the receptor target in drug effect (Jean-Soria et al., 2017). Moreover, application of the AGS Beers Criteria stresses the need for consideration of potentially inappropriate medication, particularly among older adults, as certain drugs can enhance side effects through unanticipated receptor mechanisms. Combined, these results highlight the need for an advanced understanding of receptor interactions in CNS drug therapy.

13.2.3. Pharmacokinetics of CNS Drugs

Pharmacokinetics of drugs affecting the CNS is a significant area of research due to the unique issues presented by the BBB and the physiological nature of the CNS. Information regarding the absorption, distribution, metabolism, and excretion (ADME) of CNS drugs can be critical in optimizing drug therapy. For instance, nanoparticle formulations, as demonstrated in recent studies, have enhanced the CNS pharmacokinetics of drugs already on the market, such as the CDK4/6 inhibitor palbociclib, by reducing toxicity and optimizing survival in model systems bearing brain cancers (Lim et al., 2022). Furthermore, emerging treatments like oxfendazole for neurocysticercosis highlight the importance of pharmacokinetic evaluations in the design of successful therapy. This benzimidazole anthelmintic exhibited nonlinear pharmacokinetics, affecting its bioavailability, demonstrating the necessity of patient-specific drug delivery techniques in CNS therapy (An et al., 2019). In general, a thorough understanding of pharmacokinetics is essential for optimizing CNS drug efficacy and safety (Figure 13.8).

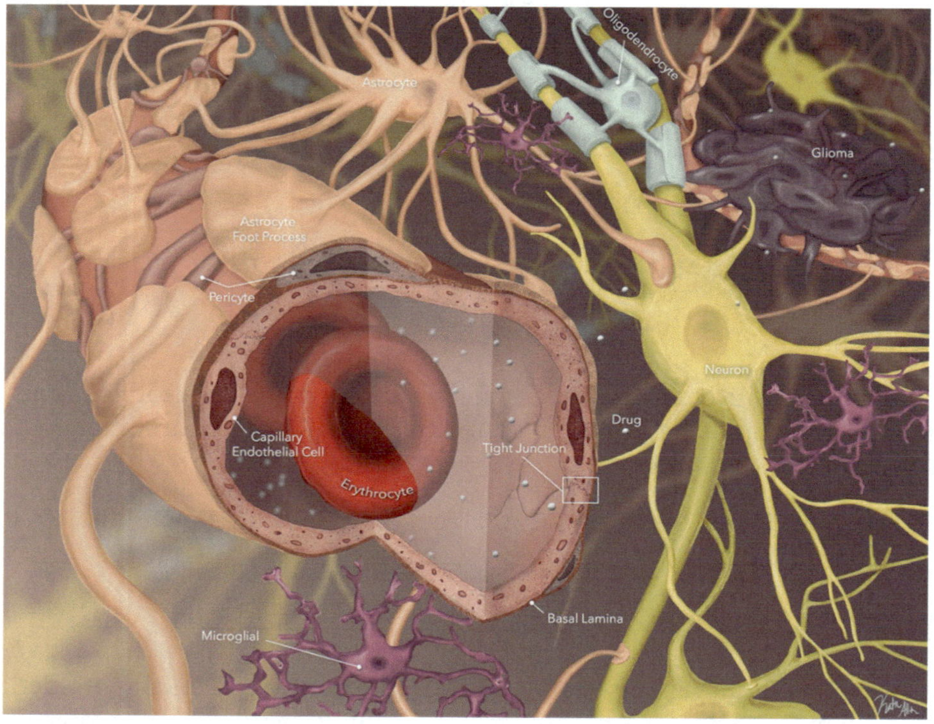

Figure 13.8. The pharmacokinetics of central nervous system (CNS) drugs is a critical area of study due to the unique challenges posed by the blood-brain barrier and the specific physiological characteristics of the CNS.

Source: https://images-provider.frontiersin.org/api/ipx/w=1200&f=png/https://www.frontiersin.org/files/Articles/365468/fonc-08-00239-HTML/image_m/fonc-08-00239-g001.jpg.

13.2.4. Pharmacodynamics and Therapeutic Outcomes

Pharmacodynamics is crucial to know in a bid to ensure optimal therapeutic effects in CNS drug therapy, particularly given the likely complexity of drug responses and interactions. Pharmacodynamics is concerned with how drugs affect the body, e.g., mechanisms of action, therapeutic effects, and potential side effects. Indeed, more recent evidence suggests that the sex variable significantly influences drug response, with evidence pointing towards various therapeutic effects and side effects of drugs in women in comparison to men. For example, women respond better to certain antipsychotics but are at higher risk for metabolic side effects (Romanescu et al.,

2022). Moreover, factors such as drug penetration through the CNS and selective permeability of the BBB also complicate such dynamics, which need advanced methodologies to make accurate exposure estimations (Rizk et al., 2017). Thus, such inclusion can contribute towards better clinical outcomes and patient-specific treatment regimens in CNS pharmacotherapy.

13.2.5. Blood-Brain Barrier and Drug Delivery

The BBB is a vital defense mechanism, tightly regulating substance transport between the blood and the CNS. While the barrier is very effective at defending the brain from toxins, it also complicates drug administration for CNS therapies. Products with the promise to ameliorate disorders such as HIV-associated neurocognitive disorders (HAND) face a long shot, considering that the compromised permeability of the BBB, which is mediated by viral proteins and neuroinflammation, limits therapeutic access to neural tissues (Said et al., 2025). Further hurdles, such as the blood-cerebrospinal fluid barrier (BCSFB), hinder drug entry, highlighting the need for novel delivery platforms (Ghosh et al., 2024). New therapies, including nasal drug administration and novel drug formulations, are working to counteract these obstacles, promising more effective CNS therapies for drugs. Thus, enhancing our knowledge of these complex interactions will be imperative in the creation of treatments that can penetrate the BBB and exhibit therapeutic effectiveness (Figure 13.9).

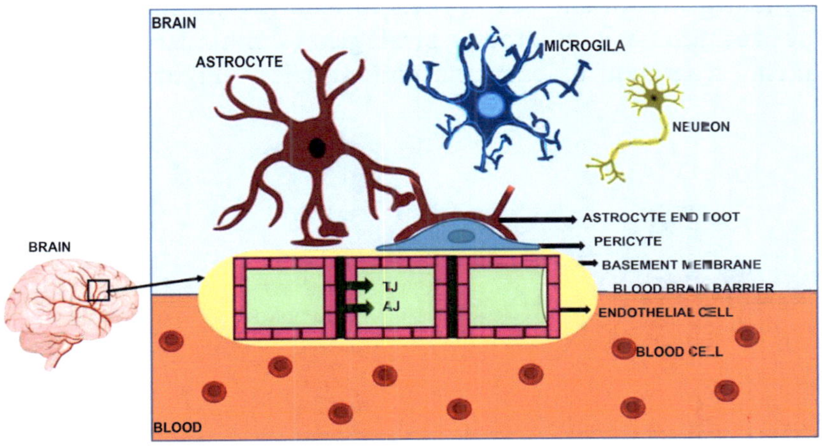

Figure 13.9. The blood-brain barrier (BBB) serves as a critical protective mechanism, meticulously regulating the passage of substances between the bloodstream and the central nervous system (CNS).

Source: https://media.springernature.com/lw1200/springer-static/image/art%3A10.1186%2Fs13041-022-00937-4/MediaObjects/13041_2022_937_Fig1_HTML.png.

13.2.6. Genetic Factors Influencing Drug Response

Identification of the genetic factors involved in drug response is necessary to achieve optimal CNS drug therapy, because variations in genes between individuals can significantly affect the effectiveness and safety of treatment. Pharmacogenomics, which is the science that investigates how genes influence drug response and metabolism, explains why certain patients experience side effects or are unresponsive to drugs. For instance, the genetic makeup may affect the metabolism of CNS drugs, such as antidepressants or antipsychotics, leading to variation in plasma concentration and therapeutic effect. This is typical in disease treatments like ALL, where relapse and treatment response are influenced by genetic rearrangements (Shertzer et al., 2020). Similarly, in HIV treatment, the inter-individual variability of drug metabolism renders compliance and long-term efficacy challenging, leading to speculation that a personalized dosing approach would optimize therapeutic effect while minimizing toxicity (Hentig et al., 2012). Through the inclusion of these genetic factors, CNS drug therapy can be optimized more particularly for the individual patient's needs.

13.2.7. Side Effects and Adverse Reactions

Treatment of CNS disorders in most cases involves long-term pharmacotherapy, which is highly complicated by side effects and ADRs. It has been documented that a high proportion of patients, including children, experience ADRs that manifest similarly to those in adults but with different severities and implications due to varying physiological conditions at various ages. For instance, in pediatric patients on monotherapy for epilepsy, gastrointestinal symptoms were observed in 32.35%, and CNS-related effects also represented 10.29% of events. Additionally, within the context of hospitals, CNS drugs were found to contribute to a high 20% of ADRs, frequently requiring extensive medical treatment due to their intensity. With these findings, it is a necessity that clinicians adopt precautionary monitoring strategies to minimize the unwanted effects of CNS drug therapy, enhancing treatment efficacy and patient safety (Figure 13.10).

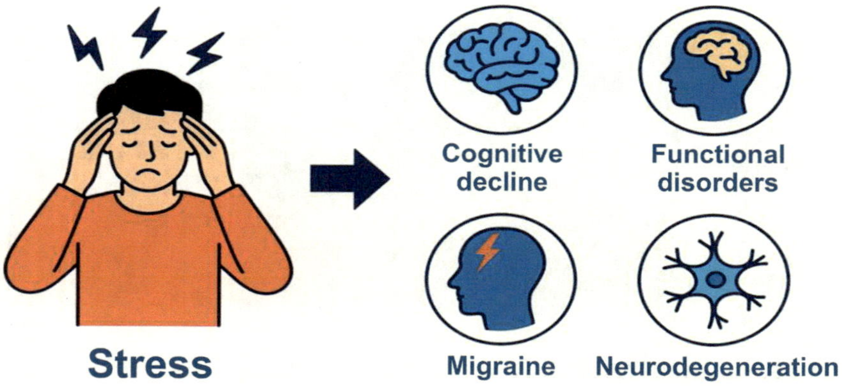

Figure 13.10. The management of central nervous system (CNS) disorders often necessitates prolonged pharmacotherapy, which can be significantly complicated by side effects and adverse drug reactions (ADRs).

Source: https://media.licdn.com/dms/image/v2/D5612AQFvY0RAXNh1SA/article-cover_image-shrink_720_1280/B56ZZanLyeHsAI-/0/1745276951040?e=2147483647&v=beta&t=40njbpsMdFj2_c_VxL0zHw5YzTee4_kYs3z5EPYLPBk.

13.2.8. Drug Interactions in CNS Therapy

The intricacy of CNS drug interactions is a significant issue for patients and clinicians alike. As the BBB restricts the passage of many therapeutic drugs, drug delivery to the brain is essential but understandably complicated; it involves invasive methods, such as direct intracerebral delivery and newer approaches like nasal mucosal engrafting, which, while promising, are fraught with dangers that are to be weighed against their benefit (Carafa et al., 2017). Additionally, the pharmacokinetic characteristics of various CNS drugs may produce clinically significant interactions. For example, triptans, which are used to treat migraine headaches, have complex interactions with CYP3A4 metabolic processes and should be carefully evaluated when used with other medications to prevent side effects like serotonin syndrome (Capi et al., 2016). Therefore, it is necessary to know such interactions for optimizing CNS drug treatment as well as patient outcomes.

13.2.9. Innovations in Drug Design and Delivery

The drug delivery and design science has made tremendous strides in enhancing the efficacy and safety of CNS therapy. More specifically, formulation technology development is crucial in addressing issues of patient compliance as well as drug abuse. For instance, recently launched products like Embeda™ and Remoxy® combine abuse-deterrent properties with pain relief efficacy. Embeda™, which is a combination of morphine and naltrexone, acts differently by inducing the release of naltrexone when the product is tried to be manipulated, thus acting as an aversion agent to deter opioid misuse (Zhao et al., 2012). Additionally, controlled release systems are increasingly being used, where drug delivery is constant and continuous, a requirement that is particularly essential in the treatment of chronic pain—a prevalent issue associated with CNS disorders (Ballet et al., 2016). These innovations both enhance patient outcomes and mitigate societal worries about opioid abuse, emphasizing the revolutionary ability of advances in drug design and delivery (Figure 13.11).

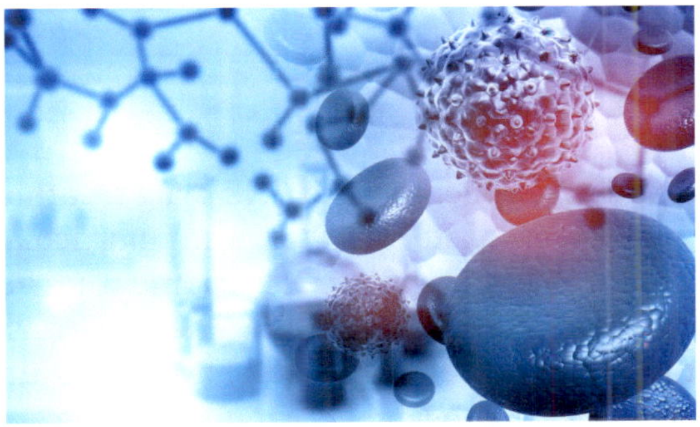

Figure 13.11. The field of drug design and delivery has seen remarkable innovations aimed at enhancing the efficacy and safety of CNS therapies.

Source: https://cdn.drugdiscoverynews.com/assets/image/3701/79154-header-image-brain-targeting-drugs-experts-have-on-their-radar-kr3-s.webp.

Test Your Knowledge

1. Name some neurotransmitters.
2. How do opioids produce analgesia and what receptors are involved?

13.3. Clinical Applications

Learning Outcome

1. Understand the treatment of depression and anxiety disorders
2. Explain the management of schizophrenia and bipolar disorder
3. Address neurodegenerative diseases
4. Focus on pain management strategies in CNS therapy
5. Describe pediatric considerations in CNS drug therapy
6. Identify CNS drug challenges in geriatric population
7. Know the role of psychotherapy in conjunction with drug therapy
8. Discuss case studies illustrating successful CNS drug therapy
9. Focus on future directions in clinical applications

The clinical applications of CNS drug treatment are pervasive and steadily increasing, particularly as researchers strive to overcome the very boundaries posed by the BBB. The BBB, a vital feature of cerebral homeostasis, renders drug delivery to the brain extremely challenging, and new approaches are being investigated. Techniques such as invasive therapies, such as direct intracranial administration or surgical implantation via nasal mucosa, are examined as delivery vehicles to guarantee drug penetration into loci of interest in the CNS (Carafa et al., 2017). Furthermore, neurorehabilitation advances have established the potential for synergistic therapies that have been used to restore function following neurological insult. Emerging evidence suggests that combining neuro-engineering solutions with individually tailored rehabilitation protocols can enhance recovery rates and even induce axonal regeneration (Edgerton et al., 2016). These developments signal a promising future of multi-modal treatments aimed not only at rectifying symptoms but also at inducing actual neural repair and long-term improvement in the patient's quality of life.

13.3.1. Treatment of Depression and Anxiety Disorders

The treatment of depression and anxiety disorders has advanced a great distance with a focus on both pharmacological and therapeutic treatment to gain maximal benefit for the patient. CNS drug treatment, particularly antidepressants and anxiolytics, plays a vital role in the treatment of these disorders. SSRIs and serotonin-norepinephrine reuptake inhibitors (SNRIs) are now first-line treatments due to their efficacy and favorable side effect profiles. Parallel to this is the role of cognitive-behavioral therapy (CBT) and other psychotherapy strategies supporting pharmacological intervention as a reaction to the overwhelming impact of psychological variables on mood disorders.

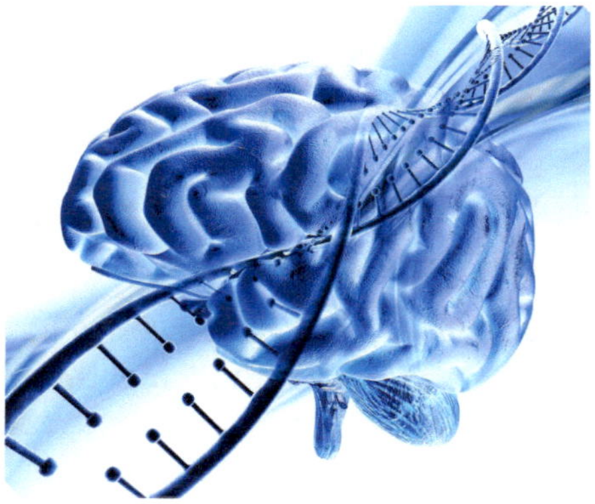

Figure 13.12. Central Nervous System (CNS) drug therapy, particularly the use of antidepressants and anxiolytics, plays a vital role in managing these conditions.

Source: https://www.marketresearchintellect.com/images/blogs/driving-innovation-in-healthcare-the-surge-of-central-nervous-system-cns-drug-market.webp.

The evidence-based treatment guidelines point towards the need for individualization of treatment protocols, respecting patient differences in response to drugs, thus demanding adaptability of therapy approaches (Group for the Advancement of Ps. Committee on Gender and Health M, 2020). Besides, ongoing research seeks to find new treatments in the form of new drug formulations and therapeutic interventions to enhance recovery and resilience in the infected subjects (Society T for Metabolism E and Diabetes of Africa S, 2018) (Figure 13.12).

13.3.2. Management of Schizophrenia and Bipolar Disorder

Both schizophrenia and BD present multifaceted challenges of clinical care and drug management, and the special nature of each demands complete understanding. Both conditions require tailored treatment management according to mood stabilizers, antipsychotics, and psychosocial interventions to bring about the best results among patients. For schizophrenia, antipsychotic medication plays a central role in management, in managing delusions and hallucinations. In contrast, for BD, mood stabilizers like lithium play a crucial role in preventing manic and depressive episodes. Other factors, such as the patient's history, potential side effects, and comorbid conditions, need to be considered while developing a management plan. The incorporation of patient-focused treatments, as noted in Society T for Metabolism E and Diabetes of Africa S (2018), into pharmacotherapy is likely to give more efficacy and compliance and, in the end, enhance the quality of life of the persons afflicted with these chronic mental illnesses, as shown in Group for the Advancement of Ps. Committee on Gender and Health M (2020).

13.3.3. Addressing Neurodegenerative Diseases

Neurodegenerative diseases (NDs) are significant challenges for contemporary healthcare, predominantly due to their progressive and multifaceted character that involves cognitive and motor functions.

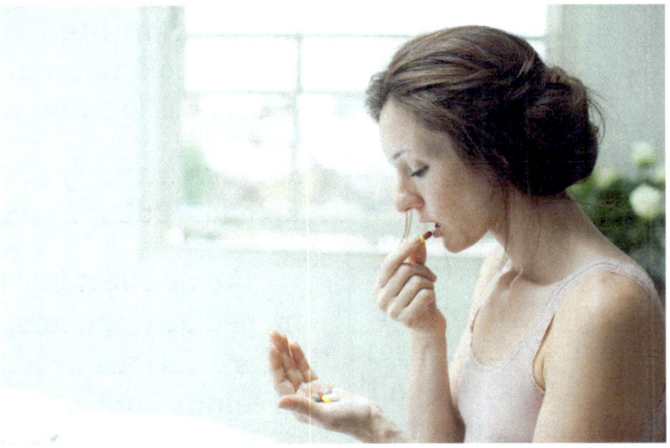

Figure 13.13. Neurodegenerative diseases (NDs) present significant challenges in contemporary healthcare, largely due to their progressive and multifaceted nature that impairs cognitive and motor functions.

Source: https://www.verywellmind.com/thmb/_grjkACIO-2guca6ndhLddWuLKI=/2121x0/filters:no_upscale():max_bytes(150000):strip_icc()/GettyImages-171631777-59f3fb32d963ac001058264b.jpg.

As the disorders more and more target the elderly population, new therapeutic approaches are crucial to control them. Developments in drug delivery systems, particularly those with nanotechnology, have recently shown promising outcomes in enhancing the efficacy of treatment by facilitating targeted delivery via the BBB. For instance, nanomaterials are employed as drug carriers to effectively boost bioavailability in the CNS and reduce side effects, thus enhancing patient treatment. Moreover, extracellular vesicles (EVs), which play a key role in intercellular communication, have been reported to be both diagnostic biomarkers and potential therapeutic targets in treating NDs. These developments reflect the ongoing advancement of CNS drug therapy modalities to overcome the complexities of neurodegenerative disorders (Xia et al., 2022; Bagherpour et al., 2025) (Figure 13.13).

13.3.4. Pain Management Strategies in CNS Therapy

Effective pain management in CNS therapy involves integrating pharmacologic and non-pharmacologic therapies. Even with the ongoing popularity of opioids as a cornerstone for managing severe pain, their administration is ridden with dependency and side effects. Other alternatives like regional anesthesia techniques and nonsteroidal anti-inflammatory drugs also offer adequate substitutes. Still, these also have limitations of their own, emphasizing the adoption of rigorous pain management practices. Non-pharmacological interventions, including patient education and mind-body approaches, have also yielded promising outcomes in reducing the intensity of pain and opioid consumption and ultimately providing improved recovery periods (Niyonkuru et al., 2024). Also, the interaction between antiretroviral drugs and illicit drug intake, in this case cocaine, illustrates the complexity surrounding CNS treatment efficacy. With this knowledge of variables, healthcare professionals can individually tailor pain control practices to enhance treatment outcomes for patients of CNS disorders (Col Rón Ortiz et al., 2024).

13.3.5. Pediatric Considerations in CNS Drug Therapy

Pediatric CNS drug therapy principles demand a knowledge of the unique pharmacokinetics in children, in addition to the potential toxicity of the therapies. Because children are not mini-adults, their maturing physiology can lead to dissimilar drug absorption, distribution, metabolism, and excretion, which must be taken into account when prescribing CNS drugs. For instance, therapies potentially valuable for the adult population may manifest with various deleterious effects in a pediatric population.

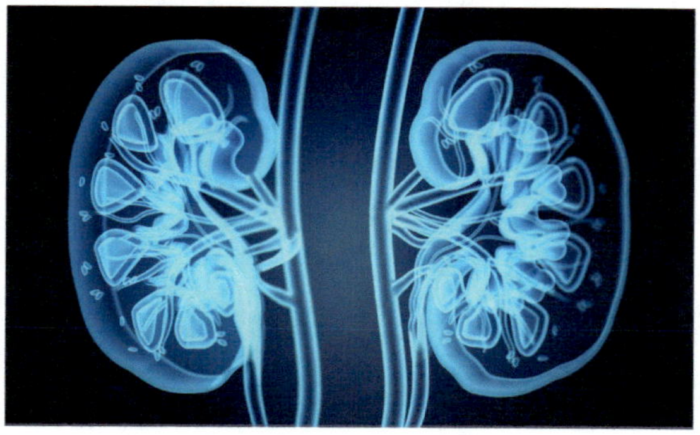

Figure 13.14. Pediatric considerations in CNS drug therapy necessitate a nuanced understanding of both the unique pharmacokinetics in children and the potential toxicity associated with these treatments.

Source: https://doseme-rx.com/wp-content/uploads/2023/11/iStock-1453826272.jpg.

Toxic effect burden is of particular interest in pediatric oncology, as in the case of ALL, where various acute poisonous effects may be developed with treatment, such as seizures and methotrexate-related stroke-like syndrome (Attarbaschi et al., 2016). Besides, the complexity of managing autoimmune and inflammatory CNS conditions in children underscores disease risk vs. treatment risk balancing, for example, in instances of neuromyelitis Optica and anti-N-methyl-D-aspartate receptor encephalitis (Dale et al., 2016) (Figure 13.14).

13.3.6. Geriatric Population and CNS Drug Challenges

The elderly population presents unique challenges in CNS drug therapy owing, in great measure, to the physiologic changes following aging. These changes entail drug distribution and metabolism changes, which complicate treatment and add to the risk of drug side effects. The BBB quite effectively protects the CNS, but the barrier becomes progressively more permeable as age goes on, leaving room for both drugs and toxins to pass more freely into the brain (Stalmans et al., 2015). So, the development of CNS drugs that are targeted for use in older patients must consider efficacy and safety equally. Moreover, evidence-based policy for enhancing care coordination and patient self-management suggests an imperative call for integrative approaches in geriatric pharmacotherapy (Morton et al., 2015). Addressing these challenges also demands not merely a more profound knowledge of the underlying biological mechanisms but stresses the need for equitable healthcare policies that are able to support this vulnerable population.

13.3.7. Role of Psychotherapy in Conjunction with Drug Therapy

The integration of psychotherapy and pharmacotherapies is a landmark part of current therapies for psychiatric disease. While drug therapy, particularly with CNS agents, yields symptomatic response, psychotherapy supports this by fixing these root emotional and cognitive issues, thus optimizing overall treatment efficacy. Research has established that the combined use of these modalities with each other can provide more benefit for the patient than either one alone. However, evidence suggests that the combined therapy does not necessarily outperform monotherapy in all patients (Curtiss et al., 2015). Further, novel psychoactive agents, so-called neuroenhancers, have potential for enhancing therapeutic benefit when combined with exposure therapies (Klempin et al., 2020). As knowledge of brain plasticity and neurogenic processes increases, it is becoming clearer that promoting an integrative model that unites psychotherapy with drug therapy can provide the most complete route to long-term recovery and better mental health (Figure 13.15).

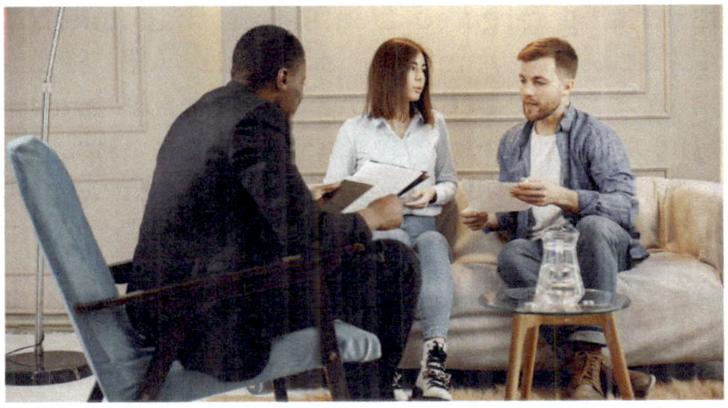

Figure 13.15. The integration of psychotherapy with pharmacological treatments represents a pivotal aspect of modern approaches to managing psychiatric disorders.

Source: https://www.elephantintheroomllc.com/wp-content/uploads/2025/02/15-Mental-Health-Counseling-Techniques-in-Therapy.jpg

13.3.8. Case Studies Illustrating Successful CNS Drug Therapy

The case study investigation highlights the promising advancement of CNS treatment for drugs, particularly through innovative therapies such as CAR-T cell therapy. An example is a 66-year-old man with diffuse large B-cell lymphoma who showed a remarkable response to CAR-T cell therapy following an isolated CNS relapse after initial treatment, such as a regimen of R-CHOP and high-dose methotrexate. This case is significant in that it evokes the therapy's ability to produce total remission, a potential paradigm shift in the therapeutic approach to secondary CNS lymphomas where the conventional drugs often fail (Takigawa et al., 2024). Further, the effectiveness of multidrug therapy in treating complex disorders is evident in the case of a woman whose secondary infertility, combined with multiple metabolic disorders, was significantly alleviated after Ayurvedic therapies. This reflects the potential of personalized drug therapies in the treatment of complicated health conditions in the CNS and other areas with the possibility for more effective treatments (Dhiman et al., 2024).

13.3.9. Future Directions in Clinical Applications

With advancements in the CNS drug therapy discipline, future clinical practice is more centered on refining targeted treatments that match the heterogeneity of neurological diseases. Refining treatments for multiple sclerosis (MS) is one promising avenue, as existing disease-modifying therapies have been limited by their inability to prevent long-term disability adequately. Advances in the understanding of immunopathogenesis are propelling research towards novel pharmacological targets with selective effects on immune responses, with reduced potential for side effects and enhanced efficacy (Rostami et al., 2015). Furthermore, exploration of neurorepair mechanisms facilitated by new rehabilitation approaches offers an alternative strategy. Researchers are now examining neurobiological and neuro-engineering solutions that promise to promote recovery from injuries such as stroke and traumatic brain injury, enhancing motor capability and the potential for neuronal regeneration (Edgerton et al., 2016). With the addition of these therapeutic pathways, future clinical applications will be more efficient and integrated therapies for CNS disorders, paving the way to improved patient outcomes (Figure 13.16).

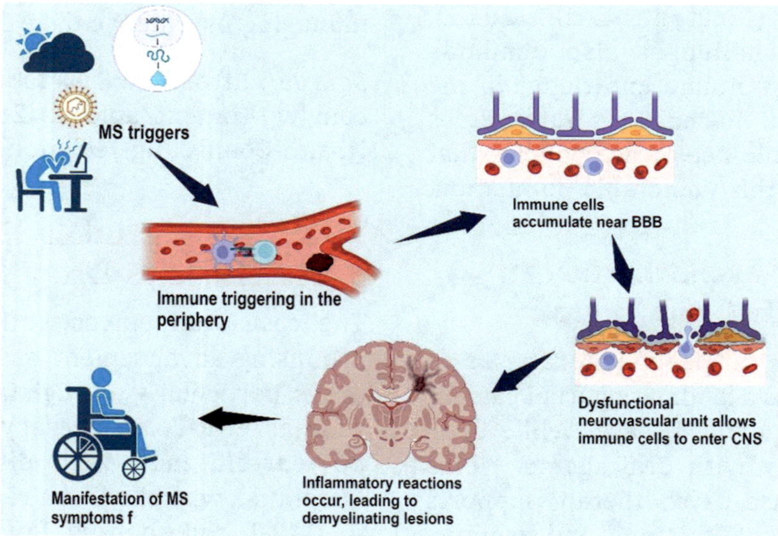

Figure 13.16. The refinement of therapies for multiple sclerosis (MS), where current disease-modifying treatments have shown limited efficacy in preventing long-term disability.

Source: https://article.imrpress.com/journal/FBL/29/11/10.31083/j.fbl2911386/2768-6698-29-11-386/fig1.jpg.

Test Your Knowledge

1. What role do stimulants like methylphenidate play in the treatment of ADHD?
2. When is general anesthesia indicated, and what drugs are commonly used for induction and maintenance?

Summary

The evolving CNS drug treatment landscape requires a comprehensive understanding of pharmacokinetics and the efficacy of treatment of diseases such as the incapacitating GBM and acute myeloid leukemia. New studies point to the potential of novel agents like WSD0628 with high radio sensitization and poor penetration across the brain, thereby resulting in enhanced treatment outcomes in GBM (Rathi et al., 2024). Simultaneously, the CPX-351 research for pediatric AML underscores the importance of novel formulations that address pharmacokinetic constraints faced by conventional chemotherapy regimens (Pollard et al., 2024). These findings reiterate that CNS drug therapy must advance not only with novel drugs but also by ensuring that their delivery across the BBB is maximized. Future research needs to be directed towards maximizing dose regimens and drug delivery schemes to ultimately enhance patient survival and quality of life in the setting of CNS malignancies.

As research in CNS drug therapy remains up to date, several notable points are emanating from contemporary debate within the academic and clinical arenas. One such advancement in HER2-positive breast cancer therapy, for instance, is the existence of MM-302, a HER2-specific antibody-liposomal doxorubicin conjugate that minimizes cardiotoxicity, a major challenge with traditional anthracyclines like doxorubicin (Cortes et al., 2016). This innovation reflects the increasing need for targeted treatments in the management of challenging diseases and the promotion of patient safety. Concurrently, recent congresses reflect the importance of learning about the brains physiological hurdles to drive drug delivery for neurological diseases, as indicated through studies by leading scientists at the CNS barrier congress in London (Brenn et al., 2017). All these findings reflect the overall trend towards safer and more personalized therapeutic strategies in CNS drug treatment.

KEY TERMS FROM THIS CHAPTER

- Acute lymphoblastic leukemia (ALL)
- Antiepileptic drugs (AEDs)
- Anxiolytics
- Bipolar disorder (BD)
- Blood-brain barrier (BBB)
- Central Nervous System (CNS)
- Chronic neurological disorder
- Delusions
- Dual cholinesterase
- Gamma-aminobutyric acid (GABA)
- Hallucinations
- Hippocampus
- Mania
- Mood stabilizers
- Non-invasive strategies
- Pharmacists
- Schizophrenia
- Seizure disorders

Critical Thinking Questions

1. **Which of the following is a commonly used selective serotonin reuptake inhibitor (SSRI)?**
   a. Amitriptyline
   b. Fluoxetine
   c. Diazepam
   d. Haloperidol
2. **Benzodiazepines act by enhancing the activity of which neurotransmitter?**
   a. Serotonin
   b. Norepinephrine
   c. Dopamine
   d. GABA (Gamma-Aminobutyric Acid)
3. **Levodopa is used in the treatment of Parkinson's disease because it:**
   a. Blocks dopamine receptors
   b. Enhances serotonin levels
   c. Is a precursor to dopamine
   d. Inhibits MAO enzymes
4. **Which of the following drugs is a typical antipsychotic?**
   a. Risperidone
   b. Haloperidol
   c. Clozapine
   d. Olanzapine
5. **What is the main mechanism of action of phenytoin?**
   a. Enhances GABA release
   b. Inhibits sodium channels
   c. Blocks calcium influx
   d. Stimulates dopamine release

Answers to Critical Thinking Questions

1. (b); 2. (d); 3. (c); 4. (b); 5. (b).

Short Answer Questions

1. What are the major classes of drugs used to treat CNS disorders?
2. How do sedative-hypnotic drugs differ from anxiolytics?
3. How do benzodiazepines enhance GABAergic activity in the brain?
4. What is the mechanism of action of selective serotonin reuptake inhibitors (SSRIs)?
5. Which CNS drugs are used to treat major depressive disorder. and how do they differ in efficacy and safety?
6. What medications are typically used in the acute and long-term treatment of schizophrenia?
7. What are the ethical concerns surrounding the overprescription of CNS stimulants in children and adolescents?

References

1. Buil, B. A., Rentsch, N. H., Weber, R. Z., Rickenbach, C., Halliday, S. J., Hotta, A., Tackenberg, C., & Rust, R. (2024). Beneath the radar: immune-evasive cell sources for stroke therapy. *Trends in Molecular Medicine, 30*(3), 223–238. https://doi.org/10.1016/j.molmed.2023.12.004Adams, M., Agrawal, S., Ahern, M., Alger, B., Armstrong, L., Arnone, D., Avraham, Y., et al. (2011). *Cannabis sativa and the Endogenous Cannabinoid System: Therapeutic Potential for Appetite Regulation*. https://core.ac.uk/download/107743.pdf (accessed on 10th June 2025).

2. Adhikari, P., Padmaja, U., & Pereira, P. (2009). *A Prospective Analysis of Adverse Drug Reactions in a South Indian hospital*. https://core.ac.uk/download/pdf/87416.pdf (accessed on 10th June 2025).

3. Agbaba, D., Alcaro, S., Bautista-Aguilera, O. M., Chioua, M., et al. (2014). *N-methyl-N-((1-methyl-5-(3-(1-(2-methylbenzyl)piperidin-4-yl)propoxy)-1H-indol-2-yl)methyl)prop-2-yn-1-amine: A new Cholinesterase and Monoamine Oxidase Dual Inhibitor*. https://core.ac.uk/download/30320284.pdf (accessed on 10th June 2025).

4. Agrawal, S., Datusalia, A. K., Dua, K., Gupta, G., et al. (2024). *Recent Developments in Intranasal Drug Delivery of Nanomedicines for The Treatment of Neuropsychiatric Disorders*. https://opus.lib.uts.edu.au/bitstream/10453/181860/3/fmed-11-1463976.pdf (accessed on 10th June 2025).

5. Almeida, N. D., Chuntova, P., Downey, K. M., Hegde, M., et al. (2018). *Genetically Engineered T-Cells for Malignant Glioma: Overcoming the Barriers to Effective Immunotherapy*. https://core.ac.uk/download/323063114.pdf (accessed on 10th June 2025).

6. Alvarez-Carbonell, D., Cannon, P. M., Chateau, M., Karn, J., et al. (2017). *HIV-1 Infection of Microglial Cells in A Reconstituted Humanized Mouse Model and Identification of Compounds That Selectively Reverse HIV Latency*. https://core.ac.uk/download/323063521.pdf (accessed on 10th June 2025).

7. An, G., Murry, D. J., Gajurel, K., Bach, T., Deye, G. A., Stebounova, L. V., Codd, E. E., et al. (2019). Pharmacokinetics, safety, and tolerability of oxfendazole in healthy volunteers: A randomized, placebo-controlled first-in-human single-dose escalation study. *Antimicrobial Agents and Chemotherapy, 63*. https://doi.org/10.1128/aac.02255-18.

8. Anand, A., Shrivastava, A., Singh, K., Barik, R., Gayakwad, D., Jailani, S., Shamim, M., et al. (2024). Neuroprotective efficacy and complementary treatment with medicinal herbs: A comprehensive review of recent therapeutic approaches in epilepsy management. *CNS & Neurological Disorders–Drug Targets*. https://www.semanticscholar.org/paper/32c6ce0253 87ea2671d0523b6f3f34995c043e97 (accessed on 10th June 2025).

9. Anderson, A., Armistead, G., Cornett, E. M., Edinoff, A. N., et al. (2022). *Phenothiazines and Their Evolving Roles in Clinical Practice: A Narrative Review*. https://core.ac.uk/download/554057814.pdf (accessed on 10th June 2025).

10. Aslund, A. K. O., Caputo, F., Ceccaldi, A., Germain, P., et al. (2020). *Delivering the Power of Nanomedicine to Patients Today*. https://core.ac.uk/download/333572117.pdf (accessed on 10th June 2025).

11. Attarbaschi, A., Barzilai, S., Escherich, G., Frandsen, T. L., et al. (2016). *Consensus Definitions of 14 Severe Acute Toxic Effects for Childhood Lymphoblastic Leukemia Treatment: A Delphi*

Consensus. https://core.ac.uk/download/42370388.pdf (accessed on 10th June 2025).

12. Bagherpour, I., Mozafari, M. R., & Naghib, S. M. (2025). Inorganic nanoparticles-based drug delivery systems for neurodegenerative diseases therapy. *Current Pharmaceutical Design*. https://www.semanticscholar.org/paper/5624dc64040d233edbdf41d5aa21c220ce609909 (accessed on 10th June 2025).
13. Ballet, S., De Baerdemaeker, A., Hoogenboom, R., Madder, A., et al. (2016). *Controlled-Release of Opioids for Improved Pain Management*. https://core.ac.uk/download/84045024.pdf (accessed on 10th June 2025).
14. Bishay, A. E., Hughes, N. C., Zargari, M., Paulo, D. L., Bishay, S., Lyons, A. T., Morkos, M. N., et al. (2024). Disparities in access to deep brain stimulation for Parkinson's disease and proposed interventions: A literature review. *Stereotactic and Functional Neurosurgery, 102*, 179–194. https://www.semanticscholar.org/paper/345d3e754db3d75cbee7cff3e928e3d50e3723ee (accessed on 10th June 2025).
15. Brenn, A., Reijerkerk, A., Zhang, B., Cerutti, C., Ridder, D. A., Duh, E. J., Lippmann, E. S., et al. (2017). *Current research Into Brain Barriers and The Delivery of Therapeutics for Neurological Diseases: A Report on CNS Barrier Congress, London, UK, 2017*. https://core.ac.uk/download/151170764.pdf (accessed on 10th June 2025).
16. Brew, B., Ellero, J., & Lubomski, M. (2017). *Interventions for Neurocognitive Dysfunction*. https://core.ac.uk/download/84111210.pdf (accessed on 10th June 2025).
17. Capi, M., Curto, M., De Andrés, F., Gentile, G., et al. (2016). *Eletriptan in the Management of Acute Migraine: An Update on The Evidence for Efficacy, Safety, And Consistent Response*. https://core.ac.uk/download/74319151.pdf (accessed on 10th June 2025).
18. Carafa, M., Di Marzio, L., Hanieh, P. N., Marianecci, C., et al. (2017). *Drug Delivery in Overcoming the Blood-Brain Barrier: Role of Nasal Mucosal Grafting*. https://core.ac.uk/download/80314980.pdf (accessed on 10th June 2025).
19. Cole, B., Kint, S., Sips, M., Van Hecke, C., et al. (2018). *Highlights from the HIV Cure and Reservoir Symposium, 11–12 September 2017, Ghent, Belgium*. https://core.ac.uk/download/237012222.pdf (accessed on 10th June 2025).
20. Colón Ortiz, R., Knerler, S. A., Fridman, L. B., Mercado, A., Price, A. S., Rosado-Franco, J. J., Wilkins, H. N., et al. (2024). Cocaine regulates antiretroviral therapy CNS access through pregnane-x receptor-mediated drug transporter and metabolizing enzyme modulation at the blood brain barrier. *Fluids and Barriers of the CNS, 21*. https://www.semanticscholar.org/paper/7a5c48f52fac234a23b1d133750471c29666cf41 (accessed on 10th June 2025).
21. Coluzzi, F., Fanelli, A., & Sacerdote, P. (2016). *Sublingual Sufentanil: A New Opportunity for the Improvement of Postoperative Pain Management in Italy*. https://core.ac.uk/download/54537561.pdf (accessed on 10th June 2025).
22. Coluzzi, F., Mattia, C., Consalvo, R., Pergolizzi, J., Raffa, R. B., et al. (2015). *The Unsolved Case of "Bone-Impairing Analgesics": The Endocrine Effects of Opioids on Bone Metabolism*. https://core.ac.uk/download/54537701.pdf (accessed on 10th June 2025).
23. Cordeiro, M. F., Hill, D., Kelada, M., Manzar, F., et al. (2021). *Innovations and Revolutions in Reducing Retinal Ganglion Cell Loss in Glaucoma*. https://core.ac.uk/download/374290618.pdf (accessed on 10th June 2025).

24. Cortes, J., Hurvitz, S. A., Krop, I. E., Miller, R. E., et al. (2016). HERMIONE: A randomized Phase 2 trial of MM-302 plus trastuzumab versus chemotherapy of physician's choice plus trastuzumab in patients with previously treated, anthracycline-naïve, HER2-positive, locally advanced/metastatic breast cancer. https://core.ac.uk/download/323076535.pdf (accessed on 10th June 2025).

25. Cortes-Flores, H., Torrandell-Haro, G., & Brinton, R. D. (2024). Clinical manifestations. *Alzheimer's & Dementia, 20*(Suppl. 3), e091759. https://www.semanticscholar.org/paper/a36515cc7146010ee293c0cbbb96dcef79d13706 (accessed on 10th June 2025).

26. Cromeens, M. G., Rowland, C., Ogbansiegbe, J., Mihas, P., Benhabbour, S. R., & Carey, E. (2023). (026) "Hoping it will be better next time:" A qualitative analysis of treatment decision-making with vulvodynia. *The Journal of Sexual Medicine*. https://www.semanticscholar.org/paper/e7390de03eba64d0befd5816fb2dcdd18b755ee5 (accessed on 10th June 2025).

27. Cruccu, G., Di Stefano, G., & Truini, A. (2018). *Current and Innovative Pharmacological Options to Treat Typical and Atypical Trigeminal Neuralgia*. https://core.ac.uk/download/188828883.pdf (accessed on 10th June 2025).

28. Cui, L., Watanabe, S., Miyanaga, K., Kiga, K., Sasahara, T., Aiba, Y., Tan, X. E., et al. (2024). A comprehensive review on phage therapy and phage-based drug development. *Antibiotics, 13*. https://www.semanticscholar.org/paper/ddfe9f2f673499d02e01d48bee8cd18291f4c542 (accessed on 10th June 2025).

29. Curtiss, J., Hofmann, S. G., & Mundy, E. A. (2015). *Neuroenhancement of Exposure Therapy in Anxiety Disorders*. https://core.ac.uk/download/215928428.pdf (accessed on 10th June 2025).

30. Dale, R. C., Lim, M., & Nosadini, M. (2016). *Therapeutic Decision Making in Autoimmune and Inflammatory Disorders of The Central Nervous System in Children*. https://core.ac.uk/download/154325209.pdf (accessed on 10th June 2025).

31. Deng, X., Li, J., He, R., Wen, Y., Lin, Y., Li, L., Ling, X., et al. (2025). High concordance of human immunodeficiency virus-1 genotypic drug resistance generated from paired cerebrospinal fluid and plasma in antiretroviral therapy-naive or -experienced patients. *Frontiers in Microbiology, 16*. https://www.semanticscholar.org/paper/476271e3b5834443455350a6cf891f412c8f6ee6 (accessed on 10th June 2025).

32. Dhiman, K., & Agarwal, P. N. (2024). Successful outcome of secondary infertility with multidrug therapy in a long-standing case of multisystem involvement. *Journal of Drug Delivery and Therapeutics*. https://www.semanticscholar.org/paper/eb6f7d492a90f51844c840de29641d545e47b987 (accessed on 10th June 2025).

33. Edgerton, V. R., Krucoff, M. O., Rahimpour, S., Slutzky, M. W., et al. (2016). *Enhancing Nervous System Recovery Through Neurobiology's, Neural Interface Training. And Neurorehabilitation*. https://core.ac.uk/download/323078214.pdf (accessed on 10th June 2025).

34. El-Hwuegi, A. S., Kumlien, E., & Sherif, F. M. (1996). *Acute Vigabatrin-Phenobarbitone Interaction on Exploratory Behavior of Rats*. https://core.ac.uk/download/286457832.pdf (accessed on 10th June 2025).

35. Elkholy, A. (2017). Nanotechnology-based drug delivery system and its applications. *Egyptian Journal of Chemistry and Environmental Health*. https://www.semanticscholar.org/paper/031d402f3ed179ba01e4de9a86c52c513c824041 (accessed on 10th June 2025).

36. Evans, D., Fernández-Bolaños Guzmán, J. M., López López, Ó., Man, A. W. C., et al. (2019). *Design and Synthesis of CNS-Targeted Flavones and Analogues with Neuroprotective Potential Against H_2O_2- and Aβ1-42-Induced Toxicity in SH-SY5Y Human Neuroblastoma Cells*. https://core.ac.uk/download/227043737.pdf (accessed on 10th June 2025).

37. Facey, K., Granados, A., Guyatt, G., Kent, D., et al. (2014). *Generating Health Technology Assessment Evidence for Rare Diseases*. https://core.ac.uk/download/42361346.pdf (accessed on 10th June 2025).

38. Gandavaram, N., & Rajalekshmi, M. (2024). A case report on tuberculosis in pregnancy revealing the need for an effective multidisciplinary approach and the importance of tailored therapy. *Indian Journal of Obstetrics and Gynecology Research*. https://www.semanticscholar.org/paper/402fc3ff271fe89829deffed58ac84ffa57dc866 (accessed on 10th June 2025).

39. Ghosh, M., Roy, D., Thakur, S., & Singh, A. (2024). Exploring the potential of nasal drug delivery for brain targeted therapy: A detailed analysis. *Biopharmaceutics & Drug Disposition, 45*. https://www.semanticscholar.org/paper/5e1c11e89836a121a1514215626c1fc22b87d45b (accessed on 10th June 2025).

40. Giubilei, F. (2016). *Beyond Cholinesterase Inhibition: Anti-Inflammatory Role and Pharmacological Profile of Current Drug Therapy for Alzheimer's disease*. https://core.ac.uk/download/98347745.pdf (accessed on 10th June 2025).

41. Group for the Advancement of Psychiatry, Committee on Gender and Mental Health. (2020). *Postpartum Mental Health Disorders: A Casebook*. https://www.semanticscholar.org/paper/88fb043f9ebeccad2fc5bfe6bfede44c15339ee2 (accessed on 10th June 2025).

42. Gutierrez, M., Osako, L., & Wincor, M. Z. (1992). *Update on Anxiolytics and Hypnotics*. https://core.ac.uk/download/215765482.pdf (accessed on 10th June 2025).

43. Haddad, H. W., Hankey, P., Ko, J., Eswani, Z., Bhatti, P., Edinoff, A. N., Kaye, A. D., et al. (2022). Viloxazine, a non-stimulant norepinephrine reuptake inhibitor, for the treatment of attention deficit hyperactivity disorder: A 3-year update. *Health Psychology Research, 10*(3), 37018. https://www.semanticscholar.org/paper/5731d470f1fbd93c1f57be9c41a01e9d00c149e2 (accessed on 10th June 2025).

44. Hirata, I., Hanaoka, S., Rokutanda, R., Funakoshi, R., & Hayashi, H. (2023). Shared decision-making practices and patient values in pharmacist outpatient care for rheumatic disease: A multiple correspondence analysis. *Journal of Pharmacy & Pharmaceutical Sciences, 26*. https://www.semanticscholar.org/paper/44ac86a38e2c9f84b0051eaa14ff16c4607e07bb (accessed on 10th June 2025).

45. Iannitelli, A., Quartini, A., & Tirassa, P. (2015). Nerve growth factor, brain-derived neurotrophic factor, and the chronobiology of mood: A new insight into the "neurotrophic hypothesis." https://core.ac.uk/download/54533223.pdf (accessed on 10th June 2025).

46. Jang, E. Y. (2019). A background of the opioid epidemic and its relationship to the Medicaid expansion. https://core.ac.uk/download/213463816.pdf (accessed on 10th June 2025).

47. Klempin, F. (2020). Signaling pathways linking behavior to neurogenesis in healthy brain and disease. https://core.ac.uk/download/322846707.pdf (accessed on 10th June 2025).

48. Knippen, S., Hildebrandt, G., Putz, F., Gossé, L. L., Ritz, J. P., & Duma, M. N. (2024). Assessing the practice of total neoadjuvant therapy for rectal cancer: An online survey among radiation

oncology departments in Germany and German-speaking regions of Austria and Switzerland. *Clinical and Experimental Medicine, 24*. https://www.semanticscholar.org/paper/5f339922809c2860d25b5ee5fa19c6e5cf769ae0 (accessed on 10th June 2025).

49. Konitsioti, A. M., Prüss, H., Laurent, S., Fink, G. R., Heesen, C., & Warnke, C. (2024). Chimeric antigen receptor T-cell therapy for autoimmune diseases of the central nervous system: A systematic literature review. *Journal of Neurology, 271*, 6526–6542. https://www.semanticscholar.org/paper/021dcc22458f85dc2b5bf6b8cf0b1a73477e4a98 (accessed on 10th June 2025).

50. Koverech, A., Martelletti, P., & Negro, A. (2018). Serotonin receptor agonists in the acute treatment of migraine: A review on their therapeutic potential. https://core.ac.uk/download/154948885.pdf (accessed on 10th June 2025).

51. Kraft, W. K. (2018). Buprenorphine in neonatal abstinence syndrome. https://core.ac.uk/download/155271558.pdf (accessed on 10th June 2025).

52. Kumari, P., Kumar, P., Ashawat, M., & Sharma, P. (2023). A comprehensive overview on phytomedicines as an upcoming/emerging candidate for the management of epilepsy. *Journal of Drug Delivery and Therapeutics*. https://www.semanticscholar.org/paper/de1fd14c10c29f8f80483d6048eadc103f979798 (accessed on 10th June 2025).

53. LeQuang, A., Bisney, J., Coluzzi, F., Gharibo, C., et al. (2018). *Gabapentin Use Disorder: Update for Clinicians*. https://core.ac.uk/download/188831513.pdf (accessed on 10th June 2025).

54. Lim, C., Dismuke, T., Malawsky, D., Ramsey, J. D., Hwang, D., Godfrey, V., Kabanov, A. V., et al. (2022). Enhancing CDK4/6 inhibitor therapy for medulloblastoma using nanoparticle delivery and scRNA-seq–guided combination with sapanisertib. *Science Advances, 8*. https://doi.org/10.1126/sciadv.abl5838.

55. McCarthy, S. (2015). Malaria prevention, mefloquine neurotoxicity, neuropsychiatric illness, and risk-benefit analysis in the Australian Defense Force. https://core.ac.uk/download/208034185.pdf (accessed on 10th June 2025).

56. Morton, S., & Dunn, W. (2015). *Addressing the Health Needs of An Aging America: New Opportunities for Evidence-Based Policy Solutions*. https://core.ac.uk/download/75783019.pdf (accessed on 10th June 2025).

57. Mudaliar, S. B., Poojary, S. S., Prasad, A. B., & Mazumder, N. (2024). Probiotics and Para probiotics: Effects on microbiota-gut-brain axis and their consequent potential in neuropsychiatric therapy. *Probiotics and Antimicrobial Proteins, 16*, 1440–1464. https://www.semanticscholar.org/paper/57abd1384a1f573d7718a86868b32f7f0f1e436b (accessed on 10th June 2025).

58. Nishad, A., Kisku, A., Datusalia, A. K., Gupta, G., Dua, K., et al. (2024). *Recent Developments in Intranasal Drug Delivery of Nanomedicines for The Treatment of Neuropsychiatric Disorders*. https://core.ac.uk/download/629701465.pdf (accessed on 10th June 2025).

59. Niyonkuru, E., Iqbal, M. A., Zhang, X., & Ma, P. (2024). Complementary approaches to postoperative pain management: A review of non-pharmacological interventions. *Pain and Therapy, 14*, 121–144. https://www.semanticscholar.org/paper/7e73de5526954cd7f5a26210457020457b40dd49 (accessed on 10th June 2025).

60. Pandarakalam, J. P. (2022). Certain aspects of immunopsychiatry. https://core.ac.uk/download/553605818.pdf (accessed on 10th June 2025).

61. Pollard, J., Alonzo, T., Gerbing, R., Kutny, M., Hirsch, B., Raca, G., Leger, K., et al. (2024). A phase 3 randomized trial for patients with *de novo* AML comparing standard therapy including gemtuzumab ozogamicin (GO) to CPX-351 with GO: A report from the Children's Oncology Group. *Blood*. https://www.semanticscholar.org/paper/0f7ff7e50c16843d7496a9019b264eca742a6070 (accessed on 10th June 2025).

62. Prabhavalkar, K. S., Bhatt, L. K., & Poovanpallil, N. B. (2015). Management of bipolar depression with lamotrigine: An antiepileptic mood stabilizer. https://core.ac.uk/download/pdf/82867856.pdf (accessed on 10th June 2025).

63. Rathi, S., Mladek, A., Xue, Z., Oh, J. H., Zhang, W., Zhang, W., Le, J., et al. (2024). Abstract B028: Systemic and CNS distributional pharmacokinetics of WSD0628, a novel radiosensitizer: Implications for the treatment of brain tumors. *Cancer Research*. https://www.semanticscholar.org/paper/1a297a15557fe65e9b22f53f8bc57ceab56d797a (accessed on 10th June 2025).

64. Rizk, M. L., Zou, L., Savic, R. M., & Dooley, K. E. (2017). Importance of drug pharmacokinetics at the site of action. *Clinical and Translational Science, 10*, 133–142. https://doi.org/10.1111/cts.12448.

65. Romanescu, M., Buda, V., Lombrea, A., Andor, M., Ledeţi, I., Suciu, M., Danciu, C., et al. (2022). Sex-related differences in pharmacological response to CNS drugs: A narrative review. *Journal of Personalized Medicine, 12*, 907. https://doi.org/10.3390/jpm12060907.

66. Rostami, A., Abrams, M., Achiron, A., Adelman, G., Allen, I., Bachmann, M., et al. (2015). *Emerging Immunopharmacological Targets in Multiple Sclerosis*. https://core.ac.uk/download/155271780.pdf (accessed on 10th June 2025).

67. Said, N., & Venketaraman, V. (2025). Neuroinflammation, blood–brain barrier, and HIV reservoirs in the CNS: An in-depth exploration of latency mechanisms and emerging therapeutic strategies. *Viruses, 17*. https://www.semanticscholar.org/paper/479a17e6d4136c8415e590320d3f9696de3b6035 (accessed on 10th June 2025).

68. Shertzer, H. (2020). *Genetic Relationships and Therapeutic Options for Relapsed Acute Lymphoblastic Leukemia*. https://core.ac.uk/download/304169063.pdf (accessed on 10th June 2025).

69. Sirgedas, L. O. (2009). Alzheimer's disease immunization strategies: A review of current research. https://core.ac.uk/download/pdf/10796822.pdf (accessed on 10th June 2025).

70. Sobczyk, M., Żuraw, D., Oleksa, P., Jasiński, K., Porzak, M., & Dacka, M. (2024). SGLT2 inhibitors and their possible use in prevention and treatment of neurological diseases. *Prospects in Pharmaceutical Sciences*. https://www.semanticscholar.org/paper/70f4bda92cf1f6afa4100aa387b23f0e7f4721c1 (accessed on 10th June 2025).

71. Soria, J. C., Ohe, Y., Vansteenkiste, J., Reungwetwattana, T., Chewaskulyong, B., Lee, K. H., Dechaphunkul, A., et al. (2017). Osimertinib in untreated *EGFR*-mutated advanced non–small-cell lung cancer. *New England Journal of Medicine, 378*, 113–125. https://doi.org/10.1056/nejmoa1713137.

72. Stalmans, S. (2015). To what extent do cell-penetrating peptides selectively cross the blood-brain barrier? https://core.ac.uk/download/55862365.pdf (accessed on 10th June 2025).

73. Styne, D. M., Arslanian, S., Connor, E. L., Farooqi, I. S., Murad, M. H., Silverstein, J., & Yanovski, J. A. (2017). Pediatric obesity—Assessment, treatment, and prevention: An Endocrine Society clinical practice guideline. *The Journal of Clinical Endocrinology & Metabolism, 102*, 709–757. https://doi.org/10.1210/jc.2016-2573.

74. Surajo, B., Khan, Z., Shadab, M., Khan, N., Sada, M., Ahmad, M., Akhter, M. S., et al. (2024). Analysis of antidiabetic drug utilization patterns in type 2 diabetes patients: A perspective on real-time prescribing practices. *International Journal of Basic & Clinical Pharmacology*. https://www.semanticscholar.org/paper/3542767115f8047c54461f80fdf65df836880290 (accessed on 10th June 2025).

75. Takigawa, K., Kawano, N., Mori, Y., Yamauchi, T., Tochigi, T., Miyawaki, K., Mori, K., et al. (2024). A case of successful CAR-T cell therapy for early isolated CNS recurrence of DLBCL with persistent CAR-T cells. *Blood Cell Therapy, 7*, 37–40. https://www.semanticscholar.org/paper/06b215215d506b09b3692ae973f273a473c6680b (accessed on 10th June 2025).

76. The Society for Endocrinology Metabolism and Diabetes of South Africa. (2018). Chapter 11: The approach to achieving glycemic control. *South African Family Practice*. https://www.semanticscholar.org/paper/d84cca25f0a3f925d3c428c6547498194a9d23b6 (accessed on 10th June 2025).

77. Torres Obando, F., Romeo, P., Vergara, D., Di Fede, G., & Soto Pardo, A. (2022). The effects of low-frequency high-intensity pulsed electromagnetic fields (diamagnetic therapy) in the treatment of rare diseases: A case series preliminary study. *Journal of Neurology and Experimental Neural Science*. https://www.semanticscholar.org/paper/2d8eb8d7a98c20787 15ef1ac49004415ce164bad (accessed on 10th June 2025).

78. von Hentig, N. (2012). *Personalizing HIV Therapy, Mission Impossible?* https://core.ac.uk/download/17028337.pdf (accessed on 10th June 2025).

79. Wijaya, I. N., Athiyah, U., Fasich, F., Rahem, A., & Hermansyah, A. (2023). The association between drug therapy problems and blood pressure control of patients with hypertension in public health center setting. *Journal of Public Health in Africa, 14*. https://www.semanticscholar.org/paper/4e0be244d2ffe8cd48ce43ad4d1bf80b6a756886 (accessed on 10th June 2025).

80. Xia, X., Wang, Y., & Zheng, J. C. (2022). Extracellular vesicles, from the pathogenesis to the therapy of neurodegenerative diseases. *Translational Neurodegeneration, 11*. https://www.semanticscholar.org/paper/c28d2bf47eefc73eb67219002cfdca0f3cf877fe (accessed on 10th June 2025).

81. Zhao, F. (2012). Innovative drug delivery and formulation designs to deter drug abuse/misuse related to suicide. https://core.ac.uk/download/84856796.pdf (accessed on 10th June 2025).

82. Zheng, Y., Liu, J., Tang, P. K., Hu, H., & Ung, C. (2023). A systematic review of self-medication practice during the COVID-19 pandemic: Implications for pharmacy practice in supporting public health measures. *Frontiers in Public Health, 11*. https://www.semanticscholar.org/paper/cb6269d6b402d3844237a28fe31e361e691e07c4 (accessed on 10th June 2025).

ENDOCRINE AND METABOLIC DISORDERS

14

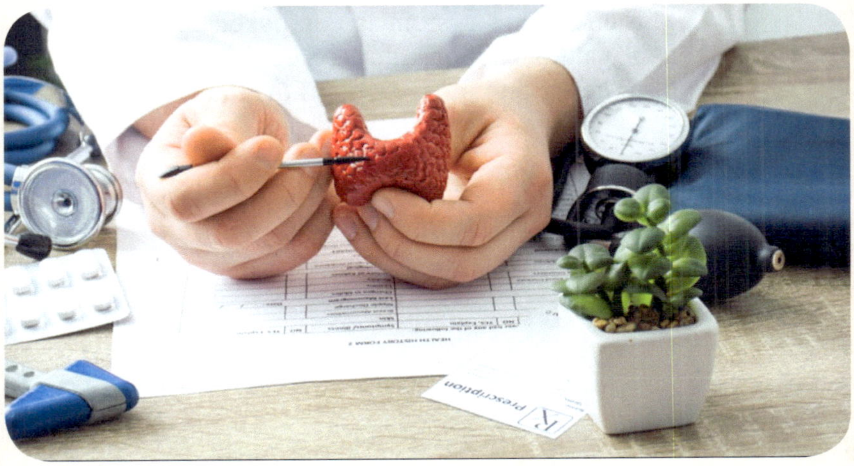

LEARNING OBJECTIVES

After studying this chapter, you will be able to:

1. Understand the overview of the endocrine system
2. Identify common endocrine disorders
3. Explain metabolic disorders
4. Discuss diagnosis and treatment approaches

Introduction

Endocrine and metabolic illnesses are a complex interplay of physiological dysregulation with profound influences on general well-being. Comprised of disruptions in hormonal regulation and metabolism, they encompass a wide array of conditions from diabetes and obesity to anorexia nervosa. That these disorders are common underscores the necessity to understand the causative mechanisms underlying such diseases and their systemic ramifications. For instance, research has indicated that type 2 diabetic patients, particularly those with metabolic syndrome, have higher serum levels of fibroblast growth factor 21 (FGF21), which is correlated with extreme body composition alterations and cardiovascular risk factors (Khoshnia et al., 2015). Similarly, anorexia nervosa is a striking example of how endocrine dysfunction may lead to extreme reproductive problems secondary to the disturbance of the hypothalamic-pituitary-ovarian axis (Ciobanu et al., 2020). A thorough evaluation of endocrine and metabolic disorders must thus be performed to develop effective treatment regimens and improve patient outcomes.

14.1. Overview of the Endocrine System

Learning Outcome

1. Understand major glands of the endocrine system
2. Explain the hormones produced by each gland
3. Discuss the role of the hypothalamus in hormone regulation
4. Know feedback mechanisms in hormone secretion
5. Explain the interaction between the endocrine and nervous systems
6. Focus on the importance of homeostasis
7. Learn standard diagnostic tests for endocrine function
8. See effects of aging on the endocrine system
9. Discuss emerging research in endocrinology

The endocrine system is essential in maintaining the body in homeostasis and in controlling body functions by secreting hormones into the bloodstream. It entails an endocrine system of glands that comprises the pituitary gland, thyroid gland, adrenal glands, and the pancreas, which in concert control several functions such as metabolism, growth, and mood. Hormones are chemical messengers that enable various organs to communicate and facilitate the body to respond appropriately to internal and external stimuli. The dysregulation of this system may lead to devastating metabolic diseases, such as diabetes and thyroid disease, with far-reaching consequences on overall health. Furthermore, the interplay between inflammation and hypoxia in these diseases highlights the complexity of hormonal regulation because hypoxic chronic states trigger proinflammatory pathways that enhance tissue injury and metabolic dysregulation (Carnevale et al., 2015). An insight into the intricate processes of the endocrine system is essential to develop successful therapeutic approaches to manage such disorders (Drew et al., 2014).

14.1.1. Major Glands of the Endocrine System

The endocrine system is composed of several large glands, each of which is crucial in controlling body functions by secreting hormones.

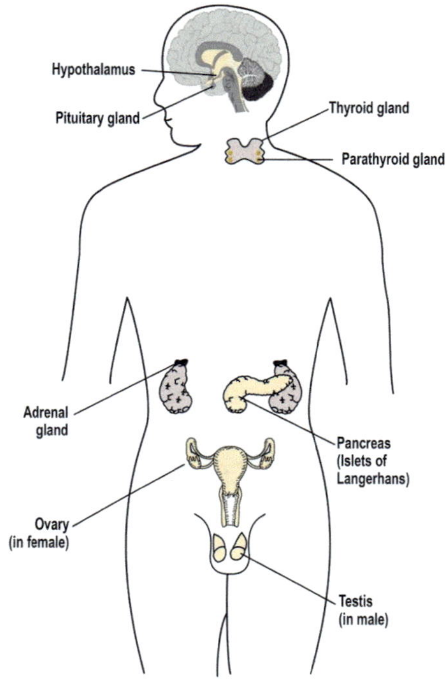

Figure 14.1. The endocrine system comprises several major glands, each playing a crucial role in the regulation of bodily functions through hormone secretion.

Source: https://europepmc.org/articles/PMC6761896/bin/arh-22-3-153f1.jpg.

The pituitary gland, which has earned the reputation as the master gland, regulates other endocrine glands and, through its secretions, evokes growth, metabolism, and stress responses. Similarly, the adrenal glands secrete hormones such as cortisol and adrenaline, which are crucial for the body's response to stress and metabolic processes. Moreover, metabolic rate is regulated by the thyroid gland through the release of thyroid hormones, influencing energy and general well-being. Notably, the skin itself is a peripheral endocrine organ with a hypothalamic-pituitary-adrenal (HPA)-like axis contributing to the production of sex and stress hormones of interest in conditions like acne and other pilosebaceous disorders (Clark et al., 2020). These contacts bear witness to the complexity of the endocrine system and its long-range implications in metabolic disease and overall health (Greenleaf et al., 2025) (Figure 14.1).

14.1.2. Hormones Produced by Each Gland

The endocrine system is made up of some glands, each of which produces distinct hormones to regulate different physiological processes. The pituitary gland, or master gland, produces hormones such as Growth Hormone (GH) and Prolactin that regulate growth and lactation, respectively. The thyroid gland releases Thyroxine (T4) and Triiodothyronine (T3), hormones that play significant roles in the regulation of metabolism and energy use; thus, their dysfunctions are the key mechanism in metabolic disorders (Kitahara et al., 2022). The adrenal glands also release corticosteroids, such as cortisol, which controls responses to stress and metabolism, and aldosterone, which governs sodium and water balance. The pancreas releases insulin and glucagon, which are key to glucose homeostasis. Furthermore, gut microbiota has also been found in recent research to affect thyroid hormone metabolism, demonstrating the fine interaction between hormones and metabolism in disease and wellness (Eöhlich et al., 2019). Such hormonal interactions are an exemplification of the fine balance required for maintaining metabolic homeostasis.

14.1.3. Role of the Hypothalamus in Hormone Regulation

Hypothalamus is central to hormone regulation as it acts as an interface between the nervous and the endocrine system to influence a number of bodily functions necessary for the maintenance of homeostasis.

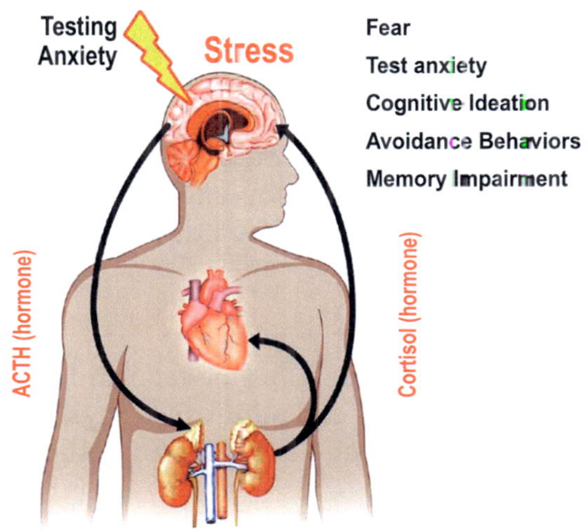

Figure 14.2. Role of the hypothalamus in hormone regulation.

Source: https://www.mdpi.com/stresses/stresses-02-00011/article_deploy/html/images/stresses-02-00011-g001.png.

It achieves this through the secretion of hormones like gonadotropin-releasing hormone (GnRH), regulating reproductive processes, and corticotropin-releasing hormone (CRH), regulating the stress response. Besides, the hypothalamus also controls metabolism, with its interaction with proopiomelanocortin (POMC) being most prominent, influencing hunger and metabolism of energy and, therefore, demonstrating its significant impact on obesity and metabolic illness (Janicka et al., 2025). Apart from this, the hypothalamus also plays a role in controlling oxidative and reductive stress, insulin release, and signal pathways, which play a critical role in diabetes and cardiovascular diseases (Mladenov et al., 2025). For this reason, it is crucial to understand the multifunctional roles of the hypothalamus to develop efficient treatments for endocrine and metabolic disorders (Figure 14.2).

14.1.4. Feedback Mechanisms in Hormone Secretion

The intricate mechanisms of feedback that regulate hormone secretion are essential in maintaining homeostasis in the endocrine system, particularly where endocrine as well as metabolic disorders are in question. These mechanisms are primarily negative feedback loops, where the effect of a hormone inhibits its secretion for balance to be maintained. For instance, in the case of polycystic ovary syndrome (PCOS), there is a hypersecretion of luteinizing hormone (LH) that is interfering with proper reproductive function due to an increased rate of pulsatile secretion of LH, indicating the neuroendocrine disturbance (Coutinho et al., 2019). Similarly, disorders like anorexia nervosa can lead to hormonal adaptation, resulting in states like functional amenorrhea, an illustration of the way that decreased caloric intake affects the hypothalamic-pituitary-ovarian axis and subsequently hormone release (Ciobanu et al., 2020). This understanding is fundamental to the development of effective treatments for endocrine diseases, an illustration of the close connection between hormones and metabolic health.

14.1.5. Interaction between the Endocrine and Nervous Systems

The intricate relationship between the nervous and endocrine systems is crucial in maintaining homeostasis and coordinating physiological reactions to internal and external stimuli. Neurotransmitters and hormones together regulate several bodily functions, including metabolism, growth, and stress.

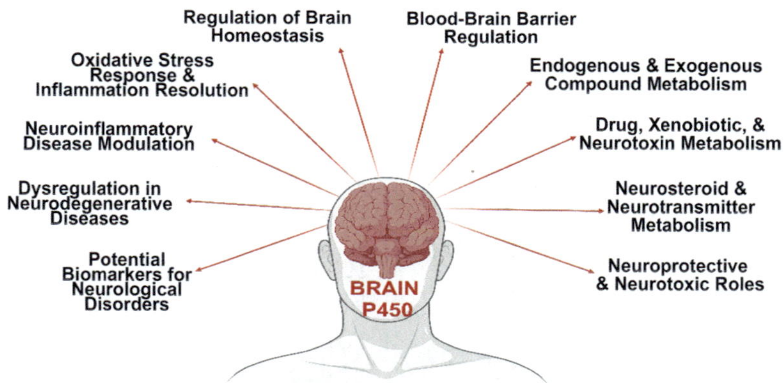

Figure 14.3. Neurotransmitters and hormones collaboratively regulate various bodily functions, including metabolism, growth, and stress responses.

Source: https://www.mdpi.com/jox/jox-15-00044/article_deploy/html/images/jox-15-00044-g001.png.

One such delicate feedback mechanism that maintains energy balance is the relationship between catecholamines released by the adrenal medulla and insulin released from the pancreas. Dysregulation of this interaction is responsible for metabolic disorders such as type 2 diabetes and hypertension, both prevalent diseases explained in current literature that illustrate their interaction and pathogenesis (Zheng et al., 2010).

Neurotoxicity, as discussed in current literature, also interrupts this delicate equilibrium with harmful neurological and metabolic consequences (Brust et al., 2014). Therefore, understanding how these systems interact is essential in developing effective treatments for endocrine and metabolic diseases and ultimately enhancing patient outcomes (Figure 14.3).

14.1.6. Importance of Homeostasis

Homeostasis is critical in maintaining a stable inner environment to allow organisms to work properly despite fluctuations in the external world. For endocrine and metabolic disease, this equilibrium is particularly critical since the disruption of homeostatic mechanisms will lead to radical physiological impacts. For instance, persistent low-grade inflammation, recently recognized as a contributor to obesity and metabolic syndrome, reduces insulin sensitivity and metabolism overall, illustrating the role of homeostatic mechanisms in the inhibition of such activities through adaptive mechanisms (Cheng et al., 2014).

In addition, the multifaceted interaction of various tissues involved in energy regulation illustrates the complexity of metabolic homeostasis. The enteroendocrine cell hormone signaling pathways, as illustrated by the Bursicon α/DLgr2 system of Drosophila, illustrate that inter-organ communication is pivotal in maintaining metabolic homeostasis as well as acquiring resistance to environmental stress (Bauer et al., 2019). Therefore, understanding the significance of homeostasis offers crucial information for the advancement of endocrine and metabolic illness regulation.

14.1.7. Common Diagnostic Tests for Endocrine Function

Evaluation of endocrine function is essential in the diagnosis of various hormonal disorders, which involves using standard diagnostic tests that often measure serum hormone levels. Such tests primarily measure major hormones such as thyroid-stimulating hormone (TSH), free thyroid hormones (FT3, FT4), and cortisol, among others, to check for conditions such as hypothyroidism and adrenal insufficiency. For instance, in patients with obstructive sleep apnea (OSA), awareness of potential thyroid dysfunction can enhance clinical practice since recent studies point towards the association of thyroid health and sleep-breathing disorders (Kumari et al., 2025).

Besides, congenital hypothyroidism is a relevant endocrine problem in genetic diseases like NKX2-1-related disorders, wherein detection during early neonatal screening and follow-up hormonal evaluation is essential for appropriate management (Carmona-Hidalgo et al., 2024). Not only do the tests facilitate accurate disease identification, but they also direct management strategies in endocrine and metabolic diseases (Figure 14.4).

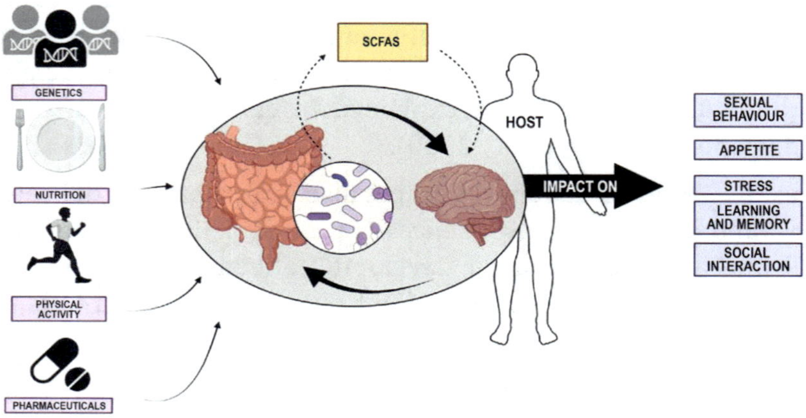

Figure 14.4. The assessment of endocrine function is crucial for diagnosing various hormonal disorders, necessitating the application of common diagnostic tests that often include serum hormone level measurements.

Source: https://www.mdpi.com/biomedicines/biomedicines-12-00221/article_deploy/html/images/biomedicines-12-00221-g001.png.

14.1.8. Effects of Aging on the Endocrine System

When individuals age, the endocrine system changes dramatically, with a significant impact on metabolic processes and overall health. The decline in the levels of hormones, particularly sex hormones such as estrogen and testosterone, is to blame for most of the diseases, including osteoporosis, cardiovascular disease, and metabolic syndrome. This loss can also be augmented by environmental factors, e.g., exposure to endocrine disruptors like bisphenol A (BPA), which interfere with hormonal signaling pathways and enhance severity of conditions like polycystic ovarian syndrome (PCOS) in premenopausal women, highlighting the intricate interaction between environmental influences and aging on endocrine function (Mukhopadhyay et al., 2022). Furthermore, endocrine secretion alterations and enhanced insulin resistance with aging can contribute to increased risk of diabetes and obesity, both of which are key components of metabolic diseases (Rinella et al., 2023). Therefore, it is crucial to understand the multifaceted effects of aging on the endocrine system to develop efficient interventions and treatment plans for the elderly.

14.1.9. Emerging Research in Endocrinology

The field of endocrinology is rapidly advancing, particularly about the relationship between metabolic disease and hormone control. Current studies highlight the intricate relationships between energy metabolism and endocrine function, with particular focus on the role of sirtuins, particularly SIRT1. This NAD+-dependent deacetylase has been found to inversely correlate with various adiposity markers, such as epicardial fat thickness, suggesting its possible functions in disorders like anorexia nervosa and obesity (Barbaro et al., 2018). Anorexia nervosa (AN) is a condition traditionally characterized by severe caloric restriction and leads to extreme endocrine adaptations affecting fertility and overall health, rendering the clinical situation even more complicated (Ciobanu et al.,

2020). Though these studies uncover the neuroendocrine pathways that bridge the link between metabolism and psychosocial determinants, unraveling these in more depth may unveil novel avenues of therapeutic interventions to treat endocrine and metabolic disorders better (Figure 14.5).

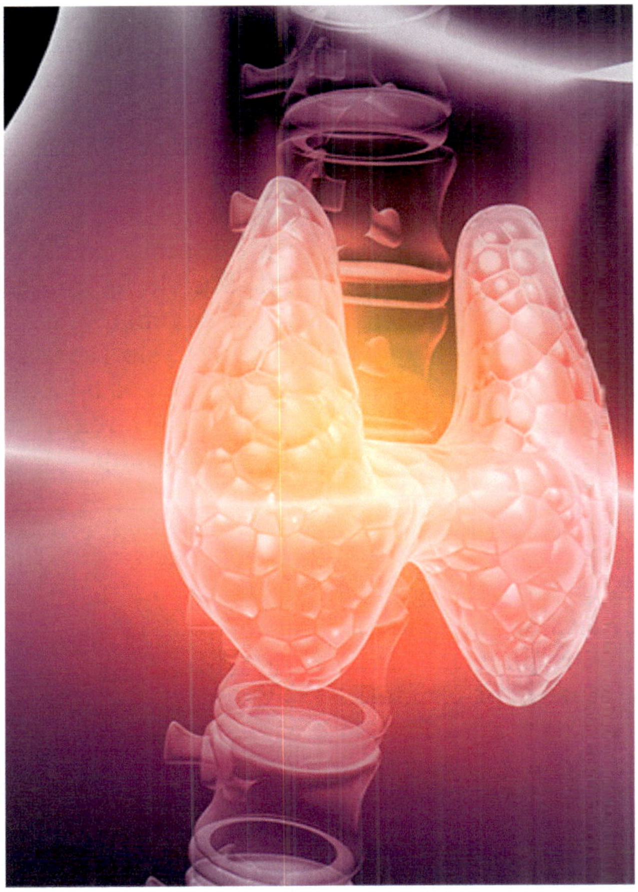

Figure 14.5. The field of endocrinology is experiencing significant advancements, particularly concerning the interplay between metabolic disorders and hormonal regulation.

Source: https://cdn.healthturkiye.com/images/endocrinology-and-metabolic-diseases_f0182b13.jpg.

Test Your Knowledge

1. What is the role of negative feedback in endocrine regulation?
2. Explain how the hypothalamus and pituitary gland coordinate endocrine activity

14.2. Common Endocrine Disorders

Learning Outcome

1. Explain types and causes of diabetes mellitus
2. Know symptoms and treatment of hypothyroidism
3. Discuss diagnosis and management of hyperthyroidism
4. Describe Cushing's syndrome
5. Focus on Addison's disease
6. Understand polycystic ovary syndrome (PCOS)
7. Explain growth hormone deficiency: causes and treatments
8. Discuss hyperparathyroidism: diagnosis and management
9. Explain the evaluation and treatment of thyroid nodules

Shared endocrine disorders are a range of hormonal imbalance conditions that have significant implications for physical and mental health. One very prominent example is PCOS, which is known to cause an array of complications, including infertility, metabolic syndrome, and psychiatric disorders like anxiety and depression. PCOS women face challenges that influence their social and personal functioning, and this calls for a multidisciplinary treatment plan that guarantees total well-being and quality of life (Annagur et al., 2018). Secondly, exposure to environmental toxicants is now a critical concern linked to endocrine diseases. Environmental toxins can interfere with hormonal action and lead to adverse effects on health, like premature delivery and developmental disabilities (Hitchcock et al., 2011). Together, these factors underscore the sheer complexity of managing endocrine diseases, wherein internal physiological mechanisms as well as external environmental influences play an important role in their etiology and progression.

14.2.1. Diabetes Mellitus: Types and Causes

Diabetes Mellitus, both Type 1 and Type 2 forms, is an example of an endocrine-metabolic disease characterized by chronic hyperglycemia resulting from insulin resistance or impaired insulin secretion. Type 1 diabetes is an autoimmune condition leading to the destruction of pancreatic beta cells responsible for insulin production and typically develops in early life. On the other hand, Type 2 diabetes, which is responsible for the majority of the disease, is most commonly associated with obesity and lack of physical activity, illustrating the epidemic of overweight in contemporary society, where barely two-thirds of adults are in the overweight or obese group.

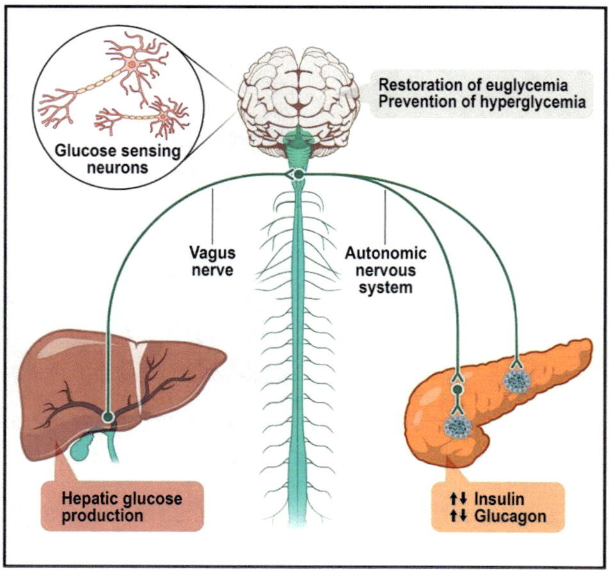

Figure 14.6. Diabetes Mellitus, encompassing Type 1 and Type 2 forms, exemplifies a spectrum of endocrine and metabolic disorders characterized by chronic hyperglycemia due to insulin resistance or inadequate insulin secretion.

Source: https://www.cell.com/cms/10.1016/j.cell.2024.06.029/asset/2842281c-1a56-461c-a625-3d122eb5f1ba/main.assets/gr2_lrg.jpg.

The interlink between obesity and insulin resistance is paramount; low-grade inflammation based on adipose tissue fuels the phenomenon, and metabolic dysregulation (Man et al., 2024). Also, there is new evidence of a distressing correlation between long COVID-19 syndrome and the onset of insulin resistance, underlining the necessity of comprehensive approaches to address viral diseases as well as metabolic disease (Man et al., 2024) (Figure 14.6).

14.2.2. Hypothyroidism: Symptoms and Treatment

Hypothyroidism, a frequent endocrine illness, has a broad spectrum of manifestations like fatigue, weight gain, and depression, with a significant impact on the quality of life of the patient. Diagnosis is typically established by elevated serum TSH levels and normal free thyroid hormones, subclinical ones having TSH levels between 4.5–10 mIU/L. Levothyroxine replacement therapy is the primary treatment, which can effectively restore thyroid hormone levels and alleviate most symptoms. However, treatment of subclinical hypothyroidism clinically is contentious, particularly when to initiate treatment; there is consensus that treatment should be tailored following patient-specific factors, as there are no strict guidelines (Aversa et al., 2016). In addition, the intricacies of thyroid function can also impact sexual health, highlighting the harmony between endocrine regulation and overall well-being, illustrating how thyroid hormones are significant not only for metabolic functions but also for considerations such as sexual desire and arousal (Aversa et al., 2016).

14.2.3. Hyperthyroidism: Diagnosis and Management

Hyperthyroidism, a condition of overproduction of the thyroid hormones, needs an appropriate and multi-modal treatment process for its proper diagnosis and handling within the overall context of endocrine and metabolic disease. A doctor prefers to employ serum testing of free thyroxine (FT4) and TSH levels, with low TSH being the marker of hyperthyroidism. The treatment may include the use of antithyroid medications, radioactive iodine, and thyroidectomy in exceptional cases. Particularly in the elderly patient, the complexity of the treatment is enhanced due to the potential presence of related conditions, as observed in studies associating chronic conditions such as primary hyperparathyroidism (PHPT) with transient thyrotoxicosis that complicates the recovery from surgical interventions (Armanini et al., 2015). Besides, research has established that subclinical hyperthyroidism heightens the risk of cardiovascular events, necessitating close observation of such patients to avert long-term complications (Auer et al., 2013). Therefore, fine management measures are crucial in averting the intricate implications of hyperthyroidism (Figure 14.7).

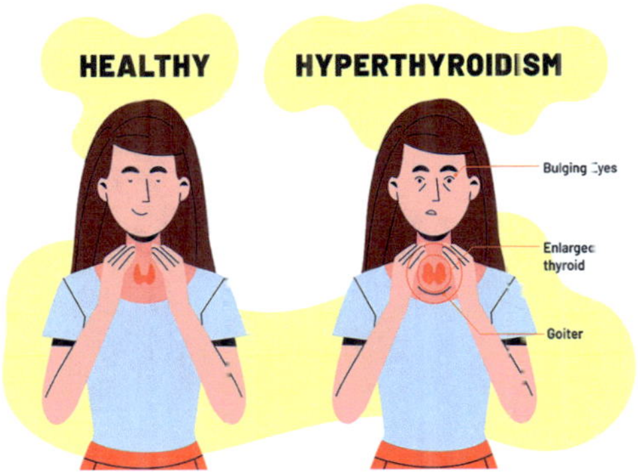

Figure 14.7. Hyperthyroidism.

Source: https://images.onlymyhealth.com/imported/images/2023/March/21_Mar_2023/Main_Hyperthyroidism.jpg.

14.2.4. Cushing's Syndrome: Causes and Effects

Cushing's syndrome, with its presenting

symptom of chronic exposure to supraphysiological concentrations of cortisol, expresses itself in a variety of metabolic and physiological derangements with a significant impact on patient health. The syndrome can present with several causes, such as pituitary adenomas (Cushing's disease), adrenal tumors, or ectopic ACTH secretion, the latter being present in approximately 15% of cases and often in association with malignancies such as small cell lung cancer, which can have sudden and aggressive impacts on metabolism (Martínez-Valles et al., 2009). The consequences of this illness reach far, and morbidity rates caused by cardiovascular disease, infection, and mental handicaps like mental exhaustion and executive functioning impairment, even after treatment, are higher (Martínez-Valles et al., 2009). Most importantly, remitted patients continue to risk greater hazards of critical complications like stroke and thromboembolism that necessitate life-long monitoring and treatment for their condition (Papakokkinou et al., 2022). Therefore, it is critical to comprehend the etiology and consequences of Cushing's syndrome in treating this multifaceted endocrine disease.

14.2.5. Addison's Disease: Symptoms and Treatment Options

Addison's disease or adrenal insufficiency is marked by a range of disabling manifestations, the most common of which are fatigue, weight loss, and hyperpigmentation of the skin. Hyponatremia and hyperkalemia are commonly seen in patients and, if left untreated, can lead to cardiovascular sequelae.

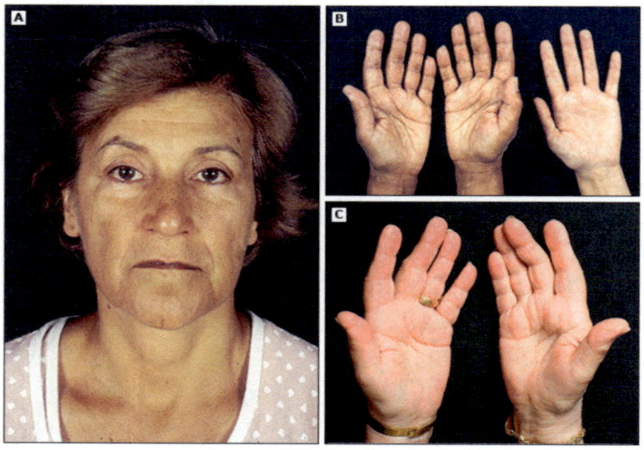

Figure 14.8. Addison's disease.

Source: https://www.uptodate.com/services/app/contents/graphic/view/ENDO/74922/HyperpigmentAddisonsdis.jpg.

The pathophysiology of Addison's disease may be autoimmune, and certain patients might also present with primary ovarian insufficiency (POI), complicating their presentation; research indicates that as many as 10.2% of women presenting with Addison's can develop POI, where sudden hormonal fall warrants proper management of reproductive status (Vogt et al., 2023). Management is usually lifelong hormone replacement therapy, initially with glucocorticoids to achieve normalization of cortisol levels, in addition to mineralocorticoids to manage aldosterone deficiency. However, corticosteroid therapy has the potential to produce side effects such as hyperglycemia, which increases the risk for metabolic dysfunction complications, and thus must be monitored closely (Barathi et al., 2011). In the end, effective treatment of Addison's disease involves a raincoat strategy that addresses both the control of symptomatology and the reconditioning of the underlying hormone (Figure 14.8).

14.2.6. Polycystic Ovary Syndrome (PCOS): Overview and Implications

PCOS is a complex endocrine and metabolic disorder that affects a high percentage of women of reproductive age. Characterized by a triad of findings of ovulatory dysfunction, hyperandrogenism, and polycystic ovaries, PCOS is associated with a range of metabolic consequences, with obesity and insulin resistance being most significant. All these etiological factors synergize to aggravate the condition, and their complications lead to infertility and long-term health consequences. Studies indicate that the impact of obesity on reproductive health is considerable, not only interfering with the hormonal balance but also creating a cycle of weight gain and psychosocial stress around fertility issues, verifying the research of Zheng et al. (2024).

In addition, new research highlights the microbiome's role in shaping reproductive disorders such as PCOS by indicating a relationship between gut health and estrogen metabolism, further pointing to the importance of understanding these relationships in effective management of PCOS, as highlighted in Elkafas et al. (2022).

14.2.7. Growth Hormone Deficiency: Causes and Treatments

Growth hormone deficiency (GHD) is a polyetiological endocrine disorder with inadequate secretion of growth hormone (GH) by the pituitary gland. GHD can be caused by multiple etiologies, including mutations, tumors, or destruction of the pituitary region as a result of trauma or radiation treatment. The effects of GHD are not limited to subnormal growth in children; in adults, it has significant metabolic implications, such as obesity, insulin resistance, and reduced bone mineral content, giving an added risk for cardiovascular disease (Smith et al., 2022).

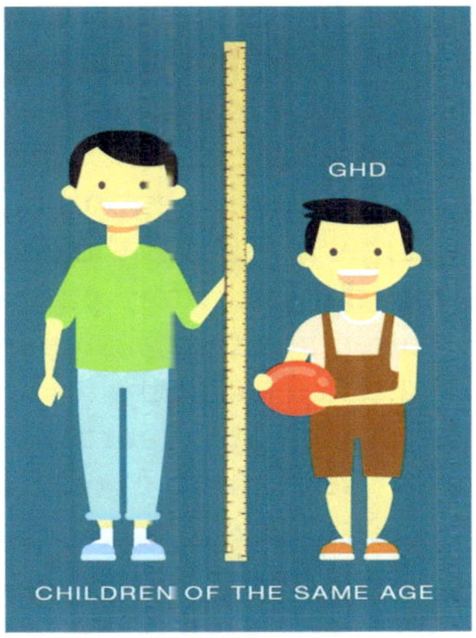

Figure 14.9. Growth hormone deficiency (GHD) is a complex endocrine disorder characterized by inadequate production of growth hormone (GH) from the pituitary gland.

Source: https://www.endocrine.org/-/media/endocrine/images/patient-engagement-webpage/condition-page-images/rare-endocrine-diseases/growth_hormone_deficiency_pe_1796x943_.jpg.

The cure depends primarily on somatropin hormone replacement therapy with a man-made growth hormone administered through once-daily injections. Despite its efficacy in improving metabolic profiles and quality of life, adherence to somatropin administration remains a challenge, particularly among adults (Smith et al., 2022). Thus, a better understanding of the etiology of GHDs and the limitations to effective management is critical in maximizing patient benefits in the field of endocrine and metabolic disorders (Figure 14.9).

14.2.8. Hyperparathyroidism: Diagnosis and Management

Diagnosis and management of hyperparathyroidism (HPTH) is an issue in endocrine and metabolic disease. Typically picked up by screening blood investigations with elevated serum calcium and parathyroid hormone, HPTH can often present asymptotically in the elderly. However, the occurrence of osteoporosis and the potential for all-cause increased mortality make an active treatment approach necessary. Effective management regimes are at times supplemented by parathyroid surgery, which is the only absolute treatment for the disorder, particularly in susceptible patients whose postoperative care requires heightened scrutiny to preventable hazards like transient hypercortisolism or thyrotoxicosis (Armanini et al., 2015). In addition, a precise knowledge of parathyroid hormone and bone health interaction is critical because abnormalities enhance osteoporotic predispositions, leading to grievous orthopedic problems (Bagimani et al., 2022). Therefore, a multidisciplinary therapeutic plan is required to achieve optimal patient outcomes.

14.2.9. Thyroid Nodules: Evaluation and Treatment

Diagnosis and management of thyroid nodules are key aspects in the treatment of endocrine and metabolic disorders. Thyroid nodules, now increasingly common among the general population, must be well evaluated to distinguish benign from malignant lesions. Ultrasound scanning plays a key role in the evaluation process, providing accurate imaging that helps characterize the nodule. Furthermore, fine-needle aspiration biopsy is usually employed to obtain cytological samples in the event of suspected malignancy. The therapeutic regimen may vary widely based on the nature of the nodules and individual factors. In subclinical thyroid disease, as in extensive reports within recent literature, the growing concern is regarding sequelae of long duration of untreated conditions, which emphasizes the need for thorough evaluation and early intervention to prevent hazards like cardiovascular complications (Biondi et al., 2008) and latent thyroid dysfunction due to treatments for diseases like Hodgkin lymphoma (Allocati et al., 2022) (Figure 14.10).

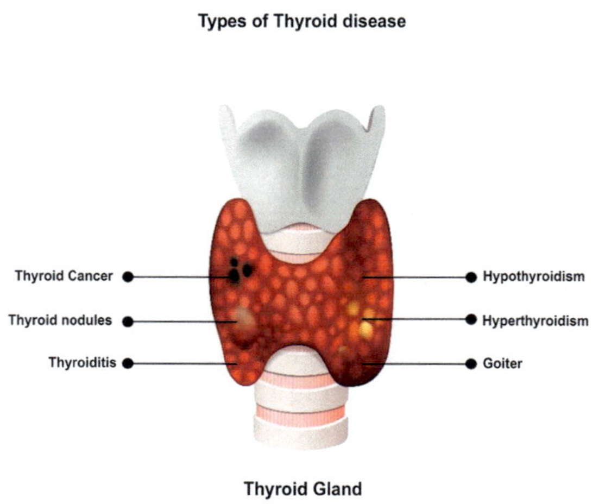

Figure 14.10. Thyroid nodules, which are increasingly common in the general population, necessitate careful assessment to distinguish between benign and malignant lesions.

Source: https://www.frontiersin.org/files/Articles/1218320/fendo-14-1218320-HTML/image_m/fendo-14-1218320-g001.jpg.

Test Your Knowledge

1. What are the hormonal abnormalities found in Cushing's syndrome?
2. What are the signs and symptoms of Addison's disease?

14.3. Metabolic Disorders

Learning Outcome

1. Learn the definition and types of metabolic disorders
2. Focus on risk factors and consequences of metabolic syndrome
3. Identify causes, health risks, and management of obesity
4. Discuss causes and treatment options for hyperlipidemia
5. phenylketonuria (PKU): genetic implications and management
6. Describe galactosemia and glycogen storage diseases
7. Understand mitochondrial disorders
8. Know the importance of nutrition in metabolic Health

Metabolic diseases are a significant juncture point between endocrine function and general health, deeply impacting multiple systems of the body. Such conditions, such as obesity, diabetes, and insulin resistance, commonly develop as the result of interactions among genetic predisposition, environmental influences, and lifestyle factors. In particular, OSA illustrates the relationship between endocrine disturbances and metabolic dysregulation, particularly because it affects the hypothalamic-pituitary-gonadal axis and contributes to some components of the metabolic syndrome, such as hypertension and glycemic dysregulation (Goswami et al., 2025). Furthermore, aging worsens metabolic challenges because elderly individuals tend to report chronic sleep issues, which also hinder metabolic wellness (Estrine et al., 2003). Thus, metabolic disorder treatment needs a multi-faceted approach that addresses both hormonal imbalance and lifestyle modification, therefore revealing the interconnectedness of endocrine and metabolic functions. Heightened awareness of these interdependencies also helps optimize the efficacy of treatments for those afflicted.

14.3.1. Definition and Types of Metabolic Disorders

Metabolic disorders include a broad group of conditions with disturbances of normal metabolic processes, which impair the body's capacity to use food for the generation of energy. These disorders can all be generalized into various types, ranging from diabetes mellitus, metabolic syndrome, and obesity-related disorders.

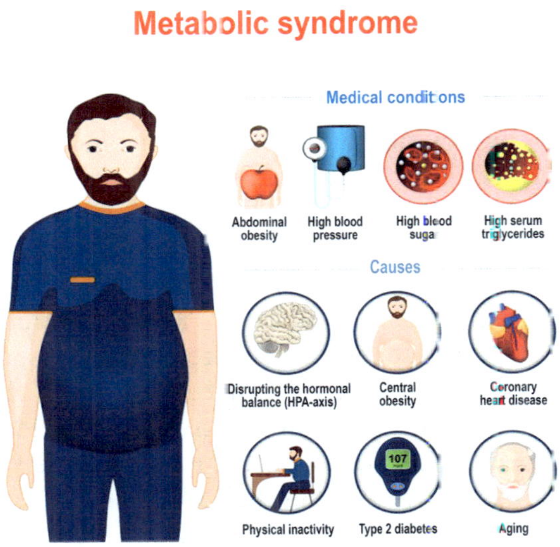

Figure 14.11. Metabolic disorders.

Source: https://relatyv.com/wp-content/uploads/2023/05/metabolic-syndrome-illustration.webp.

Diabetes mellitus is one of the common metabolic disorders that is mainly characterized by problems with insulin function and production, causing persistent hyperglycemia. Metabolic syndrome is particularly significant as it is a cluster of risk factors, such as high blood pressure, blood glucose, and triglycerides, that together elevate the risk for cardiovascular disease and diabetes (Michael et al., 2017). Additionally, lifestyle factors, including diet, are likewise determinants in managing metabolic disorders; for instance, adherence to the

Mediterranean diet, which is rich in healthy fats like extra virgin olive oil, has been shown to provide cardioprotective benefits, thereby ensuring metabolic health (Cammisotto et al., 2017). Understanding these definitions and categories is crucial for comprehensive healthcare strategies in treating endocrine and metabolic disorders (Figure 14.11).

14.3.2. Metabolic Syndrome: Risk Factors and Consequences

The presence of metabolic syndrome has become a significant health concern, in large part due to its association with multiple risk factors and potential endpoints. Central obesity, insulin resistance, hypertension, and dyslipidemia collectively characterize the syndrome, placing carriers at risk for type 2 diabetes and cardiovascular disease. The interaction of genetic predisposition and lifestyle, that is, diet and physical inactivity, increases these risks of developing systemic illness. Specifically, conditions such as PCOS demonstrate the two-dimensionality of metabolic disease because PCOS-affected women are highly prone to obesity and insulin resistance and therefore have increased cardiovascular risks (Wójcik et al., 2020). Moreover, disorders such as poor sleep and OSA can play a critical role in determining metabolic health, which accentuates the importance of overall management strategies for addressing these related issues (Nguyen et al., 2023). The management of metabolic syndrome is necessary to reduce long-term health outcomes and improve the overall quality of life.

14.3.3. Obesity: Causes, Health Risks, and Management

The increasing prevalence of obesity has stepped into the limelight due to its wide-ranging implications for health, particularly concerning endocrine and metabolic diseases. Obesity, which can result in disorders like Type II Diabetes Mellitus and PCOS, is typically the result of complex interplay between genetic, environmental, and behavioral variables rather than being a direct result of calorie intake. The rising prevalence of Type II Diabetes, previously exclusive to adults, is now desperately rising in children, and the demand for early interventions in modifiable risks such as physical activity and diet (Kapke et al., 2015). Concurrently, PCOS, also prevalent in reproductive-aged women, demonstrates the interrelation between obesity and insulin resistance, highlighting weight management as a primary intervention (Ghazeeri et al., 2021). Effective management strategies, therefore, must incorporate lifestyle modifications to the specific needs of individual cases, highlighting the pivotal role of obesity in the broader endocrine and metabolic context (Figure 14.12).

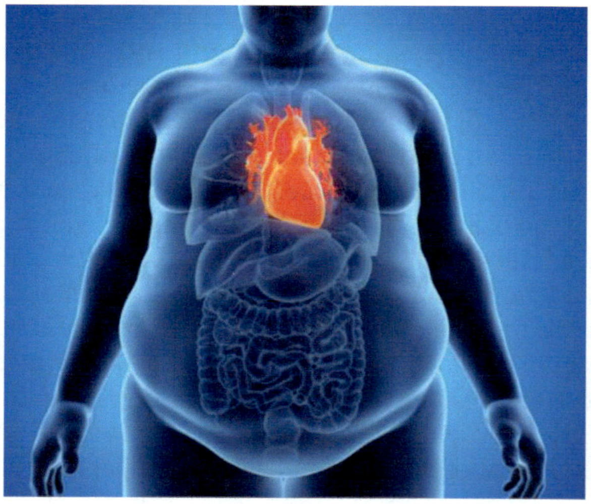

Figure 14.12. Obesity.

Source: https://www.dicardiology.com/sites/default/files/styles/content_feed_large_new/public/DAIC%20ESC%20Journal%20on%20Obesity_0.jpg?itok=jPAW5-Zw.

14.3.4. Hyperlipidemia: Causes and Treatment Options

Hyperlipidemia or elevated blood levels of

lipids is a health-damaging disorder with morbidity risks including cardiovascular disease and pancreatitis. Hyperlipidemia is a polygenic disorder, encompassing genetic syndromes such as familial hypercholesterolemia, lifestyle-related problems such as diet and physical inactivity, and metabolic disorders such as diabetes and hypothyroidism. The interplay between these variables necessitates an integrative treatment approach, in the majority of instances consisting of lifestyle modification, such as increased physical activity and diet alteration in the context of decreasing intake of saturated fats. Pharmacotherapy, and more specifically statins, is a cornerstone in the management of hyperlipidemia in lowering low-density lipoprotein (LDL) cholesterol. In addition, according to the standards for the treatment of conditions related to PCOS, an individualized treatment plan is indicated to address not just hyperlipidemia, but also associated underlying metabolic or endocrine disease (Speiser et al., 2018; Teede et al., 2018). This multifaceted approach emphasizes the necessity of individualized interventions to improve patient outcomes in treating hyperlipidemia.

14.3.5. Phenylketonuria (PKU): Genetic Implications and Management

Phenylketonuria (PKU) is a metabolic disease that is caused by genetics and involves the inability of the body to break down phenylalanine, an amino acid contained in most protein-containing food, because the enzyme phenylalanine hydroxylase is deficient in it. The result of such deficiency is the buildup of phenylalanine, which, if left untreated, will cause serious neurological impairment and mental retardation.

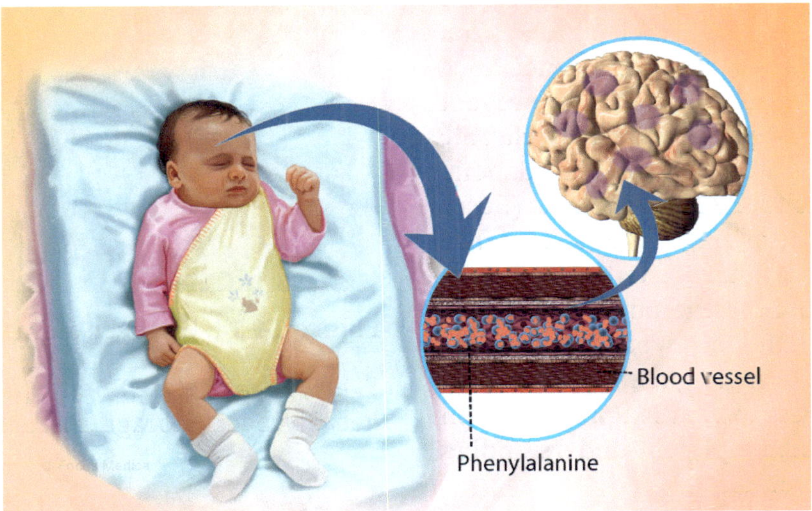

Figure 14.13. Phenylketonuria.

Source: https://th.bing.com/th?id=OCII.50AC6CE762CB97FD1F25437C8DA422C1B7941BBEBFB3D28B0D87886B989F5271&w=1606&p=0.

The genetic cause of PKU underscores the importance of early detection through newborn screening to allow for the initiation of dietary management interventions to avoid its effects. Patients are usually placed on a rigid low-phenylalanine diet, supplemented by special medical foods, to ensure adequate nutrition while not attaining neurotoxic levels of phenylalanine. Current advances in metabolic research show an integrative strategy for the management of

PKU, optimizing treatment outcome through diet, genetic counseling, and new treatments, as stressed in materials discussing the genetic, psychological, and behavioral aspects of metabolic disorders (Suárez et al., 2023) and chronic care management health care transition considerations (Dahir et al., 2021) (Figure 14.13).

14.3.6. Galactosemia: Symptoms and Dietary Management

Galactosemia, a congenital metabolic disorder resulting from galactose-1-phosphate uridylyl transferase (GALT) deficiency, is defined predominantly in the neonatal stages with symptoms such as jaundice, vomiting, and lethargy. Despite the initial dietary treatment that abolishes galactose intake being effective for reducing potentially lethal symptoms in neonates, patients typically suffer debilitating long-term sequelae such as intellectual deficiency and reproductive impairment. Research has consistently shown that adherence to a galactose-restricted diet is essential to prevent acute crises, yet most patients develop chronic sequelae, including POI and decreased bone mineral density, in about 80% of patients (Berry et al., 2019). Furthermore, the new evidence also points toward heterogeneity in clinical presentation because of differences in the time of dietary therapy and genotypes (Eissa et al., 2024). These results highlight the importance of continued studies and patient registries in enhancing galactosemia patient understanding and treatment outcomes.

14.3.7. Glycogen Storage Diseases: Overview and Treatment

Glycogen storage diseases (GSDs) are a group of inherited conditions characterized by abnormal storage of glycogen due to enzyme deficiencies in the glycogen metabolism process. GSDs present with various clinical manifestations, including hypoglycemia, weakness, and hepatomegaly, leading to interference with normal metabolic processes necessary for the production of energy. Therapeutic management of GSDs is usually symptomatic and aimed at avoiding complications, including dietary modification, enzyme supplementation, and liver transplantation in severe cases. Pathophysiology of GSDs is also essential to understand in developing new therapeutic modalities that can improve outcomes in patients. Current literature stresses the significance of accuracy in treatment to target individual enzyme deficiency. However, questions of viable patient risk stratification and management practices are still present, as indicated in recent research (Frantz et al., 2022). The complexity of the diseases is such that ongoing research and development of interventions is essential to provide alleviation from the burden of the diseases on impacted populations (Périard et al., 2021) (Figure 14.14).

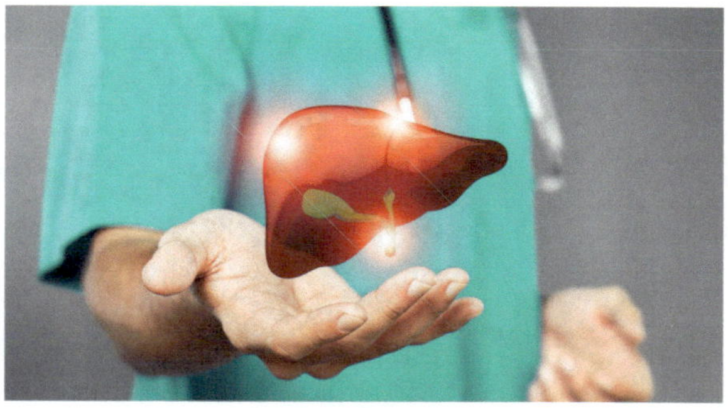

Figure 14.14. Glycogen storage diseases (GSDs).

Source: https://d35oenyzp35321.cloudfront.net/Glycogen_Storage_Disease_d665f5fdaa.jpg.

14.3.8. Mitochondrial Disorders: Causes and Effects

Mitochondrial disorders (MTDs) represent a heterogeneous collection of genetic illnesses that disrupt cellular energy metabolism with a substantial impact on multiple metabolic processes of the organism. These disorders arise from mutations in mitochondrial or nuclear DNA, resulting in defects in oxidative phosphorylation and leading to consequent ATP deficiency. Because energy deficiencies impact high-energy-demanding organs including the heart, brain, and muscles, the results can be catastrophic. Also, the evidence is mounting to link mitochondrial dysfunction with increased oxidative stress that can add to further aggravation of cellular damage and induce such disorders as genomic instability, as revealed by toxic heavy metal and pesticide exposure research (Mood et al., 2021; Alengebawy et al., 2021). The interconnection between MTDs and endocrine and metabolic dysregulations emphasizes the need for a multifaceted approach to treatment, targeting the environmental aspects involved in the production and perpetuation of these disabling disorders.

14.3.9. Importance of Nutrition in Metabolic Health

Nutrition is an essential determinant of metabolic health, with significant implications for the management and prevention of endocrine disease. Most favorable dietary habits, with macronutrient balance and sufficient fiber intake, can improve metabolic function and maintain the hormonal well-being of the body. For instance, regular physical activity, when complemented with appropriate nutritional strategies, has been observed to increase endocrine function and metabolic efficiency, primarily in those who possess multiple endocrine disorders (Tan et al., 2022). Furthermore, dietary fiber intake is required as it maintains intestinal barrier function and may reduce the risk of complications in pancreatic disorders (Badiali et al., 2019). By addressing the nutritional needs of this group, clinicians can play a crucial role in their overall metabolic health, enabling them to better manage their conditions and enhance their quality of life. This merging of healthy nutrition habits is thus central in the interplay between diet and metabolic health outcomes (Figure 14.15).

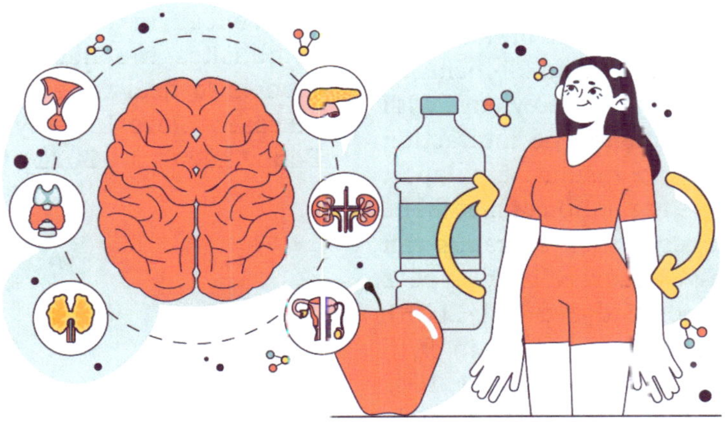

Figure 14.15. Nutrition plays a crucial role in maintaining metabolic health, significantly influencing the management and prevention of endocrine disorders.

Source: https://plminstitute.org/wp-content/uploads/2024/04/Endocrine-Function-Metabolic-Disorders.jpg.

Test Your Knowledge

1. Describe how obesity is linked to endocrine and metabolic dysregulation.
2. What genetic or lifestyle factors contribute to metabolic disorders?

14.4. Diagnosis and Treatment Approaches

Learning Outcome

1. Discuss diagnostic criteria for endocrine disorders
2. Know the role of blood tests in diagnosis
3. Learn imaging techniques for endocrine evaluation
4. Focus on pharmacological treatments for endocrine disorders
5. Understand lifestyle modifications and their impact
6. Describe surgical interventions for specific disorders
7. Know the importance of patient education and self-management
8. Explain the role of multidisciplinary teams in treatment
9. Focus on future directions in treatment and research

Accurate diagnosis and management of endocrine and metabolic disorders require an all-inclusive approach fusing newer scientific knowledge with care depending on the patient. The interaction among hormones such as insulin and leptin plays a critical role in the regulation of metabolic homeostasis, and changes in their secretion can lead to life-threatening diseases such as type 2 diabetes and obesity (Chernyadyeva et al., 2025). Also, the fight against the explosive rise in child obesity necessitates early diagnosis and mass intervention because the disease profoundly affects children's well-being in the future (Marushko et al., 2025). The use of modern diagnostic methods like body mass index (BMI) and waist circumference is a simple tool for detecting the risk group. Of similar significance is the implementation of age, social, and cultural factor-dependent tailored preventive interventions. By combining advanced diagnostic procedures with lifestyle modification methods, clinicians can enhance therapy effectiveness and reduce the long-term sequelae of these metabolic syndromes.

14.4.1. Diagnostic Criteria for Endocrine Disorders

Diagnostic criteria for endocrine disorders, particularly PCOS, are a complex and contentious subject among clinicians. PCOS is characterized by a spectrum of clinical, metabolic, and hormonal abnormalities, and it is not easy to diagnose. The most critical of these criteria is the presence of hyperandrogenism, not only identifying the disorder but also an indication for various health complications, including insulin resistance and reproductive impairment, throughout the lifetime of the individual. It is essential to know these criteria as they dictate the treatment and impact outcomes in assisted reproductive technologies. Additionally, the identification of different PCOS phenotypes establishes the need for individualized diagnosis and treatment since they are associated with differences in reproductive challenges, and establishes the need for precise diagnostic models to deal with endocrine and metabolic diseases more broadly (Gawlik et al., 2022; Badovinac et al., 2022) (Figure 14.16).

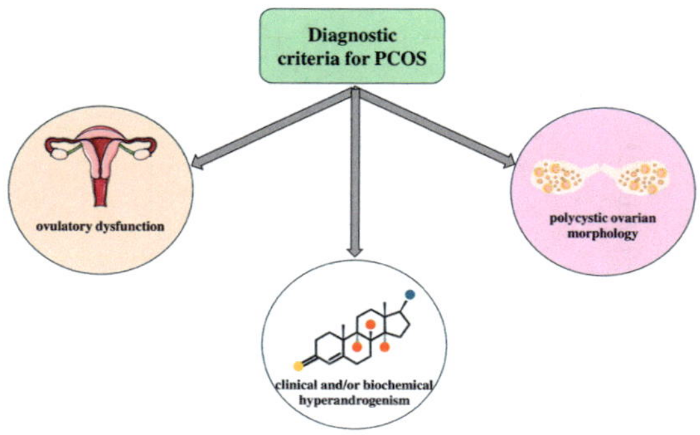

Figure 14.16. The diagnostic criteria for polycystic ovary syndrome (PCOS).

Source: https://www.mdpi.com/medicina/medicina-60-01656/article_deploy/html/images/medicina-60-01656-g001.pngs.

14.4.2. Role of Blood Tests in Diagnosis

Blood tests are a key method of diagnosis for endocrine and metabolic disorders since they can show basic information regarding hormonal levels, glucose metabolism, and the function of organs. For example, for those with MTDs, abnormal blood glucose can indicate metabolic dysfunction, with studies showing that 18.97% of MTD patient populations experienced hypoglycemia symptoms, illustrating the utility of blood testing in managing conditions (Moats et al., 2019). In addition, conditions like PCOS rely on blood testing to assess insulin resistance and hormonal imbalance, which are crucial to precise diagnosis and proper management of the condition (Bernier et al., 2012). Hence, regular blood testing not only aids in the diagnosis of these complex conditions but also enables continued management and treatment strategies, eventually improving patient outcomes and preventing associated complications.

14.4.3. Imaging Techniques for Endocrine Evaluation

Technological advancements in imaging modalities offer significantly enhanced assessment of endocrine disorders. They facilitate precise diagnosis and consequent management action. Imaging modalities such as ultrasound, computed tomography (CT), and magnetic resonance imaging (MRI) are valuable in imaging endocrine glands and identifying structural abnormalities. These consist of cysts or tumors.

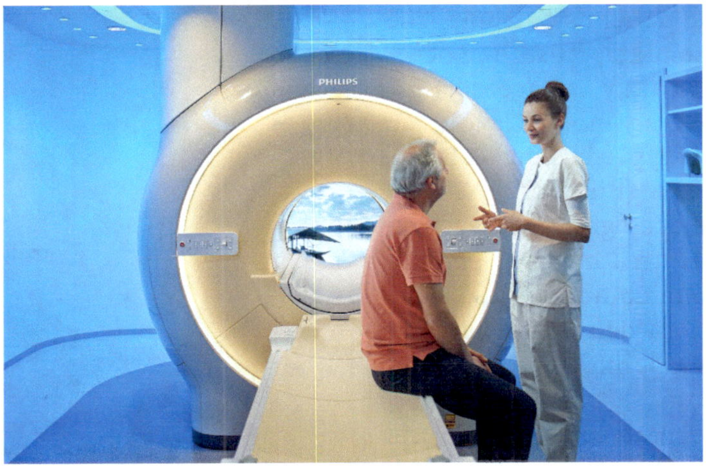

Figure 14.17. Modalities such as ultrasound, computed tomography (CT), and magnetic resonance imaging (MRI) play crucial roles in visualizing endocrine glands, allowing for the identification of structural abnormalities such as tumors or cysts.

Source: https://www.itnonline.com/sites/default/files/field/image/MRI_scanner_with_patient_Philips-Ingenia_1.5T_PR_image.jpg.

Utrad is a locum tenens and an imaging modality. In the evaluation of pituitary adenomas and adrenal tumors, for example, where significant soft tissue contrast enhances diagnostic precision, MRI is beneficial. Further, functional imaging modalities, including positron emission tomography (PET), provide information on metabolic activity, which aids in distinguishing between benign and malignant lesions. All these imaging techniques not only facilitate the diagnosis of various endocrine illnesses but also direct treatment. For instance, in conditions like Turner syndrome, the identification of related anomalies through imaging maximizes the overall treatment of the condition, as evidenced by findings showing the heterogeneous clinical presentation of affected individuals (Abacı et al., 2015) and the contribution of metabolic evaluations (Deanfield et al., 2012) (Figure 14.17).

14.4.4. Pharmacological Treatments for Endocrine Disorders

Pharmacological management of endocrine diseases is increasingly dependent on therapies that aim at the underlying hormonal imbalance as a means of mitigating secondary health complications. For example, in Cushing's syndrome, which is marked by overproduction of cortisol, early pharmacological intervention is crucial in enhancing the patient's outcome. Use of glucocorticoid receptor antagonists and other medications can significantly reduce cortisol levels, eventually reducing mortality due to comorbid conditions like hypertension, diabetes, and cardiovascular disease (Biller et al., 2016). Another facet of pharmacological intervention in endocrinology is the treatment of erectile dysfunction (ED). PDE5 inhibitors represent the initial treatment for ED, which is indicative of the synergy between endocrine regulation and sexual health (Benea et al., 2016). In each case, pharmacologic management not only corrects hormonal dysregulation but enhances overall quality of life, emphasizing the importance of individualized medical therapy in endocrine and metabolic disease.

14.4.5. Lifestyle Modifications and Their Impact

The rising prevalence of metabolic and endocrine diseases mandates a proper understanding of lifestyle changes and their immense impact on health outcomes. Current research supports the fact that even though obesity has a genetic influence, the rapid acceleration of obesity rates in recent decades can, to a considerable degree, be attributable to lifestyle, including excessive consumption of energy-dense foods and limited physical activity (Mahmoud, 2022). These changes can have profound effects on metabolic pathways, leading to obesity-related complications such as diabetes and cardiovascular disease. In addition, the new science of the gut-brain axis highlights how diet shapes the composition of gut microbiota, which can be utilized to modulate mental health and metabolic processes (Cryan et al., 2019). Hence, the use of lifestyle interventions, such as improved nutrition, improved physical activity, and stress management, can correct energy metabolism balance and avoid the risks associated with these disorders, thereby improving general well-being and health (Figure 14.18).

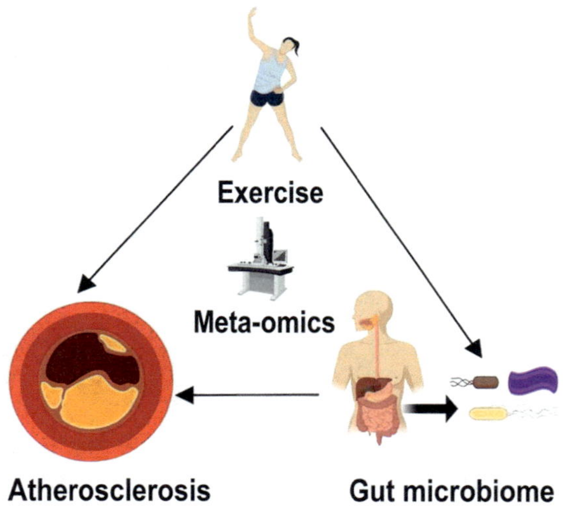

Figure 14.18. The growing prevalence of endocrine and metabolic disorders necessitates a comprehensive understanding of lifestyle modifications and their significant impact on health outcomes.

Source: https://dfzljdn9uc3pi.cloudfront.net/2024/17185/1/fig-2-full.png.

14.4.6. Surgical Interventions for Specific Disorders

Surgical interventions are a determinative factor in the treatment of some endocrine and metabolic diseases, particularly when other treatments cannot provide any relief. For example, surgeries such as adrenalectomy may be applied in situations where patients have adrenal tumors that are responsible for hormone overproduction, making it possible to restore hormonal balance. Additionally, thyroidectomy is generally done to remove malignant or hyperfunctioning thyroid tissue, eliminating conditions such as hyperthyroidism or thyroid cancer. These procedures can significantly mitigate symptoms as well as improve the patient's quality of life. Moreover, gender-affirming surgery within the transgender community showcases the importance of procedures in the therapy of hormonal imbalance related to gender dysphoria. Endocrinologists often accompany these surgical teams, as evident in Arcelus et al. (2018), providing more comprehensive patient care. Hence, surgical procedures not only assist in the cure of endocrine illnesses but also enhance the psychological well-being of the victims, thereby addressing the physiological and psychological health needs.

14.4.7. Importance of Patient Education and Self-Management

Where endocrine and metabolic disorders are being managed, the value of patient education and self-management is immeasurable. Patient empowerment with information makes them well-equipped to comprehend their condition better, ensuring better compliance with treatment and lifestyle changes.

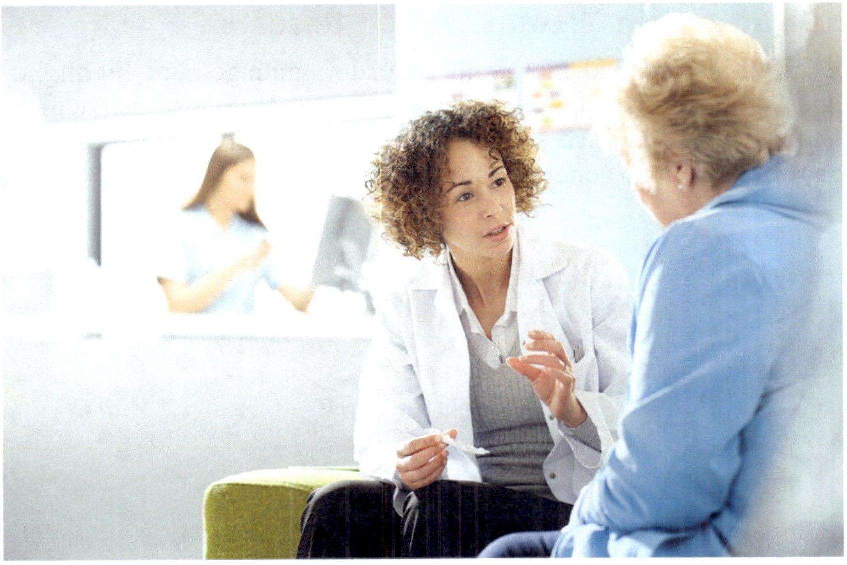

Figure 14.19. Empowering patients with knowledge equips them to better understand their conditions, leading to improved adherence to treatment regimens and lifestyle modifications.

Source: https://www.chenmed.com/sites/default/files/2023-04/Empowering%20Patients%20to%20Improve%20Care%20Plan%20Adherence.jpg.

For instance, lifestyle change, such as exercise and weight management, is critical in hypertensive patients, where drug therapy delay can be sustained through self-care intervention education

(Collard et al., 2014). Moreover, in adrenal insufficiency, a large percentage of patients fail to utilize stress dosing protocols, which can lead to adrenal crisis and hospital admission. Empirical evidence indicates that minimal patients adopt recommended stress dosing even with susceptibility to complications (Goubar et al., 2019). Hence, patient education not only improves individual health outcomes but also reduces healthcare costs by minimizing the complications resulting from endocrine conditions that are not controlled effectively (Figure 14.19).

14.4.8. Role of Multidisciplinary Teams in Treatment

Multidisciplinary teams' involvement is critical to ensuring holistic care and maximum patient outcomes in the management of endocrine and metabolic disorders. Such interdisciplinary teams comprising various healthcare professionals—like endocrinologists, nutritionists, and mental health experts—coordinate with each other to formulate individualized management plans that address the complex presentation of such disorders. For instance, in Prader-Willi syndrome management, a sophisticated genetic disorder with significant metabolic consequences, the medical professional's role as a nutritionist is fundamental in creating efficient dietary treatments and monitoring nutritional status (Barrea et al., 2022). Similarly, in polycystic ovarian syndrome patients, the multidisciplinary approach enhances symptom treatment such as anovulation and insulin resistance, with lifestyle modifications as well as drug therapies like letrozole (Akre et al., 2022). Lastly, the integration of diverse skills within multidisciplinary groups not only increases the efficacy of interventions but also ensures a holistic strategy towards patient health and welfare.

14.4.9. Future Directions in Treatment and Research

The changing face of endocrine and metabolic disorder management highlights the importance of creative strategies to maximize patient outcomes. Emerging research will take advantage of advances in precision medicine, which hold the promise of individualized therapies that account for unique hormonal profiles and genetic histories.

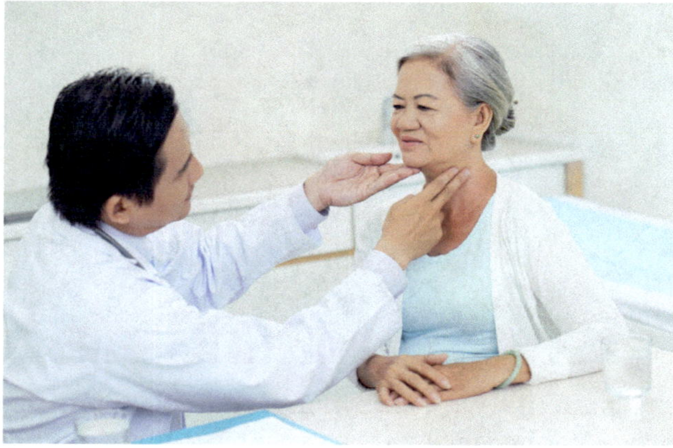

Figure 14.20. The evolving landscape of endocrine and metabolic disorder treatment underscores the need for innovative approaches to enhance patient outcomes.

Source: https://cdn.drstemcellsthailand.com/wp-content/uploads/2025/01/image-55.png.

For instance, developments in reproductive endocrinology have led to enhanced hormone control methods that significantly improve fertility rates, particularly for individuals with endocrine disorders (Laddad et al., 2023). Understanding the role of hormones such as estrogen in embryonic and postnatal health is substantial, as it may guide therapeutic interventions for metabolic illness (Arifzai et al., 2024). With technologies like biomarker-targeted strategies and artificial intelligence (AI) gaining further traction, they pave the way for improved risk stratification and management strategies. Ultimately, cross-disciplinary collaboration will become essential to align the ethics of these advancements with ensuring access to innovative therapies within the field on an equal level (Figure 14.20).

Test Your Knowledge

1. How is hormone replacement therapy used in endocrine disorders?
2. What role does lifestyle modification play in the treatment of metabolic syndrome?

Summary

In conclusion, the relationship between endocrine and metabolic illnesses highlights the complex relationship between hormonal regulation and various physiological functions, and therefore on general well-being. The relevance of lifestyle modifications, such as the intake of healthy fat diets, is emphasized by studies that show protective mechanisms from cardiovascular disease, as exemplified by the role of extra virgin olive oil in the Mediterranean diet that can decrease the incidence of myocardial infarction and stroke (Cammisotto et al., 2017). Moreover, the appearance of acanthosis nigricans in HIV/AIDS patients, which reverses with antiretroviral treatment, explains the intricate biochemical interactions produced by endocrine dysfunction (Vincentiis et al., 2020). This multifaceted view of endocrine and metabolic disease is significant, not just because it is reflected in clinical practice but also in public health policy to temper the wide-ranging consequences of such diseases.

The study of endocrine and metabolic disease reveals several fundamental themes that regulate the understanding of their intricacy. One, variations in individuals' sensitivity to hormones cause genetics to play an essential part in deciding treatment success, particularly when involving GPCR. This heterogeneity can be problematic for clinical approaches, as the contribution of individual receptors can differ between species, and that of chemical ligands is not always effective, evoking challenges in therapeutic intervention (1000 Consortium et al., 2013). Additionally, the necessity for multidisciplinary in the clinical management of hormonal treatment in transgender individuals exemplifies the profound impact of endocrine diseases on physical and mental well-being. There is evidence proving that gender-affirming hormone treatment leads to significant psychosocial improvement, including reduced depression and anxiety (Arcelus et al., 2018). So, the intricate relationship of hormonal, genetic, and psychological factors requires an integrated knowledge base to effectively manage and treat these disorders.

KEY TERMS FROM THIS CHAPTER

- Aldosterone
- Anorexia nervosa
- Bisphenol A (BPA)
- Catecholamines
- Cortisol
- Endocrine
- Endocrine dysfunction
- Endocrinology
- Equilibrium
- Fertility
- Glucagon
- Glucose homeostasis
- Growth Hormone (GH)
- Homeostasis
- Hormones

Critical Thinking Questions

1. **Which hormone is primarily responsible for lowering blood glucose levels?**
   a. Glucagon
   b. Epinephrine
   c. Cortisol
   d. Insulin
2. **Hypothyroidism is commonly treated with:**
   a. Methimazole
   b. Levothyroxine
   c. Propranolol
   d. Hydrocortisone
3. **Which of the following is a long-acting insulin?**
   a. Insulin lispro
   b. Insulin glargine
   c. Insulin aspart
   d. NPH insulin
4. **A common sign of Cushing's syndrome is:**
   a. Weight loss
   b. Hyperpigmentation
   c. Moon face
   d. Bradycardia
5. **Which of the following drugs is used to treat type 2 diabetes by increasing insulin sensitivity?**
   a. Metformin
   b. Glipizide
   c. Acarbose
   d. Sitagliptin

Answers to Critical Thinking Questions

1. (d); 2. (b); 3. (b); 4. (c); 5. (a).

Short Answer Questions

1. What are the major glands of the endocrine system and their primary functions?
2. How do hormones differ from neurotransmitters in their mechanism of action?
3. What are the key clinical features of hypothyroidism and hyperthyroidism?
4. Describe the pathophysiology of Type 1 and Type 2 diabetes mellitus.
5. What is the difference between metabolic syndrome and diabetes mellitus?
6. Explain the pathogenesis of diabetic ketoacidosis (DKA).
7. What laboratory tests are commonly used to diagnose thyroid disorders?
8. How is HbA1c used in the diagnosis and monitoring of diabetes?

References

1. Yeşilkaya, E., Bereket, A., Darendeliler, F., Baş, F., Poyrazoğlu, Ş., Aydın, B. K., Darcan, Ş., Dündar, B., Büyükinan, M., Kara, C., Sarı, E., Adal, E., Akıncı, A., Atabek, M. E., Demirel, F., Çelik, N., Özkan, B., Özhan, B., Orbak, Z., . . . Bondy, C. (2015). Turner syndrome and associated problems in Turkish children: a multicenter study. *Journal of Clinical Research in Pediatric Endocrinology*, *7*(1), 27–36. https://doi.org/10.4274/jcrpe.1771Agius, R. (2013). Review of the risks and/or benefits of thyroxine treatment in 'mild' subclinical hypothyroidism. https://core.ac.uk/download/46602445.pdf (accessed on 10th June 2025).
2. Akre, S., Sharma, K., Chakole, S., & Wanjari, M. (2022). Recent advances in the management of polycystic ovary syndrome: A review article. *Cureus.* https://doi.org/10.7759/cureus.27689.
3. Alengebawy, A., Abdelkhalek, S. T., Qureshi, S. R., & Wang, M. Q. (2021). Heavy metals and pesticides toxicity in agricultural soil and plants: Ecological risks and human health implications. *Toxics, 9*, 42. https://doi.org/10.3390/toxics9030042.
4. Allocati, E., Daniele, A., De Sanctis, V., Di Molfetta, S., Gerardi, C., Giorgino, F., Guarini, A., et al. (2022). Late endocrine and metabolic sequelae and long-term monitoring of classical Hodgkin lymphoma and diffuse large B-cell lymphoma survivors: A systematic review by the Fondazione Italiana Linfomi. https://core.ac.uk/download/541259799.pdf (accessed on 10th June 2025).
5. Annagur, B., Beck, C., Benson, A., Cronin, M., Dennett, A., Dowdy, D., et al. (2018). Polycystic ovary syndrome across the life span of women: A wellness-based integrative intervention. https://core.ac.uk/download/213088882.pdf (accessed on 10th June 2025).
6. Arcelus, J., Gooren, L., Klink, D., T'Sjoen, G., et al. (2018). Endocrinology of transgender medicine. https://core.ac.uk/download/162667742.pdf (accessed on 10th June 2025).
7. Arifzai, R., & Hewadmal, T. K. (2024). The impact of estrogen on embryonic development: A review paper. https://core.ac.uk/download/603903664.pdf (accessed on 10th June 2025).
8. Armanini, D., Bordin, L., Camozzi, V., Donà, G., et al. (2015). Transient hypercortisolism and symptomatic hyperthyroidism associated with primary hyperparathyroidism in an elderly patient: Case report and literature review. https://core.ac.uk/download/53518371.pdf (accessed on 10th June 2025).
9. Auer, R., Collet, T. H., Gencer, B., Rodondi, N., et al. (2013). Subclinical thyroid dysfunction and cardiovascular outcomes among prospective cohort studies. https://core.ac.uk/download/132562998.pdf (accessed on 10th June 2025).
10. Aversa, A., Burnett, A. L., Corona, G., Isidori, A., et al. (2016). Endocrinologic control of men's sexual desire and arousal/erection. https://core.ac.uk/download/54532167.pdf (accessed on 10th June 2025).
11. Badiali, D., Bruno, G., Ribichini, E., Rossi, M., et al. (2019). Role of fiber in nutritional management of pancreatic diseases. https://core.ac.uk/download/231748461.pdf (accessed on 10th June 2025).
12. Bagimani, P., Dadhaniya, R. K., Mahajan, N. P., Mhatre, A., et al. (2022). Case series of orthopedic complications associated with endocrine disorders presented at tertiary care center and review of literature. https://core.ac.uk/download/543133191.pdf (accessed on 10th June 2025).
13. Balali-Mood, M., Naseri, K., Tahergorabi, Z., Khazdair, M. R., & Sadeghi, M. (2021). Toxic

mechanisms of five heavy metals: Mercury, lead, chromium, cadmium, and arsenic. *Frontiers in Pharmacology, 12*, 643972. https://doi.org/10.3389/fphar.2021.643972.

14. Barathi, M. (2011). The effect of oral methylprednisolone pulse on blood sugar. https://core.ac.uk/download/235664160.pdf (accessed on 10th June 2025).
15. Barbaro, G., Basciani, S., Contini, S., Di Giorgio, M. R., et al. (2018). Inverse association of circulating SIRT1 and adiposity: A study on underweight, normal weight, and obese patients. https://core.ac.uk/download/188822504.pdf (accessed on 10th June 2025).
16. Barrea, L., Vetrani, C., Fintini, D., de Alteriis, G., Panfili, F. M., Bocchini, S., Verde, L., et al. (2022). Prader–Willi syndrome in adults: An update on nutritional treatment and pharmacological approach. *Current Obesity Reports, 11*(3), 263–276. https://doi.org/10.1007/s13679-022-00478-w.
17. Bauer, C., Cordero, J. B., Kruspig, B., Maddocks, O. D. K., et al. (2019). A neuronal relay mediates a nutrient responsive gut/fat body axis regulating energy homeostasis in adult *Drosophila*. https://core.ac.uk/download/161513999.pdf (accessed on 10th June 2025).
18. Benea, V., Georgescu, S. R., Mitran, C. I., Mitran, M., et al. (2016). The current treatment of erectile dysfunction. https://core.ac.uk/download/144552982.pdf (accessed on 10th June 2025).
19. Bernier, D. (2012). Polycystic ovary syndrome: Pathogenesis, health consequences, and treatment of PCOS in relation to insulin resistance. https://core.ac.uk/download/72048051.pdf (accessed on 10th June 2025).
20. Berry, G. T., Bosch, A. M., Burnyte, B., Cassiman, D., et al. (2019). The natural history of classic galactosemia: Lessons from the GalNet registry. https://core.ac.uk/download/286060309.pdf (accessed on 10th June 2025).
21. Biller, B. M. K., Colao, A., De Martino, M. C., Isidori, A. M., et al. (2016). Complications of Cushing's syndrome: State of the art. https://core.ac.uk/download/54532161.pdf (accessed on 10th June 2025).
22. Biondi, B., & Cooper, D. S. (2008). The clinical significance of subclinical thyroid dysfunction. https://core.ac.uk/download/54955329.pdf (accessed on 10th June 2025).
23. Brust, J. C. M., Creeley, C. E., Feldman, R., Grandjean, P., Herken, H., Panzica, G., Parent, A. S., et al. (2014). Neurotoxicity. https://core.ac.uk/download/286729125.pdf (accessed on 10th June 2025).
24. Cai, Q., & Oh, Y. (2020). The impact of IGFBP-3/IGFBP-3R system on obesity-associated insulin resistance. *Frontiers in Endocrinology, 3*, 1–4. https://www.semanticscholar.org/paper/c17c8ab07c8c03a39404a1d60c30997fe712f0d0 (accessed on 10th June 2025).
25. Cammisotto, V., Carnevale, R., Castellani, V., D'Amico, M., et al. (2017). Extra virgin olive oil and cardiovascular diseases: Benefits for human health. https://core.ac.uk/download/141695177.pdf (accessed on 10th June 2025).
26. Carmona-Hidalgo, B., Martín-Gómez, C., Herrera-Ramos, E., Rodríguez-López, R., Nou Fontanet, L., Moreno, J. C., Blasco-Amaro, J., et al. (2024). Systematic review of thyroid function in NKX2-1-related disorders: Screening and diagnosis. *PLOS ONE, 19*, Article e0283273. https://www.semanticscholar.org/paper/7824c27f676e16885cb2f338d3b0f4407fabc563 (accessed on 10th June 2025).

27. Carnevale, I., De Santis, E., Limana, F., Perrone, L., et al. (2015). One special question to start with: Can HIF/NFkB be a target in inflammation? https://core.ac.uk/download/54248898.pdf (accessed on 10th June 2025).

28. Cheng, J. X., Cho, K. W., Cozacov, Z., Hu, H. H., et al. (2014). Otopetrin 1 protects mice from obesity-associated metabolic dysfunction through attenuating adipose tissue inflammation. https://core.ac.uk/download/323066532.pdf (accessed on 10th June 2025).

29. Chernyadyeva, T. I., Bontsevich, R., & Gaus, O. V. (2025). Endocrine gastroenterological aspects of metabolic dysfunction. *Experimental and Clinical Gastroenterology.* https://www.semanticscholar.org/paper/272b746029a9d5a90ffa70074959e304362d2042 (accessed on 10th June 2025).

30. Chowdhury, S., Hossain, M. J., Akhter, S., Ahmed, M., & Nasrin, S. (2025). Assessing the prevalence and diagnosis of polycystic ovary syndrome (PCOS) in adolescents: A systematic review. *Scholars International Journal of Obstetrics and Gynecology*. https://www.semanticscholar.org/paper/988afa9b66e847604c0af50f2ee428f57619954c (accessed on 10th June 2025).

31. Ciobanu, C., Fica, S., Poterasu, M., Rowland, J., et al. (2020). Anorexia nervosa and reproduction: Connecting brain to gonads. https://core.ac.uk/download/304672903.pdf (accessed on 10th June 2025).

32. Clark, A. K., Saric-Bosanac, S., Shi, V. Y., Sivamani, R. K., et al. (2020). The role of hypothalamus-pituitary-adrenal (HPA)-like axis in inflammatory pilosebaceous disorders. https://core.ac.uk/download/288432496.pdf (accessed on 10th June 2025).

33. Clemente-Suárez, V. J., Martín-Rodríguez, A., Redondo-Flórez, L., López-Mora, C., Yañéz-Sepúlveda, R., & Tornero-Aguilera, J. F. (2023). New insights and potential therapeutic interventions in metabolic diseases. *International Journal of Molecular Sciences, 24*(13), Article 10672. https://doi.org/10.3390/ijms241310672.

34. Collard, J., Gafane, L., Nell, T., Rennie, K., et al. (2014). Physical activity and hypertension in South African adults. https://core.ac.uk/download/29852228.pdf (accessed on 10th June 2025).

35. Costa, R. M., Lobato, N. S., Neves, K. B., Tostes, R. C., et al. (2018). Perivascular adipose tissue as a relevant fat depot for cardiovascular risk in obesity. https://core.ac.uk/download/153572426.pdf (accessed on 10th June 2025).

36. Coutinho, E. A., & Kauffman, A. S. (2019). The role of the brain in the pathogenesis and physiology of polycystic ovary syndrome (PCOS). https://core.ac.uk/download/323065551.pdf (accessed on 10th June 2025).

37. Cryan, J. F., O'Riordan, K. J., Cowan, C. S. M., Sandhu, K. V., Bastiaanssen, T. F. S., Boehme, M., Codagnone, M. G., et al. (2019). The microbiota-gut-brain axis. *Physiological Reviews, 99*(4), 1877–2013. https://doi.org/10.1152/physrev.00018.2018.

38. Dahir, K., Dhaliwal, R., Simmons, J. H., Imel, E. A., Gottesman, G. S., Mahan, J. D., Prakasam, G., et al. (2021). Health care transition from pediatric- to adult-focused care in X-linked hypophosphatemia: Expert consensus. *The Journal of Clinical Endocrinology & Metabolism, 107*(2), 599–613. https://doi.org/10.1210/clinem/dgab796.

39. De Vincentiis, L., Di Paolo, M., Iacovelli, A., Mezzaroma, I., et al. (2020). A case of acanthosis nigricans in an HIV-infected patient. https://core.ac.uk/download/323192484.pdf (accessed on 10th June 2025).

40. Deanfield, J. E., Jones, A., Jones, R. W., Kowalik, J., et al. (2012). Adiposity is associated with blunted cardiovascular, neuroendocrine and cognitive responses to acute mental stress. https://core.ac.uk/download/9633186.pdf (accessed on 10th June 2025).

41. Desesquelles, A., Meslé, F., Frova, L., Pappagallo, M., Salvatore, M. A., Pace, M., & Egidi, V. (2025). Revisiting the mortality of France and Italy with the multiple-cause-of-death approach. https://core.ac.uk/download/pdf/6544416.pdf (accessed on 10th June 2025).

42. Drew, J. E. (2014). Signaling pathways implicated in obesity-associated cancers. https://core.ac.uk/download/29150956.pdf (accessed on 10th June 2025).

43. Eissa, M. E. (2024). Beyond the usual suspects: Review on exploring rare, emerging and environmentally influenced metabolic disorders. https://core.ac.uk/download/642343200.pdf (accessed on 10th June 2025).

44. Elkafas, H., Walls, M., Al-Hendy, A., & Ismail, N. (2022). Gut and genital tract microbiomes: Dysbiosis and link to gynecological disorders. *Frontiers in Cellular and Infection Microbiology, 12*, 1059825. https://doi.org/10.3389/fcimb.2022.1059825.

45. Estrine, J., & O'Brien, N. (2003). *Sleep, Health, and Aging*. https://core.ac.uk/download/71356671.pdf (accessed on 10th June 2025).

46. Evaristo-Neto, A. D., Sumner, A. E., Ziraba, A. K., Melidonis, A. M., Sadiki, A., Baleke, A., Longo-Mbenza, B., et al. (2016). Obesity and diabetes mellitus association in rural community of Katana, South Kivu, in Eastern Democratic Republic of Congo: Bukavu Observ Cohort study results. https://core.ac.uk/download/74614012.pdf (accessed on 10th June 2025).

47. Frantz, S., Hundertmark, M., Schulz-Menger, J., Bengel, F. M., & Bauersachs, J. (2022). Left ventricular remodeling post-myocardial infarction: Pathophysiology, imaging, and novel therapies. *European Heart Journal, 43*, 2549–2561. https://doi.org/10.1093/eurheartj/ehac223.

48. Fröhlich, E., & Wahl, R. (2019). Microbiota and thyroid interaction in health and disease. *Trends in Endocrinology & Metabolism, 30*(7), 479–490. https://doi.org/10.1016/j.tem.2019.05.008.

49. Gawlik, A., Skrzyńska, K., Aburto-Hernández, C., Barrera, D., Ortiz-Hernández, R., Espinoza-Simón, E., Parra-Gámez, L., et al. (2022). Impaired carbohydrate metabolism and excess of lipid accumulation in offspring of hyperandrogenic mice. *Metabolites, 12*. https://www.semanticscholar.org/paper/a6de84c075303041743981fc6500508105d55c96 (accessed on 10th June 2025).

50. Ghazeeri, G., Hmedeh, C., & Hmedeh, C. (2021). Nutritional management in polycystic ovary syndrome: Challenges and opportunities. https://core.ac.uk/download/161103740.pdf (accessed on 10th June 2025).

51. Goswami, R. (2025). Endocrine and metabolic aspects of OSA. https://core.ac.uk/download/pdf/287211085.pdf (accessed on 10th June 2025).

52. Goubar, T., McGrath, S., Rushworth, R. L., & Torpy, D. J. (2019). Pre-hospital management of acute Addison's disease: Audit of patients attending a referral hospital in a regional area. https://core.ac.uk/download/232131024.pdf (accessed on 10th June 2025).

53. Greenleaf, J. E., & Kaciuba-Uscilko, H. (2025). Acclimatization to heat in humans. https://core.ac.uk/download/pdf/42827514.pdf (accessed on 10th June 2025).

54. Hitchcock, E., & Madsen, T. (2011). *Growing Up Toxic: Chemical Exposures and Increases in*

Developmental Disease. https://core.ac.uk/download/71358334.pdf (accessed on 10th June 2025).

55. Janicka, L., Dajnowska, A., & Arciszewski, M. (2025). Role of proopiomelanocortin (POMC) derivatives in body weight regulation: A review of current knowledge and significance in the pathogenesis of obesity in mammals. *Medycyna Weterynaryjna.* https://www.semanticscholar.org/paper/e05ea4d08172099fabcfc71aacbc8a86d1fbaa0b (accessed on 10th June 2025).
56. Kapke, D. R. (2015). *Childhood Type II Diabetes: The Risks and Complications.* https://core.ac.uk/download/58826199.pdf (accessed on 10th June 2025).
57. Kaye, A., Khaled, M. E., Bembenick, K. N., Lacey, J., Tandon, A., Kelkar, R., Derouen, A. G., et al. (2024). Alkindi Sprinkle for pediatric patients with primary adrenocortical insufficiency: A narrative review. *Cureus, 16.* https://www.semanticscholar.org/paper/8ec43698d4dc8c717fdaf3d4434ea41c067a3774 (accessed on 10th June 2025).
58. Khapoli, I., Elwani, H., Khapoli, A., Dabob, K., & Khapoli, N. (2025). Prevalence of polycystic ovarian disease in Zawia Medical Center. *AlQalam Journal of Medical and Applied Sciences.* https://www.semanticscholar.org/paper/0797bfa4ff307954df11c4f97f0cbddd5084d8a4 (accessed on 10th June 2025).
59. Khoshnia, M., Marjani, A., & Shafaei, A. (2015). Serum level of fibroblast growth factor 21 in type 2 diabetic patients with and without metabolic syndrome. https://core.ac.uk/download/52205725.pdf (accessed on 10th June 2025).
60. Kitahara, C. M., & Schneider, A. B. (2022). Epidemiology of thyroid cancer. *Cancer Epidemiology Biomarkers & Prevention, 31*, 1284–1297. https://doi.org/10.1158/1055-9965.epi-21-1440 (accessed on 10th June 2025).
61. Kumari, R., Saifullah, N., Saifullah, B., Murtaza, B., Bai, K., & Yousuf, M. (2025). Assessing thyroid function in obstructive sleep apnea (OSA) patients: A correlation with sleep severity parameters. *Insights–Journal of Health and Rehabilitation.* https://www.semanticscholar.org/paper/7a71c671b85ede95b65bfb8f1f3253eb80bda7af (accessed on 10th June 2025).
62. Laddad, M., et al. (2023). Recent advances in reproductive endocrinology: Implications for fertility treatment in gynecology. https://core.ac.uk/download/596247493.pdf (accessed on 10th June 2025).
63. Mahmoud, A. M. (2022). An overview of epigenetics in obesity: The role of lifestyle and therapeutic interventions. *International Journal of Molecular Sciences, 23*, 1341. https://doi.org/10.3390/ijms23031341.
64. Man, D. E., Andor, M., Buda, V., Kundnani, N., Duda-Seiman, D., Craciun, L. M., Neagu, M. N., et al. (2024). Insulin resistance in long COVID-19 syndrome. *Journal of Personalized Medicine, 14.* https://www.semanticscholar.org/paper/f2b9eaa65fb253475e24253a3381aecf0f9c862f (accessed on 10th June 2025).
65. Martínez-Valles, M. A., Palafox-Cazarez, A., & Paredes-Avina, J. A. (2009). Severe hypokalemia, metabolic alkalosis and hypertension in a 54-year-old male with ectopic ACTH syndrome: A case report. https://core.ac.uk/download/pdf/8327271.pdf (accessed on 10th June 2025).
66. Marushko, Y., Kryvopustov, S., Khomych, O., Dmytryshyn, O., & Pysariev, A. O. (2025). Modern problems of diagnosis and prevention of obesity in children. *Child's Health.* https://www.semanticscholar.org/paper/bde8379326c8219dca739e01989be1bef64a1440 (accessed on 10th June 2025).

67. Michael, J. R. (2017). *The Relations of Metabolic Syndrome to Anxiety and Depression Symptoms in Children and Adults* [Doctoral dissertation, Indiana University of Pennsylvania]. https://core.ac.uk/download/84397711.pdf (accessed on 10th June 2025).

68. Mladenov, M., Sazdova, I., Hadzi-Petrushev, N., Konakchieva, R., & Gagov, H. (2025). The role of reductive stress in the pathogenesis of endocrine-related metabolic diseases and cancer. *International Journal of Molecular Sciences, 26*(4). https://www.semanticscholar.org/paper/cd1e5aa4c8d644cccb793f5a88aa7ea656733d1d (accessed on 10th June 2025).

69. Moats, A. (2019). *Hypoglycemia in Mitochondrial Disorders* [Master's thesis, University of Texas Medical Branch]. https://core.ac.uk/download/228022820.pdf (accessed on 10th June 2025).

70. Mukhopadhyay, R., Prabhu, N. B., Kabekkodu, S. P., & Padmalatha, S. (2022). Review on bisphenol A and the risk of polycystic ovarian syndrome: An insight from endocrine and gene expression. *Environmental Science and Pollution Research, 29*, 32631–32650. https://doi.org/10.1007/s11356-022-19244-5.

71. Nguyen, D. T., Bricout, V., Tran, H., Pham, V. H., & Duong-Quy, S. (2023). Sleep apnea in people with Down syndrome: Causes and effects of physical activity? *Frontiers in Neurology, 14*. https://www.semanticscholar.org/paper/0ebea1a4e1150ead5bc6ff736d134030dec9bac4 (accessed on 10th June 2025).

72. Papakokkinou, E. (2022). *Clinical Challenges in Cushing's Syndrome* [Thesis, National and Kapodistrian University of Athens]. https://core.ac.uk/download/491189992.pdf (accessed on 10th June 2025).

73. Périard, J. D., Eijsvogels, T. M. H., & Daanen, H. A. M. (2021). Exercise under heat stress: Thermoregulation, hydration, performance implications, and mitigation strategies. *Physiological Reviews, 101*(4), 1873–1979. https://doi.org/10.1152/physrev.00038.2020.

74. Radojčić Badovinac, A., & Smiljan Severinski, N. (2022). Polycystic ovary syndrome phenotypes and infertility treatment. In *Polycystic Ovary Syndrome*. https://www.semanticscholar.org/paper/b3995e453884010ed5145f23eb975a863d131f47 (accessed on 10th June 2025).

75. Rinella, M. E., Neuschwander-Tetri, B. A., Siddiqui, M. S., Abdelmalek, M. F., Caldwell, S. H., Barb, D., Kleiner, D. E., et al. (2023). AASLD practice guidance on the clinical assessment and management of nonalcoholic fatty liver disease. *Hepatology, 77*, 1797–1835. https://doi.org/10.1097/hep.0000000000000323 (accessed on 10th June 2025).

76. Smith, A. R., Manjelievskaia, J., Komirenko, A. S., & Morrow, C. M. (2022). PMON64 Economic burden of growth hormone deficiency in a US adult population. *Journal of the Endocrine Society, 6*, A559–A560. https://www.semanticscholar.org/paper/983e80f6f3c46c5630089b7197d815133b4e9ad6 (accessed on 10th June 2025).

77. Speiser, P., Arlt, W., Auchus, R. J., Baskin, L. S., Conway, G. S., Merke, D. P., Meyer-Bahlburg, H. F. L., et al. (2018). Congenital adrenal hyperplasia due to steroid 21-hydroxylase deficiency: An Endocrine Society clinical practice guideline. *The Journal of Clinical Endocrinology & Metabolism, 103*, 4043–4088. https://doi.org/10.1210/jc.2018-01865.

78. Tan, A., Pitt, J., McCarthy, O., Churm, R., & Bracken, R. (2022). Passing on the exercise baton: What can endocrine patients learn from elite athletes? https://core.ac.uk/download/491178312.pdf (accessed on 10th June 2025).

79. Teede, H., Misso, M., Costello, M., Dokras, A., Laven, J. S. E., Moran, L., Piltonen, T., et al. (2018).

Recommendations from the international evidence-based guideline for the assessment and management of polycystic ovary syndrome. *Clinical Endocrinology, 89*(3), 251–268. https://doi.org/10.1111/cen.13795.

80. Vogt, E. C. (2023). *Epidemiology and Etiology of Primary Ovarian Insufficiency* [Doctoral dissertation, Karolinska Institutet]. https://core.ac.uk/download/556259502.pdf

81. Wójcik, J., Obuchowska, A., Ozga, A., Standyło, A., Obuchowska, K., & Piotrowska, P. (2020). Polycystic ovary syndrome (PCOS): Risk factor, diagnostic, and current treatment. *Journal of Education, Health and Sport, 10*(8), 556–560. https://www.semanticscholar.org/paper/7cfee12f3bf4c61b1ce9e03486d4c75ab289aab7 (accessed on 10th June 2025).

82. Zheng, L., Yang, L., Guo, Z., Yao, N., Zhang, S., & Pu, P. (2024). Obesity and its impact on female reproductive health: Unraveling the connections. *Frontiers in Endocrinology, 14*, 1326546. https://doi.org/10.3389/fendo.2023.1326546.

83. Zheng, X., & Zhou, X. (2010). Neuron impairment or loss in brain may be responsible for type 2 diabetes and essential hypertension. https://core.ac.uk/download/pdf/288998.pdf (accessed on 10th June 2025).

EMERGING TRENDS IN CLINICAL PHARMACOLOGY

15

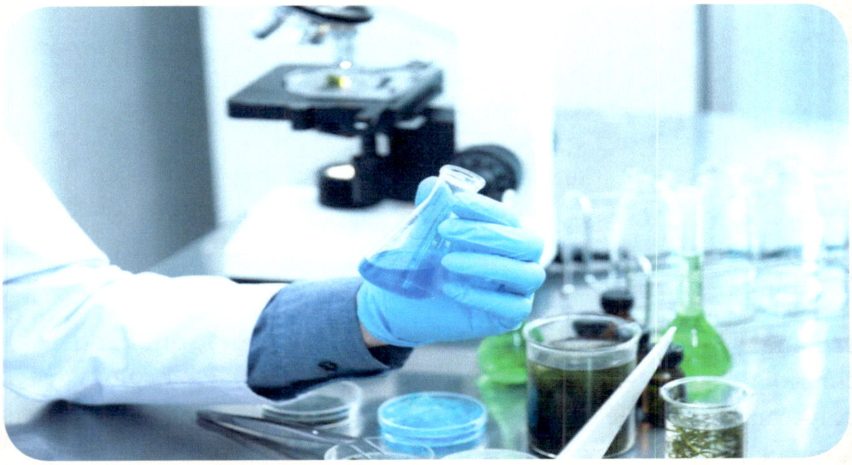

LEARNING OBJECTIVES

After studying this chapter, you will be able to:

1. Understand personalized medicine
2. Focus on digital health technologies
3. Discuss biologics and biosimilars

Introduction

Over the past decade, clinical pharmacology has undergone tremendous transformations driven by new drug development and the evolution of healthcare needs. As new therapeutic targets have emerged, such as ketamine and its enantiomers to cure resistant depression, appreciation of their influence is highly essential (Vekhova et al., 2024). Besides, the competency-based education for clinical pharmacology professionals suggests focusing on preparing professionals with skills needed as per modern demands (Johnson-Williams et al., 2024). This shift gives clinical pharmacologists the capacity to bridge between regulatory environments and the future-oriented evolution of drug therapies. Clinical pharmacology is excellently positioned to enhance patient outcomes and tackle the complex issues that are a part of contemporary medicine by learning about new trends and cultivating a workforce that is both technical and core-competent. Preparing the future generation of clinical pharmacologists is thus a strategic imperative (Figure 15.1).

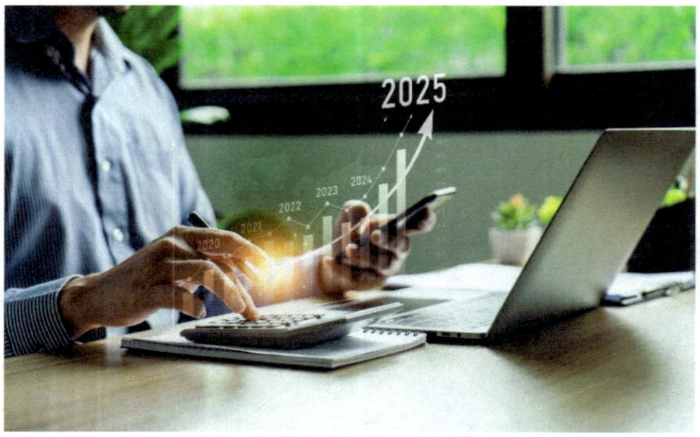

Figure 15.1. Emerging trends in clinical pharmacology.

Source: https://d1g9yur4m4naub.cloudfront.net/images/Article_Images/ImageForArticle_1407_1736348855031984.jpg.

Clinical pharmacology is also undergoing a paradigm shift with the progress in technology, research methodologies, and shifting healthcare priorities. Perhaps the most significant of such trend-setting paths is personalized medicine, where pharmacologic therapy is tailored to the individual patient's genetic, environmental, and lifestyle determinants of drug action. This evolution is supported by extensive bibliometric studies that identify the growing number of investigations for specific agents, e.g., midazolam, to which clinical application in anesthesiology and intensive care are continually being explored (Dolai et al., 2023). Additionally, the pharmaceutical nonmedical use, for example, cases of drug abuse and drug dependence involving drugs like venlafaxine and bupropion, indicate the importance of more effective pharmacovigilance and surveillance systems (Anderson et al., 2018). As these trends continue, they reveal the possibilities and challenges for clinical pharmacologists to improve drug efficacy and patient safety.

15.1. Personalized Medicine

Learning Outcome

1. Understand the definition and concept of personalized medicine
2. Explain the role of genomics in drug development
3. Focus on pharmacogenomics and patient response
4. Tailoring drug therapy to individual needs
5. Learn case studies in personalized medicine
6. Explain ethical considerations in personalized approaches
7. Identify challenges in implementation
8. Know future directions in personalized medicine
9. Learn the impact on clinical outcomes

With medical advancements, personalized medicine is a primary clinical pharmacology strategy that offers individualized therapeutic solutions compatible with the patient's profile. This is predicated on the understanding that genetic, environmental, and lifestyle factors exert tremendous influences on the efficacy and safety of therapy. Personalized medicine is centered on maximizing the choice of the right drug and dose, maximizing patient benefit, and minimizing side effects. The addition of network pharmacology principles improves this approach further, allowing for treatment development based on complex biological interactions and not a standard template (Marsh et al., 2010). The implications of personalized medicine also extend beyond practice into drug discovery and formulation, and thus redefine therapeutic innovation in healthcare (Terzic et al., 2017). They not only promise safer therapies but also result in facilitating more targeted interventions and hence making personalized medicine a cornerstone for clinical practice in the future.

15.1.1. Definition and Concept of Personalized Medicine

The concept of individualized medicine is a significant development in practice in healthcare, emphasizing therapy-guided treatment aligned with the patient's characteristics. It is a revolution growing stronger in clinical pharmacology because it facilitates changes in drug development and treatment patterns according to genetic, environmental, and lifestyle factors.

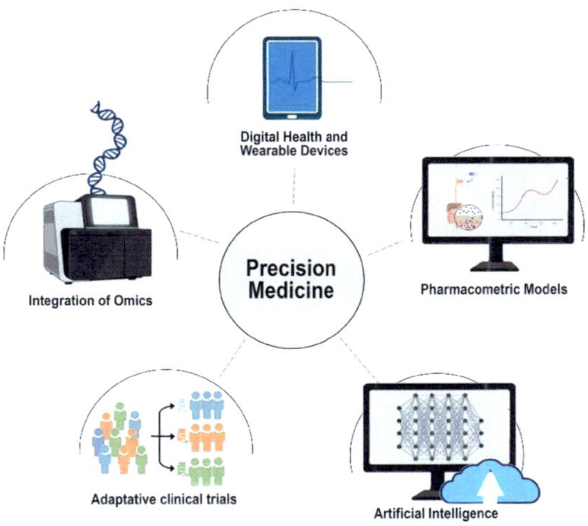

Figure 15.2. The concept of personalized medicine represents a significant evolution in the approach to healthcare, emphasizing tailored therapeutic interventions based on individual patient characteristics.

Source: https://pub.mdpi-res.com/pharmaceutics/pharmaceutics-16-00332/article_deploy/html/images/pharmaceutics-16-00332-g001.png?1709275331.

For instance, network pharmacology integration enhances personalization in therapy through identifying complex drug interactions and their potential effect on unique patients (Marsh et al., 2010). Apart from this, growing enthusiasm for systems biology has highlighted the promise of liquid biopsies with the ability to monitor tumor evolution in real-time and provide context-relevant information toward personalized therapies (Goetzl et al., 2019). These technologies not only serve to optimize therapeutic effect but also provide patients with more effective and less harmful drugs as per their individualized, distinctive biological profiles, heralding a new era for precision medicine (Figure 15.2).

15.1.2. Role of Genomics in Drug Development

Genomics in drug discovery has become the pillar in the changing scenario of clinical pharmacology. By deciphering genetic factors in disease, genomics allows for the discovery of new drug targets, making precision therapies a possibility based on personalized genetic makeup. This shift not only enhances the efficacy of treatments but also reduces the frequency of drug side effects since drugs can be tailored to match differences in genes between populations. Further, innovation in peptide therapies, which is being emphasized in recent studies, represents the growing diversity in drug discovery, calling on human genomics and natural product resources equally (Tillu et al., 2020). The expanding library of peptides in clinical trials supports the therapeutic potential of genomics to encourage innovative therapeutics (Lau et al., 2017). The future of genomics in drug development will therefore direct the direction toward more tailored and cost-effective medical interventions.

15.1.3. Pharmacogenomics and Patient Response

Pharmacogenomics is now a major driver of the optimization of therapeutic drugs for individual patients, achieving maximum efficacy while preventing adverse side effects. Pharmacogenomics translates genetic information into drug response, enabling the patient to be treated with personalized therapy according to his or her genomic constitution. Discussed in current literature is one of the practical approaches to personalized medicine, which is reconceptualizing drug development based on network pharmacology, which is preferred to identifying more effective treatments that are customized to fit patient profiles (Marsh et al., 2010). By mapping drug interactions onto biological networks, pharmacogenomics reveals avenues for innovation that promise safer and more effective therapies, hence revolutionizing clinical practice (Terzic et al., 2017). These advancements have a high potential to impact patient outcomes, taking health care out of the one-size-fits-all paradigm to a more personalized, responsive approach centered on patient-specific treatment regimens (Figure 15.3).

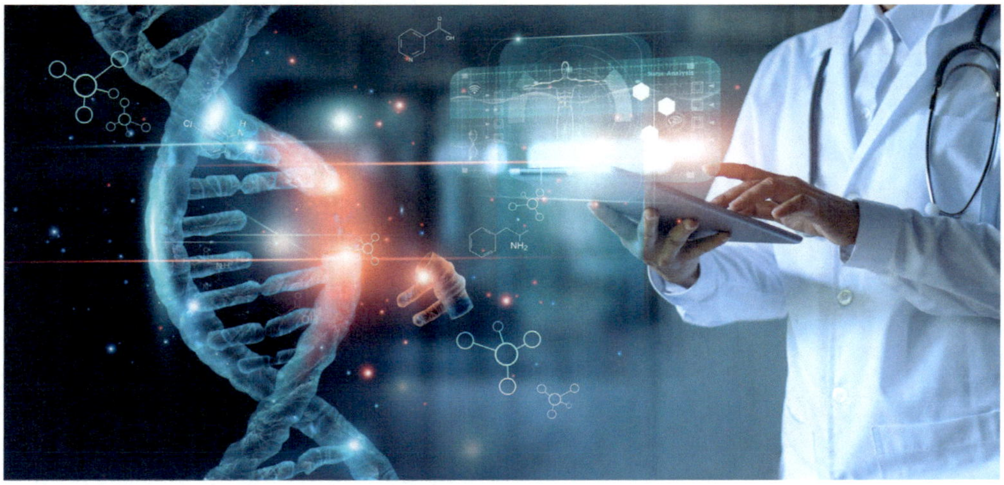

Figure 15.3. Pharmacogenomics has emerged as a pivotal element in tailoring medical treatments to individual patients, enhancing therapeutic efficacy while minimizing adverse effects.

Source: https://objective.health/wp-content/uploads/2022/01/objective-health-precision-medicine-future-of-healthcare-personalized-healthcare-scaled.jpeg.

15.1.4. Tailoring Drug Therapy to Individual Needs

The increasing recognition of individualized treatment with drugs is a salutary leap in clinical pharmacology aimed at personalizing treatment approaches to suit the unique needs of patients. This is particularly relevant to chronic conditions like type 2 diabetes mellitus (T2DM) whose more recent therapeutic agents, including glucagon-like peptide-1 receptor agonists (GLP-1 RAs), are a paradigm of personalized medicine. GLP-1 RAs not only improve glycemic control but also augment weight loss and cardiovascular risk reduction—demonstrating their general role in the management of T2DM and its complications (Chwaliszewski et al., 2024). Clinicians can personalize drug selection and dosing by integrating genetic, demographic, and clinical data. This transition to precision medicine signifies the importance of tailoring treatment methods according to individual patient conditions, substantiating the paradigm shift towards personalized therapies in modern clinical practice (Fromer et al., 2014).

15.1.5. Case Studies in Personalized Medicine

The study of case studies in personalized medicine indicates the possibility of changing the landscape of clinical pharmacology with the implementation of tailored therapeutic approaches. As technology improves, allowing us to tap into genetic and molecular data, personalized medicine allows for the development of specially crafted interventions that are matched with the individual patient profile. Present evidence supports the integration of novel diagnostic equipment, such as that outlined in new imaging technologies, to improve the precision of disease diagnosis and treatment planning (de Magalhães et al., 2025). Within oncology, for instance, high-resolution liquid biopsy techniques show compelling evidence of clinical utility in circulating tumor cells and biomarkers, exposing their potential to monitor disease progression and treatment response (Fu et al., 2024). The case studies, apart from being a demonstration of individualized style in practice, also bring into perspective the necessity to resolve such issues as cost, accessibility, and training required by healthcare practitioners. Lastly, they point towards a paradigm shift towards a personal approach to healthcare, enhancing patient outcomes and optimal therapeutic utility (Figure 15.4).

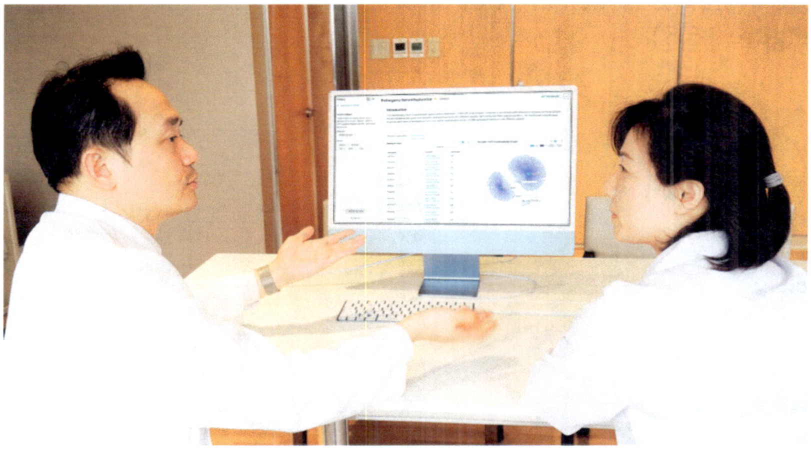

Figure 15.4. As advancements in technology enhance our ability to harness genetic and molecular insights, personalized medicine allows for the development of targeted interventions that cater to individual patient profiles.

Source: https://developer-blogs.nvidia.com/wp-content/uploads/2025/05/image1-2.png.

15.1.6. Ethical Considerations in Personalized Approaches

With the increased popularity of personalized medicine in clinical pharmacology, ethics becomes more prominent. The incorporation of AI and ML complicates issues related to data confidentiality and informed consent, as patient data is aggregated to form tailor-made treatments. Ethical problems relate to the problem of bias in algorithmic decision-making that could exacerbate health disparities among underrepresented populations. Ensuring equitable access to such advanced therapies requires sensitivity to systemic inequities in health care systems, as evidenced by the recent outcry over AI bias as a major barrier to reliable outcomes (Liu et al., 2024). Additionally, with natural products returning as potential sources of discovery for drugs, their ethical sourcing and sustainability continue to pose significant challenges that need to be tackled judiciously to maintain the integrity of pharmacological developments (Najmi et al., 2022). Therefore, resolving these ethical issues is important in order to establish public confidence in personalized strategies in clinical pharmacology.

15.1.7. Challenges in Implementation

Implementation of advanced trends in clinical pharmacology, such as model-informed precision dosing (MIPD), is faced with many challenges that prevent its widespread use in practice. Among the most critical challenges is the present lack of quantitative pharmacology knowledge required among healthcare professionals to implement MIPD principles on a successful basis. Today's curriculum in the field of education is lacking in preparing students for this need, leading to a workforce that is likely to fail in incorporating new pharmacological technologies into patient care. Regulatory policy also lags behind technological advancements, making it challenging to approve and deploy MIPD tools as medical devices, which discourages their routine application. There should be a joint effort, through an interdisciplinary collaboration between stakeholders in the academic, industry, and regulatory communities, to harmonize the language to standardize it and promote best practices that can move toward individualized therapy (Kluwe et al., 2020; Becker et al., 2020). If these systemic issues are not addressed, the therapeutic benefits of MIPD will be significantly lost (Figure 15.5).

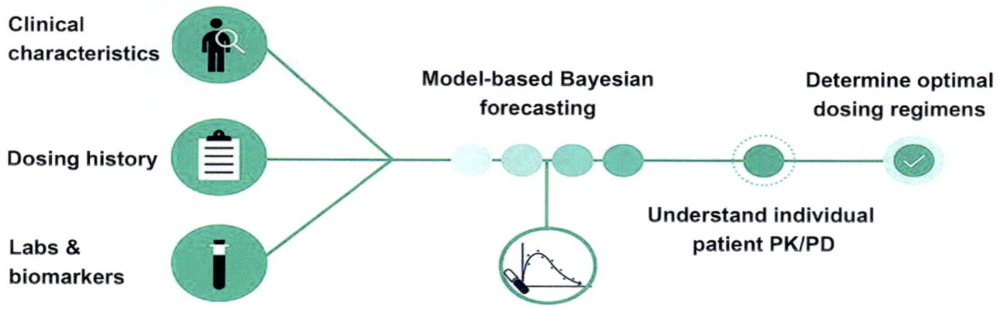

Figure 15.5. Model-informed precision dosing (MIPD).

Source: https://www.frontiersin.org/files/Articles/523256/fphar-11-00551-HTML/image_m/fphar-11-00551-g001.jpg.

15.1.8. Future Directions in Personalized Medicine

As personalized medicine matures, it essentially transforms our strategy for clinical pharmacology, especially for the treatment of chronic conditions like hypertension and cancer. The intricacies involved in such diseases call for a transition from conventional treatment models toward a more advanced appreciation of patient profiles based on genetic as well as pharmacokinetic considerations. Such a transformation would optimize treatment efficacy and minimize untoward outcomes, honoring the heterogeneity inherent in patient populations (Borghi et al., 2017). In addition, advances in biotechnology, including synthetic biology, are fostering new treatments that capitalize on engineered solutions to overcome impediments such as drug resistance, most notably in cancer therapies (Bivona et al., 2019). Through the intersection of such revolutionary advances, the future of personalized medicine can create a health ecosystem that not only responds better but is also designed more precisely to the individualized needs of every patient, ultimately improving world clinical results in an ever-changing healthcare landscape.

15.1.9. Impact on Clinical Outcomes

The evolving landscape of clinical pharmacology is an indication of the significant role that personalized medicine plays in determining clinical outcomes. As healthcare systems adapt to meet increasingly complex patient needs, the integration of network pharmacology principles becomes a critical driver of individualized therapies that enhance the effectiveness of treatment. This new direction promotes the formulation of personalized approaches that not only optimize drug discovery but also render treatment processes safer and more therapeutic following the principles of personalized medicine (Marsh et al., 2010). Moreover, the shift toward whole-person comprehension of health—incorporating social determinants and focus on population health—calls for revolutionizing healthcare professional curricula. By equipping practitioners to predict patient outcomes and requirements within the nuances of today's care environments, they can foster a culture of health that is greater than a disease model (Bouchaud et al., 2017). This nexus of practice and knowledge ultimately aims to improve clinical outcomes across diverse patient populations (Figure 15.6).

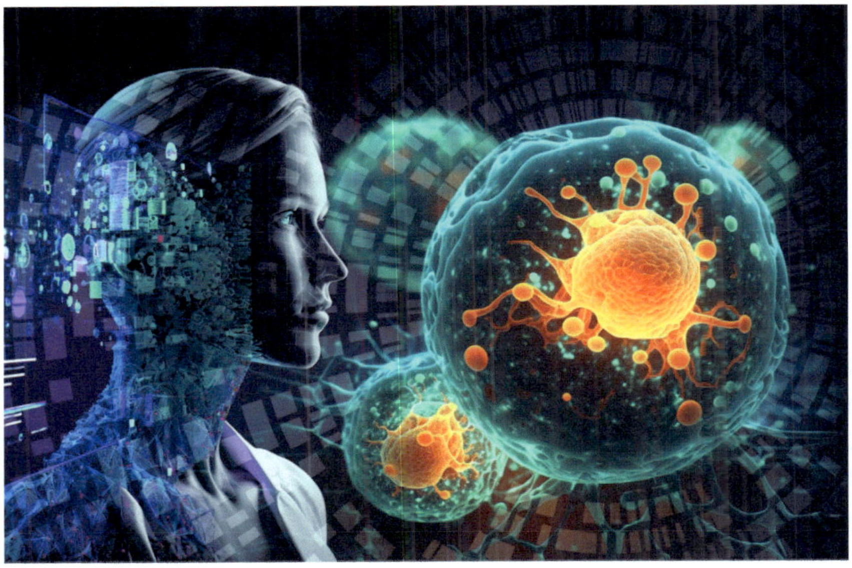

Figure 15.6. The evolving landscape of clinical pharmacology underscores the profound impact personalized medicine has on clinical outcomes.

Source: https://media.licdn.com/dms/image/D4D12AQHxiUdeISlzFw/article-cover_image-shrink_720_1280/0/1707212482462?e=2147483647&v=beta&t=PSAjBfk7UvzKywZqTV_VoRqiMtPkWMCMZGhOMVj65UQ.

Test Your Knowledge

1. What are the challenges in implementing personalized medicine in low-resource settings?
2. How does personalized medicine contribute to improving treatment outcomes and reducing adverse drug reactions?

15.2. Digital Health Technologies

Learning Outcome

1. Understand the overview of digital health in pharmacology
2. Know mobile health applications and medication management
3. Explain telepharmacy and remote patient monitoring
4. Discuss the role of artificial intelligence in drug discovery
5. Focus on data analytics in clinical decision making
6. Describe patient engagement through digital platforms
7. Identify regulatory challenges for digital health tools
8. Discuss integration of digital health into clinical practice
9. Stay informed about future trends in digital health technologies

The fast-paced technological progress of digital health is transforming the landscape of clinical pharmacology towards more effective and individualized patient care. This can be observed through the use of telehealth services and mobile health apps, which provide real-time monitoring and medication compliance. As a noteworthy example, digital technology allow doctors and other health care providers to gather and analyze data from patients with long-term conditions, resulting in prompt interventions to prevent conditions like osteoporosis and Alzheimer's disease. With an estimated 6.7 million Americans aged 65 and older afflicted by Alzheimer's, digital health technologies assist in disease control and caregivers' workload, costing an estimated $339.5 billion in 2022. Moreover, these technologies aid in osteoporosis management through adherence to antifracture medication, which in turn reduces the risk of subsequent fractures (LeBoff et al., 2022). Thus, digital health technologies are imperative for speeding up clinical outcomes in pharmacology.

15.2.1. Overview of Digital Health in Pharmacology

The introduction of digital health technologies is transforming the discipline of pharmacology, presenting new opportunities for drug discovery, development, and patient care. With data analytics, telemedicine, and mobile health apps, the pharmacological process can be optimized with enhanced patient engagement and compliance with medication.

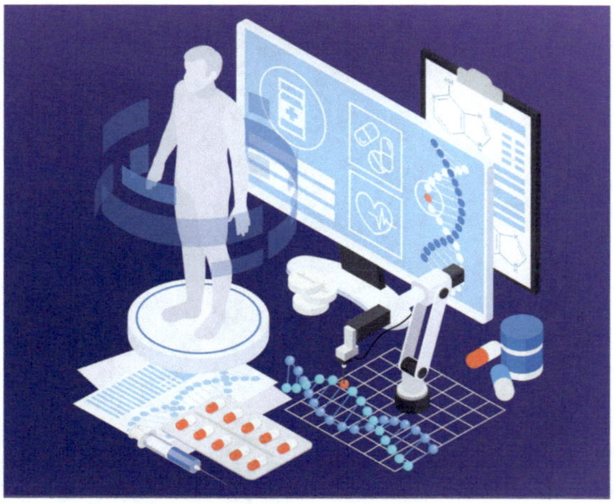

Figure 15.7. The emergence of digital health technologies is transforming the landscape of pharmacology, providing novel pathways for drug discovery, development, and patient management.

Source: https://res.cloudinary.com/dthpnue1d/image/upload/v1746010713/The_Role_of_AI_in_Drug_Discovery_and_Healthcare_8245d46c2f.webp.

For instance, machine learning (ML) models can analyze vast datasets to predict drug interactions and maximize treatment outcomes at the very core of traditional approaches to target identification and clinical trial management (Adriano et al., 2024). In addition, the integration of digital health into pharmacology enables real-time monitoring of drug action and side effects, rendering therapy more personalized and responsive (Asrar et al., 2024). With these technologies becoming more and more advanced, they usher in a new era of efficiency and precision in ensuring patient safety and therapeutic efficacy, making digital health a part of contemporary clinical pharmacology (Figure 15.7).

15.2.2. Mobile Health Applications and Medication Management

The integration of mobile health apps into medication management represents a watershed development in clinical pharmacology that maximizes patient activation and compliance with therapeutic regimens. By providing individualized reminders of medication, educational materials, and adherence monitoring, these applications enable patients to become increasingly active partners in their healthcare. Evidence indicates that educationally personalized counseling by pharmacists significantly improves medication knowledge and adherence rates among patients, proving that utilization of mobile health tools can successfully supplement conventional approaches (Mack et al., 2022). Furthermore, the prevalence of cell phones enables the development of apps designed to cater to various groups of patients, such as those with specific needs such as hearing impairments, thus broadening the scope of drug management tools (Kermani et al., 2017). As technology continues to evolve, it can revolutionize the landscape of clinical pharmacology into one where medication can be used by patients more effectively and safely.

15.2.3. Telepharmacy and Remote Patient Monitoring

The intersection of telepharmacy and remote patient monitoring is a dramatic shift in clinical pharmacology that reflects the evolving scene in patient care. Telepharmacy creates greater access to drug services, particularly in rural and underdeveloped areas, hence fostering greater patient outcomes and satisfaction via more individualized care. The pandemic of COVID-19 surfaced the immediate need for such innovations, which propelled the utilization of telepharmacy platforms that enable remote consultations and medication management (Silva et al., 2023). Additionally, the emergence of artificial intelligence-driven pharmacy practice, or pharmacointelligence, opens the potential for streamlining medication processes and enhancing clinical decision-making through data integration (Hatem, 2024). By leveraging technology and greater communication channels between health care providers and patients, telepharmacy not only addresses barriers to care but also the broader goals of public health and health care equity. As these trends further evolve, they represent profound possibilities and challenges for future clinical pharmacology (Figure 15.8).

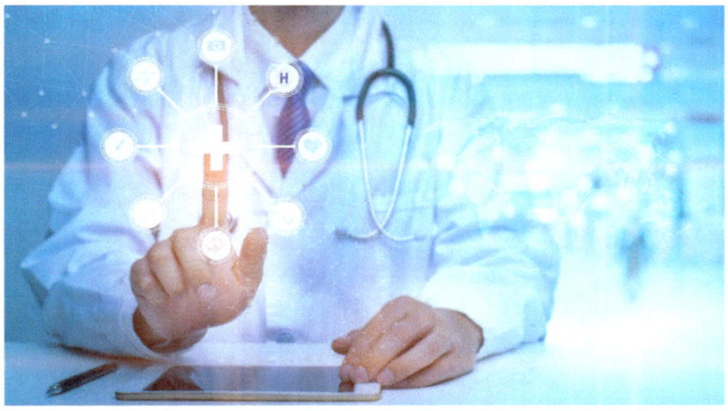

Figure 15.8. The integration of telepharmacy and remote patient monitoring signifies a pivotal shift in clinical pharmacology, highlighting the evolving landscape of patient care.

Source: https://healthsnap.io/wp-content/uploads/2024/04/e4988355-d2c5-4089-82d7-4c16099d627d.png.

15.2.4. Role of Artificial Intelligence in Drug Discovery

The use of artificial intelligence (AI) in drug discovery has been a key player in clinical pharmacology in recent years, revolutionizing traditional methods. By the integration of highly advanced algorithms and extensive data sets, AI has enhanced the identification of targets and high-throughput screening, accelerating the selection of potential drug candidates. This advancement not only streamlines the traditionally time-consuming phases of drug discovery but also introduces an efficiency heretofore beyond reach. The convergence of AI technologies and omic sciences has given rise to a rich informatics fabric that amplifies our understanding of the molecular foundation of disease. As emphasized, Big data analytics has therefore emerged to enhance the technical aspects of storage, transmission, and analysis (Alfirevic et al., 2016). Further, the achievements in AI applications in drug toxicity prediction and the optimization of clinical trials demonstrate its capability to transform therapeutic innovation with more effective and personalized treatment alternatives (Asrar et al., 2024).

15.2.5. Data Analytics in Clinical Decision Making

The integration of data analysis into clinical decision-making represents a pharmacological revolution that enables doctors to individualize therapy more optimally based on the needs of the patient. By using large amounts of patient data such as demographics, genetics, and clinical information, clinicians can utilize predictive modeling to optimize therapeutic effects and minimize side effects better.

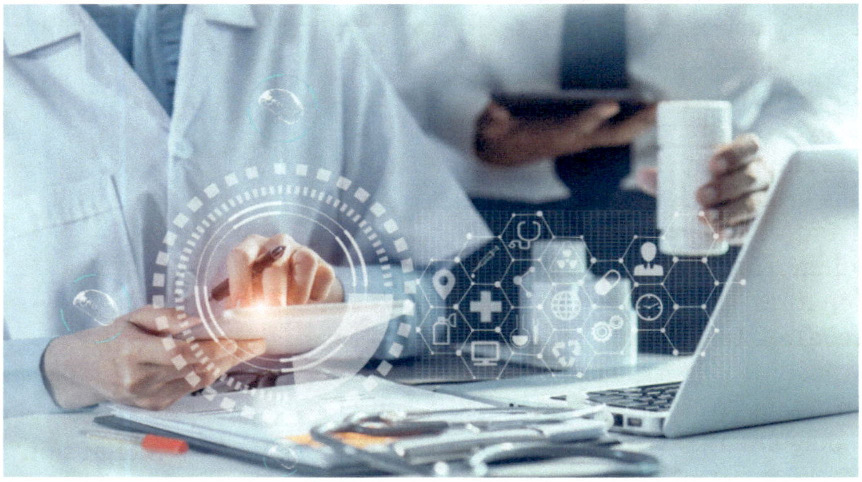

Figure 15.9. The integration of data analytics into clinical decision-making represents a transformative shift in pharmacology, enabling healthcare professionals to tailor treatments more effectively to individual patient needs.

Source: https://www.zucisystems.com/wp-content/uploads/2022/07/Data-Science-in-Healthcare-Industry-Benefits-Strategies-Applications-Tools-and-Future-Trends.png.

This trend is borne out in the emergence of MIPD, which describes the heterogeneity of patient response to treatments and facilitates personalized optimization of doses with the use of real-world evidence (Kluwe et al., 2020). Concurrently, the vigilant surveillance of disease epidemiology, such as the incidence of stroke and its contributing risk factors, highlights the importance of evidence-based decision-making towards planning and resource allocation for health interventions (Feigin et al., 2021). Ultimately, the complementarity of data analytics not only enriches clinical decision-making but also the greater goal of elevating patient care standards in the evolving context of clinical pharmacology (Figure 15.9).

15.2.6. Patient Engagement Through Digital Platforms

There has been a considerable surge in the utilization of digital platforms to improve patient engagement in clinical pharmacology over the last several years, redefining health care communication and management practices. Through a sharing of real-time data between health care providers and patients, the platforms facilitate improved adherence to drug schedules and treatment protocols, thereby improving clinical outcomes. For instance, the integration of real-time monitoring using mobile applications and wearable devices enables patients to engage actively in their care, enhancing a sense of autonomy and ownership of their treatment process. Additionally, the Pathway Platform is an exemplary case of how user design can support patient involvement and shared decision-making through enabling meaningful tracking of patient-reported outcomes, which is essential in measurement-based care (McCue et al., 2023). Besides, in recognition of the complexity of patients' needs, ongoing innovation of tailored interventions is a top priority, emphasizing the role of digital modes in defining the clinical pharmacology landscape (Panchal et al., 2025).

15.2.7. Regulatory Challenges for Digital Health Tools

The growth of e-health technologies has transformed clinical pharmacology to a large extent; however, regulatory obstacles still encumber their complete integration into healthcare systems. As the technologies, from smartphone apps to devices that allow remote monitoring, grow with further advancements, regulators are struggling to create clear guidelines that guarantee safety and efficacy without stifling innovation. The need to integrate high-dimensional biological data along with clinical, demographic, and environmental data makes the regulatory landscape challenging because existing frameworks are not in a position to keep pace with the rapid advancement of technology in health care (Alfirevic et al., 2016). In addition, while such platforms like Clinical Pharmacology & Therapeutics (CPT) provide helpful information regarding the drug discovery continuum, drug development, and use, they stress the imperative for adaptive regulatory frameworks that reflect these new tendencies (Terzic et al., 2017). Thus, eliminating such regulatory problems is central to advancing innovation without compromising patient safety and therapeutic efficacies (Figure 15.10).

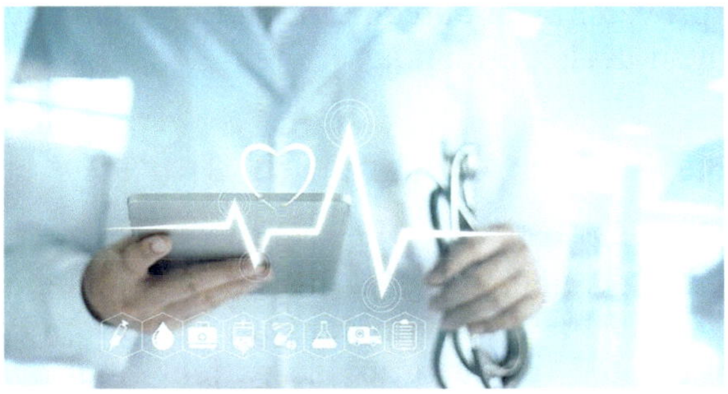

Figure 15.10. The proliferation of digital health tools has significantly transformed clinical pharmacology; however, regulatory challenges persist that hinder their optimal integration into healthcare systems.

Source: https://cdn-lipbd.nitrocdn.com/NmtxoNywbwrhgCusRjwzXqAEjXRnHzOa/assets/images/optimized/rev-a21dc4e/www.osplabs.com/wp-content/uploads/2022/04/810x435-4.jpg.

15.2.8. Integration of Digital Health into Clinical Practice

The integration of digital health into practice represents a paradigm shift within the clinical pharmacology environment, enabling the seamless incorporation of novel technologies into the care of patients. By integrating diverse data sources such as genomic information, lifestyle factors, and clinical results, practitioners can develop personalized treatment regimens that take into consideration the subtleties of a unique patient's health (Goldenberg et al., 2018). This multi-dimensional approach not only enhances the accuracy of diagnosis but also strengthens the efficacy of drug therapies, thereby addressing the intricacies of disease. Furthermore, as the nursing community argues, establishing successful models of clinical intervention and practice in response to current healthcare concerns continues to prioritize health education and practice that incorporates frontier areas of science. Lastly, the strategic application of digital health technologies will transform pharmacological practice, with improved health outcomes resulting from data-driven decision-making.

15.2.9. Future Trends in Digital Health Technologies

With advancing digital health technologies, integration into clinical pharmacology is anticipated to revolutionize patient treatment and outcomes. Projections for the future include a significant rise in the application of artificial intelligence (AI) tools to enhance diagnostic precision and therapeutic options based on data-driven knowledge, as noted in recent literature (Park et al., 2023). Additionally, mobile health interventions, particularly in chronic disease management, will allow patients to be actively engaged in self-management through surveillance of their physical activity and health indicators, which has proven promising for oncology care (Tak et al., 2023). Telemedicine will increasingly transform the provision of healthcare, facilitating real-time monitoring and individualized treatment protocols. These advancements bring into focus the need for medical education to change, to enable health professionals to use these technologies for maximum gain effectively. Collectively, these emerging digital health trends demand a move towards more patient-centered pharmacology practices, towards improved health outcomes (Figure 15.11).

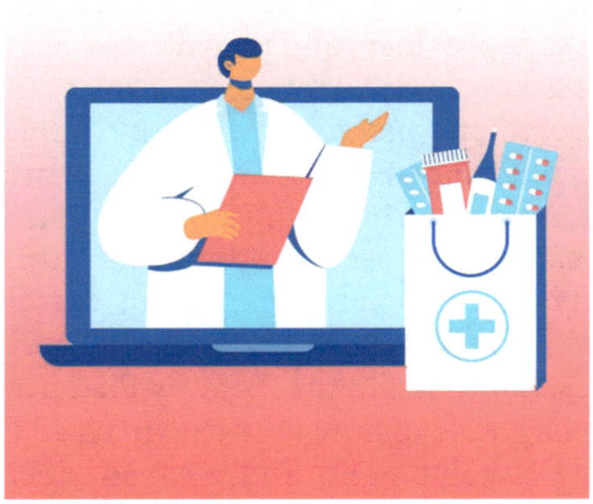

Figure 15.11. As digital health technologies continue to evolve, their integration into clinical pharmacology is poised to revolutionize patient care and treatment outcomes.

Source: https://iimtu.edu.in/blog/wp-content/uploads/2023/06/Untitled-1.jpg.

Test Your Knowledge

1. What are the benefits and limitations of using wearable devices for patient monitoring?
2. How is artificial intelligence being integrated into drug development and patient care?

15.3. Biologics and Biosimilars

Learning Outcome

1. Understand the definition and types of biologics
2. Explain the development of biosimilars
3. Discuss the regulatory framework for biologics
4. Know clinical applications of biologics
5. Focus on the cost-effectiveness of biosimilars
6. Learn safety and efficacy
7. Discuss market trends in biologics and biosimilars
8. Focus on patient access and affordability issues
9. Describe the future of biologics in clinical pharmacology

The landscape of clinical pharmacology is being revolutionized by the advent of biologics and their subsequent counterparts, biosimilars. As biological drugs—of—biological—origin—are becoming increasingly important in the treatment of chronic and complex diseases, U.S. legislation enacted in 2010 has brought a new era of competition by opening up FDA approval of biosimilars, essentially lower-cost copies of these new medicines. This policy shift should expand access to effective therapies at reduced costs (Lietzan et al., 2017). Nevertheless, compared to traditional generic drugs, biosimilar production and competition forces are much more complex, and therefore a more targeted approach to regulation as well as patent policy is required (Lietzan et al., 2017). As the marketplace continues to evolve, understanding the distinct mechanisms and implications of biosimilars versus traditional drugs becomes ever more significant to stakeholders throughout the healthcare system, from policymakers to clinicians.

15.3.1. Definition and Types of Biologics

Within the ever-evolving scenario of clinical pharmacology, biologics are a significant group of therapeutic drugs of origin from a living organism. Biologics, in general definition, represent a wide range of products such as vaccines, blood constituents, monoclonal antibodies, and genetically modified proteins, which all have significant roles in disease prevention, diagnosis, and treatment. The complexity of biologics is not only in their varied origins and applications but also in the process of producing them, which is usually reliant on sophisticated biotechnological methods. Focusing on the safety and efficacy profiles during development is another remarkable aspect of this field, where exhaustive toxicology examinations are most important in ensuring patient safety in clinical trials, particularly for first-in-human (FIH) trials (Frazier et al., 2019). In addition, advancements in technologies and methods further improve our understanding of biologics, and innovations continue to enhance therapy. As such, research on biologics is leading the way in clinical pharmacology advancements (Figure 15.12).

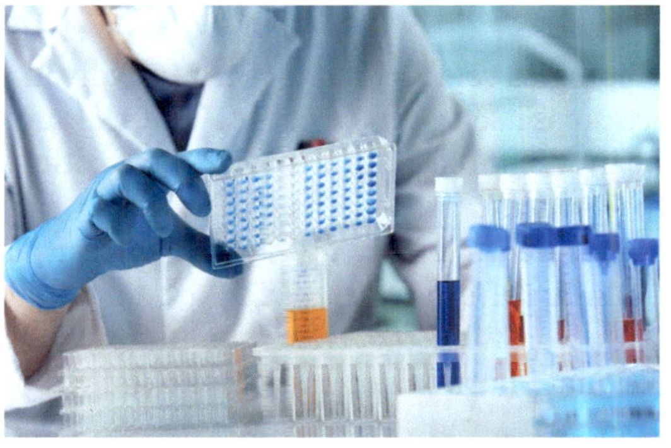

Figure 15.12. Biologics.

Source: https://www.susupport.com/uploads/media/default/02/2592-Biologics.jpg?v=1-0.

15.3.2. Development of Biosimilars

The advent of biosimilars represents a significant step forward in clinical pharmacology, making biologic therapies more widely accessible that were previously limited by the unaffordable prices of originator brand drugs. As the evolving regulatory frameworks, for example, those under the FDA, continue to take shape, the path to attaining bio-similarity is becoming clearer, and producers are now able to reproduce the complex forms of biological medications with equal safety and effectiveness. This not only sparks competition but also drives innovation within the pharmaceutical industry, pushing challenging new research that can enhance existing treatments or discover novel methods. With initiatives like the American Diabetes Association's guidelines spearheading the integration of biosimilars into treatment protocols, clinicians can make better choices on treatments for patients (ElSayed et al., 2023). Besides, information resources like Drug Bank, which provide precise details of drug interactions and drug effects, play a critical role in enabling the safe and effective use of biosimilars in clinical practice (Knox et al., 2023).

15.3.3. Regulatory Framework for Biologics

The biologics regulation system has evolved as a direct response to the rapid rate of development in the biotechnology field and the sophistication of drug formulation. The regulations play a critical role in ensuring the safety, efficacy, and quality of biologics, which are structurally and process-wise far more sophisticated than traditional pharmaceuticals. As the industry has developed to pursue new technologies, such as gene therapy and personalized medicine, making better current regulatory approaches has been increasingly critical. To illustrate, gene patent issues serve to remind us of the delicate balance regulators have to achieve; innovation is essential to spur on, but no less vital to dispel public concerns regarding access and safety (Schilling et al., 2011). Besides, the inclusion of spontaneous reporting systems (SRSs) in pharmacovigilance is indicative of the trend towards evidence-based decision-making in regulations as a response to the need for new models that are adaptive to Big Data and enhance drug safety surveillance (Antonazzo et al., 2021) (Figure 15.13).

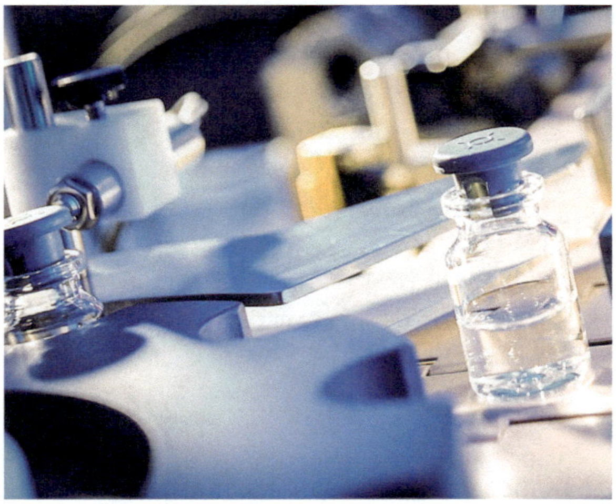

Figure 15.13. The regulatory framework for biologics has evolved in response to rapid advancements in biotechnology and the complexities of drug development.

Source: https://oakwoodlabs.com/wp-content/uploads/2023/10/vial-close-nice-5.jpg.

15.3.4. Clinical Applications of Biologics

The pharmaceutical applications of biologics are a landmark development in pharmacology since these drugs are formulated to target specific pathways involved in disease processes. By exploiting the intricacies of the biology of proteins, monoclonal antibodies, and other macromolecules, biologics are effective against many conditions from autoimmune and cancer diseases to infections and inflammatory and neurologic disorders. New technologies in therapeutic drug monitoring (TDM) mirror the potential of optimizing dosing regimens, particularly with the development of biosensors that permit real-time analysis and customization of treatment protocols. The innovation is significant since traditional approaches, such as chromatography, are prone to high economic costs and delays, thereby compromising accessibility for timely clinical intervention. With success in individualized dosing relying heavily on effective TDM, the field is poised for groundbreaking improvement that would result in enhanced patient outcomes along with reducing healthcare spending, highlighting ongoing revolutionizing of biologics in clinical pharmacology (Ates et al., 2020; Chen et al., 2020).

15.3.5. Cost-Effectiveness of Biosimilars

The cost benefits of biosimilars are increasingly widely recognized as a central factor in enhancing patient access to required biologic therapy within clinical pharmacology. When biosimilars enter the market, they offer substantial cost savings compared with their reference biologics, and that renders treatment accessible to diverse patient populations. This economic advantage is obvious in chronic diseases, such as rheumatoid arthritis, where ongoing treatment costs can exhaust health resources. More recent evidence shows that biosimilar manufacturing lines prove more cost-saving and efficient compared to traditional biologic manufacturing lines, leading to lower prices with improved patient outcomes (Angelini et al., 2020). In addition, with the growth of healthcare systems, the incorporation of biosimilars is crucial for maintaining guidelines that ensure equitable treatment across different groups, particularly as advocated in guidelines by leading diabetes care organizations (ElSayed et al., 2023). Hence, the cost-effectiveness of biosimilars not only promotes economic strategies but also facilitates enhanced clinical accessibility (Figure 15.14).

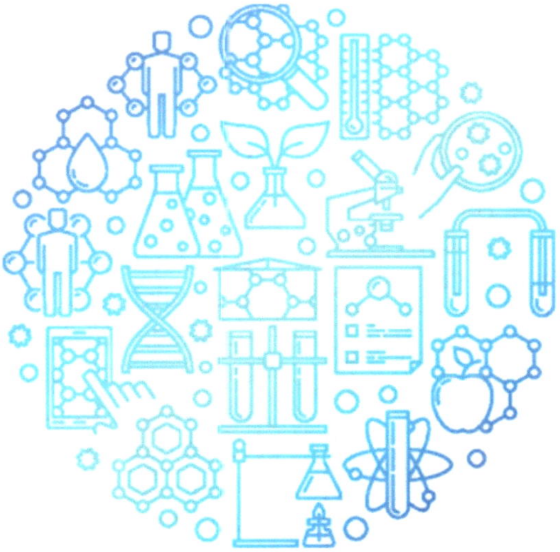

Figure 15.14. The cost-effectiveness of biosimilars is increasingly recognized as a pivotal factor in enhancing patient access to essential biologic therapies within the landscape of clinical pharmacology.

Source: https://blogs.deloitte.co.uk/.a/6a01543429fb37970c026bded304bd200c-pi.

15.3.6. Safety and Efficacy Comparisons

Assessment of safety and efficacy in novel pharmacological interventions is critical to sound clinical decision-making. Recent reports have described the contrasting profile of direct oral anticoagulants (DOACs) versus conventional anticoagulant therapies, including low-molecular-weight heparin (LMWH). These studies uncover that DOACs are very convenient with less recurrent venous thromboembolism risk but also have a higher risk of significant bleeding, particularly in patients with particular cancer-related conditions (Lee, 2021). There are also clinical trials being conducted to examine alternative therapies like the herbal formula gyejigachulbutang for the treatment of chronic diseases like knee osteoarthritis. This study will also fully assess not only pain relief but overall safety, thus providing essential data to the new treatment landscape (Sul et al., 2019). The thorough analysis of these complex therapeutic modalities brings into sharp focus the imperative of balancing treatment choices with patient profiles to optimize both safety and efficacy outcomes.

15.3.7. Market Trends in Biologics and Biosimilars

The evolving trend of market dynamics in biologics and biosimilars significantly affects clinical pharmacology, particularly in the area of targeted therapeutics. As there is greater demand for new therapies, the development of biologics—such as monoclonal antibodies and recombinant proteins—has grown significantly, spurred by their effectiveness in the treatment of multifactorial disease states such as cancer and autoimmune diseases. Meanwhile, the biosimilar market is gaining momentum as the products provide cost-effective alternatives to originator biologics, driving patient access to life-saving medicines. Success with biosimilars, though, relies on breaking through hurdles such as regulatory hurdles and physicians' trust in their efficacy and safety compared to branded drugs. Also, findings from angiogenesis studies suggest that biologics against infiltration mechanisms could be of future therapeutic potential (Liu et al., 2023). Concurrently, integrin-targeted therapeutics are broadening the inventory of biologics, and a critical understanding of their signaling pathways remains to be achieved for maximizing treatment benefit and filling unmet clinical needs (Pang et al., 2023) (Figure 15.15).

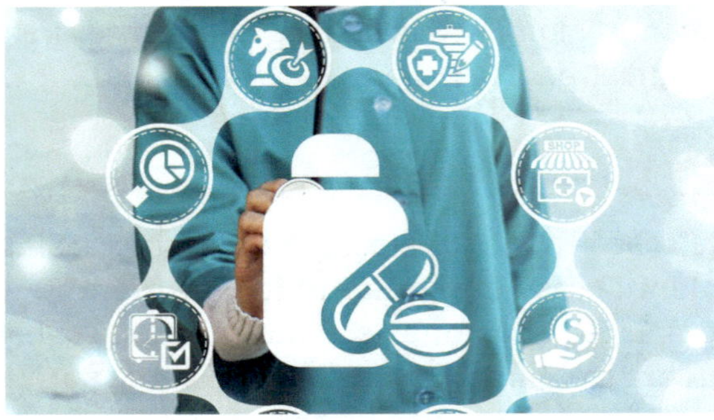

Figure 15.15. The evolving landscape of market trends in biologics and biosimilars is significantly reshaping clinical pharmacology, particularly in the realm of targeted therapies.

Source: https://www.chitkara.edu.in/blogs/wp-content/uploads/2023/11/Future-of-Pharma-Management.jpg.

15.3.8. Patient Access and Affordability Issues

Availability of affordable health care has been a necessary concern in clinical pharmacology, particularly in light of growing incidents of chronic diseases. As more and more Americans are burdened by ailments such as Alzheimer's disease, which is estimated to afflict 6.7 million individuals above the age of 65, access to care for patients is the fundamental problem that needs to be addressed. Increased healthcare spending tends to result in high out-of-pocket expenses that disproportionately burden poor people and contribute to health inequities. Compared to enhanced success in therapies such as bispecific antibodies (BsAbs) with promising treatment available, the expense might be a limitation for the majority of patients attempting to seek these new treatments (Trivedi et al., 2017). This highlights the urgent need for systems-level reform that emphasizes affordable drug pricing and expanded patient access, ensuring fair distribution of pioneering therapeutic innovations across all socio-economic levels. Overcoming these hurdles is pivotal in optimizing overall patient results within the increasingly sophisticated healthcare environment.

15.3.9. Future of Biologics in Clinical Pharmacology

With ongoing advancement in clinical pharmacology, the potential for the future of biologics is bright, particularly about increasing the precision of therapeutic interventions. Biologics, encompassing a range of products from living sources, are the focal point of medical innovation and consequent advances towards personalized medicine. The marriage of pharmacokinetics (PK) studies brings new concepts of drug absorption and metabolism, and the importance of individual variation in pharmacotherapy that genetic factors and disease states can induce (Abduljalil et al., 2019). Besides that, immune-inflammatory response regulation is one of the most critical areas for therapeutic intervention, particularly in diseases such as atherosclerosis, where available knowledge emphasizes the importance of accurate translational research to effectively utilize these biological weapons (Abbas et al., 2017). This cross-breeding of pharmaceuticals and biology not only ensures enhanced drug action but also enables customized treatment schemes for diverse patient populations, ultimately transforming the clinical therapeutics landscape (Figure 15.16).

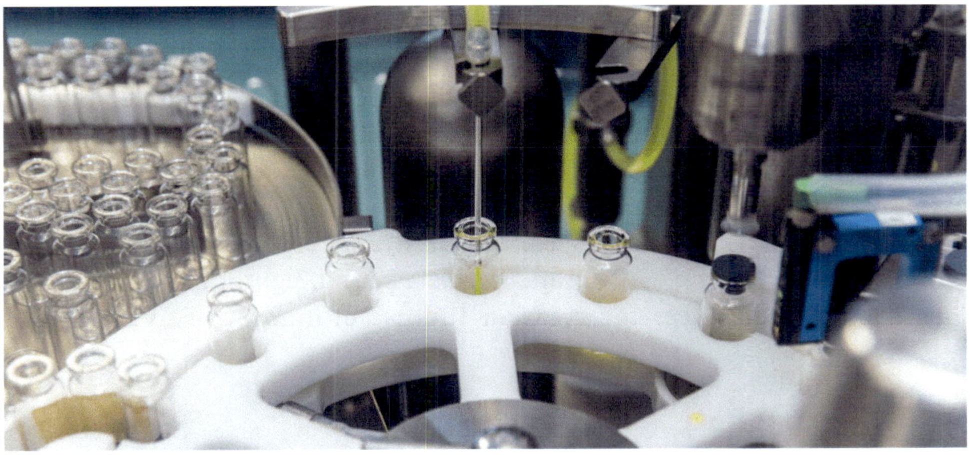

Figure 15.16. Biologics, encompassing a wide range of products derived from living organisms, are at the forefront of medical innovation, leading to advances in personalized medicine.

Source: https://adragos-pharma.com/wp-content/uploads/2024/11/Captura-de-pantalla-2024-11-21-104458-1024x480.png.

Test Your Knowledge

1. Why is immunogenicity a concern in the use of biologics and biosimilars?
2. Discuss regulatory challenges in the approval and marketing of biosimilars.

Summary

The field of clinical pharmacology is evolving in a very rapid pace, primarily driven by advances such as the applications of ketamine and non-invasive brain stimulation techniques. FDA approval of esketamine for treatment-resistant depression is a seminal milestone, justifying the therapeutic potential of ketamine uses in other psychiatric illnesses and extending pharmacologic treatment possibilities (Vekhova et al., 2024). Moreover, the advent of non-invasive brain stimulation methods, particularly on cognitive process augmentation, presents promising frontiers to multimodal treatment protocols that combine pharmacological interventions with new technologies (lópez et al., 2024). As these new trends unfold, clinicians and investigators alike will need to keep pace with developments and conform to these innovations, ultimately arriving at improved patient outcomes and a greater awareness of the pharmacological potential in these new modalities. The future of clinical pharmacology holds within it not only promises of breaching boundaries but also promises to reengineer the mental illness treatment paradigm.

Over the last few decades, clinical pharmacology has seen revolutionary changes with a number of hallmark trends, with technology advances and greater understanding of human biology being the major drivers. One trend is the development of personalized medicine, where therapeutic regimens are customized to suit unique patient profiles, thus improving efficacy with reduced adverse effects. This approach is consistent with network pharmacology that favors a systems approach to understand the influence of drugs on biological networks rather than on individual targets. This integration results in more integrated therapeutic innovations that can deliver safer and more effective therapy (Marsh et al., 2010). Interdisciplinary collaboration has also become more important, as information from genomics, bioinformatics, and data science plays an increasingly important role in informing pharmacological research and practice. Within this revolutionary environment, Clinical Pharmacology & Therapeutics is a crucial lighthouse that consistently shares insightful information that advances the creation and use of innovative treatments (Terzic et al., 2017).

KEY TERMS FROM THIS CHAPTER

Big data analytics	Biologics	Biosimilars
Blood constituents	Data confidentiality	Diagnostic precision
Digital technology	Informed consent	Mobile health
Monoclonal antibodies	Oncology	Osteoporosis
Personalized medicine	Pharmacointelligence	Pharmacologic therapy
Quantitative pharmacology	Systems biology	Telepharmacy

Critical Thinking Questions

1. **Which of the following best defines personalized medicine in clinical pharmacology?**
   a. Use of traditional medicines only
   b. Prescribing the same drug to all patients
   c. Tailoring drug therapy based on individual genetic and clinical characteristics
   d. Avoiding medications altogether
2. **Pharmacogenomics plays a key role in which of the following?**
   a. Enhancing drug solubility
   b. Understanding liver function
   c. Identifying genetic variations that influence drug response
   d. Increasing drug shelf life
3. **Which of the following is an example of a digital health tool in clinical pharmacology?**
   a. X-ray
   b. MRI
   c. Mobile health app for medication adherence
   d. CT scan
4. **Artificial intelligence (AI) is increasingly used in drug development to:**
   a. Replace doctors entirely
   b. Skip clinical trials
   c. Predict drug targets and optimize clinical trial design
   d. Reduce the need for regulatory approval
5. **Which emerging technology allows real-time monitoring of drug levels in patients?**
   a. AI modeling
   b. Pharmacogenetic screening
   c. Wearable biosensors
   d. Radiographic imaging

Answers to Critical Thinking Questions

1. (c); 2. (c); 3. (c); 4. (c); 5. (c).

Short Answer Questions

1. What is personalized medicine, and how does it differ from traditional approaches to treatment?
2. How can pharmacogenomics enhance personalized medicine?
3. What are digital health technologies and how are they transforming clinical pharmacology?
4. Describe how mobile health (mHealth) apps can improve medication adherence.
5. What are biologic drugs, and how are they different from traditional small-molecule drugs?
6. Define biosimilars and explain how they are developed and approved.

References

1. Welsh, P., Grassia, G., Botha, S., Sattar, N., & Maffia, P. (2017). Targeting inflammation to reduce cardiovascular disease risk: a realistic clinical prospect? *British Journal of Pharmacology, 174*(22), 3898–3913. https://doi.org/10.1111/bph.13818Abduljalil, K., Aghazadeh-Habashi, A., Aigrain, P., Aitman, T., Al Za'abi, M., Alegre, M. L., Alnaqeeb, M. A., et al. (2019). *Current Trends in Drug Metabolism and Pharmacokinetics* https://core.ac.uk/download/286361678.pdf (accessed on 10th June 2025).

2. Adriano, F. C. (2024). *Impact of Artificial Intelligence in The Pharmaceutical Business: A Bibliometric Analysis.* https://core.ac.uk/download/616568334.pdf (accessed on 10th June 2025).

3. Alfirevic, A., Ball, S., Chen, Y., Costa, M., Driest, S. L. V., Fang, H., Harpaz, R., et al. (2016). *Big Data Transforms Discovery-Utilization Therapeutics Continuum* https://core.ac.uk/download/46976098.pdf (accessed on 10th June 2025).

4. Anderson, K., Augustin, T., Baker, M., Baribeau, D., Bolden-Watson, C., Campagne, D., Carvalho, M., et al. (2018). *Is There a Potential of Misuse for Venlafaxine and Bupropion?* https://core.ac.uk/download/158139099.pdf (accessed on 10th June 2025).

5. Angelini, J., Talotta, R., Roncato, R., Fornasier, G., Barbiero, G., Dal Cin, L., Brancati, S., et al. (2020). JAK-inhibitors for the treatment of rheumatoid arthritis: A focus on the present and an outlook on the future. *Biomolecules, 10*(7), 1002. https://doi.org/10.3390/biom10071002.

6. Antonazzo, C. I., De Ponti, F., Moretti, U., Pariente, A., et al. (2021). Evolving roles of spontaneous reporting systems to assess and monitor drug safety. In *Pharmacovigilance: A Practical Approach* [Chapter]. https://core.ac.uk/download/478129875.pdf (accessed on 10th June 2025).

7. Asrar, S. S., Kumar, B. P., Reddy, K. S., & Revanth, K. (2024). *The Role of Artificial Intelligence and Machine Learning in Drug Discovery and Development.* https://core.ac.uk/download/621125064.pdf (accessed on 10th June 2025).

8. Ates, H. C., Roberts, J., Lipman, J., Cass, A. E. G., Urban, G., & Dincer, C. (2020). On-site therapeutic drug monitoring. *Trends in Biotechnology, 38*(11), 1262–1277. https://doi.org/10.1016/j.tibtech.2020.03.001.

9. Becker, W. C., & Fiellin, D. A. (2020). When epidemics collide: Coronavirus disease 2019 (COVID-19) and the opioid crisis. *Annals of Internal Medicine, 173*, 59–60. https://doi.org/10.7326/m20-1210.

10. Bivona, T. G., Chang, S., Hernández, A. C., & Keasling, J. (2019). *Overcoming the Challenges of Cancer Drug Resistance Through Bacterial-Mediated Therapy.* https://core.ac.uk/download/287622369.pdf (accessed on 10th June 2025).

11. Borghi, C., Grassi, G., Rosei, E. A., & Savoia, C. (2017). *Personalized Medicine—A Modern Approach for The Diagnosis and Management of Hypertension.* https://core.ac.uk/download/96884785.pdf (accessed on 10th June 2025).

12. Bouchaud, M., Brown, D., & Swan, B. A. (2017). *Creating a New Education Paradigm to Prepare Nurses for the 21st Century.* https://core.ac.uk/download/129190945.pdf (accessed on 10th June 2025).

13. Chen, C., Gao, G., Xu, Y., Pu, L., Wang, Q., Wang, L., Wang, W., et al. (2020). SARS-CoV-2–positive sputum and feces after conversion of pharyngeal samples in patients with COVID-19. *Annals of Internal Medicine, 172*, 832–834. https://doi.org/10.7326/M20-0991.

14. Chwaliszewski, K., Fikas, K., Goliszek, Z., Mazur, M., et al. (2024). *Beyond Glycemic Control: The Expanding Role of GLP-1 Analogues in Type 2 Diabetes and Metabolic Health* https://core.ac.uk/download/636385604.pdf (accessed on 10th June 2025).

15. Da Silva, J. F., Fukushima, A. R., & Nicoletti, M. A. (2023). A era digital da saúde: A necessidade da telefarmácia no Brasil e aspectos do impacto social e econômico. *Latin American Journal of Telehealth*. https://doi.org/10.32443/2175-2990(2022)427.

16. de Magalhães, A. A., & Santos, A. T. (2025). Advancements in diagnostic methods and imaging technologies in dentistry: A literature review of emerging approaches. *Journal of Clinical Medicine, 14.* https://www.semanticscholar.org/paper/c0b125d5011c819fe642f05e88b36337e7d2eaf9 (accessed on 10th June 2025).

17. Dolai, B., & Khachane, T. (2023). Unlocking the trends and patterns of midazolam research: A bibliometric criticism. https://core.ac.uk/download/578915544.pdf (accessed on 10th June 2025).

18. ElSayed, N. A., Aleppo, G., Bannuru, R. R., Bruemmer, D., Collins, B. S., Ekhlaspour, L., Gaglia, J. L., et al. (2023). 9. Pharmacologic approaches to glycemic treatment: *Standards of Care in Diabetes—2024. Diabetes Care, 47*, S158–S178. https://doi.org/10.2337/dc24-s009 (accessed on 10th June 2025).

19. Feigin, V. L., Stark, B., Johnson, C. O., Roth, G. A., Bisignano, C., Gebreheat, G., Abbasifard, M., et al. (2021). Global, regional, and national burden of stroke and its risk factors, 1990–2019: A systematic analysis for the Global Burden of Disease Study 2019. *The Lancet Neurology, 20*, 795–820. https://doi.org/10.1016/s1474-4422(21)00252-0.

20. Frazier, K. S., Greiter-Wilke, A., Grobler, A. F., et al. (2019). Drug safety Africa: An overview of safety pharmacology & toxicology in South Africa. https://core.ac.uk/download/228991477.pdf (accessed on 10th June 2025).

21. Fromer, L., Kaplan, A., Price, D., et al. (2014). Is there a rationale and role for long-acting anticholinergic bronchodilators in asthma? https://core.ac.uk/download/25497565.pdf (accessed on 10th June 2025).

22. Fu, A., Ton, M., Wang, K., Gu, W., Jin, H., Shaikh, N., Madan, S., et al. (2024). Abstract PO5-15-06: NVIGEN X® comprehensive liquid biopsy for sensitive ctDNA, circulating tumor cells (CTC), and protein detection in breast cancer: Next-generation sequencing, patient case studies, and clinical implications. *Cancer Research.* https://www.semanticscholar.org/paper/66ad54d08cbccf07c0b76d3e15fa9161eefa4f8a (accessed on 10th June 2025).

23. Goetzl, E. J., Hampel, H., Kapogiannis, D., et al. (2019). Biomarker-drug and liquid biopsy co-development for disease staging and targeted therapy: Cornerstones for Alzheimer's precision medicine and pharmacology. https://core.ac.uk/download/287624128.pdf (accessed on 10th June 2025).

24. Goldenberg, A., Hoffman, M. M., Leskovec, J., et al. (2018). Machine learning for integrating data in biology and medicine: Principles, practice, and opportunities. http://arxiv.org/abs/1807.00123 (accessed on 10th June 2025).

25. Hatem, N. A. H. (2024). Advancing pharmacy practice: The role of intelligence-driven pharmacy practice and the emergence of pharmacointelligence. *Integrated Pharmacy Research and Practice, 13*, 139–153. https://doi.org/10.2147/iprp.s466748 (accessed on 10th June 2025).

26. Johnson-Williams, B. E., Reynolds, K., Gobburu, J., & Rundio, A. (2024). A modified Delphi study to establish essential clinical pharmacology competencies. *Therapeutic Innovation & Regulatory Science, 58*, 473–482. https://www.semanticscholar.org/paper/a07bf0d5c5622bd97c0681a49fba9339d6e677f9 (accessed on 10th June 2025).

27. Kermani, F., Orooji, A., & Borhani, A. (2017). MHealth technology for deaf and hearing loss individuals. *Volume 2*, 151. https://www.semanticscholar.org/paper/9f67bf6c47fa0640ed5ac375488a1fd6968d0dfe (accessed on 10th June 2025).

28. Kluwe, F., Michelet, R., Mueller-Schoell, A., Maier, C., Klopp-Schulze, L., van Dyk, M., Mikus, G., et al. (2020). Perspectives on model-informed precision dosing in the digital health era: Challenges, opportunities, and recommendations. *Clinical Pharmacology & Therapeutics, 109*(1), 29–36. https://doi.org/10.1002/cpt.2049.

29. Knox, C., Wilson, M., Klinger, C. M., Franklin, M., Oler, E., Wilson, A. E., Pon, A., et al. (2023). DrugBank 6.0: The DrugBank knowledgebase for 2024. *Nucleic Acids Research, 52*, D1265–D1275. https://doi.org/10.1093/nar/gkad976.

30. Lau, J. L., & Dunn, M. K. (2017). Therapeutic peptides: Historical perspectives, current development trends, and future directions. *Bioorganic & Medicinal Chemistry, 26*(9), 2700–2707. https://doi.org/10.1016/j.bmc.2017.06.052.

31. LeBoff, M. S., Greenspan, S. L., Insogna, K., Lewiecki, E. M., Saag, K. G., Singer, A., & Siris, E. S. (2022). The clinician's guide to prevention and treatment of osteoporosis. *Osteoporosis International, 33*(10), 2049–2102. https://doi.org/10.1007/s00198-021-05900-y.

32. Lee, A. Y. Y. (2021). Annals for Hospitalists Inpatient Notes: Direct oral anticoagulants in patients with cancer—What hospitalists need to know. *Annals of Internal Medicine, 174*(HO2), HO2–HO3. https://www.semanticscholar.org/paper/39cd1f8a05f2774d51d9312127ecbfdf5ddcf608 (accessed on 10th June 2025).

33. Lietzan, E. (2017). The uncharted waters of competition and innovation in biological medicines. https://core.ac.uk/download/217317393.pdf (accessed on 10th June 2025).

34. Liu, Q., Joshi, A., Standing, J. F., & van der Graaf, P. H. (2024). Artificial intelligence/machine learning: The new frontier of clinical pharmacology and precision medicine. *Clinical Pharmacology & Therapeutics, 115*, 637–642. https://doi.org/10.1002/cpt.3198 (accessed on 10th June 2025).

35. Liu, Z., Chen, H., Zheng, L., Sun, L. P., & Shi, L. (2023). Angiogenic signaling pathways and anti-angiogenic therapy for cancer. *Signal Transduction and Targeted Therapy, 8*. https://doi.org/10.1038/s41392-023-01460-1 (accessed on 10th June 2025).

36. Mack, J. A., Rusu, R., Voss, E., Meg Celine, Hernández, S., Hernández-Díaz, S., Wyszynski, D., et al. (2022). Abstracts of the virtual 2nd Annual African Regional Interest Group Meeting (AfRIG), 11–13 July, 2022. *Pharmacoepidemiology and Drug Safety, 31*(7). https://www.semanticscholar.org/paper/763dc2731461f30525f7cc5730801d3d6cf13814 (accessed on 10th June 2025).

37. Marsh, A., Singer, D. R. J., Taylor, P. C., et al. (2010). Personalized medicine: The impact on chemistry. https://core.ac.uk/download/45676.pdf (accessed on 10th June 2025).

38. McCue, M., Khatib, R., Kabir, C., Blair, C., Fehnert, B., King, J., Spalding, A., et al. (2023). User-centered design of a digitally enabled care pathway in a large health system: Qualitative interview study. *JMIR Human Factors, 10*(1). https://www.semanticscholar.org/paper/ebdac79b0e386ccafdec48373327335c8ef0111d (accessed on 10th June 2025).

39. Najmi, A., Javed, S. A., Al Bratty, M., & Alhazmi, H. A. (2022). Modern approaches in the discovery and development of plant-based natural products and their analogues as potential therapeutic agents. *Molecules, 27*(2), 349. https://doi.org/10.3390/molecules27020349.

40. Panchal, N. B., & Vaghela, V. (2025). Advancements in obesity: Unravelling pathophysiology, treatment strategies, and innovative approaches. *Biosciences Biotechnology Research Asia*. https://www.semanticscholar.org/paper/7473866730962973ce35e4afa2e5fd9271270e85 (accessed on 10th June 2025).

41. Pang, X., Xu, H., Qiu, Z., Zhang, H., Xie, R., Liu, Z., Gu, Y., et al. (2023). Targeting integrin pathways: Mechanisms and advances in therapy. *Signal Transduction and Targeted Therapy, 8*. https://doi.org/10.1038/s41392-022-01259-6.

42. Park, Y. S., Lee, K. H., Jeong, H., & Kim, K. (2023). The necessity of education in response to technological advancements and future environmental changes: A comparison of Korean medicine doctors and students. *Journal of Korean Medicine*. https://www.semanticscholar.org/paper/d66906b0874b0907988087bfeee3f821bb2e63d6 (accessed on 10th June 2025).

43. Ruiz-López, I., Victoria-Montesinos, D., & Martínez-Fuentes, J. (2024). Knowledge domains and emerging trends in non-invasive brain stimulation: A bibliometric analysis via CiteSpace. *Biomédica, 44*(2), 139–150. https://www.semanticscholar.org/paper/749fd0d4710c2dd9edc58d1f8d0b92149e6d45cd (accessed on 10th June 2025).

44. Schilling, S. H. (2011). DNA as patentable subject matter and a narrow framework for addressing the perceived problems caused by gene patents. https://core.ac.uk/download/62548420.pdf (accessed on 10th June 2025).

45. Sul, J., Kim, M. K., Leem, J., Jo, H., Yoon, S., Kim, J., Lee, E., et al. (2019). Efficacy and safety of gyejigachulbutang (Gui-Zhi-Jia-Shu-Fu-Tang, Keishikajutsubuto, TJ-18) for knee pain in patients with degenerative knee osteoarthritis: A randomized, placebo-controlled, patient and assessor blinded clinical trial. *Trials, 20*(1). https://www.semanticscholar.org/paper/6dcfc255f788339ba5fa9773fc81dcbcd6162753 (accessed on 10th June 2025).

46. Tak, Y. W., Kim, J. S., Chung, H., Lee, S., Park, I., Lee, S. W., Jo, M. W., et al. (2023). Analysis of metabolic and quality-of-life factors in patients with cancer for a new approach to classifying walking habits: Secondary analysis of a randomized controlled trial. *Journal of Medical Internet Research, 27*. https://www.semanticscholar.org/paper/3875d707490ab2db82daddb3cd947559d92d5ac6 (accessed on 10th June 2025).

47. Terzic, A., & Waldman, S. A. (2017). *Clinical Pharmacology & Therapeutics*: Past, present, and future. https://core.ac.uk/download/83049656.pdf (accessed on 10th June 2025).

48. Tillu, G., Chaturvedi, S., Chopra, A., & Patwardhan, B. (2020). Public health approach of Ayurveda and Yoga for COVID-19 prophylaxis. *The Journal of Alternative and Complementary Medicine, 26*(4), 360–364. https://doi.org/10.1089/acm.2020.0129.

49. Trivedi, A., Stienen, S., Zhu, M., Li, H., Yuraszeck, T., Gibbs, J. P., Heath, T. D., et al. (2017). Clinical pharmacology and translational aspects of bispecific antibodies. *Clinical and Translational Science, 10*(3), 147–162. https://doi.org/10.1111/cts.12459.

50. Vekhova, K. A., Namiot, E. D., Jonsson, J., & Schiöth, H. (2024). Ketamine and esketamine in clinical trials: FDA-approved and emerging indications, trial trends with putative mechanistic explanations. *Clinical Pharmacology and Therapeutics, 117*(2), 374–386. https://www.semanticscholar.org/paper/6ee591816a9fe3b4322a46fd3ba331485fa52371 (accessed on 10th June 2025).

INDEX

D

E

F

G

H

N

O

P

S

T